Comprehensive Approaches to Cannabis Nursing

Kathleen Marie Pinto Araya
https://orcid.org/0009-0000-0608-7555
AZZ Medical Associates, USA & South College, USA

Rana R. Zeine
https://orcid.org/0000-0002-9485-9531
Kean University, USA

IGI Global
Scientific Publishing
Publishing Tomorrow's Research Today

Vice President of Editorial	Melissa Wagner
Director of Acquisitions	Mikaela Felty
Director of Book Development	Jocelynn Hessler
Production Manager	Mike Brehm
Cover Design	Jose Rosado

Cover painting copyright Soumaya Zeine Thompson, used with permission

Published in the United States of America by
IGI Global Scientific Publishing
701 East Chocolate Avenue
Hershey, PA, 17033, USA
Tel: 717-533-8845 | Fax: 717-533-7115
Website: https://www.igi-global.com E-mail: cust@igi-global.com

Library of Congress Cataloging-in-Publication Data

LCCN: 2026934949 (CIP Data Pending)
ISBN13: 9798337372877
Isbn13Softcover: 9798337372884
EISBN13: 9798337372891
British Cataloguing in Publication Data
A Cataloguing in Publication record for this book is available from the British Library.

Table of Contents

Detailed Table of Contents

This introductory chapter emphasizes the growing importance of comprehensive cannabis education as its use becomes increasingly widespread across communities, workplaces, and daily life. With cannabis now shifting from Schedule I to Schedule III, formally recognizing its medical use and reducing barriers to research and clinical integration, healthcare systems must adapt to a rapidly changing regulatory environment. Leaders are tasked with developing clear, evidence-informed policies for documentation, disclosure, medication reconciliation, safety monitoring, staff training, patient education, legal compliance, and quality-improvement efforts. Organizations with structured cannabis policies tend to demonstrate stronger communication, reduced liability concerns, and more consistent care delivery. By framing these emerging responsibilities and the implications of cannabis's new scheduling status, this chapter sets the foundation for the book's broader exploration of integrating cannabis into routine healthcare practice.

Cannabis nursing has become a specialty as healthcare systems face rising demand to integrate medical cannabis within complex, often contradictory regulations. This chapter examines the cannabis nurse's role in U.S. policy and advocacy to support equitable patient access and safe medical cannabis implementation. The nurse's function as a policy translator across patient, organizational, and governmental levels is emphasized. Key regulatory issues, federal-state misalignment, institutional risk management, clinician knowledge gaps, and facility access barriers are analyzed. Ryan's Law serves as a policy-to-practice example of nurse-led inpatient implementation. The chapter concludes with recommendations for governance, competency development, and structured advocacy, highlighting how the cannabis nurse connects cannabinoid science to clinical care.

Cannabis nursing leadership constitutes a critical advancement in modern nursing, integrating ethical advocacy, evidence-based care, and policy transformation across clinical and academic contexts. Anchored in the Cannabis Nursing: Scope and Standards of Practice, this chapter analyzes how nurse leaders, including hospital executives, deans, faculty, and policy advocates, advance safe and equitable integration of cannabis within healthcare and academic systems. Drawing on transformational, servant, and systems leadership frameworks, the chapter explores leadership roles, policy alignment, and translation of research into institutional and educational reform. Through case studies, ethical analysis, and research exemplars, nurse leaders are positioned as stewards of institutional change who promote healthcare consumer safety and public trust. Learning outcomes emphasize leadership competencies. The chapter concludes with applied frameworks and NCLEX-style questions, preparing leaders to advance evidence-based cannabis care grounded in ethics and human dignity.

This chapter establishes an evidence-informed framework for clinical competence in medical cannabis nursing, integrating assessment, dosing, monitoring, patient education, ethical reasoning, and professional identity formation. Drawing on the current research, regulatory guidance, and theoretical models such as the biopsychosocial approach and therapeutic stewardship, the chapter outlines the clinical and ethical complexities associated with cannabinoid-based care. It explores variability in product pharmacology, the need for structured risk stratification, the importance of shared decision-making, and the challenges posed by stigma, misinformation, and regulatory inconsistencies. By synthesising empirical findings, ethical principles, and professional standards, the chapter delineates the knowledge, skills, and reflective capabilities required to ensure safe, accountable, and context-sensitive nursing practice within an evolving therapeutic landscape.

The Cannabis Nurse Navigator is a registered nurse with specialized training in cannabis science, clinical assessment, and patient education. Functioning at the intersection of nursing care, clinical research, and patient advocacy, the Cannabis Nurse Navigator serves as a guide and liaison between patients, providers, and healthcare systems. This integrative approach allows nurses to address patient needs that often fall outside traditional care models, needs shaped by stigma, inconsistent regulation, and rapidly emerging evidence. The Cannabis Nurse Navigator does not recommend specific products, direct patients to commercial vendors, or engage in prescribing; rather, the role focuses on assessment, education, harm reduction, and systems navigation within the nursing scope of practice.

Medical cannabis consumption is expanding rapidly in the United States, yet increased access has not been accompanied by consistent clinical processes. This has created a "clinical vacuum" for patients in which cannabis is often used in unstructured settings with inconsistent outcomes. This chapter argues that these challenges reflect a failure of care delivery rather than a limitation of the cannabis plant itself. It proposes a health-focused definition of medical cannabis centered on intentionality, monitoring, and evidence-based decision-making. To operationalize this definition, a five-step clinical framework is presented: Intention, Education, Implementation, Assessment, and Adjustment. The chapter also highlights the essential role of nurses in facilitating this framework, while also recognizing that this process can be applied in self-directed use when core elements are maintained. Emphasis is placed on future research evaluating process-based cannabis care using longitudinal, patient-centered outcomes across diverse care contexts.

As cannabis nursing develops, it meets the growing demand for expert support among patients using cannabis therapeutically. This chapter outlines the Cannabis Nurse's role and practical strategies for integrating it into healthcare and communities. It covers six core knowledge areas, essential skills, workflows, and quality metrics from the National Council of State Boards of Nursing. Real-world examples highlight its impact in oncology, geriatrics, palliative care, mental health, and pain management. The chapter also discusses entrepreneurial, administrative and business opportunities, offering resources for administrators and nurse leaders, and clear pathways for nurses' education and leadership in value-based care.

Cannabis use presents complex clinical, legal, and ethical challenges within forensic nursing practice. Containing psychoactive constituents such as THC and CBD, cannabis is regulated under varying legal frameworks, including the Controlled Substances Act in the United States and the Cannabis Act in Canada, while cannabis use disorder is recognized in the DSM-5. Forensic nurses manage acute intoxication, withdrawal, and Cannabinoid Hyperemesis Syndrome, particularly among vulnerable populations such as pregnant individuals, adolescents, older adults, and persons with serious mental illness. Toxicological detection through urine and oral fluid testing, along with strict chain-of-custody procedures, supports evidence integrity in legal contexts. However, biological markers do not reliably establish real-time impairment, creating interpretive challenges.It may be concluded that cannabis-focused forensic nursing demands the integration of clinical competence, ethical accountability, and legal awareness to ensure patient-centered care, maintain evidentiary & equitable policy development.

This chapter examines cannabis nursing as an emerging specialty grounded in caring science, holistic nursing philosophy, and contemporary cannabinoid research, advancing a spirituality-first approach to clinical practice. Drawing upon Jean Watson's Theory of Human Caring, professional nursing standards, and the endocannabinoid system, the chapter asserts that spirituality is not ancillary to cannabis care but foundational to ethical, person-centered nursing practice. A Spirituality-First Clinical Model and the H.I.G.H. Framework (Hope, Inspiration, Growth, and Healing) are introduced to illustrate how cannabis-supported care may influence physical, mental, emotional, social, and spiritual domains of health. Through clinical narratives, the chapter demonstrates how presence, nonjudgment, intention, and relationship-centered care shape therapeutic outcomes. By integrating science and meaning, this work positions cannabis nursing as a relational, ethically grounded specialty that honors human dignity, supports whole-person healing, and advances holistic nursing practice.

This chapter will focus on nursing leadership, particularly nursing administration, as a critical component of fostering safety, quality, collaboration, and policy in the evolving specialties of cannabis nursing care and case management. Significant nursing administrative actions for cannabis care are from within the framework of the core values of the 2024 Cannabis Nursing Scope and Standards of Practice: Evidence-Based Practice Application Of Caring And Social Justice Ethics Cannabis Health Care Consumer-Centered Care Interprofessional Health Care Teamwork The chapter will provide cannabis nurse leaders with distinct legal, ethical, and practice considerations for navigating cannabis nursing care. Specifically, this chapter will address the conflict between federal and state laws and how these regulations continue to impact the policy landscape of cannabis healthcare operations, including regulation, administrative leadership, ethics, and advocacy, as well as the management of cannabis nursing education, competence, and stigmas.

This chapter examines medical cannabis equity through a public health lens, emphasizing how access to cannabinoid therapeutics in the United States is shaped by structural, historical, and policy-driven determinants rather than individual choice alone. Drawing on social determinants of health frameworks, the chapter analyzes how federal prohibition, state-level policy variation, financial barriers, stigma, and limited clinical guidance contribute to inequitable access and patient experiences. Particular attention is given to the role of stigma and implicit bias within healthcare settings and their effects on disclosure, clinical guidance, and trust. The chapter highlights nurses as critical actors positioned at the intersection of policy, practice, and patient experience, with unique responsibilities in advocacy, education, and harm reduction. Policy and system-level strategies, including health system integration, data surveillance, and equity-oriented reform, are presented as essential for advancing equitable medical cannabis care.

This chapter focuses on the development of curricula on medical cannabis for nursing students. It follows the National Council of State Boards of Nursing (2018) call for six essential areas of medical cannabis knowledge, attitudes, and skills to be addressed in academia. The chapter will expand on the implications of developing medical cannabis curricula for nurses that include the role of the cannabis nurse from the perspectives of the Cannabis nursing scope and standards of practice (American Nurses Association & American Cannabis Nurses Association, 2024), advocacy, ethics, safety issues, spiritual concerns, and common challenges and barriers that nurses providing care for medical cannabis patients may face.

This chapter presents an evidence-informed, ready-to-implement curriculum for integrating medical cannabis education into undergraduate and graduate nursing programs. Grounded in the NCSBN's 2018 national guidelines and the 2024 ACNA/ANA Cannabis Nursing Scope & Standards of Practice, it translates essential competencies—legal literacy, endocannabinoid system physiology, cannabinoid pharmacology, dosing principles, product literacy, a whole-person assessment, and harm-reduction strategies—into an instructional model that aligns with contemporary nursing education frameworks. Despite widespread patient use, most graduates receive no formal preparation to counsel on cannabis use, assess safety risks, or evaluate drug–drug interactions. This chapter addresses that gap by providing modular content, case-based learning tools, and competency-based evaluation methods. The curriculum equips faculty to teach confidently, supports safe and nonjudgmental patient care, and provides a scalable foundation for all programs seeking to incorporate cannabis therapeutics into modern nursing practice.

The emergence of cannabis nursing as a recognized specialty reflects a pivotal shift in healthcare policy and practice across the World. As more localities legalize cannabis for medicinal and adult use, nurses are expected to support patients who incorporate cannabis into their health and wellness choices. This chapter examines the evolving role of the cannabis nurse considering the American Nurses Association's (ANA) recognition of cannabis nursing as a specialty practice and the publication of the Cannabis Nursing Scope and Standards by the American Cannabis Nurses Association (ACNA). It emphasizes the urgent need to integrate cannabis education into academic curricula, guided by the National Council of State Boards of Nursing (NCSBN) National Guidelines for Medical Marijuana. With individuals consuming cannabis for a range of reasons, healthcare professionals must be equipped with foundational knowledge

Preface

Cannabis is rapidly reshaping modern healthcare, and nurses are at the center of this transformation. As medical cannabis moves from Schedule I to Schedule III, its therapeutic value is formally recognized, research barriers are reduced, and healthcare systems must respond with clarity, competence, and accountability. This shift demands a new level of preparedness across nursing practice, leadership, education, and policy development.

Nurses in every setting—acute care, primary care, mental health, oncology, palliative care, and community health—are increasingly caring for patients who use cannabis for symptom management, quality-of-life improvement, and supportive care. Understanding cannabinoids, including THC, CBD, and other therapeutic compounds, is now essential for safe assessment, medication reconciliation, and patient-centered care. As cannabis becomes more integrated into treatment plans, nurses must apply evidence-based practice, ethical decision-making, and clinical judgment to guide patients through benefits, risks, interactions, and appropriate use.

Healthcare systems are being challenged to build structured, evidence-informed policies that address documentation, disclosure, safety monitoring, legal compliance, and quality-improvement processes. Nursing leadership plays a critical role in shaping these policies, ensuring regulatory alignment, and promoting consistent standards across organizations. Clear regulation and thoughtful policy development reduce liability, strengthen communication, and support safer, more coordinated care.

Workforce training is now a foundational requirement. Nurses, advanced practice providers, and interprofessional teams need education in cannabis pharmacology, clinical assessment, symptom management, and ethical considerations. This includes preparing Clinical Nurse Specialists, Nurse Practitioners, and Cannabis Nurse Navigators to lead integration efforts, support complex patient needs, and guide system-level change. Nurse navigation—already central in oncology and chronic disease care—extends naturally into cannabis therapeutics, helping patients move through fragmented systems with clarity and support.

This book begins by framing the responsibilities, opportunities, and challenges created by cannabis's evolving legal and clinical landscape. It establishes the foundation for understanding cannabis nursing as a legitimate, emerging specialty grounded in evidence-based practice, patient safety, and professional standards. Through exploration of clinical practice, healthcare systems, regulation, education, leadership, and ethical care, this text prepares nurses to confidently integrate cannabis therapeutics into modern healthcare.

CHAPTER OVERVIEW

Chapter 1 establishes the foundation for this volume by examining the growing necessity of cannabis education and policy integration within contemporary nursing practice. As cannabis regulation evolves and healthcare systems confront expanding patient use, the chapter situates nurses and healthcare leaders at the center of organizational adaptation. Emphasis is placed on the implications of cannabis rescheduling, the development of evidence-informed institutional policies, and the need for comprehensive approaches to documentation, patient education, safety monitoring, and quality improvement. By framing cannabis integration as both a clinical and systems-level responsibility, this opening chapter prepares readers for the broader discussions of practice, leadership, ethics, and healthcare transformation explored throughout the book.

Chapter 2 explores the increasingly critical role of the cannabis nurse as a policy translator and advocate within the complex landscape of U.S. healthcare regulation. The chapter examines how nurses navigate tensions between federal and state laws while promoting equitable patient access to medical cannabis and safe clinical implementation. Through discussion of institutional barriers, clinician preparedness, ethical considerations, and governance strategies, the authors highlight the cannabis nurse's unique position at the intersection of law, evidence, and patient care. Practical policy examples, including nurse-led implementation initiatives, demonstrate how advocacy and systems leadership can shape access-oriented cannabis practice within modern healthcare environments.

Chapter 3 examines cannabis nursing leadership as a transformative force within healthcare systems, academic institutions, and public policy. Grounded in established nursing leadership frameworks and professional standards, the chapter positions nurse leaders as essential agents in advancing ethical, evidence-based cannabis integration. Through analysis of leadership competencies, institutional reform, research translation, and policy development, the chapter demonstrates how nursing leadership influences healthcare consumer safety, educational innovation, and public trust. Case studies and applied examples further illustrate the expanding responsibilities of cannabis nurse leaders in shaping equitable and accountable healthcare systems.

Chapter 4 presents a comprehensive framework for developing clinical competence in medical cannabis nursing. Integrating current evidence, ethical principles, and regulatory guidance, the chapter explores the multifaceted responsibilities associated with cannabinoid-based care, including patient assessment, dosing, monitoring, education, and shared decision-making. Particular attention is given to the challenges created by product variability, stigma, misinformation, and inconsistent regulation. By emphasizing reflective practice, therapeutic stewardship, and context-sensitive care, the chapter defines the professional knowledge and clinical judgment required for safe and accountable cannabis nursing practice within an evolving therapeutic landscape.

Chapter 5 introduces the Cannabis Nurse Navigator™ as an emerging model of integrative nursing practice that bridges patient advocacy, clinical assessment, education, and systems navigation. The chapter highlights the navigator's role in addressing gaps that frequently exist within traditional healthcare models, particularly those shaped by stigma, fragmented regulation, and rapidly evolving cannabis evidence. Emphasizing harm reduction, patient-centered communication, and interdisciplinary collaboration, the chapter outlines how nurses can support patients without prescribing or directing commercial cannabis use. In doing so, it presents a practical framework for enhancing continuity of care and improving patient engagement within cannabis-informed healthcare delivery.

Chapter 6 advances a structured, process-based framework for medical cannabis care that emphasizes intentionality, monitoring, and evidence-informed decision-making. Responding to the absence of standardized clinical processes surrounding cannabis use, the chapter argues that inconsistent patient outcomes often reflect gaps in care delivery rather than limitations of cannabis therapeutics themselves. Through a five-step clinical model centered on education, implementation, assessment, and adjustment, the chapter provides readers with a practical approach to patient-centered cannabis care. The discussion further underscores the critical role of nurses in facilitating structured therapeutic processes while encouraging future research focused on longitudinal and outcome-driven care models.

Chapter 7 presents the cannabis nurse as a new and evolving paradigm within patient and community care. Addressing the growing demand for knowledgeable cannabis-focused support, the chapter outlines core competencies, workflows, quality metrics, and practice applications across diverse clinical settings, including oncology, geriatrics, palliative care, mental health, and pain management. In addition to clinical practice, the chapter explores leadership, entrepreneurial, and administrative opportunities that position cannabis nurses as innovators within value-based healthcare systems. By offering practical pathways for education and professional development, the chapter reinforces the expanding influence of cannabis nursing within modern healthcare delivery.

Chapter 8 examines the complex intersection of forensic nursing, cannabis use, and legal accountability. The chapter explores the clinical, ethical, and evidentiary challenges associated with cannabis-related care, particularly in situations involving intoxication, withdrawal, toxicology testing, and vulnerable populations. Attention is given to the limitations of biological testing in determining impairment and the importance of maintaining evidentiary integrity through proper forensic procedures. By integrating legal awareness with patient-centered clinical care, the chapter demonstrates how forensic nurses contribute to ethical practice, public safety, and equitable policy development in cannabis-related contexts.

Chapter 9 approaches cannabis nursing through the lens of caring science and holistic nursing philosophy, positioning spirituality as foundational rather than peripheral to therapeutic care. Drawing from caring theory, cannabinoid science, and relationship-centered nursing practice, the chapter introduces models that integrate physical, emotional, social, and spiritual dimensions of healing. Through clinical narratives and reflective frameworks, the discussion emphasizes presence, intention, nonjudgment, and human connection as essential components of cannabis-informed nursing care. In doing so, the chapter expands the understanding of cannabis nursing as an ethically grounded specialty committed to whole-person healing and human dignity.

Chapter 10 focuses on nursing administration as a central driver of safe, ethical, and collaborative cannabis healthcare systems. Examining the regulatory tensions between federal and state law, the chapter highlights the administrative responsibilities associated with cannabis policy development, workforce competence, patient safety, and organizational leadership. Core principles from contemporary cannabis nursing standards guide discussions of evidence-based care, social justice, interprofessional collaboration, and healthcare consumer advocacy. By addressing legal complexities, stigma, and operational leadership challenges, the chapter provides nurse administrators with practical strategies for navigating the evolving cannabis healthcare landscape.

Chapter 11 examines medical cannabis equity through a public health framework that emphasizes the influence of structural, historical, and policy-driven determinants on access to care. The chapter analyzes how federal prohibition, financial barriers, stigma, policy inconsistency, and limited clinical guidance contribute to disparities in patient experiences and therapeutic access. Particular attention is given to the effects of implicit bias and healthcare stigma on disclosure, trust, and care quality. Positioning nurses as critical advocates within systems-level reform, the chapter underscores the importance of equity-oriented policy, harm reduction, and integrated healthcare strategies in advancing just and accessible cannabis care.

Chapter 12 addresses the urgent need to integrate medical cannabis education into nursing curricula. Guided by national competency recommendations and contemporary cannabis nursing standards, the chapter explores the educational implications of preparing nurses to address advocacy, ethics, safety, spirituality, and patient-centered cannabis care. It further examines the challenges and barriers faced by educators and clinicians in incorporating cannabis-related content into academic and clinical training environments. By emphasizing foundational competencies and professional preparedness, the chapter reinforces the importance of formal cannabis education in modern nursing practice.

Chapter 13 provides an evidence-informed, ready-to-implement curriculum framework designed to support the integration of medical cannabis education into undergraduate and graduate nursing programs. Aligning with national nursing guidelines and cannabis nursing standards, the chapter translates essential competencies into practical educational models that include legal literacy, pharmacology, assessment, harm reduction, and product knowledge. Through modular content, competency-based evaluation, and case-based learning strategies, the chapter equips educators with tools to confidently teach cannabis therapeutics while preparing students to deliver safe, informed, and nonjudgmental patient care in evolving healthcare settings.

Chapter 14 examines the emergence of cannabis nursing as a recognized specialty and its significance within the broader transformation of healthcare policy and practice. As legalization expands globally, the chapter emphasizes the growing expectation that nurses possess foundational knowledge of cannabis therapeutics, the endocannabinoid system, and evidence-based patient care. Attention is given to the role of professional organizations, specialty standards, and educational guidelines in shaping the future of cannabis nursing. By highlighting the importance of academic integration and ethical clinical preparation, the chapter positions cannabis nursing as an essential component of contemporary healthcare practice.

Chapter 15 concludes the volume by examining the cannabis nurse entrepreneur as an emerging leader within the rapidly evolving cannabis industry and healthcare environment. The chapter explores how nurses apply clinical insight, operational leadership, regulatory knowledge, and patient advocacy to address gaps in cannabis integration, documentation, education, and healthcare oversight. Through case studies and discussion of innovative practice models, the chapter highlights opportunities for nurses to advance health equity, improve data integrity, and support accountable cannabis care systems. The discussion ultimately positions entrepreneurship as a pathway for nursing leadership, interdisciplinary collaboration, and transformative healthcare innovation in the expanding field of cannabis therapeutics.

Acknowledgment

The development of this volume reflects the collective expertise, dedication, and vision of a diverse community of nurses, educators, clinicians, researchers, policy advocates, administrators, and healthcare leaders committed to advancing safe, ethical, and evidence-informed cannabis care. The editors extend sincere gratitude to each chapter author and contributor whose scholarship, clinical insight, and professional leadership helped shape this work into a comprehensive resource for modern nursing practice.

Chapter 1
A Contemporary Introduction to Cannabis in Nursing: Foundations for Practice

Kathleen Marie Pinto Araya
http://orcid.org/0009-0000-0608-7555
AZZ Medical Associates, USA

ABSTRACT

This introductory chapter emphasizes the growing importance of comprehensive cannabis education as its use becomes increasingly widespread across communities, workplaces, and daily life. With cannabis now shifting from Schedule I to Schedule III, formally recognizing its medical use and reducing barriers to research and clinical integration, healthcare systems must adapt to a rapidly changing regulatory environment. Leaders are tasked with developing clear, evidence-informed policies for documentation, disclosure, medication reconciliation, safety monitoring, staff training, patient education, legal compliance, and quality-improvement efforts. Organizations with structured cannabis policies tend to demonstrate stronger communication, reduced liability concerns, and more consistent care delivery. By framing these emerging responsibilities and the implications of cannabis's new scheduling status, this chapter sets the foundation for the book's broader exploration of integrating cannabis into routine healthcare practice.

FOUNDATIONS FOR PURPOSE, PRACTICE, AND POSSIBILITY

The integration of medical cannabis into contemporary healthcare systems is accelerating a significant transformation in clinical education, professional practice standards, and organizational policy. As scientific evidence expands and legalization advances across national and international jurisdictions, healthcare institutions are increasingly required to update competencies, regulatory frameworks, and models of care to address the complexities of cannabinoid therapeutics (National Academies of Sciences, Engineering, and Medicine [NASEM], 2017; Health Canada, 2022). The recent approval of Cannabis Nursing as a formal specialty by the American Nurses Association marks a pivotal development in this evolution, underscoring the need for a scientifically grounded and clinically rigorous approach to cannabis-related care (American Nurses Association [ANA], 2023). Cannabis has been moved from Schedule I to Schedule III under the federal Controlled Substances Act, based on recent executive action

DOI: 10.4018/979-8-3373-7287-7.ch001

directing the Attorney General to complete the rescheduling process. This marks the most significant shift in U.S. cannabis policy in decades and signals a move toward recognizing its medical use while reducing regulatory barriers.

This book provides a comprehensive, evidence-based foundation for understanding the role of nurses within the emerging field of cannabinoid therapeutics. It examines the scientific principles underlying cannabinoid pharmacology, conceptual dosing strategies, delivery systems, and therapeutic applications, with particular emphasis on the nurse's role in patient education and clinical assessment (Zolotov et al., 2021). The text also addresses the evaluation of symptom patterns, the determination of appropriateness for adjunctive cannabis therapy, and the integration of cannabinoid-based interventions into individualized care plans (National Academies of Sciences, Engineering, and Medicine, 2017). In addition, the book explores the broader professional responsibilities of nurses, including stigma reduction, policy development, quality assurance, and legal and regulatory compliance (Substance Abuse and Mental Health Services Administration, 2023).

Cannabis care intersects with multiple domains of healthcare, not only nurses but also the interdisciplinary teams with whom they collaborate. Physicians, pharmacists, mental health professionals, social workers, and allied health providers increasingly encounter patients who use cannabis for therapeutic, wellness, or symptom-management purposes (Murray et al., 2021; U.S. Food and Drug Administration, 2020). Bridging biomedical science, clinical practice, pharmaceutical considerations, and public health perspectives to address persistent knowledge gaps is vital to support the safe, ethical, and evidence-informed use of medical cannabis across diverse clinical environments (World Health Organization, 2023).

The chapters of this book draw upon the expertise of international clinicians representing a wide range of specialties, including medical and surgical care, anesthesia, geriatrics, emergency medicine, critical care, pediatrics, nurse-midwifery, obstetrics, family medicine, psychiatry, and palliative care. Their contributions highlight the multifaceted nature of cannabis use in clinical practice and underscore the need for specialty-specific considerations. Whether addressing neuropathic pain in adult-gerontology nursing, anxiety in psychiatric settings, symptom burden in oncology, seizure management in pediatric neurology, or comfort-focused interventions in hospice and palliative care, cannabis nursing requires a nuanced understanding of patient needs, clinical contexts, and evolving scientific evidence (Devinsky et al., 2017; Health Canada, 2022).

Establishing conceptual and professional foundations for the role of the Cannabis Nurse as a specialty extends beyond basic knowledge of plant-based therapeutics and requires proficiency in interpreting complex pharmacological interactions, understanding legal and regulatory structures, addressing stigma and misinformation, and advocating for equitable access to safe and evidence-based care (American Cannabis Nurses Association, 2023). It also demands effective collaboration within interdisciplinary teams and the ability to support patients across the lifespan, including adolescents, adults, and older adults with multiple comorbidities (Centers for Disease Control and Prevention, 2022).

The intended audience for this book reflects the broad relevance of cannabis in modern healthcare and includes nurses across all practice areas including adult-gerontology, cardiology, anesthesia, critical care, emergency medicine, family practice, forensics, geriatrics, home care, intensive care, labor and delivery, managed care, medical-surgical practice, psychiatry, military nursing, oncology, orthopedics, pediatric neurology, plastic surgery, rehabilitation, women's health, and nursing administration. Nursing students, educators, and curriculum developers will find the text valuable for integrating cannabis science into academic programs (Zolotov et al., 2021). Physicians, physician assistants, prescribers, healthcare administrators, policymakers, researchers, journalists, legislators, law enforcement professionals, and members of the general public seeking a scientifically rigorous understanding of medical cannabis will benefit from the collaborative expertise presented (World Health Organization, 2023).

This introductory chapter positions cannabis nursing as an emerging and essential specialty within the broader healthcare landscape. By synthesizing foundational scientific knowledge, clinical best practices, and interdisciplinary perspectives, scientific evidence will equip healthcare professionals with the competencies required to navigate the complexities of cannabinoid therapeutics. In doing so, it contributes to the development of a healthcare workforce capable of delivering safe, ethical, and evidence-informed cannabis care in an era of rapid scientific and regulatory change (American Nurses Association, 2023; National Academies of Sciences, Engineering, and Medicine, 2017). Furthermore, by situating cannabis within these broader contexts, educating healthcare professionals with the knowledge and critical thinking skills will assist in navigating an increasingly complex and rapidly evolving landscape.

BACKGROUND

Cannabis has re-emerged as one of the most influential forces shaping contemporary healthcare, transforming clinical practice, public health policy, patient behavior, and the responsibilities of healthcare professionals across disciplines. As legalization expands across the United States and internationally, cannabis is no longer a peripheral or stigmatized topic—it is a central component of patient care conversations, symptom management strategies, and interdisciplinary decision-making (National Academies of Sciences, Engineering, and Medicine, 2017; Health Canada, 2022). Nurses, physicians, mental health providers, pharmacists, social workers, and caregivers increasingly encounter individuals who use cannabis for therapeutic, wellness, or recreational purposes. This shift has created an urgent need for evidence-informed guidance, standardized competencies, and a shared clinical language that supports safe, ethical, and patient-centered care (American Nurses Association, 2023).

Limitations in current research pose a need for a comprehensive, scientifically grounded, and clinically relevant foundation for understanding cannabis within modern nursing and healthcare practice. Rather than focusing solely on pharmacology or clinical applications, this text examines cannabis as a multidimensional phenomenon—one that intersects with biomedical science, mental health, public health, ethics, law, social justice, and caregiving (World Health Organization, 2023). Healthcare providers across disciplines are profoundly impacted by the rise of cannabis therapeutics. Nurses, who represent the largest segment of the healthcare workforce, are often the first professionals patients consult when seeking guidance about cannabis use (Zolotov et al., 2021). They must navigate questions related to safety, symptom management, interactions with prescribed medications, and the legal and ethical dimensions of cannabis care (National Academies of Sciences, Engineering, and Medicine, 2017). Physicians and advanced practice providers face increasing pressure to understand cannabis as part of differential diagnosis, chronic disease management, and shared decision-making (National Institute on Drug Abuse, 2020). Pharmacists must evaluate potential drug interactions and counsel patients on safe use (U.S. Food and Drug Administration, 2020). Mental health professionals encounter cannabis in the context of anxiety, trauma, psychosis, and substance use disorders (Murray et al., 2021). Social workers and case managers support families navigating stigma, access barriers, and the psychosocial dimensions of cannabis use (Haug et al., 2022). Across all roles, providers must integrate emerging evidence with patient-centered communication and culturally responsive care.

Caregivers, both formal and informal, are equally affected by the growing normalization of cannabis. Family caregivers supporting individuals with chronic pain, cancer, epilepsy, dementia, or psychiatric conditions often seek guidance on whether cannabis may help alleviate symptoms or improve quality of life (Devinsky et al., 2017). Pediatric and geriatric caregivers face unique challenges related to safety, vulnerability, and ethical considerations (Centers for Disease Control and Prevention, 2022). Home health and community-based caregivers must understand how cannabis use intersects with daily functioning, medication adherence, and the management of chronic conditions (Health Canada, 2022). As cannabis becomes more widely accepted, caregivers increasingly require education, support, and resources to navigate its potential benefits and risks.

Healthcare systems and administrators are also navigating the implications of cannabis integration. Hospitals, clinics, long-term care facilities, and behavioral health organizations must develop policies for documenting cannabis use, managing impairment, ensuring patient safety, and complying with state and federal regulations (Substance Abuse and Mental Health Services Administration, 2023). Administrators must address workforce education, liability concerns, and the integration of cannabis into electronic health records, as well as quality improvement initiatives and risk management frameworks (American Nurses Association, 2023). Public health agencies must consider cannabis within broader strategies related to harm reduction, health equity, and population health (World Health Organization, 2023). These system-level considerations underscore the need for coordinated, interdisciplinary approaches to cannabis care.

This book responds to these emerging needs by offering a comprehensive exploration of cannabis from clinical, scientific, ethical, legal, and administrative perspectives. It examines the endocannabinoid system, therapeutic applications, mental health implications, public health considerations, and the evolving regulatory landscape. It highlights patients' and caregivers' experiences, healthcare professionals' responsibilities, and opportunities for innovation in nursing practice. Each chapter draws on national and international research, professional guidelines, and real-world clinical insights to equip readers with the knowledge and competencies required to navigate cannabis in contemporary healthcare (American Cannabis Nurses Association, 2023; National Academies of Sciences, Engineering, and Medicine, 2017). Ultimately, this book positions cannabis nursing as a transformative specialty that bridges biomedical science, holistic care, and social responsibility. By providing a rigorous, interdisciplinary foundation, it empowers nurses and other healthcare professionals to deliver safe, ethical, and evidence-informed care in an era where cannabis is reshaping the landscape of health and healing.

THE EMERGENCE OF CANNABIS NURSING AS A SPECIALTY

The emergence of cannabis nursing as a specialty reflects a profound transformation in healthcare, driven by shifting scientific evidence, evolving public attitudes, and expanding legalization across the United States and internationally. For decades, cannabis was marginalized within clinical practice due to restrictive policies, limited research access, and persistent stigma. However, as scientific understanding of the endocannabinoid system has advanced and patient use has increased, the need for knowledgeable, evidence-informed nursing practice has become undeniable (National Academies of Sciences, Engineering, and Medicine, 2017). The American Nurses Association's (American Nurses Association, 2023) formal recognition of cannabis nursing as a specialty marks a pivotal moment in legitimizing this field and establishing a foundation for standardized competencies, ethical practice, and professional development.

Historical Context and Shifting Paradigms

The evolution of cannabis nursing cannot be separated from the broader historical and political context surrounding cannabis regulation. In the United States, cannabis was classified as a Schedule I substance in 1970, a designation that severely restricted scientific research and reinforced public perceptions of cannabis as dangerous and medically irrelevant (National Institute on Drug Abuse, 2020). This classification limited access to standardized research materials, constrained funding opportunities, and created regulatory barriers that slowed the development of clinical evidence.

Internationally, however, several countries have advanced cannabis research more aggressively. Israel became a global leader in cannabinoid science beginning in the 1960s, with researchers identifying THC, CBD, and later the endocannabinoid system itself (Mechoulam & Parker, 2013). Canada's National Medical Cannabis Program, established in 2001, generated extensive patient registry data that informed clinical practice and policy development (Health Canada, 2022). European nations, including the Netherlands, Germany, and the United Kingdom, also contributed to the evidence base through clinical trials, observational studies, and regulatory frameworks that supported patient access.

The turning point in the United States came with the publication of the NASEM (2017) report, which systematically reviewed more than 10,000 scientific abstracts and concluded that cannabis has "conclusive or substantial evidence" for several therapeutic applications, including chronic pain, chemotherapy-induced nausea and vomiting, and multiple sclerosis-related spasticity. This authoritative review catalyzed renewed interest in cannabis research and underscored the need for healthcare professionals—including nurses—to develop competencies in cannabis therapeutics.

Professional Recognition and Specialty Development

The ANA's 2023 recognition of cannabis nursing as a specialty represents a major milestone in the evolution of nursing practice. This recognition affirms that cannabis nursing requires a distinct body of knowledge, specialized skills, and defined competencies. It also acknowledges the leadership of the American Cannabis Nurses Association (ACNA), which has spent more than a decade advocating for evidence-based cannabis education, ethical practice standards, and patient safety (American Cannabis Nurses Association, 2023).

Cannabis nursing parallels the development of other advanced practice areas such as palliative care, psychiatric-mental health nursing, and integrative health. Like these specialties, cannabis nursing requires interdisciplinary collaboration, advanced assessment skills, and a deep understanding of complex physiological systems. The endocannabinoid system, in particular, represents a foundational scientific domain that nurses must understand to provide competent care (Zou & Kumar, 2018).

Professional recognition also supports the integration of cannabis education into nursing curricula. Studies show that fewer than 10% of nursing programs currently include content on cannabinoid science or cannabis-related clinical assessment (Zolotov et al., 2021). Specialty recognition creates opportunities for academic institutions to develop standardized curricula, continuing education programs, and certification pathways that prepare nurses to meet the needs of patients who use cannabis therapeutically.

The Expanding Role of Nurses in Cannabis Care

Nurses are uniquely positioned to lead in cannabis care due to their holistic, patient-centered approach and their central role in assessment, education, and care coordination. Research shows that patients often trust nurses more than other clinicians when discussing cannabis use, particularly in stigmatized contexts such as mental health, chronic pain, and palliative care (Haug et al., 2022). Nurses frequently serve as the first point of contact for patients seeking guidance on cannabis use, and they are responsible for evaluating patient histories, identifying potential risks, and providing evidence-based education.

In mental health settings, nurses must assess for cannabis-related risks such as anxiety, psychosis, or cognitive impairment, particularly in adolescents and individuals with a family history of psychiatric disorders (Murray et al., 2021). In medical settings, nurses must evaluate the impact of cannabis on chronic disease management, medication adherence, and symptom control. In palliative care, nurses often support patients and families in navigating cannabis as part of comfort-focused care, addressing questions about symptom relief, quality of life, and ethical considerations (Health Canada, 2022).

Nurses also play a critical role in harm reduction. This includes identifying potential drug interactions, monitoring for adverse effects, and supporting patients in making informed decisions about cannabis use. As cannabis products vary widely in potency, formulation, and delivery method, nurses must help patients navigate these complexities while promoting safety and evidence-informed decision-making.

Cannabis Nursing in Contemporary Healthcare Systems

As healthcare systems adapt to increased cannabis use, nurses are essential in shaping policies, workflows, and quality assurance processes. Hospitals, clinics, long-term care facilities, and behavioral health organizations must develop protocols for documenting cannabis use, managing impairment, ensuring patient safety, and complying with state and federal regulations (Substance Abuse and Mental Health Services Administration, 2023). Administrators must address workforce education, liability concerns, and the integration of cannabis into electronic health records, as well as quality improvement initiatives and risk management frameworks.

Nurses also contribute to research and quality improvement initiatives that advance the evidence base for cannabis care. This includes participating in clinical trials, collecting patient-reported outcomes, and evaluating the impact of cannabis on symptom management, quality of life, and healthcare utilization. As cannabis becomes more integrated into mainstream healthcare, nurses will play an increasingly important role in ensuring that policies and practices reflect current evidence and support patient safety.

FOUNDATIONS OF CANNABIS SCIENCE AND THE ENDOCANNABINOID SYSTEM

Understanding cannabis within healthcare requires a foundational grasp of the biological systems through which cannabinoids exert their effects. Central to this understanding is the endocannabinoid system (ECS), a complex neuromodulatory network that plays a critical role in maintaining physiological homeostasis. Although the ECS was only formally identified in the late 20th century, it is now recognized as one of the most widespread and influential regulatory systems in the human body (Zou & Kumar,

2018). For nurses, physicians, mental health providers, and caregivers, knowledge of the ECS provides essential context for understanding why cannabis affects such a wide range of symptoms and conditions.

The Endocannabinoid System: A Central Regulator of Human Physiology

The ECS consists of three primary components: endogenous cannabinoids (endocannabinoids), cannabinoid receptors, and metabolic enzymes. The two primary endocannabinoids—anandamide (AEA) and 2-arachidonoylglycerol (2-AG)—bind to cannabinoid receptor type 1 (CB1) and type 2 (CB2), influencing processes such as pain perception, mood regulation, immune function, appetite, memory, and stress response (Mackie, 2020). CB1 receptors are highly concentrated in the central nervous system, particularly in regions associated with cognition, emotion, and motor control. CB2 receptors are primarily expressed in immune cells and peripheral tissues, where they modulate inflammation and immune responses.

The ECS operates as a homeostatic regulator, helping the body maintain internal balance in response to stress, injury, or environmental changes. This regulatory function explains why cannabis may influence such diverse conditions as chronic pain, anxiety, epilepsy, inflammatory disorders, and neurodegenerative diseases (National Academies of Sciences, Engineering, and Medicine [NASEM], 2017). It also underscores why healthcare providers across disciplines must understand the ECS, even if they do not directly recommend or authorize cannabis use.

Phytocannabinoids and Their Interaction With the ECS

Cannabis produces more than 120 phytocannabinoids, each with unique chemical structures and biological effects. The two most extensively studied are Δ9-tetrahydrocannabinol (THC) and cannabidiol (CBD). THC binds directly to CB1 receptors, producing psychoactive effects, including analgesia, appetite stimulation, and muscle relaxation (Pertwee, 2015). CBD interacts more indirectly with the ECS, influencing serotonin receptors, TRPV1 channels, and inflammatory pathways, which contribute to its anxiolytic, anti-inflammatory, and neuroprotective properties (Ibeas Bih et al., 2015).

International research has expanded understanding of additional cannabinoids such as cannabigerol (CBG), cannabinol (CBN), and tetrahydrocannabivarin (THCV), each of which may have therapeutic potential. Israel, Canada, and several European nations have led much of this research, contributing to a growing global evidence base (Mechoulam & Parker, 2013; Health Canada, 2022). As this science evolves, healthcare providers must remain informed about emerging findings and their implications for patient care. Table 1 demonstrates key research studies on the endocannabinoid system.

Table 1. Key research studies on the Endocannabinoid System (ECS)

Section	Study/Authors	Year	Focus of Study	Key Findings Related to ECS	Relevance to Cannabis Science
Foundational ECS Research	Mechoulam & Parker	2013	Identification and characterization of the ECS	Described the ECS as a neuromodulatory system regulating mood, appetite, pain, and cognition	Established the biological basis for cannabinoid activity and therapeutic potential
Receptor Function & Physiology	Mackie	2020	Distribution and function of CB1 and CB2 receptors	Demonstrated high CB1 density in CNS regions governing memory, motor control, and emotion; CB2 in immune tissues	Clarified why THC produces psychoactive effects and why cannabinoids modulate inflammation
Receptor Function & Physiology	Zou & Kumar	2018	Comprehensive review of ECS physiology	Identified ECS as a homeostatic regulator influencing multiple organ systems	Provided foundational framework for understanding broad therapeutic applications of cannabis
Clinical Applications	Devinsky et al.	2017	CBD in treatment-resistant epilepsy	Showed CBD reduces seizure frequency via ECS-related and non-ECS pathways	Supported FDA approval of CBD-based medications and validated ECS involvement in seizure modulation
Clinical Applications	Russo	2016	Clinical Endocannabinoid Deficiency (CED) hypothesis	Proposed that low endocannabinoid tone may contribute to migraine, fibromyalgia, and IBS	Suggested rationale for cannabinoid-based therapies in chronic, treatment-resistant conditions
Clinical Applications	Bergamaschi et al.	2011	CBD and anxiety modulation	Demonstrated CBD reduces anxiety through 5-HT1A and ECS-related mechanisms	Provided evidence for anxiolytic properties of cannabinoids
Population-Level Insights	Di Forti et al.	2019	High-potency cannabis and psychosis risk	Found association between high-THC exposure and increased psychosis incidence	Highlighted ECS involvement in dopaminergic and neuropsychiatric pathways
Population-Level Insights	NASEM Report	2017	Systematic review of >10,000 cannabis studies	Concluded substantial evidence for cannabis in chronic pain, spasticity, and nausea	Reinforced ECS as a therapeutic target across multiple conditions
Population-Level Insights	Health Canada Registry Data	2022	Real-world outcomes of medical cannabis use	Documented patient-reported improvements in pain, sleep, and quality of life	Provided population-level evidence supporting ECS-mediated symptom relief

Importance of the ECS for Healthcare Providers and Caregivers

The ECS is relevant to nearly every area of healthcare because it intersects with systems that providers routinely assess and manage. In pain management, the ECS modulates nociceptive signaling, making it central to understanding chronic pain and neuropathy (National Academies of Sciences, Engineering, and Medicine, 2017). Within mental health, dysregulation of the ECS has been implicated in anxiety, depression, post-traumatic stress disorder, and psychosis, highlighting its importance in psychiatric assessment and treatment planning (Murray et al., 2021). Neurologically, the ECS influences seizure activity, neuroinflammation, and neuroprotection, which helps explain why CBD has demonstrated efficacy in the treatment of treatment-resistant epilepsy and other neurological conditions (Devinsky et al., 2017). In geriatric care, age-related changes in ECS function may affect cognition, fall risk, and medication interactions, requiring careful evaluation in older adults. Pediatric considerations are equally important, as the developing ECS plays a significant role in neurodevelopment and raises unique concerns regarding adolescent cannabis exposure (Centers for Disease Control and Prevention, 2022). In palliative care, the ECS contributes to appetite, sleep, mood, and overall comfort—domains that are essential to supporting quality of life at the end of life (Health Canada, 2022). Because the ECS influences so many physiological systems, providers across disciplines must be prepared to assess how cannabis use may interact with existing conditions, medications, and treatment plans.

The ECS and the Concept of Clinical Endocannabinoid Deficiency

One emerging area of research is the hypothesis of "clinical endocannabinoid deficiency" (CED), which proposes that certain chronic conditions may be associated with insufficient or dysregulated endocannabinoid signaling. Early evidence suggests that disorders such as migraine, fibromyalgia, and irritable bowel syndrome may involve ECS dysfunction (Russo, 2016). Although this theory remains under investigation, it has gained attention because it may help explain why some patients report symptom relief with cannabinoid-based therapies.

For healthcare providers, the CED hypothesis highlights the importance of understanding the ECS not only as a target of cannabis but as a fundamental physiological system that may contribute to chronic illness. This perspective encourages a more nuanced approach to patient assessment and supports integrating ECS-related knowledge into nursing and medical education.

Global Contributions to ECS and Cannabis Science

While the United States has historically lagged in cannabis research due to federal restrictions, international contributions have significantly advanced the field. Israel's pioneering work in cannabinoid chemistry and clinical trials has shaped global understanding of cannabis therapeutics (Mechoulam & Parker, 2013). Canada's national medical cannabis program has generated large-scale patient registry data, offering insights into real-world patterns of use, symptom outcomes, and safety considerations (Health Canada, 2022). European agencies, such as the National Institute for Health and Care Excellence (NICE), have published clinical guidelines for cannabis-based medicines, further strengthening the evidence base (National Institute for Health and Care Excellence, 2019). These global efforts underscore the importance of viewing cannabis science through an international lens. For nurses and other healthcare professionals, staying informed about global research enhances clinical decision-making and supports culturally competent care for diverse patient populations.

CLINICAL ASSESSMENT, NURSING CONSIDERATIONS, AND SAFETY MONITORING

As cannabis use becomes increasingly prevalent across clinical populations, healthcare providers must rely on rigorous scientific evidence to guide assessment, safety monitoring, and patient education. Randomized control trials (RCTs), systematic reviews, and epidemiological studies have clarified both the therapeutic potential and the risks associated with cannabis use. Nurses, who frequently serve as the primary point of contact for patients, must integrate this evidence into comprehensive assessments that consider biological, psychological, and social dimensions of health. The scientific literature consistently emphasizes that cannabis assessment must be individualized, evidence-informed, and grounded in an understanding of the endocannabinoid system and its interactions with disease processes (Zou & Kumar, 2018; National Academies of Sciences, Engineering, and Medicine, 2017).

A comprehensive assessment begins with a detailed exploration of the patient's cannabis use history. Research indicates that up to 30–40% of adults with chronic pain report using cannabis for symptom management, often without disclosing this to their healthcare providers (Boehnke et al., 2016). Studies also show that patients frequently self-titrate cannabis based on perceived symptom relief, which underscores the importance of understanding not only frequency and duration of use but also product characteristics, including cannabinoid ratios and terpene profiles (Cuttler et al., 2018). Nurses must assess how patients perceive the effects of cannabis on pain, sleep, mood, and daily functioning, while also evaluating for adverse effects such as cognitive impairment or anxiety. Evidence from observational studies suggests that patients often report improvements in quality of life and reductions in opioid use when incorporating cannabis into their symptom management strategies (Campbell et al., 2018), though scientific interpretation is important as variability in the study design is noted.

The assessment is a critical component of cannabis-related care, supported by a substantial body of research. RCTs have demonstrated a reduction in anxiety with the use of CBD for individuals who have social anxiety disorder, as CBD modulates the limbic system activity (Bergamaschi et al., 2011). Conversely, high-potency THC has been associated with increased risk of psychosis, particularly among adolescents and individuals with genetic vulnerability (Murray et al., 2021). A large case-control study across 11 European sites found that daily use of high-THC cannabis increased the odds of psychotic disorder nearly fivefold (Di Forti et al., 2019). Nurses must therefore assess for psychiatric history, family history of psychosis, and current mental health symptoms, recognizing that cannabis may have differential effects depending on individual vulnerability. Screening tools such as the PHQ-9, GAD-7, and CUDIT-R have demonstrated reliability in identifying co-occurring mental health concerns and problematic cannabis use patterns (Substance Abuse and Mental Health Services Administration, 2023). These tools can be particularly practical for nurses, enabling them to efficiently assess mental health status and substance use. Implementing these tools involves brief, structured interviews or questionnaires that can be easily integrated into routine assessments, allowing nurses to make informed clinical decisions with greater confidence.

Medication reconciliation is an essential component of cannabis assessment, supported by extensive pharmacokinetic research. CBD is a potent inhibitor of cytochrome P450 enzymes, particularly CYP2C19 and CYP3A4, which can significantly increase serum levels of medications such as clobazam, warfarin, and certain antidepressants (U.S. Food and Drug Administration, 2020). RCTs in pediatric epilepsy populations have demonstrated that CBD can elevate clobazam metabolite levels by more than 60%, necessitating careful monitoring and dose adjustments (Devinsky et al., 2017). THC also interacts with CYP enzymes, though its effects are less pronounced. Nurses must collaborate with pharmacists and prescribers to identify potential interactions and ensure safe medication management.

Safety monitoring must be continuous and evidence-based. Clinical trials and observational studies consistently report that cannabis may cause sedation, dizziness, impaired concentration, and orthostatic hypotension, all of which can affect daily functioning and increase risk of injury (National Academies of Sciences, Engineering, and Medicine, 2017). Longitudinal studies have shown that heavy, long-term cannabis use may be associated with cognitive decline, particularly when use begins in adolescence (Meier et al., 2012). Nurses must monitor for changes in cognition, mood, and functional status, and assess whether cannabis use aligns with the patient's goals and improves quality of life. In palliative care settings, observational studies have shown that cannabis may improve appetite, sleep, and overall comfort, though evidence remains mixed and requires individualized assessment (Health Canada, 2022).

Education and harm reduction are central to nursing practice in cannabis care. Research shows that patients who receive evidence-based counseling are more likely to use regulated products, understand and comply with avoidance of high-risk behaviors such as driving under the influence, and recognize early signs of problematic use (Haug et al., 2022). Nurses must provide clear, nonjudgmental information about potential risks and benefits, emphasizing the importance of product quality, safe consumption practices, and open communication with the healthcare team. By integrating scientific evidence into patient education, nurses help individuals navigate cannabis use safely and effectively, contributing to improved outcomes and quality of life.

The Significance of Cannabis in Non-Healthcare Settings

Cannabis is gaining increasing significance beyond clinical and healthcare environments, influencing a wide range of social, economic, cultural, and regulatory domains. As legalization expands across multiple jurisdictions, cannabis has become embedded in sectors such as agriculture, commerce, criminal justice reform, workplace policy, education, and community development (National Academies of Sciences, Engineering, and Medicine [NASEM], 2017; World Health Organization [WHO], 2023). Understanding these broader contexts is essential for nurses and other professionals who must navigate the intersection of medical cannabis use with societal norms, legal structures, and public perceptions.

In the economic sector, cannabis has emerged as a major agricultural and commercial commodity. The expansion of regulated cultivation, manufacturing, and retail industries has generated substantial employment opportunities and tax revenues in many regions (Health Canada, 2022). These developments have stimulated innovation in plant science, product formulation, and supply-chain logistics, while also raising questions about sustainability, environmental impact, and equitable participation in emerging markets. The increasing economic visibility of cannabis contributes to shifting public attitudes, reducing stigma, and normalizing its presence in everyday life (Centers for Disease Control and Prevention [CDC], 2022).

Cannabis also plays a significant role in legal and social justice contexts. Decades of prohibition disproportionately affected marginalized communities, resulting in inequities in arrest rates, incarceration, and long-term socioeconomic outcomes (Centers for Disease Control and Prevention, 2022). Contemporary legalization efforts increasingly incorporate restorative justice measures, such as expungement of prior convictions and community reinvestment initiatives. These policy shifts reflect a broader societal recognition of the need to address historical harms and promote equitable access to the benefits of legalization

(Substance Abuse and Mental Health Services Administration, 2023). For healthcare professionals, awareness of these dynamics is essential for providing culturally responsive and trauma-informed care.

Workplace environments represent another important non-healthcare setting influenced by cannabis. Employers must navigate complex regulatory landscapes involving occupational safety, impairment assessment, and employee rights (Substance Abuse and Mental Health Services Administration, 2023). The coexistence of legal cannabis use with workplace drug-testing policies creates challenges for both employers and employees, particularly in safety-sensitive industries. Nurses working in occupational health, case management, or administrative roles may encounter situations in which cannabis use intersects with disability accommodations, workers' compensation claims, or return-to-work evaluations. A nuanced understanding of these issues supports fair, evidence-informed decision-making.

Educational settings are also affected by the evolving cannabis landscape. Schools, universities, and community organizations increasingly require evidence-based curricula addressing cannabis science, harm reduction, and legal considerations (World Health Organization, 2023). Adolescents and young adults represent a population with heightened vulnerability to the neurocognitive effects of cannabis, making prevention and education efforts essential (Centers for Disease Control and Prevention, 2022). Nurses who work in school health, public health, or community outreach roles contribute to these initiatives by providing accurate information and supporting early intervention strategies.

Cannabis further influences cultural and social practices, including wellness trends, spiritual traditions, and recreational activities. The normalization of cannabis in media, advertising, and consumer culture shapes public perceptions and may influence patterns of use across demographic groups (National Academies of Sciences, Engineering, and Medicine, 2017). These cultural shifts have implications for healthcare providers, who must navigate conversations with patients whose beliefs, expectations, or motivations for cannabis use are shaped by non-medical influences.

Overall, the significance of cannabis in non-healthcare settings underscores the importance of interdisciplinary awareness and societal context in cannabis nursing. Nurses must understand how economic forces, legal reforms, workplace policies, educational initiatives, and cultural narratives shape patient experiences and influence patterns of cannabis use (American Nurses Association, 2023). This broader perspective enables healthcare professionals to provide informed, culturally competent, and ethically grounded care in an era where cannabis extends far beyond the boundaries of clinical practice. Table 2, Key Non-Healthcare Sectors Influenced by Cannabis and Their Implications synthesizes major non-healthcare sectors influenced by cannabis legalization and commercialization. It highlights the interdisciplinary implications for nursing practice, public health, and policy development. Representative sources reflect foundational literature and governmental reports that inform current understanding of cannabis-related societal impacts.

Table 2. Key non-healthcare sectors influenced by cannabis and their implications

Sector	Key Areas of Influence	Context and Scope	Implications for Society	Relevance to Health Care Professionals	Representative Sources
Economic and Commercial Sector	Cultivation, manufacturing, retail markets, taxation	Legal cannabis has become a multibillion-dollar industry, driving growth in agriculture, biotechnology, retail, and supply-chain logistics. Market expansion has increased employment opportunities and stimulated innovation in product development and agricultural science (Health Canada, 2022).	Increased tax revenue, job creation, and economic diversification; concerns regarding sustainability, environmental impact, and equitable market participation.	Nurses benefit from understanding product variability, potency, and consumer trends that influence patient use and expectations.	Health Canada (2022); NASEM (2017)
Legal and Criminal Justice Systems	Decriminalization, expungement, enforcement practices, restorative justice	Cannabis policy reform has prompted major shifts in policing, sentencing, and criminal record expungement. These reforms aim to address decades of disproportionate enforcement affecting marginalized communities (Centers for Disease Control and Prevention, 2022).	Reduction in cannabis-related arrests; improved social equity; increased community trust; ongoing disparities in enforcement.	Awareness of legal status and patient rights supports culturally responsive, trauma-informed care.	CDC (2022); Substance Abuse and Mental Health Services Administration (2023)
Workplace and Occupational Settings	Drug testing, impairment standards, employee rights, safety-sensitive roles	Employers must balance legal cannabis use with occupational safety requirements. The absence of validated impairment tests complicates policy development, particularly in transportation, construction, and healthcare (SAMHSA, 2023).	Evolving workplace policies; challenges in ensuring safety; potential conflicts between employee rights and employer liability.	Occupational health nurses navigate return-to-work evaluations, disability accommodations, and safety assessments.	Substance Abuse and Mental Health Services Administration (2023); World Health Organization (2023)

continued on following page

Table 2. Continued

Sector	Key Areas of Influence	Context and Scope	Implications for Society	Relevance to Health Care Professionals	Representative Sources
Educational Institutions	Prevention programs, curriculum development, youth education	Schools and universities increasingly require evidence-based cannabis education. Adolescents remain vulnerable to neurocognitive effects, making prevention and early intervention essential (Centers for Disease Control and Prevention, 2022).	Improved public health literacy; reduced youth risk behaviors; need for standardized curricula.	School and public health nurses support prevention, early identification, and accurate information dissemination.	CDC (2022); WHO (2023)
Community and Cultural Environments	Social norms, media representation, wellness trends	Cannabis is increasingly normalized through media, advertising, and consumer culture. Public narratives influence perceptions of safety, therapeutic value, and recreational use (National Academies of Sciences, Engineering, and Medicine, 2017).	Shifts in cultural attitudes; increased visibility of cannabis in daily life; potential for misinformation.	Nurses must understand cultural influences shaping patient beliefs, expectations, and motivations.	NASEM (2017); WHO (2023)
Environmental and Agricultural Systems	Water use, energy consumption, sustainability practices	Cannabis cultivation—especially indoor growing—requires significant water and energy resources. Environmental impacts include soil degradation, pesticide use, and carbon emissions (Health Canada, 2022).	Need for sustainable agricultural practices; environmental regulation; ecological monitoring.	Environmental health nurses may address exposure risks and sustainability concerns.	Health Canada (2022)

continued on following page

Table 2. Continued

Sector	Key Areas of Influence	Context and Scope	Implications for Society	Relevance to Health Care Professionals	Representative Sources
Technology and Innovation	Biotechnology, extraction science, laboratory testing	Advances in extraction methods, analytical chemistry, and product engineering have improved product consistency and safety. Technology also supports contaminant testing and cannabinoid profiling (National Academies of Sciences, Engineering, and Medicine, 2017).	Improved product quality; enhanced consumer safety; rapid innovation in cannabis science.	Clinicians must understand product types, formulations, and testing standards to guide patient education.	NASEM (2017)
Public Safety and Transportation	Impaired driving policies, roadside testing, law enforcement training	Cannabis legalization requires updated impaired-driving laws and reliable roadside testing tools. Current assessments remain limited and inconsistent (Substance Abuse and Mental Health Services Administration, 2023).	Public safety concerns; need for validated impairment measures; evolving enforcement strategies.	Emergency and trauma nurses frequently encounter cannabis-related motor vehicle incidents.	Substance Abuse and Mental Health Services Administration (2023); CDC (2022)
Housing and Community Planning	Zoning laws, public housing regulations, landlord policies	Cannabis use intersects with housing policies, including restrictions in public housing and zoning for dispensaries. These policies influence community access and equity (World Health Organization, 2023).	Community disparities in access; neighborhood-level policy variation; potential for housing insecurity.	Nurses working in community health must understand how housing policies affect patient access and stability.	World Health Organization (2023)

continued on following page

Table 2. Continued

Sector	Key Areas of Influence	Context and Scope	Implications for Society	Relevance to Health Care Professionals	Representative Sources
Tourism and Hospitality	Cannabis tourism, hospitality services, recreational travel	Legalization has led to cannabis-focused tourism, influencing hospitality, travel, and recreational industries. This trend raises public health and safety considerations (Health Canada, 2022).	Increased tourism revenue; need for public health messaging; cross-jurisdictional legal challenges.	Nurses may encounter tourists seeking medical guidance or experiencing adverse effects.	Health Canada (2022)
Ethics, Governance, and Social Responsibility	Corporate ethics, equity programs, community reinvestment	Cannabis industries increasingly adopt social responsibility frameworks addressing equity, transparency, and community impact (Substance Abuse and Mental Health Services Administration, 2023).	Improved accountability; opportunities for community reinvestment; ethical considerations in commercialization.	Nurses contribute to ethical policy development and advocate for equitable access to care.	Substance Abuse and Mental Health Services Administration (2023); ANA (2023)

Policy Implications of Cannabis Use in Non-Healthcare Settings

The expanding significance of cannabis across non-healthcare sectors carries important policy implications that affect public health, regulatory oversight, and clinical practice. Policymakers must balance economic opportunity, social justice priorities, and public safety concerns while ensuring that regulatory frameworks support equitable and evidence-informed approaches to cannabis use (National Academies of Sciences, Engineering, and Medicine, 2017). As commercial markets grow, policies governing product quality, contaminant testing, labeling accuracy, and consumer protection become essential to safeguard public health and ensure individuals have access to safe, standardized cannabis products (Health Canada, 2022).

Legal reforms related to decriminalization and expungement reflect efforts to address the disproportionate impact of prohibition on marginalized communities. These policies aim to reduce inequities in arrest rates, incarceration, and long-term socioeconomic outcomes (Centers for Disease Control and Prevention, 2022). For healthcare professionals, awareness of these reforms is essential for providing culturally competent care and understanding the social determinants that shape patient experiences with cannabis.

Workplace policy development remains a complex area due to the coexistence of legal cannabis use and workplace safety requirements. The absence of universally accepted impairment standards complicates employer decision-making, particularly in safety-sensitive industries (Substance Abuse and Mental

Health Services Administration, 2023). Occupational health nurses and administrators must interpret evolving regulations and support fair, evidence-based implementation of workplace policies.

Educational policy is another critical domain. Schools and universities require clear guidelines for prevention, early intervention, and youth education, given the heightened vulnerability of adolescents to cannabis-related neurocognitive effects (Centers for Disease Control and Prevention, 2022). Evidence-informed curricula and prevention strategies can support healthier decision-making and reduce potential harms.

Regulatory agencies must continue refining policies related to cultivation, distribution, taxation, and product oversight. Effective regulation requires coordination across public health, agriculture, law enforcement, and economic development sectors (World Health Organization, 2023). As cannabis becomes increasingly integrated into society, policies must remain adaptable to emerging scientific evidence, technological advancements, and evolving patterns of use. For nurses and other healthcare professionals, understanding these policy landscapes is essential for providing informed guidance, advocating for patient safety, and contributing to interdisciplinary policy development.

Foundational Knowledge in Cannabinoid Pharmacology, Dosing Strategies, Delivery Methods, and Symptom Management

Cannabinoid science has advanced rapidly over the past several decades, transforming cannabis from a stigmatized substance into a subject of rigorous biomedical inquiry. Foundational knowledge in cannabinoid pharmacology, conceptual dosing principles, delivery systems, and symptom management is essential for nurses, clinicians, and caregivers who support patients navigating cannabis therapeutics. Understanding these core concepts enables healthcare professionals to evaluate patient needs, anticipate therapeutic responses, identify potential risks, and guide evidence-informed decision-making across diverse clinical settings.

Cannabinoid pharmacology begins with the recognition that cannabis contains more than 120 phytocannabinoids, with Δ9-tetrahydrocannabinol (THC) and cannabidiol (CBD) being the most extensively studied. These compounds exert their effects primarily through the endocannabinoid system (ECS), a neuromodulatory network that regulates homeostasis across multiple physiological domains, including pain perception, mood, appetite, immune function, and neuroprotection (Zou & Kumar, 2018). THC acts as a partial agonist at CB1 receptors, which are densely concentrated in the central nervous system. This interaction produces psychoactive effects, analgesia, appetite stimulation, and muscle relaxation, but may also contribute to anxiety, tachycardia, impaired cognition, and psychosis in vulnerable individuals (Murray et al., 2021). THC also binds to CB2 receptors in peripheral tissues, influencing inflammation and immune activity.

CBD, in contrast, has low affinity for CB1 and CB2 receptors and instead modulates multiple non-cannabinoid pathways, including serotonin 5-HT1A receptors, TRPV1 channels, and adenosine signaling (Ibeas Bih et al., 2015). These mechanisms contribute to CBD's anxiolytic, anti-inflammatory, anticonvulsant, and neuroprotective properties. Importantly, CBD may mitigate some of THC's adverse effects, such as anxiety or cognitive impairment, although findings vary across studies. Beyond THC and CBD, emerging cannabinoids such as cannabigerol (CBG), cannabinol (CBN), and tetrahydrocannabivarin (THCV) are gaining scientific attention. Early evidence suggests potential roles in inflammation, sleep regulation, metabolic function, and neurodegeneration, though research remains preliminary (Mechoulam & Parker, 2013).

The pharmacokinetics of cannabinoids are influenced by route of administration, product formulation, individual metabolism, and genetic factors. Cannabinoids are highly lipophilic, distribute into fatty tissues, and exhibit prolonged elimination phases. Metabolism occurs primarily through hepatic cytochrome P450 enzymes, creating potential for drug–drug interactions—particularly with CBD, which inhibits CYP2C19 and CYP3A4 (U.S. Food and Drug Administration, 2020). These interactions underscore the importance of comprehensive medication reconciliation and interdisciplinary collaboration.

Dosing recommendations for cannabinoid-based therapeutics rely on principles of individualized, gradual titration rather than fixed numerical guidelines. The variability in patient physiology, cannabinoid sensitivity, metabolic rate, prior cannabis exposure, and comorbid conditions necessitates a cautious, patient-centered approach. Evidence-informed frameworks consistently emphasize beginning with the lowest feasible dose, introducing cannabinoids slowly, and adjusting incrementally based on therapeutic response and tolerability (National Academies of Sciences, Engineering, and Medicine, 2017). This strategy is particularly important given the biphasic effects of THC—where low exposures may alleviate symptoms such as pain or anxiety, while higher exposures may exacerbate them—and the potential for CBD to influence serum levels of concomitant medications through cytochrome P450 interactions (U.S. Food and Drug Administration, 2020). Effective dosing requires ongoing assessment of functional outcomes, including changes in sleep, mood, pain interference, appetite, and daily functioning, rather than relying solely on symptom intensity. Nurses play a central role in guiding patients through this process by monitoring for adverse effects, evaluating therapeutic benefit, and supporting informed decision-making as part of a comprehensive, interdisciplinary care plan. benefit from systematically tracking their responses, noting both therapeutic effects and adverse reactions.

Delivery methods further shape cannabinoid pharmacokinetics and clinical effects. Inhalation through smoking or vaporization delivers cannabinoids rapidly to the bloodstream via pulmonary absorption, producing effects within minutes and lasting two to four hours (Centers for Disease Control and Prevention, 2022). This route allows for rapid symptom relief and easier self-titration but carries respiratory risks, particularly with combustion. Vaporization reduces exposure to harmful byproducts but still requires caution in individuals with pulmonary disease.

Oral ingestion through capsules, edibles, or oils undergoes first-pass metabolism, resulting in delayed onset and prolonged duration. This route is useful for sustained symptom control but increases the risk of delayed overconsumption due to slow onset. Metabolic conversion of THC to 11-hydroxy-THC may intensify psychoactive effects. Sublingual and buccal administration, such as tinctures and sprays absorbed through the oral mucosa, offers an intermediate onset and more predictable effects than edibles, making these products common choices for chronic pain, anxiety, and sleep disturbances. Topical products provide localized relief without systemic psychoactivity, making them useful for musculoskeletal pain or inflammation. Transdermal patches deliver cannabinoids systemically over extended periods and may benefit patients requiring steady plasma levels. Emerging delivery systems, including nanotechnology-enhanced formulations and metered-dose inhalers, aim to improve bioavailability and dosing precision, potentially enhancing safety and consistency in clinical settings.

Cannabis is used to manage a wide range of symptoms, though evidence varies by condition. Chronic pain is one of the most common indications, with moderate evidence supporting cannabis for neuropathic pain and patient-reported improvements in sleep and quality of life (National Academies of Sciences, Engineering, and Medicine, 2017). Anxiety and mood disorders represent another area of interest. CBD shows promise for reducing anxiety, particularly in social anxiety disorder, while high-THC products may worsen anxiety or trigger panic in susceptible individuals (Bergamaschi et al., 2011).

Sleep disturbances may improve with THC, which can reduce sleep latency, and with CBD, which may enhance sleep quality by reducing anxiety or pain. In epilepsy, high-quality evidence supports CBD for treatment-resistant pediatric epilepsies such as Dravet and Lennox-Gastaut syndromes (Devinsky et al., 2017). In oncology, cannabis may alleviate chemotherapy-induced nausea and vomiting, stimulate appetite, and improve overall well-being, though evidence varies across formulations. In palliative and end-of-life care, cannabis may support comfort, appetite, sleep, and mood, aligning with holistic care goals (Health Canada, 2022).

Across all symptom domains, healthcare providers must balance patient-reported outcomes with scientific evidence, recognizing that cannabis responses are highly individualized. Effective symptom management requires ongoing assessment, open communication, and a commitment to evidence-informed, patient-centered care. By integrating foundational knowledge in cannabinoid pharmacology, conceptual dosing strategies, delivery methods, and symptom management, clinicians and caregivers can support safe, ethical, and effective cannabis use in diverse clinical contexts.

Legal, Ethical, and Administrative Considerations in Cannabis Care

The integration of cannabis into healthcare practice occurs within a complex and rapidly evolving legal and ethical landscape. Providers, caregivers, and healthcare systems must navigate conflicting federal and state regulations, emerging professional standards, and significant ethical considerations related to patient autonomy, safety, and equity. As cannabis becomes increasingly normalized, the need for clear administrative policies and evidence-informed ethical frameworks has become essential. This section synthesizes national and international research, regulatory guidance, and professional standards to support healthcare providers in delivering safe, ethical, and legally compliant cannabis care.

The Legal Landscape: Federal–State Tensions and Global Variability

Cannabis regulation in the United States is characterized by a fundamental tension between federal prohibition and state-level legalization. Under the U.S. Controlled Substances Act, cannabis remains a Schedule I substance, defined as having "no accepted medical use" and a "high potential for abuse" (National Institute on Drug Abuse, 2020). This classification restricts research, limits interstate commerce, and creates legal ambiguity for healthcare providers. At the same time, more than 38 states have legalized medical cannabis, and 24 have legalized adult-use cannabis, creating a patchwork of policies that vary widely in terms of qualifying conditions, product regulations, and provider responsibilities (Centers for Disease Control and Prevention, 2022).

Internationally, regulatory frameworks differ substantially. Canada legalized medical cannabis nationally in 2001 and adult-use cannabis in 2018, creating one of the most comprehensive regulatory systems in the world (Health Canada, 2022). Germany, Israel, Australia, and the United Kingdom have established medical cannabis programs supported by national guidelines and standardized products. These international models provide valuable insights into how centralized regulation can support product quality, patient safety, and research infrastructure.

For healthcare providers, understanding the legal context is essential for safe practice. Nurses and clinicians must be aware of their state's scope-of-practice laws, documentation requirements, and institutional policies. They must also understand the implications of federal law, particularly in federally funded institutions such as Veterans Affairs (VA) hospitals, where cannabis remains prohibited despite widespread patient use (National Academies of Sciences, Engineering, and Medicine, 2017).

Ethical Considerations: Autonomy, Beneficence, and Harm Reduction

Ethical considerations are central to cannabis care, particularly given the historical stigma, evolving evidence base, and diverse patient motivations for use. The principles of autonomy, beneficence, nonmaleficence, and justice provide a framework for ethical decision-making. Respect for autonomy requires that providers support patients in making informed decisions about cannabis use. Research shows that patients often turn to cannabis after experiencing inadequate relief from conventional treatments, particularly for chronic pain, anxiety, and cancer-related symptoms (Boehnke et al., 2016). Nurses must provide accurate, evidence-based information while respecting patient values and preferences. Beneficence and nonmaleficence require providers to balance potential benefits with known risks. Systematic reviews indicate that cannabis may offer therapeutic benefits for certain conditions, but also carries risks such as cognitive impairment, psychiatric symptoms, and drug interactions (National Academies of Sciences, Engineering, and Medicine, 2017). Ethical practice requires careful assessment, monitoring, and patient education to minimize harm. Justice requires equitable access to safe, regulated cannabis products and unbiased care. Research shows that racial and socioeconomic disparities persist in cannabis-related arrests, access to medical cannabis programs, and participation in the legal cannabis industry (World Health Organization, 2023). Healthcare providers must be aware of these inequities and work to ensure that all patients receive fair, stigma-free care. Harm reduction requires providers and administrators to ensure compliance with documentation, liability, and institutional policy to ensure consumer and workplace safety.

Documentation, Liability, and Institutional Policy

Healthcare institutions must develop clear policies to guide cannabis-related care, including documentation standards, safety protocols, and risk management strategies. Documentation should include the patient's cannabis use history, perceived benefits and risks, potential interactions, and any education provided. Accurate documentation protects both patients and providers, particularly in settings where cannabis use may affect treatment decisions, medication management, or safety protocols.

Liability concerns are significant, particularly in states where cannabis remains illegal at the federal level. Providers must practice within their scope, follow institutional policies, and avoid making unsupported claims about cannabis efficacy. Research shows that inconsistent institutional policies contribute to provider uncertainty and may discourage open communication with patients (Haug et al., 2022). Clear administrative guidance is essential for supporting safe, consistent practice.

Workplace Safety and Impairment Considerations

Cannabis use raises important questions about workplace safety, particularly in safety-sensitive occupations such as transportation, construction, and healthcare. Evidence indicates that cannabis can impair reaction time, coordination, and short-term memory, though impairment varies widely based on product type, individual tolerance, and timing of use (Health Canada, 2022). Healthcare providers must assess whether cannabis use may affect a patient's ability to perform daily activities safely, including driving, operating machinery, or managing medications.

Institutions must also address cannabis use among healthcare staff. While off-duty cannabis use may be legal in many states, impairment during work hours is prohibited. Administrators must develop clear policies that balance employee rights with patient safety, informed by evidence on impairment detection and workplace risk (Centers for Disease Control and Prevention, 2022).

Administrative Leadership and System-Level Integration

Healthcare administrators play a critical role in integrating cannabis into organizational practice by creating clear policies that guide documentation and disclosure, medication reconciliation, safety monitoring, staff training, patient education, legal compliance, and quality improvement efforts. Evidence suggests that healthcare institutions with well-defined cannabis policies benefit from stronger communication, reduced liability concerns, and more consistent patient care (Substance Abuse and Mental Health Services Administration, 2023). Administrators are also responsible for supporting workforce education, which is essential given that many nurses and clinicians report feeling underprepared to address cannabis-related questions or provide guidance to patients (Zolotov et al., 2021).

The Role of Professional Organizations

Professional organizations such as the American Nurses Association (ANA), American Cannabis Nurses Association (ACNA), and National Council of State Boards of Nursing (NCSBN) have begun issuing guidance on cannabis care. The ANA's 2023 recognition of cannabis nursing as a specialty underscores the need for standardized competencies and ethical frameworks. The NCSBN (2018) has issued guidelines for nurses working with medical cannabis patients, emphasizing assessment, education, and safety monitoring. These professional standards provide a foundation for evidence-informed practice and support the integration of cannabis into nursing education and certification pathways.

Stigma Reduction, Health Equity, and Public Health Implications

Cannabis use exists at the intersection of science, culture, law, and public health. Despite growing legalization and an expanding body of scientific evidence, stigma surrounding cannabis remains deeply embedded in healthcare systems, public policy, and societal attitudes. This stigma influences patient disclosure, provider communication, access to care, and the equitable distribution of health resources. A substantial body of research demonstrates that stigma—both structural and interpersonal—continues to shape patient experiences and health outcomes, particularly among marginalized populations (Hathaway et al., 2018). As cannabis becomes increasingly integrated into healthcare, reducing stigma and addressing inequities are essential components of ethical, evidence-informed practice.

The roots of cannabis stigma can be traced to decades of political rhetoric, racialized criminalization, and misinformation. Early 20th-century U.S. federal campaigns portrayed cannabis as dangerous and morally corrupting, often targeting immigrant and minority communities (Musto, 1999). The 1970 Controlled Substances Act classified cannabis as a Schedule I substance, reinforcing the perception that it lacked medical value and posed significant risks (National Institute on Drug Abuse, 2020). These policies contributed to widespread public fear, limited scientific research, and punitive legal consequences that disproportionately affected Black and Latinx communities (World Health Organization, 2023). Even as scientific understanding has evolved, the legacy of these policies continues to influence public attitudes and healthcare practices. Studies show that many healthcare providers still hold negative or outdated beliefs about cannabis, often due to limited education and exposure to biased information (Zolotov et al., 2021). This stigma can discourage patients from discussing cannabis use openly, leading to missed opportunities for assessment, safety monitoring, and harm reduction.

Stigma within healthcare settings has significant implications for patient care. Research indicates that patients who perceive judgment or disapproval from providers are less likely to disclose cannabis use, even when it is medically relevant (Haug et al., 2022). This lack of disclosure can compromise clinical decision-making, particularly in areas such as medication reconciliation, mental health assessment, and chronic disease management. Providers may underestimate the therapeutic potential of cannabis or overestimate its risks due to limited training and exposure to outdated information (Zolotov et al., 2021). This knowledge gap can contribute to implicit bias, affecting how providers interpret patient symptoms, assess risk, and offer guidance. Nurses, who often serve as patient advocates and educators, play a critical role in counteracting stigma by fostering open communication, providing evidence-based information, and supporting patient autonomy.

Health equity is a central concern in cannabis policy and practice. Despite widespread legalization, access to medical cannabis remains uneven across demographic groups. Research shows that individuals from lower socioeconomic backgrounds, rural communities, and minority populations face greater barriers to accessing regulated cannabis products, medical certifications, and cannabis-competent healthcare providers (World Health Organization, 2023). These disparities reflect broader inequities in healthcare access, insurance coverage, and social determinants of health. Racial disparities are particularly pronounced. Although cannabis use rates are similar across racial groups, Black individuals in the United States have historically been arrested for cannabis-related offenses at nearly four times the rate of white individuals (ACLU, 2020). These disparities have long-term consequences for employment, housing, education, and health. Even in states with legalized cannabis, individuals with prior convictions may face barriers to employment in the legal cannabis industry or may be excluded from medical cannabis programs. Healthcare providers must recognize how these inequities shape patient experiences and access to care. Nurses and clinicians can promote equity by advocating for inclusive policies, supporting expungement initiatives, and ensuring that cannabis-related education and services are accessible to diverse populations.

Cannabis legalization has broad public health implications, both positive and negative. On the positive side, legalization has been associated with increased access to regulated products, reduced reliance on illicit markets, and improved product safety through standardized testing and labeling (Health Canada, 2022). Some studies suggest that legalization may reduce opioid-related harms by providing an alternative for pain management, though findings remain mixed and require further investigation (Campbell et al., 2018). However, legalization also raises concerns about increased use among adolescents, impaired driving, and the commercialization of high-potency products. Epidemiological studies indicate that adolescent cannabis use has remained relatively stable in many legalized jurisdictions, though perceptions of harm have decreased (Centers for Disease Control and Prevention, 2022). Research on cannabis-impaired driving shows that THC can impair reaction time and coordination, though the relationship between THC levels and impairment is complex and not directly comparable to alcohol (National Academies of Sciences, Engineering, and Medicine, 2017). Public health agencies must balance these risks and benefits by implementing evidence-based policies, including public education campaigns, impaired driving prevention strategies, and regulations on product potency and marketing. Nurses, who often serve as trusted sources of health information, play a vital role in disseminating accurate, evidence-based guidance to patients and communities.

Healthcare providers are uniquely positioned to reduce cannabis-related stigma and promote equitable care. Research shows that provider education is one of the most effective strategies for reducing stigma and improving patient outcomes (Zolotov et al., 2021). By integrating cannabis science into nursing and medical curricula, institutions can equip future providers with the knowledge and skills needed to deliver compassionate, evidence-informed care. Providers can also reduce stigma by adopting nonjudgmental communication strategies, acknowledging the historical context of cannabis criminalization, and validating patient experiences. Studies indicate that patients who feel respected and supported are more likely to disclose cannabis use, adhere to treatment plans, and engage in shared decision-making (Haug et al., 2022).

A comprehensive public health approach to cannabis must address prevention, education, harm reduction, and equity. This includes ensuring access to accurate, evidence-based information; supporting research on therapeutic and adverse effects; reducing barriers to medical cannabis programs; addressing racial and socioeconomic disparities; promoting safe consumption practices; and integrating cannabis into chronic disease management and mental health care. International models, such as Canada's public health-oriented cannabis framework, demonstrate how regulation, education, and harm reduction can work together to support population health (Health Canada, 2022). Nurses and other healthcare professionals play a central role in implementing these strategies at the clinical and community levels, helping to build a more equitable and evidence-informed approach to cannabis care.

FUTURE DIRECTIONS IN CANNABIS NURSING AND HEALTHCARE INNOVATION

The rapid evolution of cannabis science, clinical practice, and public policy signals a transformative moment for healthcare. As research expands and societal attitudes shift, cannabis nursing is poised to play a central role in shaping the future of patient care, interdisciplinary collaboration, and health system innovation. The next decade will likely bring significant advancements in clinical research, precision medicine, digital health, workforce education, and global policy alignment. Understanding these emerging trends is essential for preparing nurses, healthcare providers, and caregivers to meet the evolving needs of diverse patient populations.

One of the most significant future directions in cannabis care is the expansion of rigorous clinical research. Although the evidence base has grown substantially in recent years, many questions remain about long-term safety, therapeutic efficacy, and optimal clinical applications. International research hubs—particularly in Israel, Canada, and parts of Europe—continue to lead large-scale clinical trials examining cannabinoids for chronic pain, neurodegenerative diseases, psychiatric disorders, and inflammatory conditions (Mechoulam & Parker, 2013; Health Canada, 2022). In the United States, recent policy shifts have begun to ease research restrictions, enabling more universities and health systems to conduct randomized controlled trials and longitudinal cohort studies (National Institute on Drug Abuse, 2020). As the evidence base expands, nurses will play a critical role in translating research findings into clinical practice, patient education, and policy development.

Advances in precision medicine represent another promising frontier. Emerging research suggests that genetic variations in cannabinoid receptors, metabolic enzymes, and endocannabinoid signaling pathways may influence individual responses to cannabis (Zou & Kumar, 2018). Pharmacogenomic testing, already used in psychiatry and oncology, may eventually help clinicians predict which patients are most likely to benefit from cannabinoid-based therapies and which may be at higher risk for adverse effects. Precision medicine approaches could also support personalized treatment plans that consider patient genetics, comorbidities, medication profiles, and symptom patterns. Nurses, who are central to patient assessment and care coordination, will be essential in implementing these personalized approaches and educating patients about their implications.

Digital health technologies are also poised to transform cannabis care. Mobile health applications, wearable devices, and remote monitoring tools are increasingly used to track symptoms, sleep patterns, mood, and medication adherence. Early studies suggest that digital platforms can help patients monitor their responses to cannabis, identify adverse effects, and engage more actively in their care (Cuttler et al., 2018). Telehealth has expanded access to cannabis-competent providers, particularly in rural and underserved communities. As digital health tools become more sophisticated, nurses will play a key role in interpreting patient-generated data, integrating it into care plans, and supporting patients using technology safely and effectively.

Workforce education and professional development will be critical to the future of cannabis nursing. Studies consistently show that most nurses and clinicians feel underprepared to address cannabis-related questions due to limited formal education (Zolotov et al., 2021). The American Nurses Association's recognition of cannabis nursing as a specialty (American Nurses Association, 2023) provides a foundation for developing standardized curricula, certification pathways, and continuing education programs. Academic institutions will need to integrate cannabis science, clinical assessment, and policy literacy into nursing and medical education. Professional organizations such as the American Cannabis Nurses Association (ACNA) will continue to play a central role in defining competencies, supporting research, and advocating for evidence-informed practice.

Health systems will also need to adapt to the growing integration of cannabis into patient care. This includes developing clear policies for documentation, safety monitoring, medication reconciliation, and staff education. As cannabis becomes more widely used, hospitals and clinics will need to address questions related to impairment, workplace safety, and liability. Administrators will need to ensure that electronic health records incorporate cannabis-related data fields, that staff receive ongoing training, and that quality improvement initiatives address cannabis-related outcomes. Research suggests that institutions with clear cannabis policies experience improved communication, reduced risk, and more consistent patient care (Substance Abuse and Mental Health Services Administration, 2023).

Global policy alignment represents another important future direction. As more countries legalize medical or adult-use cannabis, international collaboration will be essential for harmonizing research standards, product regulations, and clinical guidelines. Organizations such as the World Health Organization (WHO) and the International Association for Cannabinoid Medicines (IACM) are increasingly involved in shaping global cannabis policy and supporting cross-national research initiatives (World Health Organization, 2023). Nurses and healthcare providers will need to stay informed about global trends, particularly as patients access information and products across borders.

Finally, the future of cannabis nursing will be shaped by a growing emphasis on health equity and social justice. Addressing the legacy of cannabis criminalization, reducing disparities in access to medical cannabis programs, and ensuring that marginalized communities benefit from cannabis-related research and economic opportunities will be essential. Nurses, who are often at the forefront of advocacy and community engagement, will play a vital role in promoting equitable access, supporting policy reform, and ensuring that cannabis care is grounded in compassion, respect, and cultural humility.

Taken together, these emerging trends point to a future in which cannabis nursing is deeply integrated into mainstream healthcare, supported by robust scientific evidence, advanced technologies, and interdisciplinary collaboration. As the field continues to evolve, nurses will remain central to ensuring that cannabis care is safe, ethical, equitable, and grounded in the best available evidence.

CONCLUSION

Cannabis is reshaping the landscape of modern healthcare in ways that are both profound and far-reaching. As legalization expands and scientific evidence grows, cannabis has moved from the margins of clinical practice to a central position in conversations about symptom management, chronic disease care, mental health, public health, and health equity. This chapter has outlined the foundational knowledge, interdisciplinary considerations, and emerging trends that define cannabis nursing as a rapidly evolving specialty. It has also highlighted the essential role of nurses, caregivers, and healthcare systems in navigating the complexities of cannabis use with scientific rigor, ethical clarity, and cultural humility.

The integration of cannabis into healthcare requires a deep understanding of the endocannabinoid system, the therapeutic and adverse effects of cannabinoids, and the diverse ways in which patients use cannabis to manage symptoms and improve quality of life. Research demonstrates that cannabis may offer meaningful benefits for conditions such as chronic pain, epilepsy, anxiety, and cancer-related symptoms, while also posing risks related to cognitive impairment, psychiatric vulnerability, and drug interactions (National Academies of Sciences, Engineering, and Medicine, 2017; Devinsky et al., 2017; Murray et al., 2021). Nurses and clinicians must therefore conduct comprehensive assessments, monitor safety concerns, and support patients in making informed decisions grounded in evidence rather than stigma or misinformation.

Legal, ethical, and administrative considerations further shape the landscape of cannabis care. The tension between federal prohibition and state-level legalization in the United States creates ongoing challenges for providers, institutions, and patients (National Institute on Drug Abuse, 2020). Ethical practice requires balancing patient autonomy with beneficence and nonmaleficence, while also addressing longstanding inequities rooted in the history of cannabis criminalization (World Health Organization, 2023). Healthcare systems must develop clear policies, documentation standards, and workforce education strategies to ensure safe, consistent, and legally compliant care.

Stigma reduction and health equity are central to the future of cannabis nursing. Research shows that stigma continues to influence patient disclosure, provider communication, and access to care, particularly among marginalized populations (Hathaway et al., 2018; Haug et al., 2022). Nurses, as trusted patient advocates, play a critical role in challenging stigma, promoting culturally responsive care, and supporting equitable access to evidence-based cannabis information and services. Public health frameworks that emphasize harm reduction, education, and community engagement will be essential for addressing both the benefits and risks of cannabis legalization.

Looking ahead, the future of cannabis nursing will be shaped by advances in clinical research, precision medicine, digital health technologies, and global policy alignment. As the evidence base expands, nurses will be central to translating research into practice, supporting interdisciplinary collaboration, and advocating policies that promote patient safety and health equity. The recognition of cannabis nursing as a specialty by the American Nurses Association (American Nurses Association, 2023) marks a pivotal step in formalizing this field and underscores the need for standardized competencies, academic curricula, and professional development pathways.

Ultimately, cannabis nursing represents a transformative opportunity to integrate biomedical science, holistic care, and social responsibility. By embracing evidence-informed practice, fostering open communication, and addressing the historical and structural factors that shape cannabis use, nurses and healthcare providers can help build a more equitable, compassionate, and scientifically grounded approach to cannabis care. As cannabis continues to influence healthcare systems, patient experiences, and public health, the role of nurses will remain indispensable in guiding this evolving field with integrity, expertise, and a commitment to patient well-being.

REFERENCES

American Cannabis Nurses Association. (2023). *Cannabis nursing scope and standards of practice.* ACNA.

American Civil Liberties Union. (2020). *A tale of two countries: Racially targeted arrests in the era of marijuana reform.* https://www.aclu.org

American Nurses Association. (2023). *Recognition of cannabis nursing as a specialty practice.* ANA.

Bergamaschi, M. M., Queiroz, R. H. C., Chagas, M. H. N., de Oliveira, D. C. G., De Martinis, B. S., Kapczinski, F., Quevedo, J., Roesler, R., Schröder, N., Nardi, A. E., Martín-Santos, R., Hallak, J. E. C., Zuardi, A. W., & Crippa, J. A. S. (2011). Cannabidiol reduces the anxiety induced by simulated public speaking in treatment-naïve social phobia patients. *Neuropsychopharmacology : Official Publication of the American College of Neuropsychopharmacology, 36*(6), 1219–1226. DOI: 10.1038/npp.2011.6 PMID: 21307846

Boehnke, K. F., Litinas, E., & Clauw, D. J. (2016). Medical cannabis use is associated with decreased opiate medication use in a retrospective cross-sectional survey of patients with chronic pain. *The Journal of Pain, 17*(6), 739–744. DOI: 10.1016/j.jpain.2016.03.002 PMID: 27001005

Campbell, G., Hall, W., Peacock, A., Lintzeris, N., Bruno, R., Larance, B., Nielsen, S., Cohen, M., Chan, G., Mattick, R., Blyth, F., Shanahan, M., & Degenhardt, L. (2018). Effect of cannabis use in people with chronic non-cancer pain prescribed opioids: Findings from a 4-year prospective cohort study. *The Lancet. Public Health, 3*(7), e341–e350. DOI: 10.1016/S2468-2667(18)30110-5 PMID: 29976328

Centers for Disease Control and Prevention. (2022). *Cannabis and public health.* CDC.

Cuttler, C., Spradlin, A., Cleveland, M. J., & Craft, R. M. (2018). Short- and long-term effects of cannabis on symptoms of post-traumatic stress disorder. *Journal of Affective Disorders, 227*, 298–304. DOI: 10.1016/j.jad.2017.10.049 PMID: 32469819

Devinsky, O., Cross, J. H., Laux, L., Marsh, E., Miller, I., Nabbout, R., Scheffer, I. E., Thiele, E. A., & Wright, S. (2017). Trial of cannabidiol for drug-resistant seizures in the Dravet syndrome. *The New England Journal of Medicine, 376*(21), 2011–2020. DOI: 10.1056/NEJMoa1611618 PMID: 28538134

Di Forti, M., Quattrone, D., Freeman, T. P., Tripoli, G., Gayer-Anderson, C., Quigley, H., Rodriguez, V., Jongsma, H. E., Ferraro, L., La Cascia, C., La Barbera, D., Tarricone, I., Berardi, D., Szöke, A., Arango, C., Tortelli, A., Velthorst, E., Bernardo, M., Del Ben, C., & Murray, R. M. (2019). The contribution of cannabis use to variation in the incidence of psychotic disorder across Europe. *The Lancet. Psychiatry, 6*(5), 427–436. DOI: 10.1016/S2215-0366(19)30048-3 PMID: 30902669

Hathaway, A. D., Mostaghim, A., Erickson, P. G., Kolar, K., & Osborne, G. (2018). A nuanced view of normalisation: Attitudes of cannabis non-users in a study of undergraduate students. *Drugs: Education Prevention & Policy, 25*(1), 68–77. DOI: 10.1080/09687637.2017.1290780

Haug, N. A., Padula, C. B., Sottile, J. E., Vandrey, R., Heinz, A. J., & Bonn-Miller, M. O. (2022). Cannabis use patterns and motives: A comparison of younger, middle-aged, and older medical cannabis dispensary patients. *Addictive Behaviors, 125*, 107–110. DOI: 10.1016/j.addbeh.2021.107110 PMID: 28340421

Health Canada. (2022). *Canadian cannabis survey*. Government of Canada.

Ibeas Bih, C., Chen, T., Nunn, A. V. W., Bazelot, M., Dallas, M., & Whalley, B. J. (2015). Molecular targets of cannabidiol in neurological disorders. *Neurotherapeutics; the Journal of the American Society for Experimental NeuroTherapeutics*, *12*(4), 699–730. DOI: 10.1007/s13311-015-0377-3 PMID: 26264914

Mackie, K. (2020). Cannabinoid receptors: Where they are and what they do. *Journal of Neuroendocrinology*, *32*(1), e12805. DOI: 10.1111/jne.12805 PMID: 18426493

Mechoulam, R., & Parker, L. A. (2013). The endocannabinoid system and the brain. *Annual Review of Psychology*, *64*(1), 21–47. DOI: 10.1146/annurev-psych-113011-143739 PMID: 22804774

Meier, M. H., Caspi, A., Ambler, A., Harrington, H., Houts, R., Keefe, R. S. E., McDonald, K., Ward, A., Poulton, R., & Moffitt, T. E. (2012). Persistent cannabis users show neuropsychological decline from childhood to midlife. *Proceedings of the National Academy of Sciences of the United States of America*, *109*(40), E2657–E2664. DOI: 10.1073/pnas.1206820109 PMID: 22927402

Murray, R. M., Englund, A., Abi-Dargham, A., Lewis, D. A., Di Forti, M., Davies, C., Sherif, M., McGuire, P., & D'Souza, D. C. (2021). Cannabis-associated psychosis: Neural substrate and clinical impact. *Nature Reviews. Neuroscience*, *22*(11), 691–702. DOI: 10.1038/s41583-021-00509-8

Musto, D. F. (1999). *The American disease: Origins of narcotic control* (3rd ed.). Oxford University Press. DOI: 10.1093/oso/9780195125092.001.0001

National Academies of Sciences, Engineering, and Medicine. (2017). *The health effects of cannabis and cannabinoids: The current state of evidence and recommendations for research*. National Academies Press. https://doi.org/DOI: 10.17226/24625

National Institute for Health and Care Excellence. (2019). *Cannabis-based medicinal products: NICE guideline [NG144]*.

National Institute on Drug Abuse. (2020). *Marijuana research report*. NIH.

Pertwee, R. G. (2015). Endocannabinoids and their pharmacological actions. *Handbook of Experimental Pharmacology*, *231*, 1–37. DOI: 10.1007/978-3-319-20825-1_1 PMID: 26408156

Russo, E. B. (2016). Clinical endocannabinoid deficiency reconsidered: Current research supports the theory in migraine, fibromyalgia, irritable bowel, and other treatment-resistant syndromes. *Cannabis and Cannabinoid Research*, *1*(1), 154–165. DOI: 10.1089/can.2016.0009 PMID: 28861491

Substance Abuse and Mental Health Services Administration. (2023). *Clinical guidance for treating cannabis use disorder*. SAMHSA.

U.S. Food and Drug Administration. (2020). *FDA regulation of cannabis and cannabis-derived products*.

World Health Organization. (2023). *Cannabis and cannabinoids: Public health considerations*. WHO.

Zolotov, Y., Vulfsons, S., Zarhin, D., & Sznitman, S. (2021). Medical cannabis: An oxymoron? Physicians' perceptions of medical cannabis. *The International Journal on Drug Policy*, *88*, 103–112. DOI: 10.1016/j.drugpo.2020.103112 PMID: 29653439

Zou, S., & Kumar, U. (2018). Cannabinoid receptors and the endocannabinoid system: Signaling and function in the central nervous system. *International Journal of Molecular Sciences*, *19*(3), 833. DOI: 10.3390/ijms19030833 PMID: 29533978

KEY TERMS AND DEFINITIONS

Cannabis: A therapeutic plant containing cannabinoids that interact with the endocannabinoid system to influence pain, mood, inflammation, and neurological function. In healthcare, it refers to regulated medical products used to support symptom management and improve quality of life.

Education: The structured process of building foundational and advanced knowledge so clinicians, students, and the public can understand cannabinoid science, safe use, risks, benefits, and legal responsibilities.

Rescheduling: A federal policy action that moves cannabis from one controlled substance category to another, changing restrictions on research, prescribing, access, and regulatory oversight.

Healthcare: The integrated system of professionals, services, and settings that deliver patient-centered care. In cannabis practice, this includes assessment, treatment planning, monitoring, and interdisciplinary collaboration.

Policy: The rules, standards, and organizational decisions that guide how cannabis is used, documented, regulated, and integrated into clinical and educational settings.

Regulation: The legal and administrative framework governing how cannabis is produced, tested, labeled, dispensed, and monitored to ensure product quality, patient safety, and compliance with state and federal laws.

Clinical Practice: The day-to-day application of evidence-based assessment, treatment, monitoring, and patient education. In cannabis care, this includes evaluating appropriateness, dosing strategies, delivery methods, interactions, and symptom response.

Workforce Training: The development of competencies for nurses, prescribers, pharmacists, and allied health professionals to safely integrate cannabinoid therapeutics into care, including pharmacology, assessment, documentation, and legal considerations.

Patient Safety: The commitment to minimizing harm through accurate assessment, safe dosing, monitoring for adverse effects, preventing interactions, and ensuring product quality.

Integration: The coordinated incorporation of cannabis therapeutics into mainstream healthcare systems, including workflows, electronic health records, interdisciplinary communication, and policy alignment.

Chapter 2
Policy and Advocacy Roles of the Cannabis Nurse in U.S. Healthcare Systems:
Translating Law, Ethics, and Evidence Into Access-Oriented Practice

Laura Barrett
http://orcid.org/0009-0004-0183-3861
University of Maryland, Baltimore, USA

ABSTRACT

Cannabis nursing has become a specialty as healthcare systems face rising demand to integrate medical cannabis within complex, often contradictory regulations. This chapter examines the cannabis nurse's role in U.S. policy and advocacy to support equitable patient access and safe medical cannabis implementation. The nurse's function as a policy translator across patient, organizational, and governmental levels is emphasized. Key regulatory issues, federal-state misalignment, institutional risk management, clinician knowledge gaps, and facility access barriers are analyzed. Ryan's Law serves as a policy-to-practice example of nurse-led inpatient implementation. The chapter concludes with recommendations for governance, competency development, and structured advocacy, highlighting how the cannabis nurse connects cannabinoid science to clinical care.

INTRODUCTION

As medical cannabis programs expand across the United States, nurses increasingly encounter patients who use cannabis therapeutically for symptom management, chronic illness, and severe or life-limiting conditions (National Academies of Sciences, Engineering, and Medicine, 2017). Patients seek cannabis-based therapies for pain, chemotherapy-related nausea, neurological disorders, epilepsy, palliative symptom relief, and a growing range of chronic health conditions. This clinical reality has accelerated

DOI: 10.4018/979-8-3373-7287-7.ch002

rapidly in parallel with state-level legalization efforts, positioning cannabis as an increasingly visible component of therapeutic care.

Despite growing public acceptance and state authorization, healthcare systems remain constrained by federal prohibition. Cannabis continues to be classified as a Schedule I substance under the Controlled Substances Act (Drug Enforcement Administration [DEA], n.d.), a designation indicating no accepted medical use and high abuse potential. This federal classification produces regulatory discord across healthcare environments, particularly those reliant on federal funding, accreditation, or controlled substance governance structures.

This discord is not a singular barrier but generates a cascade of operational challenges. Regulatory ambiguity contributes to institutional risk aversion, inconsistent policy development, and limited clinical guidance. Healthcare organizations, navigating legal uncertainty and perceived liability exposure, frequently default to restrictive practices that prohibit cannabis entirely rather than operationalize structured access frameworks. The result is a paradox in which therapies authorized by law remain inaccessible within the very systems responsible for delivering patient care.

Clinicians often lack clear guidance regarding documentation, safety monitoring, and continuation of cannabis use during hospitalization. Patients may experience abrupt discontinuation of therapies that have been effective in managing symptoms. Families report distress when symptom management regimens are interrupted upon admission, and in some cases, patients resort to unsupervised or undisclosed use to maintain symptom control. These experiences demonstrate that access barriers are not abstract policy concerns but have direct implications for safety, autonomy, and quality of life.

Within this evolving landscape, cannabis nursing has been formally recognized as a specialty practice. The American Nurses Association's recognition affirms that therapeutic cannabis requires dedicated clinical knowledge, ethical competence, and policy literacy (American Nurses Association [ANA], 2023). The publication of Cannabis Nursing: Scope and Standards of Practice further establishes competencies spanning patient education, harm reduction, legal navigation, and advocacy (American Cannabis Nurses Association & ANA, 2024).

Unlike chapters that focus on cannabinoid pharmacology or therapeutic dosing, this chapter examines the policy and advocacy domain of cannabis nursing. Its emphasis is structural rather than biochemical, analyzing how nurses translate statutory authorization into operational practice across healthcare settings.

To improve clarity and reduce repetition across sections, this chapter advances a central organizing concept: the cannabis nurse as a policy translator. This role operates across micro (patient), meso (organizational), and macro (legislative) levels, bridging law, ethics, and clinical practice to ensure that legal authorization results in meaningful, safe, and equitable patient access.

Nursing's Structural Role in Health Policy and Legislative Systems

The evolution of nursing practice into policy and advocacy roles reflects a broader shift within healthcare toward interdisciplinary and systems-level engagement. Nursing scholarship increasingly recognizes policy involvement as a core dimension of professional practice, rather than an optional extension of clinical work.

The author's trajectory from bedside nursing into policy and advocacy mirrors pathways described in contemporary nursing scholarship on health policy engagement. The American Journal of Nursing framework conceptualizes this evolution as a progression of influence, beginning with clinical observation and expanding through partnership, organizational engagement, and legislative reach (Zalon et al., 2024).

Nurses represent the largest segment of the healthcare workforce and maintain sustained contact with patients across care continuums. From acute care hospitals to long-term care facilities, hospice, and community settings, nurses function as the primary interface between patients, providers, and institutional systems.

Because of this proximity, nurses frequently identify care barriers before they are visible to policymakers or administrators. They observe interruptions in therapy, unmanaged symptoms, documentation gaps, and ethical tensions arising from regulatory constraints. In this sense, nursing practice generates practice-informed policy intelligence derived from lived clinical realities.

Legislative and regulatory systems depend on this insight. Laws that authorize therapies without addressing implementation logistics risk remaining symbolic rather than operational. Nurses therefore function as policy translators, bridging statutory language and clinical workflow. Their role includes identifying safety considerations, defining scope boundaries, designing documentation structures, and ensuring alignment with institutional governance frameworks.

Professional ethics reinforce this responsibility. Provision 8 of the ANA Code of Ethics affirms nursing's obligation to collaborate across sectors to influence health policy, reduce disparities, and protect human rights. (American Nurses Association, 2015/2021). Legislative advocacy is therefore not ancillary to nursing practice but embedded within its ethical mandate.

Cannabis Policy as a Catalyst for Legislative Nursing Engagement

In the author's professional experience, repeated exposure to gaps between legally authorized cannabis therapies and institutional practice served as an inflection point for policy engagement. Hospitalized patients were frequently required to discontinue cannabis despite therapeutic benefit and legal authorization. Families reported distress when symptom management regimens were abruptly interrupted upon admission. Patients admitted to secretly having family bring medicine from home. Clinicians expressed uncertainty regarding liability, storage, and documentation.

These discontinuities revealed a systemic disconnect between legalization and implementation. Advocacy efforts initially focused on clarifying institutional barriers, engaging risk management departments, and educating interdisciplinary teams. Over time, this work expanded into formal policy engagement, including participation in legislative initiatives, regulatory consultation, and institutional governance planning.

Among these initiatives was engagement in advocacy related to the foundational Ryan's Law bill in California. Designed to protect access for terminally ill patients within healthcare facilities, Ryan's Law became a landmark example of policy translation. Nurse advocates, beginning with those affiliated with the Cannabis Nurses Network, contributed to stakeholder education, legislative dialogue, and implementation planning. This work demonstrated how nursing insight could shape statutory frameworks that were both compassionate and operationally feasible.

From Clinical Observation to Systems-Level Advocacy

Clinical experiences repeatedly reveal a disconnect between legalization and implementation. Hospitalized patients are often required to discontinue cannabis despite therapeutic benefit and legal authorization. Families report distress when symptom management regimens are interrupted, and clinicians' express uncertainty regarding liability, storage, and documentation.

These discontinuities reflect a broader system-level gap: legalization alone does not ensure access. Implementation requires translation, interpretation of policy into practice, which falls disproportionately to nurses operating at the intersection of patient care and institutional systems.

This progression, from bedside awareness to legislative engagement, reflects a broader trend within cannabis nursing and the profession at large. Nurses do not disengage from clinical practice when entering policy arenas; rather, they extend clinical advocacy into system-level domains.

Policy engagement includes drafting institutional guidelines, advising legislators, participating in regulatory workgroups, and contributing to model legislation. It also involves negotiating stakeholder concerns related to liability, diversion prevention, impairment monitoring, and federal compliance.

Through these activities, nurses ensure that policy reforms translate into meaningful patient access rather than remaining aspirational. Their role is particularly critical in therapeutic areas like cannabis, where scientific advancement, legal reform, and institutional readiness evolve at different paces.

Translating Law, Ethics, and Evidence Into Practice

As medical cannabis legalization continues to expand, and as federal rescheduling discussions evolve, healthcare systems face increasing pressure to reconcile regulatory frameworks with patient need. Institutional accommodation of cannabis use will require governance structures, education models, risk mitigation protocols, and ethical guidance.

Nurses stand at the center of this transition. Their ability to integrate endocannabinoid system and cannabinoid science with patient advocacy, legislative awareness, and institutional policy design positions them as indispensable leaders in shaping the future of cannabis access in healthcare.

The sections that follow examine this role in depth, beginning with the historical and regulatory background of medical cannabis policy and progressing through implementation challenges, legislative case studies, and future policy directions.

Understanding the contemporary advocacy and policy role of the cannabis nurse requires situating this work within the broader historical and regulatory architecture that governs medical cannabis access. The tensions observed in institutional implementation, federal prohibition, state authorization, liability concerns, and fragmented operational guidance, are not isolated phenomena but the product of decades of evolving legislation, scientific discovery, and public health discourse. To fully appreciate how nurses function as translators of law into practice, it is necessary to examine the policy foundations that shape cannabis integration within healthcare systems. The following section therefore explores the historical trajectory of U.S. medical cannabis policy, the emergence of cannabis nursing as a specialty, and the structural access gaps that have positioned nurses at the forefront of legislative advocacy and institutional policy development.

Chapter's Policy and Advocacy Objectives

Grounded in these structural and ethical foundations, this chapter examines the cannabis nurse's role in shaping policy, advocacy, and implementation across U.S. healthcare systems. Specifically, the chapter aims to:

- Examine the federal and state policy landscape governing medical cannabis access.
- Define advocacy roles of cannabis nurses across institutional and legislative domains.
- Analyze controversies and operational barriers affecting facility-based cannabis policy adoption.
- Present evidence-informed implementation models and policy solutions.

By situating cannabis nursing within broader health policy frameworks, the chapter highlights how nurses function as catalysts for equitable access, patient safety, and regulatory translation.

BACKGROUND

United States Cannabis Policy and Healthcare

A persistent federal–state divide characterizes United States cannabis policy. While a majority of states authorize medical cannabis, federal law continues to classify cannabis as a controlled substance under the Controlled Substances Act (DEA, n.d.). This lack of alignment has historically restricted research, constrained reimbursement pathways, and fostered institutional caution, particularly in hospitals, long-term care facilities, and other federally regulated settings (National Academies of Sciences, Engineering, and Medicine, 2017; Moritz College of Law, Ohio State University, 2025).

Public health analyses consistently emphasize that legalization alone does not guarantee access. Implementation depends on regulatory clarity, supply-chain controls, workforce education, and equity-oriented safeguards (Griffith et al., 2025; Woodbridge et al., 2024). In practice, healthcare organizations must interpret overlapping legal, clinical, and operational considerations without standardized guidance.

Uncertainty regarding liability, diversion, impairment, and documentation frequently results in restrictive institutional policies that prohibit cannabis use altogether, even when such use is legally authorized. These policies disproportionately affect hospitalized, institutionalized, and medically complex patients who are least able to self-advocate (Americans for Safe Access, 2025; McKaig et al., 2025).

Importantly, these barriers are not independent. Regulatory ambiguity drives institutional risk aversion, which is further amplified by workforce knowledge gaps and the absence of standardized implementation frameworks. When considered together, these forces function as an interconnected system that constrains operational access within healthcare environments.

Advocacy Engagement Pathway

Cannabis nursing advocacy operates across interconnected system levels:

- Institutional Advocacy: Policy drafting, governance participation, staff education, and implementation oversight
- Legislative and Professional Advocacy: Testimony, coalition building, advisory roles, and engagement with professional organizations

Rather than functioning as separate domains, these levels represent a continuum of influence. Bedside observations inform institutional policy development, which in turn shapes legislative priorities and regulatory evolution.

Common Institutional Barriers

Healthcare organizations routinely encounter recurring barriers:

- Unclear legal interpretation
- Fear of diversion or liability
- Concerns regarding federal funding implications
- Lack of standardized staff education
- Absence of documentation frameworks

These barriers reinforce one another. For example, insufficient education increases perceived clinical and legal risk, which in turn supports restrictive policy decisions.

High-Impact Nursing Advocacy Actions

Cannabis nurses address these barriers through:

- Translating statutes into operational policies
- Leading interdisciplinary governance structures
- Providing evidence-informed testimony and stakeholder education
- Embedding equity considerations into access policies

These actions represent the translation of policy intent into clinical and organizational practice.

Facility-Level Policy Implementation Stages

The implementation of medical cannabis policies within healthcare facilities typically follows structured stages:

1. Identify applicable state law and institutional obligations
2. Define patient eligibility criteria and exclusions
3. Establish governance structures and interdisciplinary oversight
4. Develop workflow tools and documentation templates
5. Train staff and validate competencies
6. Monitor outcomes and revise policy through quality improvement processes
7. Bridge communication between executive leadership, clinical teams, and patient-centered care needs

These stages are best understood as iterative rather than linear, forming a continuous cycle in which policy, practice, and evaluation inform one another.

Cannabis nurses can respond to these barriers by:

- Translating statutes into operational policies.
- Leading interdisciplinary governance structures.
- Providing evidence-informed testimony and stakeholder education.

- Embedding equity considerations into access policies.

Solutions and Recommendations

Healthcare systems are urged to incorporate structured, nurse-led policy-to-practice frameworks that concentrate on clarity, safety, and access, including:

- Formal governance models with embedded nursing leadership.
- Competency-based education aligned with national nursing guidance.
- Standardized documentation integrated into electronic health records.
- Risk mitigation protocols addressing impairment, mobility, and adverse effects.
- Ongoing quality monitoring and iterative policy refinement.

Professional Foundations of Cannabis Nursing Advocacy

Nursing has a long-standing ethical obligation to advocate for patient-focused, evidence-informed care (American Nurses Association [ANA], 2016). This mandate extends to therapeutic cannabis through:

- Recognition of cannabis nursing as a specialty practice by the American Nurses Association in collaboration with the American Cannabis Nurses Association (American Nurses Association, 2023).
- National regulatory guidance outlining nursing responsibilities related to patient education, safety monitoring, documentation, and advocacy (National Council of State Boards of Nursing, 2018; American Cannabis Nurses Association, & American Nurses Association, 2024).
- Professional position statements supporting the therapeutic use of cannabinoids and calling for expanded research and policy reform (American Nurses Association, 2016; National Academies of Sciences, Engineering, and Medicine, 2017).
- Nurse-led advocacy organizations, such as the Cannabis Nurses Network, which have operationalized (put into practice) professional standards through legislative engagement (participation in lawmaking), policy drafting (creating organizational rules), and implementation guidance (direction for putting policy into effect), most notably contributing to the development and dissemination (widespread distribution and adoption) of Ryan's Law and similar frameworks for medical cannabis access in healthcare settings (Cannabis Nurses Network, n.d.; see subsequent Ryan's Law sections).

Together, these foundations authorize all nurses to engage in policy development, organizational governance, and legislative advocacy while remaining within professional scope and regulatory boundaries (American Cannabis Nurses Association, & American Nurses Association, 2024).

Figure 1. Ethical and professional alignment of cannabis nursing policy and advocacy with Provision 8.2 of the American Nurses Association Code of Ethics and the Cannabis Nursing: Scope and Standards of Practice (Developed by the author based on professional standards (American Nurses Association, 2015/2021; American Cannabis Nurses Association & American Nurses Association, 2024; Cannabis Nurses Network, n.d.)

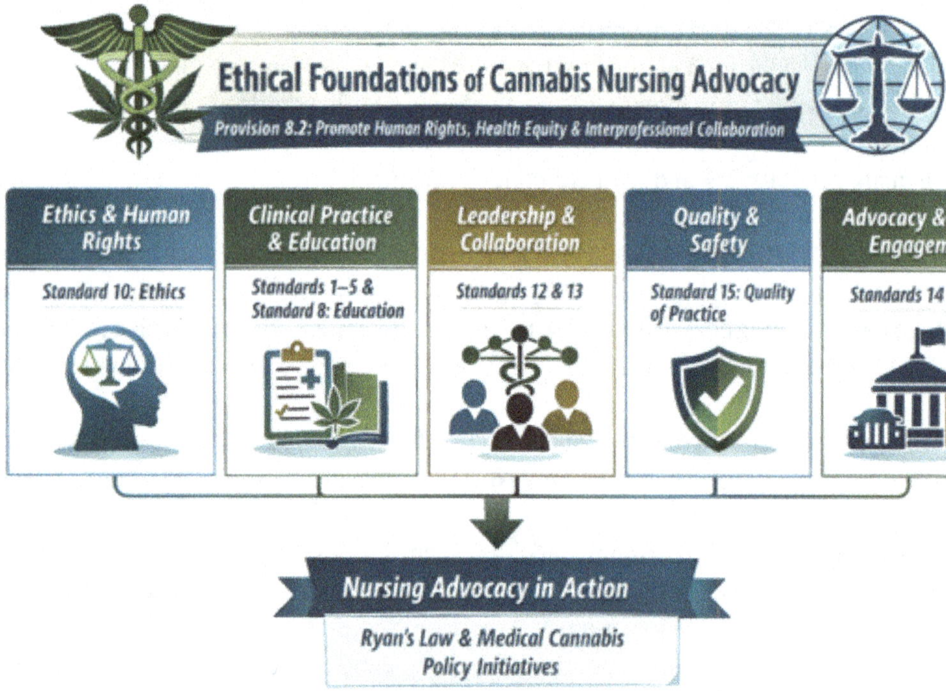
Ethical Foundations of Cannabis Nursing Advocacy
Provision 8.2: Promote Human Rights, Health Equity & Interprofessional Collaboration
Ethics & Human Rights
Standard 10: Ethics
Clinical Practice & Education
Standards 1–5 & Standard 8: Education
Leadership & Collaboration
Standards 12 & 13
Quality & Safety
Standard 15: Quality of Practice
Advocacy & Policy Engagement
Standards 14 & 16
Nursing Advocacy in Action
Ryan's Law & Medical Cannabis Policy Initiatives

Ethical Foundations: Applying ANA Code of Ethics Provision 8.2 to Cannabis Nursing and Health Advocacy

Provision 8.2 of the American Nurses Association (ANA) Code of Ethics for Nurses affirms nurses' ethical obligation to collaborate across disciplines and sectors to protect human rights, address social determinants of health, and reduce health disparities (American Nurses Association [ANA], 2015/2021). This ethical mandate provides a core framework for cannabis nursing practice. It aligns directly with the professional expectations articulated in Cannabis Nursing: Scope and Standards of Practice, particularly Standard 10: Ethics and Standard 14: Advocacy (American Cannabis Nurses Association & ANA, 2024).

Within cannabis nursing, Provision 8.2 supports interprofessional collaboration among nurses, physicians, pharmacists, dispensary clinical leadership, administrators, and community stakeholders to promote equitable access to evidence-informed cannabis care and to reduce stigma associated with its use (American Nurses Association, 2015/2021). The Scope and Standards identify advocacy, patient education, harm reduction, and care coordination as core competencies of cannabis nursing practice (Standards 1–5: Assessment through Implementation; Standard 8: Education), particularly in contexts shaped by historical criminalization, regulatory inconsistency, and health inequities (American Cannabis Nurses Association, & American Nurses Association, 2024). Education related to safe use, routes of administration, monitoring for adverse effects, and respect for patient autonomy reflects nursing's responsibility to mitigate disparities and promote population health.

Provision 8.2 also provides clear ethical justification for nursing leadership in hospitals and facility-based access initiatives. The Scope and Standards explicitly recognize nurses' roles in organizational governance, policy development, and systems-level quality improvement (Standards 12, 13, and 15: Leadership; Collaboration; Quality of Practice) (American Cannabis Nurses Association, & American Nurses Association, 2024). Collaboration with hospital leadership, ethics committees, legal counsel, pharmacy, and risk management to develop medical cannabis access policies constitutes systems-level advocacy consistent with both the Code of Ethics and specialty practice standards. Restricting access to a legally authorized and clinically beneficial therapy during hospitalization may exacerbate symptom burden, undermine patient autonomy, and contribute to inequitable care, raising ethical concerns related to justice, beneficence, and non-maleficence, core nursing values reinforced by Standard 10: Ethics.

Finally, Provision 8.2 affirms nurses' engagement in health policy and advocacy beyond the clinical setting. The Scope and Standards explicitly support nurse participation in legislative advocacy, professional organizations, and public policy initiatives aimed at improving access, safety, and regulatory clarity for cannabis-based care (Standard 14: Advocacy; Standard 16: Professional Practice Evaluation) (American Cannabis Nurses Association, & American Nurses Association, 2024). Within this ethical and professional framework, cannabis-related advocacy is not political activity, but a legitimate extension of nursing practice grounded in human rights, public health, and health equity. These principles are operationalized in subsequent sections through national and state case examples, including the implementation of Ryan's Law and the development of hospital-based medical cannabis policies.

Why Implementation Falls to Nurses

In most healthcare settings, nurses serve as the primary interface between patients, clinicians, and institutional systems (Zalon et al., 2024). As such, nurses are uniquely positioned to:

- Identify access to medical cannabis barriers at the bedside (Schauer et al., 2021).
- Translate statutory and regulatory language into clinical workflows (Americans for Safe Access, 2025).
- Align patient advocacy with organizational risk management and compliance requirements (McKaig et al., 2025).
- Educate interdisciplinary teams on safe, ethical, and legally compliant cannabis-related practice (American Cannabis Nurses Association, & American Nurses Association, 2024; Philpot et al., 2019).

The Cannabis Educated Nurse as a Policy and Advocacy Leader

The cannabis nurse's role in policy and advocacy may be conceptualized across three interconnected levels:

- **Micro-Level (Patient and Caregiver):**

Education, harm reduction counseling, access navigation, documentation support, and advocacy for patient autonomy within institutional policy constraints.

- **Meso-Level (Organization):**

Development and implementation of facility policies, staff education programs, clinical workflows, quality monitoring systems, and interdisciplinary governance structures.

- **Macro-Level (State and Federal):**

Legislative testimony, coalition participation, professional association leadership, and public health advocacy focused on access, equity, and safety.

This multilevel engagement positions cannabis nursing as both a clinical and policy-oriented specialty.

MAIN FOCUS OF THE CHAPTER

This chapter focuses on the policy and advocacy functions of the cannabis nurse within United States healthcare systems, stressing the translation of statutory authorization into operational access for patients. While medical cannabis has been legalized at the state level across much of the country, institutional implementation within hospitals, long-term care facilities, schools, and other regulated settings remains inconsistent and frequently restrictive. These access gaps are not solely legal in nature; they arise from regulatory ambiguity, institutional risk aversion, workforce knowledge deficits, and the absence of standardized governance frameworks.

The chapter advances the concept of the cannabis nurse as a "policy translator", a role situated at the intersection of clinical practice, organizational governance, and legislative action. Rather than functioning solely as educators or bedside clinicians, cannabis nurses are positioned as intermediaries who interpret law, ethics, and evidence into implementable policies and workflows that preserve patient safety while advancing equity and autonomy.

Using practice-based vignettes drawn from national and Maryland-specific advocacy efforts, the chapter illustrates how nurses influence policy across multiple system levels. Ryan's Law is presented as a national exemplar of nurse-informed legislative action that enabled facility-based access for terminally ill patients in California. Maryland case examples further demonstrate how incremental legislative successes, nonprofit advocacy, and voluntary institutional policy development can advance compassionate access even when comprehensive legislation does not pass.

By placing these experiences within established nursing theory, professional scope and standards, and emerging federal policy developments, including cannabis rescheduling, the chapter highlights the expanding responsibility of nurses to lead access-oriented implementation in evolving therapeutic domains. The focus remains on the practical mechanisms by which nurses translate policy intent into lived patient experience within healthcare systems.

ISSUES, CONTROVERSIES, AND PROBLEMS

Federal–State Misalignment

Healthcare institutions must reconcile state medical cannabis laws with ongoing federal prohibition, particularly when federal funding, accreditation requirements, or controlled substance regulations are implicated (Drug Enforcement Administration [DEA], n.d.; Moritz College of Law, Ohio State University, 2025). This lack of alignment often leads to conservative institutional interpretations that restrict patient access despite legal authorization, even in the absence of explicit federal prohibitions related to patient use of medical cannabis within healthcare facilities (Americans for Safe Access, 2025; Centers for Medicare and Medicaid Services, as cited in McKaig et al., 2025).

Knowledge Gaps and Safety Concerns

Clinician discomfort with cannabis, inconsistent education, and concerns related to impairment, falls, and potential drug–drug interactions add to variable counseling and risk management practices across healthcare settings (Philpot et al., 2019; Schauer et al., 2021). Without standardized competencies and institutional guidance, facilities struggle to balance patient safety with equitable access to therapeutic cannabis (National Council of State Boards of Nursing, 2018; American Cannabis Nurses Association, & American Nurses Association, 2024).

Equity Implications

Patients who are hospitalized, disabled, or institutionalized are often least able to self-advocate and most affected by restrictive cannabis policies (National Academies of Sciences, Engineering, and Medicine, 2017). Advocacy efforts that fail to incorporate equity considerations risk reinforcing disparities in symptom control, autonomy, and quality of life, particularly among patients with serious illness or complex care needs (Americans for Safe Access, 2025; McKaig et al., 2025).

1. Core Policy Implementation Domains (CPID)

The successful integration of medical cannabis into healthcare settings depends on coordinated attention to multiple, interdependent policy domains that transcend legal authorization alone (Americans for Safe Access, 2025; McKaig et al., 2025).

a. Governance and Accountability

Strong governance structures are essential to ensure consistent policy interpretation, oversight of implementation, and alignment with institutional risk management frameworks (Griffith et al., 2025).

i. **Executive Sponsorship and Clinical Leadership**

Visible executive support, paired with nursing and medical leadership, legitimizes policy adoption and facilitates interdisciplinary cooperation (Zalon et al., 2024).

ii. **Defined Staff Roles and Escalation Pathways**

Clear delineation of nursing, provider, and administrative responsibilities reduces scope-of-practice ambiguity and mitigates liability concerns (National Council of State Boards of Nursing, 2018; American Cannabis Nurses Association, & American Nurses Association, 2024).

b. Clinical Workflow and Documentation

Embedding medical cannabis processes into existing clinical workflows promotes safety, consistency, and compliance (McKaig et al., 2025).

i. **Eligibility and Contraindication Screening**

Structured screening processes support appropriate continuation or discontinuation decisions and align cannabis use with individualized treatment goals (National Academies of Sciences, Engineering, and Medicine, 2017; MacCallum & Russo, 2018).

ii. **Standardized Documentation and Incident Reporting**

Documentation of cannabis use, observed effects, and adverse events is critical for continuity of care, quality monitoring, and organizational accountability (Philpot et al., 2019; American Cannabis Nurses Association, & American Nurses Association, 2024).

2. Advocacy Engagement Pathway (AEP)

Nursing advocacy operates across multiple system levels, requiring strategic engagement consistent with professional ethics and policy mechanisms (American Nurses Association, 2016; Zalon et al., 2024).

a. Institutional Advocacy (Policy Drafting and Education)

Within organizations, cannabis nurses contribute to policy development, staff education, and governance committees to ensure access policies are evidence-informed and operationally feasible (Americans for Safe Access, 2025; McKaig et al., 2025).

b. Legislative and Professional Advocacy (Testimony and Coalition Work)

At the state and national levels, nurses engage in legislative testimony, professional coalitions, and advisory roles to shape statutes and regulatory guidance that reflect patient-centered care and clinical realities (American Nurses Association, 2016; American Cannabis Nurses Association, & American Nurses Association, 2024).

Common Institutional Barriers

Healthcare organizations commonly experience recurring barriers that impede medical cannabis policy adoption and implementation (Griffith et al., 2025; Moritz College of Law, Ohio State University, 2025):

- **Unclear Legal Interpretation**

Misunderstanding of federal oversight and state authorization contributes to overly restrictive institutional policies (DEA, n.d.).

- **Fear of Diversion or Liability**

Concerns related to substance control and adverse events frequently exceed evidence of manageable clinical risk (McKaig et al., 2025).

- **Lack of Standardized Staff Education**

Inconsistent clinician knowledge undermines safe counseling, monitoring, and documentation (Philpot et al., 2019; Schauer et al., 2021).

- **Absence of Documentation Frameworks**

Without clear documentation standards, facilities struggle to integrate cannabis use into clinical records and quality systems (American Cannabis Nurses Association, & American Nurses Association, 2024).

High-Impact Nursing Advocacy Actions

Cannabis nurses can address these barriers through targeted, high-impact advocacy actions grounded in professional standards and implementation science (American Nurses Association, 2016; American Cannabis Nurses Association, & American Nurses Association, 2024):

- Translate statutory and regulatory language into operational policies aligned with institutional workflows
- Lead interdisciplinary governance and policy committees
- Provide evidence-informed testimony and stakeholder education
- Embed equity considerations into access policies to protect at-risk populations (National Academies of Sciences, Engineering, and Medicine, 2017; Americans for Safe Access, 2025)

Steps for Facility-Level Policy Implementation

1. Identify applicable state law and facility obligations (APIS, n.d.; DEA, n.d.).
2. Define patient eligibility and exclusions based on clinical and legislative criteria (National Academies of Sciences, Engineering, and Medicine, 2017).
3. Establish governance structures and interdisciplinary oversight mechanisms (Zalon et al., 2024).

4. Develop workflow tools and documentation templates (McKaig et al., 2025).
5. Train staff and validate competencies using standardized education models (NCSBN, 2018; American Cannabis Nurses Association, & American Nurses Association, 2024).
6. Monitor outcomes and revise policy through ongoing quality improvement processes (Griffith et al., 2025).

PRACTICE-BASED VIGNETTES

Facility-Based Access and Ryan's Law

Ryan's Law in California requires eligible healthcare facilities to permit qualified patients to use medical cannabis under defined conditions (Americans for Safe Access, 2025). While jurisdiction-specific, Ryan's Law illustrates national implementation challenges, including eligibility screening, storage procedures, staff role clarification, documentation, and risk mitigation (McKaig et al., 2025). Published inpatient oncology implementation research demonstrates that successful adoption depends on nurse-led coordination, interdisciplinary collaboration, and alignment with institutional safety protocols (McKaig et al., 2025).

Practice-Based Vignette 1: National Nurse-Led Advocacy, Ryan's Law, and the Emergence of Policy Blueprints for Facility-Based Access

Context: Facility-Based Access as a National Policy Gap

Prior to the passage of Ryan's Law in California, access to medical cannabis within healthcare facilities remained largely unresolved across the United States. Even in states with established medical cannabis programs, hospitalized and institutionalized patients frequently lost access to therapeutically authorized cannabis upon admission due to institutional prohibition, regulatory uncertainty, and conservative interpretations of federal law (National Academies of Sciences, Engineering, and Medicine, 2017). This gap was particularly consequential for patients with serious or terminal illness, whose symptom burden often intensifies during inpatient or hospice care (McKaig et al., 2025).

This policy vacuum has been widely recognized across advocacy and professional domains. In 2023, Doctors for Drug Policy Reform (D4DPR) published a white paper explicitly identifying that, despite widespread legalization of medical cannabis, more than half of U.S. states and the majority of healthcare facilities lack clear legal or administrative frameworks governing patient use of medical cannabis within healthcare settings (Doctors for Drug Policy Reform, 2023).

Foundational Development of Ryan's Law and Legislative Architecture

The legislative foundation of Ryan's Law emerged from nurse-led advocacy networks seeking to address this continuity-of-care gap. Prior to the bill's introduction, healthcare facilities routinely prohibited cannabis use within inpatient and residential care environments, even when such use was legally authorized at the state level.

The Cannabis Nurses Network played a central role in identifying this disparity and mobilizing clinical advocacy to address it. As documented through the organization's Ryan's Law Action Center, members contributed directly to the authorship, policy framing, and legislative advancement of California Senate Bill 311 (Cannabis Nurses Network, n.d.). Nurse advocates collaborated with legal experts, patient families, and interdisciplinary stakeholders to ensure statutory language reflected both patient rights and operational feasibility.

A defining feature of the bill's development was its clinical framing. Advocacy efforts positioned facility-based cannabis access as an issue of symptom management, palliative care ethics, and continuity of treatment rather than broader legalization policy. Educational briefings and legislative testimony emphasized:

- Patient dignity at end of life
- Safe storage and administration safeguards
- Staff role delineation
- Documentation and liability frameworks
- Alignment with hospice and palliative care standards

Legal collaboration further supported statutory viability. Ryan's Law co-author Ken Sobel, Esq., a legal counsel and educator affiliated with the Cannabis Nurses Network, contributed expertise in cannabis law and regulatory interpretation, strengthening legislative drafting and institutional acceptability (Cannabis Nurses Network, n.d.).

Author's Role: Committee-Based Advocacy and Multistate Coordination

As part of professional membership in the Cannabis Nurses Network, the author joined the Ryan's Law advocacy team in 2021 during the legislative effort to advance Senate Bill 311. Participation occurred within a coordinated, nurse-led advocacy infrastructure emphasizing clinical credibility, patient safety, and implementation feasibility.

Following enactment, signed September 28, 2021, and effective January 1, 2022, the advocacy focus expanded nationally to address similar facility-based access barriers in other legalized states (Cannabis Nurses Network, n.d.; McKaig et al., 2025).

The author engaged in a structured multistate committee model leveraging virtual collaboration. Regular videoconference meetings were used to:

- Identify key legislators
- Share model statutory language
- Coordinate testimony
- Align advocacy strategy
- Support state-specific policy drafting

This model relied on nurses who were "boots on the ground" within each jurisdiction, enabling localized policy translation while maintaining fidelity to core access and safety principles (American Nurses Association [ANA], 2016; Zalon et al., 2024).

Outcome: Legislative Diffusion, Policy Blueprints, and Implementation Readiness

Ryan's Law established a statutory requirement for California healthcare facilities, including acute care hospitals, skilled nursing facilities, congregate living health facilities, and hospice providers, to permit the use of medical cannabis by terminally ill patients with valid physician recommendations (Cannabis Nurses Network, n.d.).

The law defines terminal illness as a prognosis of one year or less if disease follows its natural course and requires no additional physician authorization beyond the standard medical cannabis recommendation (Cannabis Nurses Network, n.d.; McKaig et al., 2025).

As national advocacy expanded, attention shifted toward transferable implementation frameworks. The D4DPR white paper introduced legislative and administrative guidelines intended to function as blueprints for states and healthcare systems (Doctors for Drug Policy Reform, 2023). Nurses, the author, participated in introducing these models to policymakers and institutional stakeholders.

Educational initiatives addressed:

- Legal interpretation
- Staff role boundaries
- Documentation standards
- Storage procedures
- Risk mitigation strategies

Insight: Nursing as a Driver of Policy Diffusion and Implementation

This experience illustrates how nurses influence health policy beyond single-jurisdiction advocacy by functioning as connectors between legislation, clinical practice, and institutional governance. The nurse-led committee model used to advance Ryan's Law principles reflects an evolving approach to policy diffusion grounded in clinical credibility and professional ethics (American Nurses Association, 2016; Doctors for Drug Policy Reform, 2023; Zalon et al., 2024).

Importantly, nursing influence extended beyond legislative authorship. Through sustained advocacy, policy adaptation, and implementation planning, nurses ensured that statutory authorization translated into operational access for patients.

In rapidly evolving therapeutic domains such as medical cannabis, this translational role remains essential to bridging the divide between law and lived patient experience (American Cannabis Nurses Association, & American Nurses Association, 2024; McKaig et al., 2025).

Practice-Based Vignette 2: Maryland's Legislative Pathway From School-Based Access to Compassionate Care Continuity

Context: School-Based Barriers to Medical Cannabis Access

In Maryland, early legislative efforts addressing medical cannabis access within institutional settings emerged not from hospitals, but from public schools. Before 2021, students who were certified medical cannabis patients, including children with complex and chronic medical conditions, were required to leave school premises to receive their medication. This practice necessitated daily parental presence and off-campus administration, disrupting education, increasing caregiver burden, and undermining continuity of care. These barriers reflected a larger institutional reluctance to integrate medical cannabis into regulated environments, even when use was legally authorized and clinically indicated.

Legislative Precedent: HB 331 (Maryland General Assembly, 2021)

In response to these challenges, Maryland enacted House Bill 331, commonly known as Connor's Courage Act, in 2021. The legislation permitted qualifying medical cannabis patients, including minors, to receive their cannabis medication during school hours through the school nurse's office, rather than requiring administration off school property (Maryland General Assembly, 2021). The law established an organized framework for school nurses to oversee administration, aligning cannabis access with existing medication management and nursing practice standards within educational settings.

HB 331 functioned as a critical legislative precedent by affirming that medical cannabis could be safely integrated into institutional care models when supported by nursing oversight, clear documentation, and defined administrative processes. Importantly, the law reframed cannabis not as an exception requiring exclusion, but as a therapeutic agent subject to the same continuity-of-care principles applied to other prescribed treatments.

Operationalization: Clinical Authorization and Documentation

Implementation of Connor's Courage Act required the development of formal authorization mechanisms to ensure clinical appropriateness and regulatory compliance. As part of this process, the Maryland Medical Cannabis Commission (now the Maryland Cannabis Administration) established a physician-completed form authorizing medical cannabis use in the school setting. This documentation verified patient certification, outlined permitted administration parameters, and enabled school nurses to integrate cannabis administration into routine medication workflows while maintaining compliance with state regulations (Maryland Medical Cannabis Commission, n.d.).

The use of standardized physician authorization reinforced the role of nurses as gatekeepers of safe medication administration and positioned cannabis within established clinical governance structures. This approach mitigated institutional concerns related to liability and diversion while preserving access for pediatric patients who would otherwise experience treatment disruption.

Insight: Legislative Sequencing and the Expansion of Compassionate Access

The passage and implementation of HB 331 revealed an essential insight for subsequent advocacy efforts in Maryland: incremental, setting-specific legislation can serve as a foundation for broader access reforms. By demonstrating that medical cannabis could be administered safely in schools under nursing supervision, Connor's Courage Act challenged assumptions that institutional cannabis access was inherently unmanageable or unsafe.

This legislative experience directly informed later attempts to extend medical cannabis access into healthcare facilities. It also highlighted limitations in existing policy frameworks, particularly the reliance on setting-specific statutes rather than comprehensive continuity-of-care protections. For nurse advocates, HB 331 highlighted the strategic value of grounding cannabis legislation in nursing practice, patient safety, and operational feasibility rather than in abstract debates over drug policy.

More broadly, the Maryland experience illustrates how early successes in pediatric and educational settings can catalyze subsequent efforts to address access gaps across the healthcare continuum. As later sections of this chapter will demonstrate, these lessons became central to efforts to advance compassionate access legislation for hospitalized and institutionalized patients beyond the school environment (American Nurses Association, 2016; Doctors for Drug Policy Reform, 2023).

Practice-Based Vignette 3: HB1135/SB587 (2023) and the Limits of Legislative Success in Advancing Compassionate Access

Context: From Educational Settings to Healthcare Facilities

Following the enactment of HB 331 (Connor's Courage Act) in 2021, attention in Maryland shifted toward broader continuity-of-care challenges affecting medical cannabis patients outside the school environment. While Connor's Courage Act established a precedent for nurse-mediated cannabis administration within schools, patients continued to face access disruptions upon admission to hospitals, skilled nursing facilities, and other regulated healthcare settings. These disruptions mirrored the national policy gap identified in emerging scholarship and policy analyses, which note that legalization alone does not ensure access within institutional care environments (National Academies of Sciences, Engineering, and Medicine, 2017; Doctors for Drug Policy Reform, 2023).

Advocacy Infrastructure: Formation of the Connor Sheffield Foundation

In parallel with legislative efforts, the Connor Sheffield Foundation, a Maryland-based nonprofit organization, was formed to support cannabis advocacy, patient education, and research, with a particular focus on continuity of care for pediatric and young adult patients. The foundation emerged directly from the implementation experience of Connor's Courage Act and the recognition that statutory access alone was insufficient without sustained advocacy and policymaker engagement.

Through the foundation, nurses, caregivers, and patient advocates, including the author, engaged in intensive legislative outreach efforts. These efforts included hours, days, and weeks spent meeting with Maryland lawmakers, committee staff, and regulatory stakeholders to provide testimony, respond to concerns, and explain the clinical and ethical implications of interrupted access to medical cannabis. Advocacy extended beyond formal hearings to include direct, door-to-door engagement with legislators, reflecting a deliberate strategy to humanize policy discussions and ground them in patients' lived experiences.

Legislative Effort: HB1135/SB587 (2023)

In 2023, Maryland lawmakers introduced House Bill 1135 and Senate Bill 587, legislation designed to address facility-based access to medical cannabis for patients admitted to healthcare facilities (Maryland General Assembly, 2023). Informed by earlier successes in school-based access, national models such as California's Ryan's Law, and sustained advocacy through the Connor Sheffield Foundation, the proposed bills sought to prevent medically authorized cannabis from being discontinued solely due to hospitalization or institutionalization.

The author participated in advocacy efforts supporting HB1135/SB587, contributing clinical and policy insight to stakeholder discussions with legislators, professional associations, and healthcare system representatives. Testimony and legislative engagement emphasized continuity of care, patient safety, and the ethical implications of forcing patients to choose between hospitalization and symptom control. Lawmakers raised concerns about implementation logistics, liability exposure, federal regulatory ambiguity, and the absence of standardized institutional frameworks, which advocates addressed through repeated engagement and education.

Notably, the bills garnered substantial bipartisan support and were favorably received in both the House and Senate, reflecting growing legislative recognition of the issue's clinical and humanitarian dimensions.

Outcome: Legislative Support Without a Floor Vote

Despite strong committee engagement and broad conceptual support, HB1135/SB587 did not advance to a floor vote during the 2023 legislative session. The absence of a final vote was not attributable to opposition to the underlying principles of access, but rather to unresolved concerns regarding implementation, institutional liability, and regulatory complexity, barriers commonly identified in national analyses of facility-based cannabis policy (Doctors for Drug Policy Reform, 2023; Moritz College of Law, Ohio State University, 2025).

Nevertheless, the legislative process itself generated significant secondary effects. Committee hearings, extended stakeholder meetings, and sustained advocacy efforts created formal and informal spaces for healthcare leaders, regulators, and nursing advocates to participate extensively with the practical realities of cannabis use in healthcare facilities. These dialogues clarified areas of consensus, such as the need for clear governance structures, documentation standards, and defined staff roles, even as statutory resolution remained elusive.

Insight: Legislative Process as a Catalyst for Policy Change

The experience of HB1135/SB587 illustrates a critical insight for nurse advocates: legislative success cannot be measured solely by passage into law. Even when bills fail to reach a floor vote, the process of drafting, debating, and refining legislation, supported by sustained nonprofit advocacy and direct legislator engagement, can surface institutional barriers, educate decision-makers, and catalyze alternative pathways to implementation.

For nurses engaged in policy advocacy, this case stresses the value of persistence, relationship-building, and multi-modal engagement beyond formal legislative calendars. The advocacy efforts of the Connor Sheffield Foundation, coupled with the strong support HB1135/SB587 received in both chambers, laid the groundwork for subsequent off-session collaboration, including the development of internal hospital policies addressing medical cannabis access in the absence of a statutory mandate.

In this way, HB1135/SB587 functioned as an essential transitional effort, bridging earlier successes in school-based access and later policy achievements within healthcare systems. The bill's trajectory highlights the distinct and influential role nurses play in sustaining momentum, translating legislative intent into operational dialogue, and ensuring that patient-centered access remains a visible priority even when formal statutory change is deferred (American Nurses Association [ANA], 2016; Zalon et al., 2024).

Practice-Based Vignette 4: Voluntary Hospital Policy Development Following Legislative Impasse in Maryland

Context: Policy Development Following Legislative Impasse

Following the conclusion of the 2023 legislative session, during which HB1135/SB587 failed to advance to a floor vote despite broad support, Maryland healthcare institutions remained without a statutory framework governing patient use of medical cannabis within hospitals. As in many states, the absence of clear legislation resulted in continued institutional prohibition or inconsistent decision-making, leaving medically authorized patients vulnerable to abrupt discontinuation of therapy upon hospitalization (Doctors for Drug Policy Reform, 2023; National Academies of Sciences, Engineering, and Medicine, 2017).

Rather than allowing the legislative impasse to halt progress, nurse advocates recognized an opportunity to pursue an alternative pathway: voluntary, institutionally adopted policy. This method aligns with national policy analyses, which emphasize that healthcare facilities often have the authority to implement access policies independent of legislative mandate, provided that such policies are structured to address safety, governance, and risk management concerns (Doctors for Drug Policy Reform, 2023).

Author's Role: Off-Session Stakeholder Engagement and Consensus Building

During the non-session months following the 2023 legislative cycle, the author engaged in sustained stakeholder meetings with representatives from Maryland hospitals, healthcare associations, and regulatory partners. These discussions focused on identifying common concerns raised during the legislative process, liability exposure, staff role clarity, storage and administration safeguards, and federal regulatory uncertainty, and translating them into policy language acceptable to healthcare systems.

Drawing on experience from Ryan's Law implementation efforts and informed by the legislative dialogue surrounding HB1135/SB587, the author contributed to the development of a Maryland Hospital Medical Cannabis Use Policy Template. This template was designed to be voluntary, allowing individual hospitals to opt in or opt out based on institutional readiness, while ensuring coherence across systems that chose to participate. The inclusion of an explicit opt-out clause mirrored provisions found in Ryan's Law–inspired frameworks, acknowledging institutional autonomy while preserving patient access where feasible (Cannabis Nurses Network, n.d.; McKaig et al., 2025).

Policy Design: Voluntary Access With Defined Safeguards

The policy template established two primary options for hospitals:

(1) to prohibit medical cannabis use within the facility, or
(2) to permit patient self-administration of medical cannabis under defined conditions.

For facilities electing to permit access, the policy delineated eligibility criteria, verification requirements, storage protocols, documentation expectations, and clear boundaries around nursing and staff responsibilities. Consistent with national guidance, the policy prohibited staff administration or handling of cannabis, restricted routes of administration to non-combustible forms, and required that medical cannabis remain a continuation of patient-directed therapy rather than a hospital-supplied medication (American Cannabis Nurses Association & American Nurses Association, 2024; Doctors for Drug Policy Reform, 2023).

By embedding these safeguards, the policy addressed concerns repeatedly raised during legislative hearings while preserving the core ethical principle articulated in HB1135/SB587: that medically authorized cannabis should not be discontinued solely due to hospitalization.

Outcome: Voluntary Adoption and Implementation Readiness

Following stakeholder review, the policy template was approved by the Maryland Hospital Association for voluntary use, allowing individual healthcare systems to implement medical cannabis access policies by choice rather than by compulsion. This outcome represented a significant shift from blanket prohibition toward structured accommodation, achieved without statutory enforcement.

Significantly, the policy's voluntary nature reduced institutional resistance while enabling early adopters to pilot implementation, generate internal data, and refine procedures. This approach is closely aligned with the recommendations outlined in the Doctors for Drug Policy Reform white paper, which emphasized incremental adoption, model policies, and administrative guidance as viable pathways in jurisdictions where legislation has stalled (Doctors for Drug Policy Reform, 2023).

Insight: Nursing Leadership Beyond Statute

This experience illustrates a central theme of cannabis nursing policy work: when legislation fails to advance, nursing advocacy does not stop; it adapts. By shifting focus from statutory mandate to institutional consensus, nurse leaders were able to operationalize access principles debated during the legislative process and translate them into actionable policy.

The Maryland hospital policy initiative demonstrates how nurses function as intermediaries between law, ethics, and healthcare operations. Through off-session engagement, policy drafting, and negotiation, the author and collaborating stakeholders advanced patient-centered access while respecting institutional autonomy and regulatory constraints. This case reinforces the argument that meaningful policy change in healthcare often occurs through voluntary adoption and professional leadership, particularly in emerging therapeutic domains where law has yet to fully catch up with clinical practice (American Nurses Association [ANA], 2016; Zalon et al., 2024).

SOLUTIONS AND RECOMMENDATIONS

A peer organization in the field, Doctors for Drug Policy Reform (D4DPR), published a 2023 white paper titled Legislative and Administrative Guidelines for Regulating Cannabis Use in Healthcare Facilities that explicitly identified a persistent policy gap. Despite the legalization of medical cannabis in many U.S. states, more than half of the states and the majority of healthcare facilities lack clear legal or administrative frameworks governing patient use of medical cannabis within healthcare settings (Doctors for Drug Policy Reform, 2023). The white paper was developed as a practical blueprint for lawmakers, healthcare administrators, and other stakeholders seeking to create or refine statutes and institutional policies that regulate medical cannabis use in hospitals, long-term care facilities, and other regulated settings (Doctors for Drug Policy Reform, 2023).

In response to these findings, nurses, including the author, have joined collaborative efforts with D4DPR to introduce these legislative and administrative blueprints to policymakers, healthcare systems, and professional stakeholders. This emerging interprofessional collaboration reflects a growing recognition that nurse involvement is essential to translating policy frameworks into operationally feasible, patient-centered practices within healthcare facilities (American Nurses Association, 2016; American Cannabis Nurses Association & American Nurses Association, 2024).

Healthcare systems should adopt structured, nurse-led policy-to-practice frameworks that center on clarity, safety, and equitable access (Americans for Safe Access, 2025; American Cannabis Nurses Association, & American Nurses Association, 2024). Recommended strategies include:

- Formal governance models with nursing leadership embedded in decision-making structures (Zalon et al., 2024).
- Competency-based education in accordance with national nursing guidance (National Council of State Boards of Nursing, 2018; American Cannabis Nurses Association, & American Nurses Association, 2024).
- Standardized documentation integrated into electronic health records (Philpot et al., 2019).
- Risk mitigation protocols addressing impairment, mobility, and adverse effects (MacCallum & Russo, 2018; National Academies of Sciences, Engineering, and Medicine, 2017).
- Ongoing quality monitoring and iterative policy refinement (Griffith et al., 2025).

Cannabis nurses should also engage in external advocacy using public health framing, emphasizing patient safety, equity, and evidence rather than ideology (American Nurses Association, 2016; Americans for Safe Access, 2025).

FUTURE RESEARCH DIRECTIONS

Additional research needs to examine:

- Outcomes of inpatient and long-term care cannabis policy implementation (McKaig et al., 2025).
- Effectiveness of nursing-led education on safety, quality of documentation, and clinician confidence (Philpot et al., 2019; Zolotov, 2025).

- Impact of federal policy reform and rescheduling on healthcare access and institutional practice (Moritz College of Law, Ohio State University, 2025).
- Equity outcomes associated with facility-based cannabis access policies, particularly for hospitalized and vulnerable populations (National Academies of Sciences, Engineering, and Medicine, 2017; Americans for Safe Access, 2025).

Federal Rescheduling of Cannabis and the Evolving Role of Healthcare Facilities and Nursing Practice: A Theoretical Nursing Framework Perspective

The proposed federal rescheduling of cannabis from Schedule I to Schedule III under the Controlled Substances Act represents a significant inflection point in U.S. health policy with direct implications for access, legitimacy, and clinical integration within healthcare facilities. Under Schedule I, cannabis has been legally defined as having no accepted medical use, a designation that has historically constrained research, reinforced institutional risk aversion, and limited formal engagement by healthcare systems despite widespread state-level legalization (Congressional Research Service [CRS], 2023). Reclassification to Schedule III would formally acknowledge accepted medical use and reduce administrative and regulatory barriers to clinical research, thereby strengthening the evidence base necessary for informed institutional policy development and patient-centered care (American Bar Association [ABA], 2024; U.S. Department of Health and Human Services [HHS], 2023).

For hospitals, long-term care settings, and assisted living communities, particularly those operating in states with legalized medical or adult-use cannabis, Schedule III status may reduce perceived federal enforcement risk and facilitate more transparent internal governance around accommodating patient or resident use. Although rescheduling alone would not federalize state cannabis markets, authorize prescribing absent U.S. Food and Drug Administration approval, or require healthcare facilities to dispense cannabis, it would materially reduce the legal discord between federal drug policy and state-regulated patient access (CRS, 2024). In assisted living settings, where residents often self-administer medications and facilities are regulated primarily at the state level, the impact may be especially pronounced, supporting cannabis accommodation as a lawful personal health decision rather than an exceptional or high-risk activity. Accordingly, the practical effect of rescheduling is likely to manifest not as immediate operational expansion, but as increased institutional willingness to develop policies that normalize cannabis alongside other symptom-management modalities.

Within this evolving policy landscape, nurses are uniquely positioned to shape the transition toward more acceptable and clinically integrated cannabis use, a role well supported by established nursing theory. The American Nurses Association's formal recognition of cannabis nursing as a specialty practice, along with the publication of Cannabis Nursing: Scope and Standards of Practice, establishes a professional framework for evidence-based, ethical, and patient-centered engagement with cannabis therapeutics (American Nurses Association [ANA], 2023, 2024). These standards are closely aligned with Person-Centered Care Theory, which emphasizes respect for individual values, autonomy, and lived experience, positioning patients as active partners in decision-making rather than passive recipients of care (McCormack & McCance, 2017).

Principles of Harm Reduction Theory further inform nursing engagement with cannabis in healthcare and assisted living settings. Harm reduction prioritizes minimizing adverse outcomes rather than enforcing abstinence and is particularly applicable in contexts where patients or residents are already using cannabis legally under state law. Nurses operationalize harm reduction by assessing patterns of use, educating on safer routes of administration, monitoring for potential interactions or impairment, and advocating for policies that reduce risk without denying autonomy. The ANA Scope and Standards explicitly support this approach through competencies related to assessment, patient education, ethical advocacy, and interprofessional collaboration (American Nurses Association, 2024).

From a holistic nursing theory perspective, the integration of cannabis into care reflects nursing's commitment to addressing the physical, psychological, social, and spiritual dimensions of health. Holistic nursing recognizes symptom relief, quality of life, and meaning making as legitimate therapeutic goals, particularly in chronic illness, palliative care, and aging populations commonly served in assisted living communities. As federal rescheduling reduces structural barriers to research and legitimizes medical cannabis within the regulatory hierarchy, nurses are positioned to translate emerging evidence into holistic care plans that acknowledge cannabis as one component of a broader integrative strategy.

In practice, nurses function as critical boundary-spanners between evolving policy, institutional risk management, and patient experience. This role includes educating patients and residents on potential benefits and risks, documenting cannabis use within care plans, monitoring for impairment or drug–drug interactions and advocating for policies that respect patient autonomy while maintaining safety and regulatory compliance. In assisted living communities, where self-administration predominates, nurses play a central role in operationalizing theoretical principles, ensuring that cannabis use remains resident-directed while integrating its consideration into assessments of function, fall risk, cognition, and quality of life.

Collectively, the convergence of federal rescheduling, expanding state legalization, and theoretically based nursing practice suggests a gradual but meaningful shift toward normalized medical cannabis use within healthcare systems. While further regulatory action, particularly from the U.S. Food and Drug Administration, will be required to fully integrate cannabis into prescribing and reimbursement frameworks, nursing leadership grounded in person-centered, harm-reduction, and holistic care theories, as codified through the ANA Scope and Standards, will be fundamental in shaping ethically sound, evidence-informed, and patient-centered access across healthcare facilities.

The conceptual relationship between federal cannabis rescheduling, nursing theory, and facility-level policy integration is illustrated in Figure 1. The model demonstrates how federal regulatory change creates conditions for clinical legitimacy, which are operationalized through nursing theory and professional standards, ultimately informing healthcare facility policies and practice frameworks.

Figure 2. Conceptual framework linking federal cannabis rescheduling, nursing theory, and healthcare facility policy integration

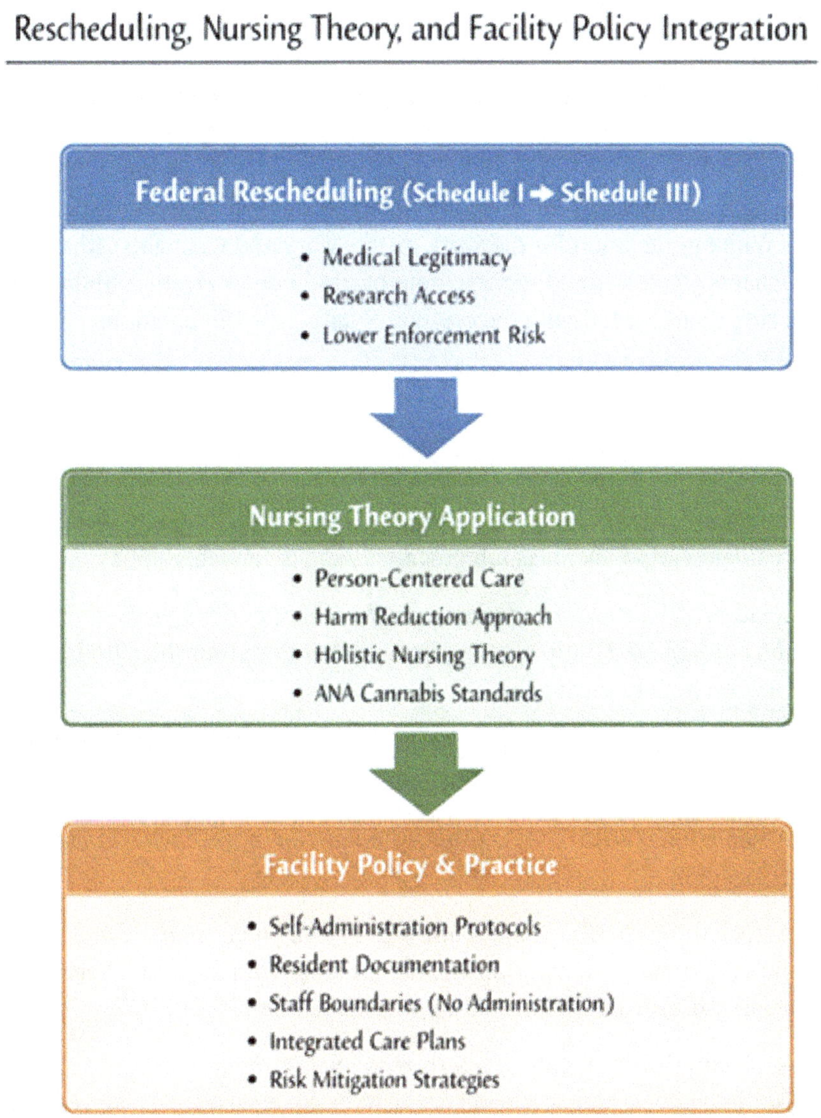

ACKNOWLEDGMENT

The author acknowledges the contributions of nurses, patients, caregivers, legal advocates, healthcare stakeholders, and advocacy organizations whose collaborative efforts informed the policy and advocacy initiatives described in this chapter. Special recognition is extended to nursing colleagues and advocacy partners engaged in the Cannabis Nurses Network, American Cannabis Nurses Association, Society of Cannabis Clinicians, Doctors for Drug Policy Reform, Americans for Safe Access, Connor's Courage, Connor Sheffield Foundation, and the National Clinical Director Consortium, whose commitment to patient-centered care and professional integrity continues to shape access to medical cannabis within healthcare systems. With appreciation for the work of the Maryland Cannabis Administration and the Maryland State legislators. And lastly, a specific note of gratitude to Heather Manus, Ken Sobel, and Jim Bartell for honoring Ryan Bartell with the original Ryan's Law bill creation.

REFERENCES

Alcohol Policy Information System. (n.d.). *About cannabis policy*. National Institute on Alcohol Abuse and Alcoholism. https://alcoholpolicy.niaaa.nih.gov/about/about-cannabis-policy

American Bar Association. (2024). *Rescheduling cannabis: Implications for health law, research, and regulation. The Health Lawyer, 36*(3). https://www.americanbar.org/groups/health_law/resources/health-lawyer/2024-february/rescheduling-cannabis/

American Cannabis Nurses Association, & American Nurses Association. (2024). *Cannabis nursing: Scope and standards of practice* (2nd ed.). American Nurses Association.

American Nurses Association. (2015/2021). *Code of ethics for nurses with interpretive statements*. American Nurses Association.

American Nurses Association. (2016). *Therapeutic use of marijuana and related cannabinoids* [Position statement]. https://www.nursingworld.org/practice-policy/nursing-excellence/official-position-statements/id/therapeutic-use-of-marijuana-and-related-cannabinoids/

American Nurses Association. (2023). *ANA officially recognizes cannabis nursing as a specialty nursing practice* [News release]. https://www.nursingworld.org/news/news-releases/2023/ana-officially-recognizes-cannabis-nursing-as-a-specialty-nursing-practice/

Americans for Safe Access. (2025). *Healthcare facility guide to implementing Ryan's Law*. https://www.safeaccessnow.org/ryanslaw_facilityresources

Cannabis Nurses Network. (n.d.). *Ryan's Law Action Center: Guidance for nurses and health care professionals on California Senate Bill 311*. https://www.cannabisnursesnetwork.com/ryans-law-action-center/

Congressional Research Service. (2023). *The Controlled Substances Act (CSA): A legal overview for the 118th Congress* (LSB11105). https://crsreports.congress.gov

Congressional Research Service. (2024). *Federal marijuana policy: Rescheduling and implications* (R48048). https://crsreports.congress.gov

Doctors for Drug Policy Reform. (2023, February 17). *Legislative and administrative guidelines for regulating cannabis use in healthcare facilities* [White paper]. https://www.d4dpr.org/post/d4dpr-publishes-white-paper-on-legislating-cannabis-use-in-healthcare-facilities

Drug Enforcement Administration. (n.d.). *Drug scheduling*. U.S. Department of Justice. https://www.dea.gov/drug-information/drug-scheduling

Griffith, S., Kreider, R., & Leung, J. (2025). *A coordinated approach to cannabis policy and product safety. Issues in Science and Technology*. https://issues.org/coordinated-approach-cannabis-policy-safety-griffith-kreider-leung

MacCallum, C. A., & Russo, E. B. (2018). Practical considerations in medical cannabis administration and dosing. *European Journal of Internal Medicine*, *49*, 12–19. DOI: 10.1016/j.ejim.2018.01.004 PMID: 29307505

Maryland General Assembly. (2021). *House Bill 331: Connor's Courage Act*. https://mgaleg.maryland.gov

Maryland General Assembly. (2023). *House Bill 1135 / Senate Bill 587*. https://mgaleg.maryland.gov

Maryland Medical Cannabis Commission. (n.d.). *Medical cannabis use in schools: Physician authorization form*. Maryland Department of Health. https://www.marylandpublicschools.org/about/Documents/DSFSS/SSSP/SHS/SHSGuidelines/StudentMedicalCannabisAuthForm.pdf

McCormack, B., & McCance, T. (2017). *Person-centered practice in nursing and health care: Theory and practice* (2nd ed.). Wiley-Blackwell.

McKaig, A., Ridad, A. R. V., Bell, A., McParlane, R., & Quirch, M. (2025). Implementing Ryan's Law on an inpatient medical oncology unit. *Clinical Journal of Oncology Nursing*, *29*(1), 86–90. DOI: 10.1188/25.CJON.86-90 PMID: 39933092

Moritz College of Law, Ohio State University. (2025). *Federal marijuana rescheduling: Process and impact*. Drug Enforcement and Policy Center. https://moritzlaw.osu.edu/faculty-and-research/drug-enforcement-and-policy-center/research-and-grants/policy-and-data-analyses/federal-marijuana-rescheduling

National Academies of Sciences, Engineering, and Medicine. (2017). *The health effects of cannabis and cannabinoids: The current state of evidence and recommendations for research*. National Academies Press. https://doi.org/DOI: 10.17226/24625

National Council of State Boards of Nursing. (2018). The NCSBN national nursing guidelines for medical marijuana. *Journal of Nursing Regulation*, *9*(2), 19–26. DOI: 10.1016/S2155-8256(18)30094-2

Philpot, L. M., Ebbert, J. O., & Hurt, R. T. (2019). A survey of the attitudes, beliefs, and knowledge about medical cannabis among primary care providers. *BMC Family Practice*, *20*(1), 17. DOI: 10.1186/s12875-019-0906-y PMID: 30669979

Schauer, G. L., Njai, R., & Grant, A. M. (2021). Clinician beliefs and practices related to cannabis. *Cannabis and Cannabinoid Research*, *7*(4), 508–515. DOI: 10.1089/can.2020.0165 PMID: 33998899

U.S. Department of Health and Human Services. (2023). *Basis for the recommendation to reschedule marijuana from Schedule I to Schedule III*. https://www.hhs.gov

Woodbridge, M., Sarma, N., & Vaillencourt, D. (2024). *Cannabis quality: The need for science-based global harmonization of standards.* U.S. Pharmacopeia. https://www.usp.org/sites/default/files/usp/document/our-work/DS/uspastm-cannabis-quality-recommendations.pdf

Zalon, M. L., Ludwick, R., & Patton, R. M. (2024). Strengthening nurses' influence in health policy. *The American Journal of Nursing*, *124*(9), 28–36. https://journals.lww.com/ajnonline/fulltext/2024/09000/strengthening_nurses__influence_in_health_policy.17.aspx. DOI: 10.1097/01.NAJ.0001028316.80475.bf PMID: 39115377

Zolotov, Y., Mendoza Temple, L., Isralowitz, R., Gorelick, D. A., Abraham, R., Abrams, D. I., Barich, K., Boehnke, K. F., Dahmer, S., Friedman, J., Frye, P., Haramati, A., Isaac, J., Mathre, M. L., McNabb, M. E., Ring, M., Russo, E. B., Slawek, D. E., Temple, B. R., & Kogan, M. (2025). Developing medical cannabis competencies: A consensus statement. *JAMA Network Open*, *8*(1), e2839750. https://jamanetwork.com/journals/jamanetworkopen/fullarticle/2839750. DOI: 10.1001/jamanetworkopen.2025.35049 PMID: 41055914

KEY TERMS AND DEFINITIONS

Advocacy: Professional actions undertaken to influence policies, practices, and systems to promote patient welfare, equity, safety, and access to evidence-informed healthcare.

Cannabis Nursing: A recognized specialty nursing practice focused on the clinical, educational, ethical, legal, and advocacy dimensions of therapeutic cannabis use across healthcare settings.

Controlled Substances Act (CSA): A United States federal statute that regulates the manufacture, distribution, and use of certain substances and establishes drug scheduling classifications that directly impact cannabis policy and research.

Equitable Access: The principle that all patients, particularly those who are hospitalized, disabled, or institutionalized, should have fair and consistent access to medically authorized therapies without discrimination or undue barriers.

Institutional Policy: Formal rules, procedures, or guidelines adopted by healthcare organizations to govern clinical practice, operational workflows, and meet regulatory requirements within specific care environments.

Policy Implementation: The process of translating laws, regulations, or organizational directives into operational practices, including governance structures, workflows, education, and evaluation mechanisms.

Regulatory Misalignment: A condition in which federal, state, and institutional laws or policies conflict or lack clarity, resulting in inconsistent application and barriers to healthcare access.

Ryan's Law: California legislation enacted to permit eligible terminally ill patients to use medical cannabis within certain healthcare facilities, serving as a model for facility-based access policies nationwide.

Scope of Nursing Practice: The legally and professionally defined boundaries of nursing roles and responsibilities include clinical care, education, documentation, advocacy, and participation in policy development.

Stakeholder Engagement: Collaborative involvement of individuals or organizations, including nurses, patients, administrators, regulators, and policymakers, in the development, negotiation, and implementation of healthcare policy.

Chapter 3
Cannabis Nursing Leadership:
Clinical, Academic, and Policy Transformation in Healthcare Systems

Deanna Marie Collins Sommers
http://orcid.org/0009-0007-6499-0882
American Cannabis Nurses Association, USA

Llewellyn Dawn Smith
http://orcid.org/0009-0000-1217-6992
American Cannabis Nurses Association, USA

ABSTRACT

Cannabis nursing leadership constitutes a critical advancement in modern nursing, integrating ethical advocacy, evidence-based care, and policy transformation across clinical and academic contexts. Anchored in the Cannabis Nursing: Scope and Standards of Practice, this chapter analyzes how nurse leaders, including hospital executives, deans, faculty, and policy advocates, advance safe and equitable integration of cannabis within healthcare and academic systems. Drawing on transformational, servant, and systems leadership frameworks, the chapter explores leadership roles, policy alignment, and translation of research into institutional and educational reform. Through case studies, ethical analysis, and research exemplars, nurse leaders are positioned as stewards of institutional change who promote healthcare consumer safety and public trust. Learning outcomes emphasize leadership competencies. The chapter concludes with applied frameworks and NCLEX-style questions, preparing leaders to advance evidence-based cannabis care grounded in ethics and human dignity.

OBJECTIVES

1. Analyze how transformational, servant, and systems leadership theories inform clinical, academic, and policy roles in cannabis nursing.
2. Evaluate strategies for developing hospital and academic policies that ensure safe, ethical, and compliant cannabis care.
3. Apply evidence-based and ethical frameworks from the Cannabis Nursing Scope & Standards of Practice and ANA Code of Ethics to leadership decision-making.

DOI: 10.4018/979-8-3373-7287-7.ch003

4. Design educational or policy initiatives that advance institutional readiness, staff competency, and interprofessional collaboration.
5. Reflect on future leadership competencies aligned with the ANA 2040 Vision, including technology, equity, and global health integration.

BACKGROUND

The legalization of medical and adult-use cannabis across most of the United States and increasingly worldwide which has transformed healthcare consumers expectations, therapeutic options, and professional responsibilities in healthcare (Centers for Disease Control and Prevention (CDC), 2025). Nurses, as the largest and most trusted profession (Gallup Poll, 2026) .

The recognition of Cannabis Nursing as a specialty by the American Nurses Association (ANA) and the American Cannabis Nurses Association (ACNA) in 2023 formally acknowledged that cannabis care is grounded in specialized knowledge, competencies, and ethical leadership.

In addition, National Council of State Boards of Nursing (NCSBN) provided medical marijuana guidelines which included six essentials for nurses (NCSBN, 2018). However, despite this milestone and nurse guidelines, the integration of cannabis content and policy within healthcare institutions remains sparse. Many hospitals lack clear administrative policies, and most nursing curricula provide limited education on the endocannabinoid system, cannabinoid pharmacology, ethical dilemmas, and cannabis healthcare consumer safety standards.

This gap emphasizes the urgent need for leadership across clinical and academic institutions. Nurse leaders: deans, nurse executives, faculty, and cannabis nurses are responsible for creating the structures, policies, and learning environments that support safe, informed, and equitable cannabis care.

This chapter addresses that need by providing a comprehensive, systems-level exploration of cannabis nursing leadership. It demonstrates how nurse leaders operationalize professional standards in hospital policy, academic curriculum design, and advocacy initiatives that influence legislation and global collaboration.

Significance to Nursing Practice and Education

The chapter contributes to the growing body of nursing leadership scholarship by situating cannabis nursing within the broader framework of 21st-century health transformation. It reinforces nursing's identity as a moral, evidence-based profession while offering a model for interdisciplinary collaboration and policy engagement.

Clinical significance. Nurse leaders in hospitals are often the first to navigate complex questions about cannabis use in palliative care, pain management, psychiatric, neurology and oncology, settings. Their leadership determines whether cannabis care occurs safely and ethically or remains fragmented and inconsistent.

Academic significance. Deans and program directors hold the authority to embed cannabis education within nursing curricula, ensuring graduates develop the knowledge and confidence needed to practice in evolving clinical environments. Academic leaders also collaborate with clinical partners and engage with state boards of nursing to align educational content and institutional policies related to cannabis use by nurses and nursing students with regulatory expectations. In parallel, faculty advance research and scholarship that inform evidence-based practice and contribute to the development of national standards (Parmelee, 2025; King et al., 2024).

Policy significance. Nurse leaders advocate local, state, national, and international levels for legislation and institutional policy that reflect nursing ethics, cannabis healthcare consumer rights, and public safety. Their policy engagement elevates nursing's voice within health governance and aligns with ANA's Imagining the American Nurses Enterprise (ANE) into 2040 (American Nurses Association, 2023).

The chapter bridges these domains, demonstrating how academic and clinical leadership intersect through research, policy translation, and mentorship to create a sustainable leadership pipeline.

Alignment with ANA 2040 and the Cannabis Nursing Scope & Standards of Practice

The ANA 2040 Vision positions nursing as a globally engaged, technologically enabled profession grounded in equity and social justice (American Nurses Association, 2023). Cannabis nursing reflects this trajectory through its holistic, person-centered approach and its commitment to advancing health equity (Clark C. M., 2019). Compare the alignment domains matrix in Table 1.

Table 1. ANA 2040 vision alignment domains matrix

ANA 2040 Priority	Cannabis Nursing Contribution
Equity & Access	Addresses disparities in access to cannabis therapeutics, particularly among communities disproportionately affected by historical criminalization.
Technological Innovation	Integrates informatics, telehealth, and emerging AI tools to enhance cannabis care delivery, clinical decision-making, and data analysis (Shepherd, 2024; Cawthorn, 2024)
Global Citizenship	Engages in cross-national collaborations that promote shared ethical principles and consistent standards for cannabis care.
Lifelong Learning	Demonstrates ongoing professional development, reflective practice, and mentorship among faculty and clinical educators.

Positioning cannabis nursing within the ANA 2040 framework reinforces that it is not a peripheral specialty, Instead, it represents a forward-looking evolution of nursing leadership, ethics, and professional identity, fully aligned with the nursing profession's envisioned future.

Audience and Pedagogical Design

This chapter is intended for nurse executives and managers engaged in developing institutional cannabis policy including academic leaders (deans, directors, and faculty) revising nursing curricula; nurse educators prepare continuing education or certification programs. In addition, advanced practice nurses are engaged in clinical leadership and cannabis healthcare consumer education. Moreover, policy advocates, researchers, and doctoral students in nursing leadership.

Pedagogically, the chapter integrates reflective questions, real-world case exemplars, and evidence tables that align with learning objectives and the American Cannabis Nurses Association (ACNA) Scope and Standards of Practice competencies. Each major section can serve as a foundation for classroom discussion, continuing education, or leadership development workshops.

Scholarly and Practical Contributions

This chapter advances nursing knowledge and leadership in five key methods:

1. Bridging Research and Policy: Demonstrates how nurse leaders translate clinical evidence into institutional and legislative reform.
2. Creating Educational Infrastructure: Provides templates for curriculum and faculty development in cannabis nursing.
3. Elevating Ethical Standards: Integrates ANA and ACNA frameworks to guide moral decision-making in uncertain regulatory contexts.
4. Promoting Global Dialogue: Aligns U.S. cannabis nursing leadership with international nursing priorities for 2040.
5. Empowering Nurse Leaders: Establishes a replicable model of mentorship, resilience, and professional advocacy.

Collectively, these contributions strengthen nursing's role as a global leader in emerging therapeutics, public health, and health systems transformation.

Evaluation, Dissemination, and Outcomes

The effect of this chapter may be measured through both educational and organizational outcomes. Nursing programs and hospital systems adopting these frameworks can evaluate effectiveness through increased faculty and staff competence in cannabis nursing concepts; enhanced policy compliance and ethical documentation practices; growth in research and scholarship output related to cannabis nursing care; active mentorship participation and leadership succession; alignment with institutional diversity, equity, and inclusion goals.

Dissemination strategies include presentations at ANA, ACNA, AACN and other national nursing conferences; integration into ACNA continuing education modules; and publication within leadership and holistic nursing journals.

This chapter proposal situates cannabis nursing leadership at the union of education, practice, and policy reform. Drawing on the principles of ethical leadership, evidence-based practice, and systems thinking, it provides an integrated model for guiding healthcare transformation. Furthermore, the content in this chapter is in alignment with the *ANA 2040 Vision.* Cannabis nurse leaders will continue to redefine what it means to lead building systems that are technologically adept, globally connected, and deeply compassionate. This chapter invites nurse leaders to not only envision that future but to lead in its development into nursing practice.

INTRODUCTION

The Expanding Role of Cannabis Nursing Leadership

The legalization and medical acceptance of cannabis across the United States and globally have initiated one of the most significant paradigms shifts in contemporary nursing practice. As healthcare consumers increasingly consume cannabis for symptom management, pain control, and wellness, nurses have been recognized as the most trusted professional in health care (Gallup Poll, 2026). They are at the intersection of clinical evidence, policy reform, and advocacy for healthcare consumers who use cannabis (American Cannabis Nurses Association & American Nurses Association, 2024; NCSBN, 2018).

The recognition of *Cannabis Nursing* as a specialty by the American Nurses Association (ANA) and the American Cannabis Nurses Association (ACNA) in 2023 formally positioned nurses as leaders in cannabis care delivery, education, and policy. This designation affirmed that cannabis nursing requires unique competencies in pharmacology, ethics, cultural humility, and health systems leadership. It also confirmed what many pioneering nurses had already demonstrated in practice that leadership is not confined to the boardroom or academic office, but occurs wherever nurses influence policy, guide ethical decisions, and empower others to provide safe, informed, and compassionate care.

Within hospitals and clinical systems, nurse leaders play a central role in establishing institutional readiness through policy development, education, and ethical oversight. They must navigate the evolving discrepancies between federal prohibition and state legalization, while implementing hospital policies that protect cannabis healthcare consumers, staff, and organizations. Leadership at this level involves creating and implementing protocols for documentation, administration, and cannabis healthcare consumer education; establishing competency frameworks; and fostering interprofessional collaboration with pharmacy, medicine, and risk management. The nurse leader becomes a systems navigator by balancing safety, compliance, and advocacy to create environments where cannabis care can occur ethically, safely and effectively.

Furthermore, academic leaders: deans, directors, and faculty chairs guide the next generation of nurses toward cannabis literacy. Their leadership extends beyond curriculum design to encompass faculty development, research mentorship, and institutional accreditation. By embedding cannabis content across nursing curricula, academic leaders ensure that graduates enter the workforce prepared to provide evidence-based care in an increasingly cannabis-inclusive health system (NCSBN, 2018; American Cannabis Nurses Association & American Nurses Association, 2024).

Clinical and academic leaders, jointly shape the future of cannabis nursing through a shared vision and collaboration. Their collective efforts form the foundation of a profession capable of addressing health equity, reducing stigma, and aligning nursing holistic philosophy with the realities of contemporary therapeutics. This chapter examines how leadership across hospitals, universities, and policy environments advances the ethical integration of cannabis nursing across the healthcare continuum.

Foundations of Cannabis Nursing Leadership

The trajectory of cannabis nursing leadership reflects a broader historical transformation in both nursing and society from prohibition and stigma to the gradual recognition of cannabis as a therapeutic and public health consideration (NCSBN, 2018; American Cannabis Nurses Association & American Nurses Association, 2024). During much of the twentieth century, cannabis was viewed solely through the lens of criminalization, its potential medical applications largely suppressed by federal policy and social prejudice (National Academies of Sciences, Engineering, and Medicine, 2017). Despite these barriers, nurses consistently encountered cannabis healthcare consumers who used cannabis for symptom relief, long before its medical legitimacy was formally acknowledged. This proximity to cannabis healthcare consumer experience positioned nurses as early observers and, eventually, advocates for evidence-based cannabis care.

The emergence of the American Cannabis Nurses Association (ACNA) in 2010 marked a pivotal moment in the professionalization of cannabis nursing. Early ACNA leaders, many of whom were advanced practice nurses, educators, and policy advocates, sought to ground cannabis nursing in science, ethics, and public health principles (American Cannabis Nurses Association & American Nurses Association, 2024). Their leadership laid the foundation for formal specialty recognition by the American Nurses Association (ANA) in 2023, a milestone that validated the role of nursing in advancing cannabis-related education, policy, and clinical standards. This recognition symbolized not only a disciplinary advancement but also a cultural shift toward embracing the nurse's role in shaping compassionate, evidence-informed cannabis care.

The Nurse as Advocate and Systems Leader

Cannabis nursing leadership emerges from the intersection of advocacy, ethics, and evidence. Nurse leaders often act as the bridge between health care systems bound by complex regulations and cannabis healthcare consumers seeking relief through cannabis therapeutics. This dual accountability to the institution and to the cannabis healthcare consumer requires nurses to exercise advocacy that is both ethical and strategic. Leadership, therefore, is not merely positional but moral and relational (American Nurses Association, 2025). It calls upon the nurse to balance institutional compliance with the commitment to protect and empower the "cannabis health care consumer," the inclusive term endorsed in the .

Effective advocacy leadership demands literacy in regulatory frameworks, institutional risk, and cannabis healthcare consumer rights. It also requires moral courage in hospital environments marked by regulatory ambiguity and persistent stigma. Cannabis nurse leaders embody a form of servant leadership that prioritizes cannabis healthcare consumer well-being while engaging in policy discussions that shape the broader delivery of care. Whether testifying before a policy board, advising an ethics committee, or educating interdisciplinary teams, these leaders translate evidence and values into actionable policy.

Theoretical Foundations of Cannabis Nursing Leadership

Several leadership theories provide conceptual grounding for cannabis nursing practice across hospital, academic, and policy domains: See table 2, Theoretical foundations of cannabis nursing leadership.

Table 2. Theoretical foundations of cannabis nursing leadership

Leadership Theory	Core Emphasis	Application in Cannabis Nursing
Transformation Leadership	Vision, empowerment, cultural change	Challenges stigma, drives policy development, fosters psychological safety, and frames cannabis care as holistic, evidence-based practice (Bass, 2006; Doody, Transformational leadership in nursing practice, 2012).
Servant Leadership	Compassion, justice, community needs	Prioritizes health care consumers, advances equitable access, and models empathy and integrity to build trust (Spears, 2010; Sherman, 2010).
Systems Leadership	Collaboration across adaptive networks	Aligns hospitals, universities, regulators, and community partners to harmonize protocols and standards (Senge, 2006; Shirey, 2013).
Ethical Leadership	Integrity, autonomy, justice	Confronts misinformation, addresses discriminatory policies, and protects scientific integrity in evolving evidence landscapes (American Nurses Association, 2025; Gallagher, 2010).

Alignment with Professional Standards

The *Cannabis Nursing: Scope and Standards of Practice* (ANA & ACNA, 2023) and the *ANA Code of Ethics for Nurses* (2025) together establish the professional framework that guides cannabis nursing leadership. These documents affirm that nurses are responsible for advancing health equity, scientific inquiry, and public policy that safeguard human dignity. Leadership in cannabis nursing therefore involves not only operational skill but adherence to professional values: beneficence, autonomy, and justice.

Hospital based nurse leaders use these standards to guide institutional readiness. They integrate policy language that supports safe documentation, storage, and administration of cannabis within the constraints of state and federal law. Academic leaders apply the same standards to curriculum design and faculty development, ensuring that nursing education reflects ethical and evidence-based approaches to cannabis care. At the policy level, these standards provide a unified voice for nurses advocating within professional and governmental systems.

Holistic and Integrative Perspectives

Cannabis nursing leadership is also rooted in the philosophy of holistic nursing, which views health as the balance of body, mind, and spirit. This integrative perspective aligns with the therapeutic potential of cannabinoids and the individualized nature of cannabis healthcare consumer-centered care. Holistic nurse leaders recognize that cannabis therapeutics intersect with social, cultural, and emotional dimensions of health. By integrating holistic and biomedical perspectives, they promote comprehensive care models that respect cannabis healthcare consumer autonomy while grounding practice in safety and science (Clark C., 2021).

In summary, the foundations of cannabis nursing leadership rest upon three interdependent pillars: ethical advocacy, theoretical grounding, and systems integration. From early pioneers in cannabis advocacy to contemporary hospital administrators and academic deans, nurse leaders have continually shaped the trajectory of cannabis care through courage, scholarship, and collaboration. Leadership in this field requires fluency in clinical science, institutional policy, and compassionate care, qualities that reflect the core values of the nursing profession.

The following sections build upon these foundations, examining how leadership manifests across clinical, academic, and policy settings, and how nurse leaders operationalize these principles to transform health care delivery.

CLINICAL AND HOSPITAL LEADERSHIP IN CANNABIS NURSING

Clinical and hospital leadership in cannabis nursing reflects the integration of professional standards, ethical responsibility, and evidence-informed practice. Guided by the *Cannabis Nursing: Scope and Standards of Practice* (ANA & ACNA, 2023) and grounded in the ACNA's mission pillars, nurse leaders shape the structures that support safe cannabis care across the health system. Their work spans the clinical, unit, and organizational levels where they translate policy into practice, prepare staff for emerging responsibilities, and ensure that cannabis health care consumers receive care rooted in safety, equity, and professional integrity. This multilevel leadership framework provides the foundation for examining how nurses influence cannabis care at the micro, meso, and macro levels of the health system.

Nurse managers and Clinical Nurse Leaders (CNLs) play a pivotal role in translating safe-consumption cannabis policies into bedside practice. Their work occurs within a dual compliance framework that requires careful balance between clinical best practice and institutional liability protection. Most nurses have not received formal instruction in cannabis therapeutics, which creates a knowledge gap that influences documentation, communication, and safe-use practices. This leadership assumes a transformative character as nurse leaders guide the ethical and operational integration of cannabis therapeutics into institutional systems while safeguarding cannabis health care consumer safety and professional integrity. Together, these leadership roles form a continuum that extends from clinical implementation to systemic transformation, grounded in the *Cannabis Nursing: Scope and Standards of Practice* and aligned with ACNA's mission to promote cannabis nursing excellence.

Policy development in cannabis nursing requires coordinated leadership across the clinical unit and organizational levels of the health system. At the micro level, nurses identify gaps in education, documentation, communication, and workflow that influence cannabis health care consumer safety. At the meso level, nurse managers and Clinical Nurse Specialists collaborate with pharmacy, compliance, and interprofessional partners to shape procedures that reflect ethical and legal expectations. At the macro level, directors and advanced practice nurses guide the creation of institutional policies that align with state regulations, organizational priorities, and cannabis nursing standards. See Table 3 describing the differences in Micro-Meso-Macro Leadership Roles in Cannabis Policy Development

Table 3. Micro-meso-macro leadership roles in cannabis policy development

Level of Leadership	Primary Focus	Key Responsibilities in Cannabis Policy Development	Alignment with ACNA Mission Pillars
Micro (Clinical/Bedside	Direct care and workflow integration	Identify gaps in documentation and communication. Support safe-use practices during care. Provide feedback on policy feasibility and workflow impact	Promote safety and clarity in care delivery. Support equitable access to evidence-informed information
Meso (Unit/Department)	Operational coordination and staff readiness	Collaborate with pharmacy, compliance, and interprofessional partners. Orient staff to legal and ethical expectations. Standardized documentation and communication procedures	Strengthening team-based practice Advance consistent accountable cannabis care
Macro (Organizational/Systems	Institutional policy creation and strategic alignment	Develop and approve cannabis policies. Align institutional procedures with state regulations and professional standards. Guide to risk management and ethical oversight	Shape structures that support safe, equitable cannabis care Promote systems-level advocacy and professional integrity

Policy Creation and Implementation in Hospital Systems

Policy creation and implementation in hospital systems require nurse leaders to demonstrate both policy literacy and procedural agility. Developing cannabis related policies involves navigating overlapping domains of law, ethics, pharmacology, and nursing regulation, often within environments where federal and state expectations diverge. Nurse leaders frequently chair or co-chair policy task forces that include pharmacy directors, physicians, compliance officers, and legal counsel, ensuring that institutional procedures reflect scientific evidence and organizational safety priorities. Because cannabis can interact with other medications, potentially altering therapeutic effects or increasing adverse risks, nursing policies must include robust assessment and documentation protocols to support clinical decision-making and cannabis health care consumer safety. This includes performing accurate and nonjudgmental medication reconciliation that explicitly accounts for cannabis consumption, whether prescribed, recommended, or self-directed. Through this interdisciplinary and clinically grounded approach, nurse leaders help shape policies that are both operationally all feasible and aligned with cannabis nursing standards of practice.

Key components of hospital cannabis policies typically address eligibility and verification, administration and storage, documentation and communication, education and competency, and risk mitigation. These domains form the structural backbone of safe use infrastructure and parallel the Six Right of Medication Administration: right cannabis health care consumer, right product, right dose, right route, right time, and right documentation. Cannabis introduces unique complexities within each of these rights. For example, the "right product" may require navigating cultivar-specific effects, labeling inconsistencies, and formulation variability, while the "right dose" often involves titration guidance and individualized education to support safe use. One Midwestern teaching hospital developed a nurse-led "Medical Cannabis Care Pathway" in 2024 to support cannabis use among oncology and palliative care cannabis health care consumers (Braun, 2023). Co-authored by nursing leadership and the pharmacy department, the policy aligned state law with institutional ethics standards and established clear documentation and education guidelines. Early evaluation demonstrated improved interdisciplinary communication, greater staff confidence in addressing cannabis-related questions, and increased cannabis health care consumer satisfaction with symptom-management options. Together, these elements illustrate the foundational policy domains that guide safe and consistent cannabis care across hospital systems. See the Policy Spotlight 1 box for a concise overview of the core components that anchor hospital cannabis policies. These domains reflect common elements of hospital cannabis policy development informed by current nursing leadership practice. While these policy components establish the structural foundation for safe cannabis care, their success depends on strong interprofessional collaboration.

Spotlight 1., Policy Spotlight: Core Components of Hospital Cannabis Policies

1. **Eligibility and Verification** – defining how cannabis health care consumers with valid state medical cannabis certifications are identified and documented in the electronic health record.
2. **Administration and Storage** – establishing protocols for securing, labeling, and storing cannabis health care consumer-owned cannabis products; clarifying staff roles in administration or self-administration.
3. **Documentation and Communication** – ensuring accurate charting of cannabis use and consistent communication across the care team.
4. **Education and Competency** – mandating annual staff education on cannabis pharmacology, drug interactions, and consumer counseling.
5. **Risk Mitigation** – outlining procedures for incidents, adverse events, or suspected impairment among consumers or staff.

Interprofessional Collaboration and Leadership Influence

Effective cannabis nursing leadership within hospital systems is inherently interprofessional. Nurse leaders function as integrative partners, bridging frontline nursing staff, pharmacy services, medical providers, compliance teams, and executive administration to ensure coordinated, evidence-informed care. Their role includes facilitating communication across disciplines, especially in complex cases where cannabis use intersects with prescribed medications, symptom-management strategies, or regulatory constraints. By grounding discussions in evidence, ethical reasoning, and institutional policy, nurse leaders help teams navigate uncertainty, reduce stigma, and align care plans with both clinical realities and consumer needs. This collaborative approach strengthens decision-making, enhances safety, and reinforces nursing's vital role in shaping equitable cannabis care.

Workforce Education and Competency Development

This section will explore how cannabis nursing leaders design and implement staff education programs that build clinical competency, reduce stigma, and align with institutional policy. Competency-based cannabis training ensures that nurses and allied professionals understand the endocannabinoid system (ECS), cultivar-specific effects, dosing strategies, and documentation protocols. Continuing education (CE) modules offer scalable pathways for skill development, often integrating case studies, legal updates, and consumer-centered care models. Stigma reduction is a critical component—requiring intentional dialogue, myth-busting, and values-based reflection to shift attitudes shaped by decades of prohibition and misinformation.

Workforce education represents one of the most powerful levers of hospital-based leadership, particularly as providers remain underinformed about cannabis therapeutics. Knowledge gaps surrounding the endocannabinoid system (ECS), product options and effects, consumer-centered care are compounded by stigma and federal scheduling barriers (Russo, 2016). In contrast, nurses are often better prepared to support cannabis health care consumers, offering education, advocacy, and clinical insight grounded in professional standards and lived experience. Clinical nurse leaders and educators therefore play a critical role in preparing staff to address cannabis use with accuracy, empathy, and confidence. Effective continuing education programs and in-service trainings include core elements such as cannabinoid and terpene pharmacology, safety considerations related to dosing and drug interactions, documentation standards for cannabis health care consumer-reported consumption and informed consent, communication strategies to counter stigma and misinformation, and awareness of legal and institutional policies that shape safe practice. Collaboration with providers becomes both clinical and educational, requiring nurse leaders to navigate resistance, build trust, and advocate for evidence-informed care while coordinating with compliance teams to reinforce documentation integrity and regulatory adherence. Hospitals that invest in structured cannabis education programs consistently report improved nursing confidence and stronger cannabis health care consumer engagement. For example, a large urban academic medical center integrated a mandatory cannabis competency course into its nursing orientation program, led by nurse educators certified in cannabis therapeutics, resulting in great consistency in consumer education and a reduction in medication-error reports involving cannabis products (Zolotov, 2021; Balneaves, 2018). Effective cannabis education programs address three essential competency clusters: 1) clinical knowledge, including cannabinoid pharmacology and safety considerations; 2) professional practice skills, such as documentation standards and informed-consent processes; and 3) communication and regulatory literacy, including stigma-reduction strategies and awareness of legal and institutional policies. Grounded in the Cannabis Nursing Scope and Standards of Practice, ACNA's mission pillars, and emerging models of team-based care, this educational leadership style strengthens institutional readiness and elevates the quality of cannabis care across hospital systems.

> "A well-prepared nursing workforce requires mastery of cannabis pharmacology, safety documentation, communication, and regulatory literacy" – Llewellyn

Figure 1. Nurses play a central role in educating and empowering cannabis health care consumers

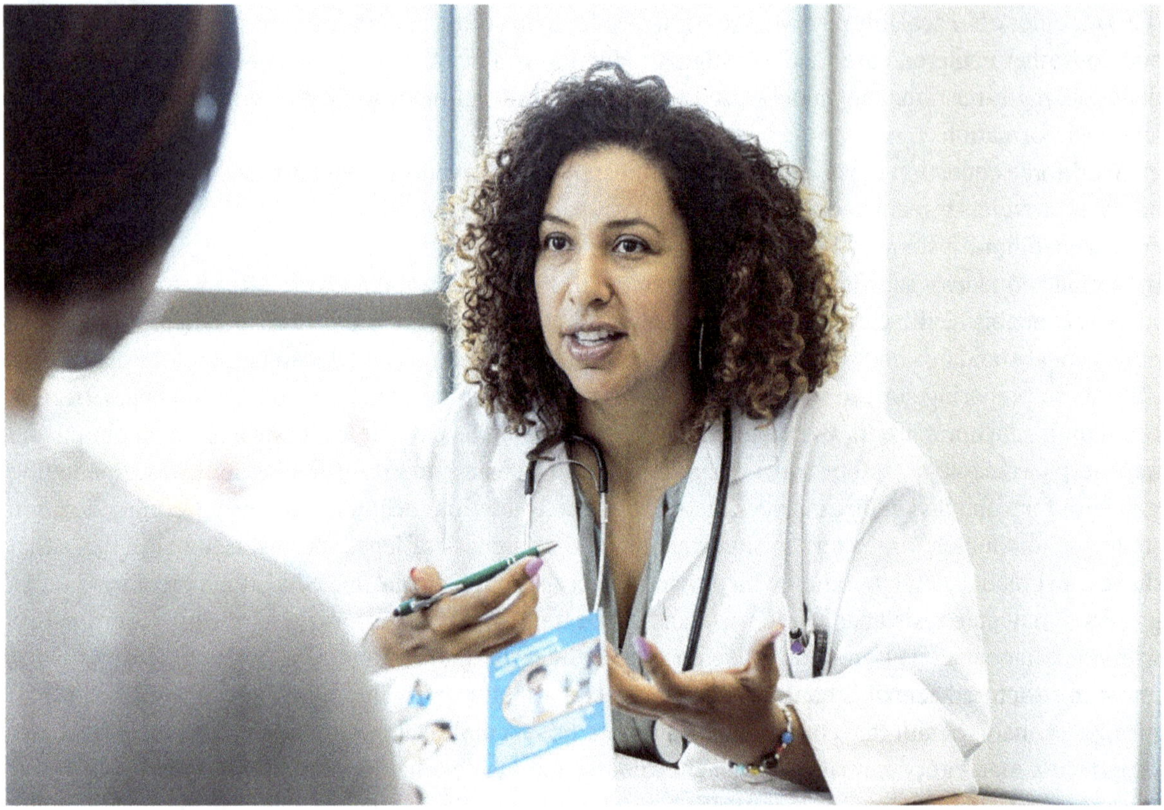

Ethical Leadership and Risk Navigation

Ethical leadership in hospital-based cannabis care requires nurse leaders to navigate complex tensions between consumer autonomy, clinical safety, and regulatory constraints. Cannabis health care consumers have the right to make informed decisions about their health, including the use of cannabis therapeutics, nevertheless nurses must also uphold institutional, state, and federal regulations, which may remain outdated, inconsistent, or punitive. These tensions surface in everyday practice: a physician may hesitate to acknowledge cannabis use due to federal scheduling, or a palliative care consumer may wish to self-administer cannabis for symptom relief despite institutional policies that prohibit consumption. In such scenarios, the ethical nurse leader mediates discussion using evidence-based data and ethical reasoning grounded in the *ANA Code of Ethics* (2025), safeguarding autonomy while promoting a culture of mutual respect and learning across the interprofessional team. Ethical practice requires balancing respect for consumer choice with risk mitigation, transparent documentation, and collaboration with hospital ethics committees. Nurse leaders may also advocate for policy revisions, presenting peer-reviewed evidence on safety, efficacy, and quality-of-life outcomes to align institutional practice with contemporary clinical realities. Guided by the cannabis nursing practice standards of care, nurse leaders serve as ethical stewards, advocating for justice, reducing harm, and ensuring that consumer-centered care remains uncompromised within evolving legal and organizational landscapes.

Change Management and Stigma Reduction

Effective change management in cannabis nursing leadership requires collaboration across organizational, industrial, regulatory, and healthcare sectors. Nurse leaders must engage with CE providers, dispensary networks, compliance teams, and regulatory bodies to ensure that evolving practice remain evidence informed, legally sound, and operationally feasible. This cross-sector approach supports the development of unified competencies, shared language, and scalable implementation strategies that help staff adapt confidently to new expectations and workflows. Grounded in the *Cannabis Nursing Scope and Standards of Practice*, ACNA's mission pillars, and ANA's Professional Development Standards, this systems-level work established the foundation for sustainable integration of cannabis care within hospital environment.

Introducing cannabis into a hospital's care model is not only a policy shift but a cultural transformation. Resistance often emerges from fear of liability, limited clinical knowledge, or deeply ingrained stigma shaped by decades of prohibition. Nurse leaders serve as change managers in these moments, drawing on principles of organizational psychology to guide staff through the stages of awareness, acceptance, and adaptation. Effective strategies include early stakeholder engagement, transparent communication that addresses misconceptions, incremental implementation through pilot units, and continuous feedback loops that allow staff to shape refinements based on real-world experience. By modeling openness, compassion, and evidence informed practice, nurse leaders normalize cannabis discussion within professional settings, strengthening trust and fostering a more inclusive, stigma-free environment for cannabis health care consumers.

Leadership Outcomes and Quality Indicators

Cannabis nursing leadership in hospitals contributes to measurable outcomes that extend far beyond policy compliance. Effective leadership shapes clinical practice, strengthens interdisciplinary communication, and enhances the overall experience for cannabis health care consumers. By establishing clear expectations, modeling evidence-informed care, and supporting staff through education and change management, nurse leaders create the conditions for safe, consistent, and ethically ground cannabis integration across the health system.

Leadership effectiveness can be evaluated through indicators such as increased staff competence and confidence in discussing cannabis use; improved cannabis health care consumer satisfaction scores related to symptom management; reduced incidents of unreported cannabis use or adverse interactions; enhanced interdisciplinary collaboration and documentation accuracy; and a strengthened institutional reputation for innovation and ethical, consumer centered care. Together, these outcomes reinforce the role of nurse leaders as essential architects of safe, equitable cannabis integration within hospital environments.

Taken together, these leadership outcomes and quality indicators demonstrate how cannabis nursing leadership shapes not only staff readiness and clinical safety but also the broader culture and performance of the health system. To illustrate how these principles translate into real-world practice, the following case studies offer concrete examples of nurse leaders navigating policy implementation, interdisciplinary collaboration, stigma reduction, and healthcare consumer-centered care within diverse hospital environments.

Examples in Cannabis Nursing Leadership

Cannabis nursing leadership emerges across diverse clinical, policy, and community settings, often driven by nurses who recognize unmet needs and advocate for safer more compassionate models of care. The following examples illustrate three distinct catalysts for change: clinical evidence, legislative advocacy, and patient narrative. These examples demonstrate how nurses translate emerging knowledge into practice, influence institutional policy, and elevate the voices of patients and families. Together, these examples highlight the multifaceted nature of cannabis nursing leadership and the essential role nurses play in shaping ethical, evidence-informed approaches to cannabis integration within modern health systems.

Example 1. Nurse-Led Research as a Catalyst for Clinical Innovation

In 2019, an endoscopy nurse deeply engaged in cannabis nursing encountered Twardowski's 2019 study on cannabis use and sedation requirements. Recognizing similar patterns in her own practice, she pursued her hospital's Magnet research benefit to replicate the study within a Magnet-designated community hospital. After securing approval from colleagues, unit leadership, the research committee, and the Chief Nursing Officer, this nurse partnered with a nurse data analyst and seasoned DNP research mentor from the systems research department. Together, they collaborated with informatics specialist to modify the EPIC pre-operative history tool, enabling nurses to systematically document cannabis consumption habits consistently.

The study, conducted from November 2020 through March 2022, evaluated 1,018 adult outpatients undergoing upper and lower GI endoscopic procedures. A single endoscopist and a consistent anesthesia team ensured procedural standardization. Findings validated Twardowski's study and demonstrated that cannabis-consuming patients required significantly higher weight- and time-adjusted propofol doses to achieve and maintain adequate sedation, aligning with emerging national literature. Importantly, recovery times did not differ between groups, indicating that increased sedation requirements did not lead to oversedation or prolonged recovery. Published in *Gastroenterology Nursing* (July/August 2024), this study provided actionable evidence for anesthesia planning, pre-procedure assessment, and consumer safety protocols. It also exemplified how one cannabis nurse scientist translates bedside observations into rigorous inquiry, influence documentation standards, and advance institutional readiness in an evolving clinical landscape.

Example 2. Ryan's Law – Advocacy and Interdisciplinary Leadership in Action

Ryan's Law (California Senate Bill 311), enacted in 2021, represents a landmark example of how interdisciplinary advocacy can transform institutional norms and expand compassionate access to cannabis for terminally ill health care consumers. The law gained momentum through the dedicated efforts of cannabis activists. A cannabis nurse leader and advocate along with an attorney worked alongside

Ryan's family to elevate their story, mobilize professional networks, and engage lawmakers in addressing the ethical tension between patient comfort and restrictive hospital policies.

Ryan's Law requires California hospitals and certain healthcare facilities to allow medicinal cannabis consumption for terminally ill patients under defined conditions. For nurse leaders, the law emphasizes the profession's responsibility to advocate for dignity, autonomy, and compassionate symptom management. Implementation demands thoughtful policy development, staff education, interdisciplinary collaboration, and stigma-conscious communication strategies. This case demonstrates how nurses, attorneys, and families can work together to transform individual suffering into systemic change, reinforcing the essential role of nursing leadership in shaping cannabis consumer centered policy in institutions and public domains.

Example 3. Charlotte Figi – Patient Narrative as Driver of National Awareness

Patient narratives often catalyze shifts in public perception, clinical curiosity, and legislative action. One of the most influential stories in moder cannabis history is that of Charlotte Figi, a young girl with Dravet syndrome whose severe, treatment-resistant seizures dramatically improved with high-CBD, low-THC extract later cultivated as Charlotte's Web™. Her family's decision to explore cannabidiol as an adjunct therapy led to profound reduction in seizure frequency, capturing national attention and challenging long-standing stigma surrounding cannabis therapeutics.

Charlotte's story, shared widely through advocacy networks, documentaries, and educational forums, helped humanize science and inspire a wave of research into cannabinoid-based therapies. Although Charlotte tragically passed away from complications related to COVID-19 years later, her legacy continues to influence clinical practice, research priorities, and public policy. For nurse leaders, her story signifies the importance of honoring patient and family experiences as legitimate sources of knowledge and remaining open-minded, informed and ethically grounded when discussing cannabis therapeutics with health care consumers exploring alternative or adjunctive therapies.

Together, these three case studies illustrate the breadth and depth of cannabis nursing leadership. From generating clinical evidence and shaping institutional policy to amplifying health care consumers narratives that transform public understanding, nurses play a pivotal role in advancing safe, ethical, and compassionate cannabis integration across the healthcare continuum. These examples demonstrate how leadership emerges at the bedside, in the boardroom, and within communities. And, how nurses, guided by professional standards and a commitment to health care consumer care, are uniquely positioned to drive meaningful changes in this rapidly evolving specialty nursing practice.

Clinical and hospital leadership in cannabis nursing embodies the synthesis of ethics, advocacy, and evidence-based management. Nurse leaders serve as the driving force behind policy creation, staff education, and interdisciplinary collaboration that ensure safe and compassionate cannabis care. Their influence extends beyond institutional walls, shaping public perception, informing legislative action, and modeling professional courage in an evolving healthcare landscape. In this work, nurses navigate the complexities of stigma, regulatory ambiguity, and rapidly emerging science while remaining steadfastly committed to patient dignity and safety.

By embracing transformational, servant, and systems-level leadership principles, cannabis nurse leaders do more than implement policy, they humanize it. They ensure that each regulation, protocol, and guideline reflects the lived realities of cannabis health care consumers and the ethical obligations of the nursing profession. Nursing leadership exhibits what it means to practice at the forefront of modern nursing: ethically grounded, scientifically informed, and socially responsive. As a result, they chart a path for future generations of nurses who will continue to advance equitable evidence-informed cannabis care across the healthcare continuum.

ACADEMIC LEADERSHIP: DEANS, DIRECTORS, AND FACULTY ADVOCATES

Academic Nursing Leadership in a Changing Healthcare Landscape

Academic leaders: deans, associate deans, program directors, and faculty are instrumental in the role of shaping the future of nursing practice through curriculum design, institutional culture and policy, and faculty development. As cannabis therapeutics gain recognition within clinical practice, nursing schools increasingly are responsible for preparing graduates who are competent, ethical, and confident in providing cannabis-informed care. The academic leader therefore becomes not only an administrator but a visionary, responsible for aligning education with evolving societal and healthcare realities.

The inclusion of cannabis content in nursing education remains inconsistent across programs in the United States. Many curricula continue to omit formal instruction on the endocannabinoid system, cannabis pharmacology, or the ethical and legal aspects of cannabis care. This omission leaves a significant knowledge gap among new graduates, often resulting in clinical discomfort and missed opportunities for cannabis healthcare consumer advocacy (Spector, 2018; Parmelee, 2025; Clark C., 2021). Academic leaders who recognize this deficiency act as catalysts for change in developing curricular strategies that reflect the specialty of cannabis nursing and align with the *Cannabis Nursing: Scope and Standards of Practice* (ANA & ACNA, 2023).

The Dean as a Strategic Visionary

The dean of a nursing college occupies a unique position of influence balancing institutional priorities and policies, accreditation requirements, and professional leadership. The dean's leadership and authority determine whether a nursing program remains reactive to policy shifts or becomes proactive in shaping cannabis policies and cannabis education in curriculum.

Strategic deans lead with a systems perspective, recognizing cannabis education as integral to holistic, evidence-based nursing. They allocate resources for faculty development, encourage scholarly inquiry into cannabis therapeutics, and initiate partnerships with clinical and policy organizations such as the American Cannabis Nurses Association (ACNA) and state boards of nursing.

Deans also play a critical role in ensuring alignment between nursing education and licensure requirements. As advocacy continues for inclusion of cannabis-related competencies in the National Council Licensure Examination (NCLEX), deans must anticipate these changes by embedding cannabis science, ethics, and cannabis health care consumer . The National Council of State Boards of Nursing (NCSBN, 2018) outlined six essential guidelines to support safe and accountable nursing care related to medical cannabis consumers. These guidelines established foundational expectations for nursing knowledge, clinical judgment, and professional conduct in jurisdictions where medical cannabis is legal. Academic deans may also advocate for continuing education programs for alumni and clinical partners, positioning their institutions as leaders in cannabis-informed professional development.

Program Directors and Associate Deans: Operationalizing Change

If the dean provides vision, program directors and associate deans translate that vision into structure and implementation. These leaders oversee curriculum mapping, course revision, and faculty development and support to ensure that cannabis content is woven throughout nursing programs. Systematic integration of cannabis therapeutics and the endocannabinoid system involve more than adding isolated lectures. It requires a systematic approach that connects cannabis content to anatomy, pathophysiology, pharmacology, advance medical surgical, pediatrics, mental health, ethics, community health, and leadership courses. For example, a director may lead a curriculum committee to introduce the *Cannabis Nursing Scope and Standards* within leadership and policy courses, emphasizing advocacy, cannabis healthcare consumer safety, and clinical documentation.

Drawing on practice-informed academic leadership experience, the author, in an associate dean role, has observed that practice-based nursing programs benefit from coordinated partnerships with clinical sites to ensure students encounter real-world applications of cannabis nursing. These experiences may occur through community health, hospice, oncology, integrative medicine, or regulated medical dispensary placements. Such experiential learning deepens student understanding of the clinical, ethical, and regulatory dimensions of cannabis care while strengthening readiness for practice within institutional frameworks.

Faculty Champions and the Role of Educator as Advocates

Faculty champions often represent the first line of cannabis nursing leadership within academia. These educators inspired by their own clinical experiences or professional development through ACNA, attend continuing education programs or college courses, and introduce cannabis topics into existing courses.

The leadership of faculty champions is characterized by innovation and persistence. In many cases, they must navigate institutional resistance rooted in stigma, misinformation, or administrative caution. By grounding their advocacy in evidence and ethics, faculty leaders can gradually shift perceptions and establish legitimacy for cannabis nursing as a necessary component of modern education.

Faculty champions also contribute to scholarship through research, publications, and presentations at conferences (Sommers, 2023). Their academic work not only informs evidence-based practice but also raises the visibility of nursing leadership in cannabis care. Faculty members who publish in peer-reviewed journals or collaborate on national research initiatives reinforce the credibility of the field and support academic policy reform.

Faculty Development and Institutional Readiness

A major responsibility of academic leaders is ensuring that faculty members possess the knowledge and confidence to teach cannabis-related content competently. Parmalee and Clark describes that most nursing faculty report minimal formal training in cannabis pharmacology or endocannabinoid science (Parmelee R. C., 2021). In addition, the research describes faculty bias cite (Parmelee & Clark, 2022; King, et al., 2024). This deficit accentuates the need for structured professional development. Deans and directors can implement faculty readiness initiatives by implementing strategies for cannabis nursing education as found in Spotlight 2.

Spotlight 2. Faculty Readiness Strategies for Cannabis Nursing Education

Access to Professional Learning

Providing faculty with ACNA webinars, continuing education modules, and certificate programs that build foundational and advanced cannabis nursing knowledge.

Internal Capacity Building

Hosting workshops focused on the *Cannabis Nursing: Scope and Standards of Practice* to ensure consistent understanding of professional expectations.

National Engagement

Supporting faculty participation in national conferences where cannabis nursing, policy, and regulatory developments are discussed.

Interdisciplinary Collaboration

Encouraging partnerships with colleagues in science, pharmacology, psychology, ethics, and public health to strengthen curricular integration and shared expertise.

Mentorship Pathways

Establishing structured mentorship programs that pair experienced cannabis nurse educators with novice faculty to support growth, confidence, and pedagogical alignment.

These initiatives strengthen faculty knowledge and cultivate collaboration, intellectual openness, and academic courage, reinforcing a compassionate and inclusive approach to curricular innovation.

Accreditation, Governance, and Policy Alignment

Academic leaders must navigate regulatory and accreditation guidelines that govern curriculum content and program evaluation. Integrating cannabis nursing within existing frameworks requires strategic advocacy with institutional committees, boards of trustees, and regional accreditors.

During curriculum revision, program directors can align cannabis-related learning outcomes with established educational standards, including the Quality and Safety Education for Nurses (QSEN) competencies (QSEN Institute, 2013) and the American Association of Colleges of Nursing (AACN) Essentials (American Association of Colleges of Nursing, 2021). This alignment positions cannabis nursing education within widely accepted frameworks that emphasize healthcare consumer safety, quality improvement, and interprofessional collaboration.

At the governance level, nursing school leaders may propose formal policy statements that affirm the ethical and scientific foundations of cannabis nursing education. These policies establish institutional legitimacy, safeguard faculty for academic freedom, and demonstrate alignment with national nursing standards. Additionally, they offer structured guidance for navigating complex deliberations within governing boards and community stakeholder forums.

For example, when revising curricula, directors may align new cannabis-related outcomes with existing program standards, such as Quality and Safety Education for Nurses (QSEN) competencies, QSEN Institute. (2013) or the American Association of Colleges of Nursing (AACN) *Essentials* (2021) (QSEN Institute, 2020; American Association of Colleges of Nursing, 2021). Doing so situates cannabis education within widely accepted paradigms of cannabis healthcare consumer safety, quality improvement, and interprofessional collaboration.

Academic–Clinical Partnerships

Sustainable cannabis nursing education depends on robust partnerships between nursing schools and clinical institutions. Academic leaders play a key role in forging these relationships, ensuring that nursing students engage in cannabis-informed care within practice environments that are legally compliant, educationally rigorous, and supportive of competency-based learning outcomes.

These partnerships are mutually beneficial: hospitals gain access to emerging evidence and faculty expertise, while nursing programs strengthen clinical placement opportunities and collaborative policy development. Academic and clinical partnerships further support the establishment of joint governance structures focused on cannabis care, resulting in standardized policy frameworks and shared educational resources for both staff and students.

This collaboration exemplifies systems leadership, demonstrating how academic and clinical leaders can co-create infrastructures that normalize cannabis care as part of comprehensive health practice.

Example: College / University-Led Cannabis Curriculum Integration

The following composite example illustrates how academic leadership can support the phased integration of cannabis nursing education in alignment with guidance from the National Council of State Boards of Nursing (NCSBN). Under the leadership of a dean, program director, and curriculum chair, a college of nursing conducted a formal needs assessment that identified strong student interest and gaps in cannabis-related content. In response, a faculty task force developed longitudinal learning modules embedded across multiple semesters, addressing the endocannabinoid system, clinical safety, ethical decision-making, and population health.

The initiative incorporated community partnerships with palliative care organizations to support observational learning experiences. Over a two-year implementation period, program evaluation may demonstrate increased student self-efficacy in cannabis healthcare consumer education and improved faculty confidence in teaching cannabis-related content. Curricular integration also supports student preparation for emerging licensure expectations, including potential future NCLEX content related to cannabis therapeutics. This leadership-driven approach contributes to measurable cultural and curricular transformation within the institution.

Challenges and Future Directions

Academic leaders must contend with numerous challenges in cannabis nursing education:

- **Regulatory ambiguity:** Federal prohibition complicates funding and curriculum approvals.
- **Stigma and bias:** Persistent misconceptions among faculty, administrators, and community partners.
- **Faculty workload:** Limited time and resources for professional development.
- **Evidence gaps:** Need more robust nursing-specific research to inform curriculum design.

Incorporating cannabis nursing into the curriculum aligns with nursing's ethical responsibility to ensure competent, evidence-based care.

Academic leadership in cannabis nursing represents both an opportunity and a professional obligation. Deans, directors, and faculty champions stand at the forefront of preparing nurses to meet the realities of contemporary healthcare. By fostering faculty readiness, aligning policy with ethics, and modeling scholarly integrity, these leaders ensure that cannabis nursing is not a marginal topic but a core competency within nursing education.

Academic nurse leaders drive a future in which evidence-based cannabis care is standard practice and where the principles of compassion, justice, and science guide every dimension of nursing education.

LEADERSHIP AT THE INTERSECTION OF CLINICAL POLICY AND ACADEMIA

Bridging Two Worlds: The Convergence of Academia and Practice

Cannabis nursing leadership increasingly depends on the ability to integrate academic vision with clinical practicality. Hospitals and universities no longer operate as separate spheres; rather, they form a continuum where knowledge generation, skill development, and cannabis healthcare consumer care inform one another. The rise of cannabis nursing is situated at the intersection of ethics, policy, and therapeutics which has accelerated the need for stronger academic and practice partnerships.

Deans, nursing directors, and hospital chief nursing officers (CNOs) are uniquely positioned to facilitate this alignment. Together, they form a leadership triad that drives both educational reform and institutional readiness for cannabis integration. In this collaboration, the academic leader ensures curricular relevance and scholarly rigor, while the hospital leader implements evidence-informed policy and staff education. When this synergy is achieved, the result is a healthcare system that not only trains competent practitioners but also enacts policies rooted in nursing ethics and science.

Collaborative Governance and Shared Accountability

Collaborative governance between hospitals and nursing schools provides a framework for joint decision-making around policy and education. Nursing deans and hospital nurse executives may co-chair cannabis policy or education task forces designed to synchronize learning outcomes, clinical competencies, and institutional standards.

One illustrative governance model is the joint academic and clinical council, advisory council which brings nursing faculty together with health system executives as part of ongoing AACN accreditation processes focused on curriculum alignment, practice partnerships, and continuous quality improvement (American Association of Colleges of Nursing, 2021). Within this structure, academic and clinical leaders collaboratively review emerging legislation, evaluate current evidence, and develop unified educational and clinical protocols. This shared governance approach supports alignment between program outcomes and clinical practice expectations, ensuring that curricular standards and institutional policies evolve in a coordinated and intentional manner. The council also provides a formal mechanism to address regulatory complexity, manage institutional risk, and support professional advocacy consistent with accreditation expectations.

Collaborative councils may also focus on faculty practice appointments, where academic faculty hold active clinical roles within hospital systems. These dual roles strengthen the bidirectional translation of knowledge between academic instruction and clinical practice. The nurse who teaches cannabis therapeutics in the academic setting may simultaneously lead clinical policy development within the hospital, ensuring alignment between education and practice.

Translating Evidence into Policy

Cannabis nursing research often originates within academic environments but achieves impact only when translated into policy and practice. Academic nurse leaders serve as primary conduits of new evidence to hospital leadership. Results from university-driven research on cannabinoid use in symptom management can inform updates to institutional pain management policies.

Clinical nurse leaders provide structured feedback to academic partners regarding practice-based challenges, including patient hesitancy related to cannabis care, documentation variability, and interprofessional coordination concerns. This reciprocal exchange of knowledge between clinical practice and academic inquiry reflects a systems leadership approach in which continuous integration of evidence and application informs curricular refinement, research priorities, and health system improvement.

Collaborative dissemination mechanisms including joint grand rounds, research symposiums, and continuing education conferences further reinforce this translation. Through these venues, faculty and clinical leaders present case studies, policy updates, and emerging evidence to both students and practicing clinicians, creating a culture of shared learning and professional development.

Policy Alignment and Institutional Readiness

Hospital policies governing cannabis use are effective only to the extent that they are supported by comprehensive education. Academic leaders play a critical role in preparing graduates who are equipped to navigate these policies safely and ethically in clinical practice. When academic and hospital leaders collaborate, institutional policy language can be intentionally reflected within educational competencies, thereby creating continuity between nursing education and clinical expectations.

Within this collaborative framework, clinical documentation requirements related to patient-reported cannabis use can be integrated into simulation experiences and clinical coursework, enabling students to develop proficiency in assessment, documentation, and therapeutic communication. In addition, distinctions between nurse administration and cannabis healthcare consumer, self-administration of cannabis products can be addressed through structured ethical analysis, case-based learning, and guided debriefing activities.

This deliberate alignment between policy and pedagogy strengthens institutional readiness by minimizing knowledge gaps, reducing the potential for legal or ethical missteps, and enhancing confidence among both new graduates and practicing nurses.

The Role of Joint Appointments and Academic Practice Partnerships

Joint faculty appointments between colleges / universities and health systems represent a potential strategy for strengthening practice and academic partnerships in cannabis nursing leadership, consistent with AACN expectations for integrated education, practice, and continuous quality improvement. Although not yet widely implemented, these roles may enable nurse leaders to contribute across education, research, and clinical policy domains in a coordinated manner. Within this model, a faculty member holding concurrent responsibilities in academic instruction and health system education leadership could support the bidirectional translation of cannabis-related policies and evidence into both curricular design and clinical practice.

These dual appointments have the potential to enhance professional credibility across academic and clinical settings while facilitating timely dissemination of evidence-informed practices. They may also expand research capacity by improving access to clinical data for academic inquiry and accelerating the application of emerging findings within health systems. When intentionally structured, these partnerships can function as practice–academic learning laboratories that support innovation in cannabis nursing education and clinical governance.

Implementation of joint faculty appointments requires careful consideration of governance structures, role delineation, workload expectations, and funding mechanisms. Clear institutional agreements and shared accountability frameworks are essential to ensure sustainability and alignment with accreditation standards. Addressing these considerations proactively may support the successful integration of joint appointments as a leadership strategy within cannabis nursing.

Example: Collaborative Policy and Curriculum Reform

The following illustrative example demonstrates how coordinated leadership between academic and clinical administration can support alignment of cannabis nursing education and institutional policy, consistent with AACN accreditation expectations.

A large academic health center may initiate a coordinated partnership between its college of nursing and affiliated hospital system to standardize cannabis nursing education and clinical policy. Under the joint leadership of the Dean of Nursing and the system's Chief Nursing Officer, a dual academic and clinical cannabis task force can be established to support shared governance and continuous quality improvement. The task force may conduct a comprehensive review of state statutes, institutional risk management guidance, and national nursing standards, comparing these sources with existing organizational policies. In parallel, the college of nursing may revise leadership and ethics coursework to integrate cannabis-related policy analysis, ethical reasoning, and advocacy-focused learning activities. These curricular enhancements can be intentionally aligned with AACN Essentials domains, including Knowledge for Nursing Practice, Professionalism, Interprofessional Partnerships, and Systems-Based Practice.

Within a defined implementation period, such a partnership could result in the development of a unified cannabis policy adopted across multiple hospital campuses and embedded within undergraduate and graduate nursing curricula. Program evaluation may indicate increased staff confidence in addressing cannabis-related patient inquiries and improved consistency in clinical documentation practices. This illustrative scenario highlights the potential benefits of coordinated leadership and shared accountability between academic and clinical settings in advancing ethically grounded, evidence-informed cannabis nursing practice.

Leadership Implications

This case underscores the critical role of integrated academic and clinical leadership in operationalizing cannabis nursing standards across education and practice environments. By aligning curricular outcomes with institutional policy and accreditation expectations, nurse leaders can reduce variability, mitigate legal and ethical risk, and enhance workforce readiness. The use of shared governance structures enables timely translation of emerging evidence and policy changes into both educational preparation and clinical care delivery. For academic deans, program directors, and health system executives, this model highlights the importance of sustained collaboration, clear role delineation, and continuous evaluation in advancing cannabis nursing leadership within complex healthcare systems.

Evaluation Metrics and Outcome Measurement

To sustain progress, academic and clinical collaborations require measurable outcomes. Nurse leaders must evaluate not only the success of policy implementation but also the educational and clinical impacts of these initiatives.

Key metrics include:

- Faculty and staff competency assessments on cannabis-related care.
- Student and new-graduate self-efficacy scores.
- Policy compliance and documentation accuracy rates.
- Reduction in clinical incidents or ethical consultations related to cannabis use.
- Growth in interdisciplinary research and publication of results.

Continuous quality improvement (CQI) frameworks, commonly used in hospitals, can also be applied to academic–practice partnerships. Regular audits, debriefs, and data reviews ensure that policies remain current and responsive to emerging evidence and legislation.

Ethical Synergy and Leadership Identity

At the intersection of academic preparation and clinical policy is a shared ethical responsibility fundamental to cannabis nursing leadership. Academic leaders establish the moral, intellectual, and professional foundations necessary to prepare nurses for practice, while clinical leaders enact these values through the delivery of safe, patient-centered, and evidence-informed cannabis care. This reciprocal relationship reflects the ethical obligations articulated in the *Code of Ethics for Nurses with Interpretive Statements* (American Nurses Association, 2025) particularly the duty to practice with compassion and respect for the inherent dignity, worth, and rights of all individuals (American Nurses Association [ANA], 2025, Provision 1) and the responsibility to promote health, prevent harm, and protect patient safety across all settings (ANA, 2025, Provision 3).

The integrity of cannabis nursing leadership is sustained through intentional alignment between theory and practice. When academic curricula reflect current evidence and regulatory realities, and institutional policies are informed by scholarly inquiry and ethical reasoning, nurse leaders collectively uphold professional accountability, competence, and responsibility for ongoing self-regulation (ANA, 2025, Provision 5). This alignment affirms nursing's obligation to respond to emerging health needs in ways that are scientifically grounded, ethically justified, and socially responsible.

Academic and clinical nurse leaders also share a professional identity rooted in nursing's broader social responsibility to advance health equity, reduce stigma, and protect public trust. Whether engaged in curriculum design, faculty development, or organizational policy formation, cannabis nurse leaders function as moral agents committed to collaboration and systems-level change that promotes human rights and health diplomacy (ANA, 2025, Provision 8). Within this shared ethical framework, cannabis-informed care is positioned not as peripheral, but as a legitimate and ethically grounded component of holistic, person-centered healthcare.

Leadership at the intersection of academia and clinical policy exemplifies nursing's ethical mandate to integrate knowledge, practice, and advocacy in service of the public good. Through collaboration among deans, program directors, and nurse executives, durable infrastructures emerge that support educational excellence, clinical safety, and ethical accountability. These partnerships reinforce nursing's central role in shaping cannabis education and policy in ways that protect patients, strengthen professional integrity, and advance population health (ANA, 2025).

Through shared governance, mutual accountability, and evidence-informed collaboration, cannabis nurse leaders extend traditional conceptions of leadership. Their work demonstrates that the most enduring advances in healthcare occur where education and practice converge guided by ethical principles, professional standards, and a collective commitment to public trust.

Policy and Advocacy Leadership in Cannabis Nursing

Nurses as Policy Change Agents and Advocates

Advocacy has been woven within the moral fabric of nursing. The cannabis nurse's responsibility extends beyond the cannabis healthcare consumer care to the transformation of systems and policies that affect health outcomes. As legislative reform and clinical science and research evolve, nurse leaders occupy a unique position to shape ethical, evidence-based frameworks for cannabis use in healthcare consumers which has recently become more urgent.

Policy leadership in cannabis nursing encompasses a spectrum of activities from organizational policy development to legislative testimony and coalition building. Cannabis nurse leaders translate bedside experience and population health evidence into policy language that informs lawmakers, boards of nursing, and healthcare institutions. Their advocacy is grounded in the *ANA Code of Ethics for Nurses* (2025 revision), which affirms that nurses must "participate in the advancement of the profession through contributions to practice standards, education, administration, and policy." Therefor hospital administrators, deans, or organizational presidents, cannabis nurse leaders act as policy change agents to ensure that nursing's voice remains central in the national dialogue on cannabis therapeutics.

Institutional and Organizational Policy Development

Institutional policy functions as a critical lever of systems leadership through which broader regulatory reform is informed and advanced. Hospital and academic nurse leaders routinely participate in internal governance and policy committees responsible for establishing cannabis-related guidelines applicable to both clinical staff and nursing students. These policies delineate the operational, legal, and ethical parameters of cannabis care, addressing patient possession, nursing education and staff development, and documentation practices while upholding nursing's obligations to promote health, prevent harm, and protect patient rights (American Nurses Association [ANA], 2025, Provisions 1 and 3).

Within healthcare systems, nurse executives collaborate with compliance and risk management leaders to develop policies that clarify professional responsibilities for documenting patient-reported cannabis use, establish procedures for storage and self-administration, and ensure adherence to applicable laws and regulations. In academic settings, deans and program directors enact institutional policies that safeguard faculty academic freedom, thereby supporting ethical scholarship and evidence-based teaching in alignment with nursing's responsibility for professional integrity, competence, and accountability (ANA, 2025, Provision 5).

These institutional policies exemplify systems leadership by aligning education, practice, and governance across organizational boundaries. Grounded in the Cannabis Nursing: Scope and Standards of Practice (American Nurses Association & American Cannabis Nurses Association, 2023), they demonstrate how evidence-informed cannabis care can be integrated within regulatory frameworks while advancing equity, transparency, and public trust. This coordinated approach reflects nursing's broader social responsibility to influence health policy and promote justice at the systems level (ANA, 2025, Provision 8).

Building on this foundation of institutional policy leadership, nurse leaders are positioned to extend their influence beyond organizational boundaries, translating internal governance practices into broader advocacy, regulatory engagement, and leadership development initiatives that shape the future of cannabis nursing.

Local and State Advocacy

At the local and state levels, nurse leaders are well positioned to serve as educators and trusted advisors to policymakers on matters related to cannabis nursing practice. Their sustained engagement with patients, families, and communities provides a practice-informed perspective that can strengthen policy dialogue and enhance the relevance of regulatory decision-making. Through structured engagement with legislative bodies, regulatory agencies, and advisory groups, nurse leaders may contribute to the development of medical cannabis policy in ways that reflect clinical realities, ethical obligations, and public health priorities, consistent with nursing's responsibility to promote health and prevent harm (American Nurses Association [ANA], 2025, Provisions 1 and 3).

Collaborative efforts between academic and clinical nurse leaders and state regulatory entities can further support the development of position statements or guidance documents that clarify nursing roles in cannabis care. These documents may articulate expectations related to patient assessment, education, documentation, and ethical practice, thereby promoting greater consistency for nurses, educators, and employers. When informed by both academic expertise and clinical leadership, such initiatives illustrate how coordinated nursing leadership can influence policy development while upholding professional integrity and accountability (ANA, 2025, Provision 5).

Beyond formal regulatory engagement, nurse leaders may extend their advocacy through public health education initiatives, community-based forums, and interprofessional collaboration with colleagues in pharmacy, medicine, and social work. These efforts reflect nursing's broader social responsibility to address stigma, advance health equity, and support informed, evidence-based use of cannabis therapeutics across diverse populations (ANA, 2025, Provision 8).

Through sustained engagement in policy education, regulatory collaboration, and community advocacy, cannabis nurse leaders extend their ethical responsibility beyond individual institutions, contributing to the development of just, evidence-based policies that support safe and equitable cannabis care across healthcare systems.

National Policy and Professional Collaboration

At the national level, collaboration with professional organizations strengthens nursing's collective voice and amplifies the impact of leadership in cannabis policy and practice. The American Cannabis Nurses Association (ACNA) serves as a national forum for advancing cannabis nursing practice and policy, working in partnership with the American Nurses Association (ANA), the National Council of State Boards of Nursing (NCSBN), and other allied stakeholders, such as Patients Out of Time and Society of Cannabis Clinicians. As a participant in the ANA Membership Assembly, ACNA contributes directly to national dialogue and professional governance. Through these collaborations, nurse leaders engage in collective action to influence health policy, promote ethical practice, and advance the health and well-being of the public, consistent with nursing's social responsibility (American Nurses Association [ANA], 2025, Provision 8).

Within these national organizations, nurse leaders contribute to the development of position statements, policy briefs, and professional guidance that inform nursing education, clinical practice, and licensure. A central area of advocacy involves advancing the inclusion of cannabis-related content within licensure examinations and continuing professional development frameworks. Aligning educational and licensure standards with emerging evidence supports nursing's obligation to ensure competence, protect the public, and uphold professional accountability (ANA, 2025, Provisions 3 and 5). Inclusion of cannabis content within licensure expectations promotes foundational competence in areas such as pharmacology, patient safety, ethical decision-making, and regulatory compliance.

National collaboration has also supported the formal recognition of cannabis nursing as a specialty practice, reinforcing the legitimacy of this area of care within the broader nursing enterprise. This recognition reflects nursing's commitment to evidence-based practice, ethical leadership, and responsiveness to evolving healthcare needs. It further establishes a foundation for continued policy development related to licensure protection, workforce preparation, research access, and reimbursement considerations.

In addition, nurse leaders engaged in national advocacy work to promote greater policy coherence across jurisdictions. Through participation in policy forums, interdisciplinary roundtables, and professional advisory groups, they contribute to the development of evidence-informed frameworks that address regulatory variability, safeguard patient safety, and enable nurses to practice to the full extent of their education and competence. Collectively, these efforts exemplify nursing's ethical mandate to lead at the systems level and to address complex health challenges through collaboration, advocacy, and stewardship of the profession (ANA, 2025, Provision 8).

Ethical and Legal Considerations in Policy Leadership

Cannabis policy advocacy presents a complex leadership challenge that requires nurse leaders to navigate ethical obligations within evolving legal and regulatory frameworks. Ongoing federal restrictions continue to introduce uncertainty for healthcare organizations, academic institutions, and individual practitioners. Within this context, nurse leaders are called to exercise moral courage by engaging in advocacy that advances cannabis healthcare consumers welfare and public health while maintaining adherence to professional standards, institutional policy, and applicable law.

The *Code of Ethics for Nurses with Interpretive Statements* provides essential ethical direction for navigating the complexities of cannabis policy advocacy. Provisions affirming nursing's obligations to promote health, prevent harm, and advance social justice establish a clear ethical framework for leadership engagement in this area (American Nurses Association [ANA], 2025, Provisions 1, 3, and 8). Within this framework, nurse leaders are called to act as advocates for conditions that support safe, equitable, and evidence-based care.

When nurse leaders engage in efforts to expand research access, reduce policy barriers, or address gaps in insurance coverage related to medical cannabis, such advocacy reflects nursing's ethical commitment to the protection of human dignity and the reduction of health inequities. These actions are grounded not in personal or political ideology, but in professional responsibility to ensure that care decisions are informed by science, guided by compassion, and responsive to the needs of individuals and communities. As cannabis policy continues to evolve, ethical leadership grounded in the ANA Code of Ethics remains central to nursing's role in shaping just and accountable health systems (American Cannabis Nurses Association & American Nurses Association, 2024).

Building Advocacy Capacity and Political Competence

To sustain progress, nurse leaders must cultivate the next generation of advocates. Academic programs play an essential role in developing students' policy literacy and civic engagement skills. Faculty can integrate cannabis policy analysis into leadership and community health courses, teaching students how to evaluate legislation, communicate with policymakers, and craft evidence-based policy statements and white papers.

Hospital leaders can complement this preparation through mentorship and staff development programs that encourage participation in professional organizations and advocacy initiatives. Nurse executives may support nurses attendance on legislative days or sponsor workshops on policy writing and testimony preparation.

Political competence, the ability to navigate power structures and influence decision-making is a critical component of leadership development. Cannabis nurse leaders who understand policy processes and coalition building are better equipped to translate cannabis healthcare consumer stories and clinical evidence into systemic change.

Example: Nurse-Led Policy Reform Through Coalition Building

The following illustrative example highlights how nurse-led coalition building may be leveraged to advance ethical and policy reform related to cannabis nursing practice. A regional coalition composed of nurse leaders, nursing educators, and patient advocates may be formed to address inconsistencies between state medical cannabis statutes and hospital-level policy. Co-led by an academic dean and a hospital chief nursing officer, such a coalition could focus on developing clearer pathways for accommodating registered medical cannabis patients within acute care settings under defined safety considerations.

Through a collaborative and evidence-based approach, the coalition may collect and analyze data related to patient experience, staff perceptions, and clinical workflow considerations associated with cannabis care. Nursing faculty could contribute to the development of policy statements, synthesizing these findings, which nurse leaders may then present to state policymakers as part of legislative or regulatory consultation processes.

As a result of these coordinated efforts, state-level guidance or statutory language could emerge that permits healthcare organizations to establish institutional policies addressing cannabis healthcare consumers, self-care within nurse guided safety protocols. This illustrative scenario demonstrates how nurse led coalition is grounded in research, education, and ethical advocacy which may serve as a strategic mechanism for influencing policy reform while aligning professional standards with cannabis healthcare consumer centered care.

The Global Dimension of Policy Leadership

As cannabis reform advances globally, nurse leaders are increasingly engaged in international policy dialogue. Through participation in global conferences, virtual collaborations, and partnerships with international nursing organizations, U.S. cannabis nurse leaders contribute expertise in advocacy, ethics, and systems leadership. These cross-national exchanges support policy coherence and the dissemination of evidence-informed best practices, consistent with nursing's ethical responsibility to address health concerns that transcend national boundaries (American Nurses Association [ANA], 2025, Provision 8).

Global collaboration also provides critical ethical insight into issues of decriminalization, health equity, and access to palliative care. In alignment with international nursing frameworks advanced by organizations such as the International Council of Nurses, nurse leaders advocate for globally relevant competencies that respect cultural diversity while upholding shared commitments to patient safety, human rights, and compassionate care (International Council of Nurses, n.d.).

Policy and advocacy leadership demonstrates professional influence in cannabis nursing. Bridging clinical practice, academic inquiry, and legislative engagement, nurse leaders ensure that cannabis integration advances within ethical and evidence-based frameworks. Their advocacy transforms policy but positively influences culture by redefining cannabis from a source of stigma to a domain of healing.

Through strategic partnerships, ethical conviction, and scholarly rigor, cannabis nurse leaders embody the nursing profession's enduring commitment to the health and wellbeing of the public. This leadership ensures that as cannabis policy continues to evolve, nursing serves as it moral compass and scientific authority.

RESEARCH, QUALITY IMPROVEMENT, AND EVIDENCE-BASED LEADERSHIP IN CANNABIS NURSING

The Imperative for Research Leadership

Evidence-based practice constitutes a foundational element of nursing professionalism, and cannabis nursing. The expanding clinical application of cannabinoid therapeutics necessitates rigorous and methodologically, statistically significant research to inform safe, ethical, and effective cannabis nursing care. Nurse leaders across clinical, academic, and policy environments play a central role in advancing this scientific foundation.

Leadership in cannabis nursing research begins with scholarly inquiry that addresses clinically relevant questions related to dosing, safety, symptom management, and patient experience. However, research leadership extends beyond study design to include the development of supportive infrastructures, mentorship of emerging scholars, and the systematic translation of findings into education, policy, and clinical practice. In this capacity, nurse leaders function as both investigators and change agents, ensuring that the evolving evidence base for cannabis care remains aligned with nursing's core commitments to patient safety, compassion, equity, and social justice (Clark C., 2021).

Research Priorities in Cannabis Nursing

To strengthen the evidence base, nurse leaders are increasingly identifying priority areas of inquiry aligned with the *Cannabis Nursing: Scope and Standards of Practice* (ANA & ACNA, 2023):

1. **Clinical Outcomes Research:** Investigating the effects of medical cannabis on pain, anxiety, nausea, sleep, and quality of life across the lifespan and diverse populations.
2. **Safety and Pharmacology Studies:** Evaluating drug interactions, dosage forms, and adverse effects relevant to nursing practice.
3. **Nursing Education and Competency Research:** Assessing the effectiveness of cannabis curricula, continuing education programs, and certification pathways.
4. **Policy and Ethics Research:** Exploring nurses' attitudes, workplace policies, and ethical challenges related to cannabis care.
5. **Population Health and Health Equity:** Studying disparities in access to cannabis therapeutics, particularly among marginalized or chronically ill populations.

These research domains establish a framework through which nurse leaders can advance a nursing focused evidence-based cannabis care.

The Nurse Leader as Researcher and Collaborator

Nurse leaders often bridge the gap between clinical practice and academic or scientific support. Hospital based nurse scientists or directors of nursing research may lead pilot studies exploring cannabis interventions for symptom relief in oncology or palliative care. Academic deans and faculty researchers design longitudinal studies examining educational outcomes or cannabis healthcare consumer safety implications.

Ongoing federal policy discussions regarding cannabis rescheduling and research reform have the potential to alter the national research landscape. Any shift in federal classification or enforcement priorities would expand opportunities for scientific inquiry, funding, and clinical translation, with direct implications for patient access, safety, and evidence-based care. Consistent with nursing's ethical mandate to influence health policy and protect the public (American Nurses Association [ANA], 2025, Provision 8), nurse leaders must remain informed and prepared to guide research agendas and institutional responses as federal policy evolves ensuring that emerging evidence continues to serve the health and well-being of cannabis healthcare consumers.

Research collaboration increasingly extends beyond national boundaries, as U.S. nurse researchers engage with colleagues in Canada, Israel, and Europe; regions with more established cannabis research infrastructures (Health Canada, 2018; Meiri, 2021; Hoch et al., 2025). These international partnerships facilitate knowledge exchange, comparative studies, and methodological rigor, while strengthening the professional legitimacy of cannabis nursing science. Global engagement reflects nursing's ethical commitment to international collaboration and shared responsibility for advancing health and human rights, consistent with the Code of Ethics for Nurses and principles advanced by the International Council of Nurses (American Nurses Association [ANA], 2025, Provision 8).

Translating Evidence Based Research into Practice and Policy

Research leadership in cannabis nursing extends beyond publication to the intentional translation of evidence into clinical practice, education, and policy. Nurse leaders function as knowledge translators, synthesizing research findings for application by clinicians, administrators, and policymakers. Through this role, nurse-led research informs clinical guidelines, institutional protocols, and educational resources, supporting safe and effective cannabis care.

The process, from inquiry to application to education reflects the principles of evidence-based nursing and aligns with the ethical obligations outlined in the Code of Ethics for Nurses with Interpretive Statements, including the responsibilities to promote health, ensure professional competence, and advance practice through the integration of evidence (American Nurses Association [ANA], 2025, Provisions 3 and 5)

Quality Improvement and Data-Driven Leadership

Quality improvement (QI) initiatives represent an important avenue for nurse leadership in cannabis care environments and directly support the AACN Essentials domains of Quality and Safety, Systems-Based Practice, and Scholarship for Nursing Practice. Distinct from formal research, QI focuses on the systematic evaluation and optimization of existing clinical processes to improve patient outcomes and organizational performance. Nurse leaders apply structured methodologies including Plan, Do, Study, Act (PDSA) cycles, root cause analysis, benchmarking, and Six Sigma frameworks to evaluate cannabis related policies, workforce competencies, and cannabis healthcare consumers outcomes.

Within cannabis care settings, Six Sigma informed QI initiatives may include evaluation of clinical documentation related to cannabis healthcare consumer reported cannabis use, route of administration, and symptom response; assessment of nurse adherence to institutional cannabis policies; measurement of nursing knowledge and confidence following targeted education; and analysis of patient-reported outcomes related to symptom management. These activities reflect the AACN emphasis on data-driven decision-making, risk reduction, and continuous quality improvement across care systems.

QI initiatives generate actionable internal data that support continuous practice refinement and inform future research priorities, aligning with the Essentials' focus on integrating evidence into practice and improving system performance. When implemented within cannabis-inclusive healthcare systems, Six Sigma driven QI efforts provide quantifiable evidence of nursing leadership's contribution to safety, quality, and innovation.

Examples of cannabis focused QI activities consistent with the AACN Essentials include auditing electronic health record documentation of patient-reported cannabis use, evaluating compliance with institutional cannabis policies, measuring changes in staff knowledge and confidence following educational interventions, and monitoring patient satisfaction related to symptom management in settings that provide cannabis education or support patient self-administration protocols (American Society for Quality, n.d.).

Data Ethics, Inclusion, and Health Equity

Leadership in cannabis research and QI carries ethical responsibilities that extend beyond methodology. Nurse leaders must safeguard participant rights, ensure data accuracy, and address equity in study design.

Historically, cannabis criminalization has disproportionately affected communities of color; therefore, equitable research must intentionally include diverse populations and acknowledge historical injustices (King et al., 2024; National Academies of Sciences, Engineering, and Medicine, 2017.

Ethical data stewardship includes transparency in funding sources, avoidance of commercial bias, and publication of both positive and negative results. Nurse leaders model these standards through open data practices and adherence to institutional ethics guidelines. Moreover, this reinforces nursing's role as an ethical compass within cannabis nursing care which can be commercially influenced.

Mentorship and Capacity Building in Research Leadership

Sustaining cannabis nursing research requires deliberate mentorship and infrastructure. Academic leaders cultivate research pipelines by embedding inquiry into undergraduate and graduate education. Clinical leaders foster nurse led research councils or evidence-based practice committees that empower nurses to propose and conduct projects.

Formal mentorship programs, such as pairing DNP or PhD students with clinical researchers, create pathways for scholarly development and strengthen collaboration between academia and practice. Nurse leaders also advocate for institutional research funding, partnerships with external foundations, and inclusion of cannabis topics in federal grant portfolios.

Mentorship embodies servant and transformational leadership: experienced scholars guide emerging investigators while reinforcing nursing's collective commitment to advancing knowledge. Example 4 conveys how nurse led academic and clinical partnerships can advance cannabis research and inform practice and policy.

Example 4. Academic-Clinical Partnership Advancing Cannabis Nursing Research

A nurse-let academic-clinical partnership demonstrated how collaborative leadership can advance cannabis research and inform practice and policy. In this initiative, a college of nursing and a hospital palliative care service jointly examined the effects of medical cannabis on pain and anxiety among health care consumers receiving end-of-life care. Academic and clinical nurse leaders coordinated Institutional Review Board approval, staff education, and interdisciplinary collaboration with pharmacy and social work.

Findings showed meaningful improvements in reported pain and reductions in opioid use among cannabis health care consumers. These outcomes supported revisions to institutional palliative care guidelines and contributed to broader policy discussions related to symptom management.

This example illustrates the AACN Essentials domains of **Knowledge for Nursing Practice**, **Scholarship for Nursing Practice**, and **Systems-Based Practice**, and reflects nursing's ethical obligations to promote health, alleviate suffering, and integrate evidence into care delivery in alignment with the Code of Ethics for Nurses with Interpretive Statements 9ANA, 2025, Provisions 1, 3, and 5).

Dissemination and Professional Impact

Dissemination of cannabis nursing research is itself an act of leadership. Cannabis nurse scholars present findings through peer-reviewed journals, ACNA conferences, ANA policy briefs, and interdisciplinary symposia. By contributing to the scholarly record, they elevate nursing's credibility and influence in the broader cannabis science community.

Effective dissemination strategies include publishing open-access scholarship; presenting findings in legislative and regulatory forums; developing continuing education modules; leading change management initiatives that integrate evidence into organizational policy and practice; and engaging in responsible media communication to support public understanding. Collectively, these approaches advance the AACN Essentials domains of Scholarship for Nursing Practice, Systems-Based Practice, Knowledge for Nursing Practice, Professionalism, and Quality and Safety, while aligning with nursing's ethical obligations to share knowledge, promote health, prevent harm, and advance the public good (American Nurses Association [ANA], 2025, Provisions 3, 5, 7, and 8).

These activities reinforce nursing's ethical mandate to share knowledge that advances public health and strengthens clinical safety. Cannabis nursing research and quality improvement leadership integrate nursing science, ethical accountability, and professional advocacy. Through evidence generation, policy evaluation, and mentorship of emerging scholars, nurse leaders strengthen the legitimacy of cannabis-informed care and ensure that clinical decisions are guided by empirical evidence rather than stigma or uncertainty. Through inquiry, interdisciplinary collaboration, and purposeful dissemination, cannabis nurse leaders advance practice in ways that support the safe, equitable delivery of cannabis therapeutics in alignment with nursing's professional standards and societal obligations.

LEADERSHIP DEVELOPMENT AND MENTORSHIP PIPELINES IN CANNABIS NURSING

Building the Leadership Continuum

The evolution of cannabis nursing from advocacy movement to recognized specialty practice has created an urgent need for intentional leadership development. As the field expands into hospitals, academia, community health, and policy arenas, sustaining this growth depends on preparing future leaders equipped with clinical expertise, policy fluency, and ethical grounding.

Leadership development in cannabis nursing must be viewed as a continuum, beginning with student exposure, advancing through mentorship and continuing education, and culminating in national and international leadership roles. The goal is not only to create individual leaders but also to establish a self-sustaining professional culture where mentorship, collaboration, and advocacy are embedded in everyday practice.

Mentorship and the Development of Future Nurse Leaders

Mentorship remains a cornerstone of nursing leadership development and holds particular importance in cannabis nursing, an emerging specialty shaped by regulatory complexity and persistent stigma. Through formal organizational programs, academic advising, clinical coaching, and peer networks, experienced nurse leaders support professional growth while fostering leadership self-efficacy and ethical resilience. Effective mentors model integrity, collaboration, and moral courage, guiding nurses in translating policy into practice and advancing cannabis-informed care. In this way, mentorship functions as both a developmental and transformational process, sustaining leadership capacity and extending professional influence across generations.

Continuing Education and Leadership Competency Building

Cannabis nursing requires lifelong learning due to its rapidly evolving legal, pharmacological, and policy landscape. Nurse leaders must therefore commit to ongoing professional development to maintain competence and credibility.

Continuing education (CE) offerings through ACNA, ANA, and other organizations provide essential opportunities for leadership skill-building. Programs may include:

- **Advanced cannabis pharmacology** and symptom management.
- **Legal and ethical leadership** for institutional policy design.
- **Advocacy and health policy training**, preparing nurses to engage effectively with legislators and boards of nursing.
- **Research and data analytics**, enabling leaders to interpret evidence for practice and policy.
- **Communication and media engagement**, equipping nurse leaders to serve as credible public educators.

Academic deans and hospital educators can further support leadership development by offering tuition reimbursement or dedicated professional development time for nurses pursuing certification or graduate education in leadership or cannabis nursing.

The exploration of specialty credentialing and micro-credentialing pathways aligned with American Nurses Credentialing Center (ANCC) frameworks represents a potential milestone for professional recognition in cannabis nursing. ANCC, aligned approaches emphasize competency-based validation, continuing professional development, and outcomes focused on assessment. Applied to cannabis nursing leadership, these frameworks could support standardized expectations for knowledge, ethical practice, and leadership competence while promoting consistency and accountability across clinical, academic, and policy roles.

The development of ANCC, credentials or micro-credentials would further align cannabis nursing with established models of specialty recognition, lifelong learning, and professional excellence, positioning nurse leaders to meet evolving practice demands while maintaining public trust.

Creating Institutional Pathways for Leadership

Institutions play a pivotal role in cultivating leadership capacity by creating intentional pathways for nurses to engage in governance, scholarship, and policy development. Nurse executives and academic administrators may support emerging cannabis nurse leaders through leadership fellowships, research-focused learning opportunities, shared governance structures, and succession planning frameworks. These approaches expand access to leadership development beyond formal titles, reinforcing that influence within cannabis nursing is grounded in professional competence, ethical commitment, and engagement with evidence-informed practice.

Professional Networking and Community of Practice

Professional community reinforces leadership identity. Through networking opportunities, conferences, and committees, nurses gain mentorship, visibility, and collective power.

The ACNA provides a vital platform for leadership development. Committees dedicated to education and research, policy, and diversity, equity, and inclusion provide structured environments for leadership development and mentorship of cannabis nurse leaders. Participation exposes nurses to governance processes, strategic planning, and collaboration with national organizations such as ANA, Organizations as part of the ANA Membership Accessibly, NCSBN and Student Nurses Association.

Academic institutions can mirror this approach by fostering structured scholarly communities within nursing programs, where students engage in collaborative projects, policy dialogue, and research focused on cannabis nursing leadership. These experiences cultivate a sense of professional purpose and prepare graduates to assume leadership roles immediately upon entering nursing practice.

Resilience, Self-Care, and Sustainable Leadership

Leadership in cannabis nursing often requires navigating controversial and emotionally charged territory. Nurse leaders must advocate for evidence-based practice while managing resistance from colleagues, administrators, or policymakers. Without deliberate self-care and boundary setting, leaders risk compassion fatigue or burnout.

Sustainable leadership in cannabis nursing requires intentional attention to personal well-being and resilience. Evidence related to the endocannabinoid system (ECS) (Russo, 2016) which demonstrates a role in stress regulation, mood, sleep, and physiological homeostasis which underscores the importance of balance, recovery, and self-regulation for individuals in demanding leadership roles (Clark C., 2021). Within this context, nurse leaders are ethically obligated to model practices that support both personal well-being and professional effectiveness while navigating complex clinical, academic, and policy environments.

Leadership development initiatives that integrate resilience-building strategies support ethical longevity and clarity in decision-making. These strategies may include structured peer support or reflective practice groups, intentional scheduling of rest periods or sabbaticals when feasible, and engagement in restorative practices such as mindfulness, movement, or time in nature. Maintaining clear professional boundaries and healthy work–life integration further aligns with nursing's responsibility to preserve personal integrity and competence.

Resilient leadership strengthens organizational stability and trust. Consistent with the Code of Ethics for Nurses with Interpretive Statements, which affirms the nurse's duty to self as foundational to ethical practice (American Nurses Association [ANA], 2025, Provision 5), attention to well-being enhances leaders' capacity to act ethically, sustain perspective, and lead effectively within complex institutional and political contexts.

Mentorship Outcomes and the Ripple Effect

Mentorship and leadership development extend their influence beyond individual nurses, strengthening organizational stability, advancing scholarly collaboration, and reinforcing evidence-informed practice across academic and clinical settings. Through intentional guidance and professional community, nurse leaders sustain the growth of cannabis nursing as an ethical, inquiry-driven discipline. Investment in mentorship pathways and leadership infrastructures supports the evolution of cannabis nursing from an emerging specialty into a durable professional field which is defined by compassionate, competent, and courageous leadership.

FUTURE DIRECTIONS AND GLOBAL INTEGRATION IN CANNABIS NURSING LEADERSHIP

Envisioning the Future of Cannabis Nursing Leadership

The next two decades will define how cannabis nursing is integrated into mainstream healthcare, public health policy, and global education. As the profession matures from advocacy to institutionalization, leadership will evolve from pioneering individual efforts to collective, system-level transformation.

The American Nurses Association's *Imagining the American Nurses Enterprise into 2040* (ANE 2040) initiative articulates a vision for nursing that is equitable, innovative, interprofessional, and globally engaged. Cannabis nursing leadership naturally aligns with this vision. Its roots in cannabis healthcare consumer advocacy, evidence-based care, and social justice mirror the ANA's call for future nursing to "shape health care that is both technologically advanced and compassionately human."

Cannabis nurse leaders are not merely specialists in a niche field; they represent a leading expression of nursing's evolution toward holistic, person-centered, equity-driven, and globally informed healthcare leadership.

Global Policy Harmonization and International Collaboration

As more countries legalize or decriminalize medical and adult-use cannabis, international collaboration becomes both a necessity and an ethical imperative. Cannabis nurse leaders are increasingly participating in multinational research, education, and policy development initiatives.

Global collaboration fosters the exchange of best practices and accelerates the standardization of cannabis nursing competencies. Partnerships between the American Cannabis Nurses Association (ACNA), the International Council of Nurses (ICN), and global nursing organizations can support the creation of an *International Framework for Cannabis Nursing Education and Practice*. This framework would ensure consistency in safety standards, ethics, and cannabis healthcare consumer care across borders.

International policy harmonization also holds potential to address disparities in research access. In countries where cannabis remains heavily restricted, global nursing advocacy can help influence public health agendas, promote ethical research access, and support compassionate use programs. Cannabis nurse leaders, informed by the ANA 2040 emphasis on global citizenship, will play a critical role in shaping these dialogues.

Leadership in Technology, Informatics, and Telehealth

The integration of technology and telehealth into cannabis nursing represents one of the most promising frontiers for leadership innovation. The ANA 2040 framework envisions nursing as a data-driven, technology-enabled profession that harnesses artificial intelligence (AI), machine learning, and digital health tools to enhance clinical outcomes and cannabis healthcare consumer engagement.

Cannabis nurse leaders are uniquely positioned to guide the ethical use of these technologies. For example, AI algorithms can analyze cannabis healthcare consumer-reported outcomes related to cannabis use, enabling personalized care recommendations while maintaining privacy and cultural sensitivity. Telehealth platforms expand access to cannabis nursing consultation in rural or underserved communities, advancing health equity, a central principle of both ACNA's mission and ANA 2040's equity agenda.

Leadership in digital transformation requires nurses to be not only users of technology but architects of its ethical integration. Academic leaders will need to prepare students to navigate digital documentation, data ethics, and telehealth protocols related to cannabis care, ensuring that nursing remains the moral and clinical anchor within increasingly technological systems.

Value-Based and Integrative Healthcare Models

The future of cannabis nursing is also tied to the rise of value-based care models that prioritize outcomes, prevention, and cannabis healthcare consumer satisfaction. Cannabis nurse leaders can play a decisive role in integrating cannabinoid therapeutics within these frameworks by demonstrating measurable improvements in quality of life, symptom burden, functional status, sleep quality, appetite, anxiety management, and overall patient-reported outcomes.

Hospitals and insurers are increasingly evaluating cannabis-informed interventions through cost benefit frameworks. In parallel, policy discourse has intensified following public statements by Donald Trump expressing interest in expanding Medicare coverage for certain cannabis-related therapies through executive action. While regulatory pathways remain evolving, nurse leaders can leverage quality improvement data and clinical outcomes research to demonstrate how cannabis-informed care supports the Triple Aim of healthcare improving cannabis healthcare consumers experience, advancing population health, and reducing costs.

Moreover, cannabis nursing aligns with the integrative and holistic care models central to ANA 2040's vision. The future nurse leader will bridge traditional medicine and emerging therapies, ensuring that evidence, empathy, and ethics guide all aspects of care delivery. Integrating cannabis within interprofessional wellness models in conjunction with nutrition, mindfulness, and complementary therapies represents a paradigm shift toward whole-person care.

Leadership Competencies for 2030 and Beyond

As cannabis nursing leadership continues to evolve, success will depend on a core set of competencies that reflect systems thinking, ethical accountability, and global engagement. Guided by the ANA and ACNA standards, future nurse leaders will be expected to integrate policy literacy with digital fluency, collaborate across disciplines, advocate for equity, and steward innovation responsibly. Central to this work is mentorship, ensuring the transfer of knowledge, values, and leadership capacity across generations.

These competencies reflect the ANA 2040 Vision of nurses as architects of care systems, policy, and technology, grounded in evidence and guided by human dignity. Cannabis nurse leaders are uniquely positioned to lead this transformation: advancing safe, equitable, and evidence-informed care while preserving the relational essence of nursing.

This is not merely the future of cannabis nursing. It reflects the future direction of nursing where ethical leadership, scientific rigor, and social responsibility converge to shape health systems that serve individuals, communities, and the public good.

The ANA 2040 Vision: Ethical and Technological Leadership in Nursing

The *Imagining the American Nurses Enterprise into 2040* framework envisions nurses as co-creators of health policy, social change, and innovation. It calls for "unity across enterprise, advocacy for all people, and leadership that advances health and equity in every setting."

Cannabis nursing embodies this vision in practice. It unites advocacy with science, compassion with evidence, and micro-level cannabis healthcare consumer care with macro-level policy engagement. As healthcare becomes more technologically sophisticated and globally interconnected, cannabis nurse leaders exemplify the type of adaptive, ethically grounded leadership that ANA 2040 describes.

By 2040, cannabis nursing may be fully normalized within curricula, licensure examinations, and healthcare policy which would be a testament to the sustained leadership of nurses who advocated for safe, evidence-informed integration long before it was mainstream.

A Global Call to Leadership

Looking ahead, cannabis nurse leaders will continue to expand their influence beyond borders and bureaucracies. They will collaborate with policymakers, educators, and researchers to dismantle stigma, improve access to care, and advance global health literacy about cannabis therapeutics.

As articulated by Angela Beddoe, Chief Executive Officer of the American Nurses Enterprise, the ANA 2040 Vision calls for a generation of nurse leaders who are prepared not only to adapt to change, but to actively shape the future of healthcare. Nurses educated within ANA 2040 aligned frameworks are positioned to ensure that as medicine and technology continue to evolve, nursing remains anchored in ethical leadership, public trust, and a commitment to advancing health and well-being.

In this global context, cannabis nursing leadership extends beyond plant-based therapeutics. It reflects a model of adaptive, equity-driven leadership aligned with the future of nursing: evidence-based, digitally literate, globally informed, and grounded in respect for human dignity, ethical practice, and the advancement of health and well-being.

Future directions in cannabis nursing leadership are defined by convergence of technology and ethics, science and compassion, local advocacy and global collaboration. Guided by the ANA 2040 vision and grounded in the ACNA's commitment to excellence, nurse leaders will continue to champion policies, education, and research that align safety with innovation.

By 2040, cannabis nursing leadership will stand as a symbol of nursing's capacity to transform healthcare uniting systems thinking, social justice, and scientific rigor to create a future where all cannabis healthcare consumers have access to informed, compassionate, and equitable care.

CONCLUSION

Leadership in cannabis nursing represents one of the most significant evolutions in contemporary nursing practice. It bridges clinical expertise, academic innovation, and policy leadership, demonstrating how nurses drive systemic change from the bedside to the boardroom. Through the collaborative efforts of hospital executives, academic leaders, faculty, and policy advocates, cannabis nursing has moved from the margins of healthcare discourse to a position of professional recognition and ethical inquiry.

Within hospital systems, nurse leaders have established policies that promote patient safety, documentation integrity, and nursing education related to cannabinoid therapeutics. Their leadership reflects transformational practice integrating compassion with regulatory compliance and advocacy with accountability. In academic settings, deans, directors, and faculty champions have advanced curricular standards that incorporate cannabis pharmacology, ethics, and research literacy, preparing graduates to practice confidently within an increasingly complex therapeutic landscape.

At the policy level, cannabis nurse leaders have shaped legislation, licensure frameworks, and public dialogue, ensuring that nursing remains both the ethical and scientific compass of healthcare reform. Through evidence-informed advocacy, they have elevated professional guidance and reinforced nursing's social contract to advance human dignity, health equity, and ethical care.

The integration of the ANA 2040 Vision situates cannabis nursing leadership within the broader future of the profession. By aligning innovation, interprofessional collaboration, and global engagement, nurse leaders affirm that cannabis nursing is not a departure from mainstream practice but a vital expression of nursing's evolution. This leadership demonstrates what is possible when empathy, scientific rigor, and social justice converge, advancing technologically sophisticated care systems grounded in respect for human dignity, ethical accountability, and the promotion of health and well-being.

As the cannabis landscape progresses toward 2040, nurse leaders must sustain this momentum through mentorship, scholarship, and policy engagement. Leaders must continue to advocate for investment in education, ethical practice, international collaboration, and professional resilience will be essential to strengthening leadership capacity across generations.

Leadership in cannabis nursing transcends administrative authority; it is a moral commitment. It reflects the courage to envision healthcare systems where every patient receives safe, informed, and respectful care; where stigma gives way to science; and where nursing continues to shape the conscience of healthcare. This is not merely the future of cannabis nursing; it is the future of nursing.

Artificial Intelligence Disclosure Statement

Artificial intelligence (AI) tools were utilized solely to support text-based elements during the preparation of this chapter, including narrative refinement, grammatical and structural editing, organizational guidance, citation formatting, and summarization of publicly available, appropriately cited sources. No AI tools were used to generate tables, figures, graphs, diagrams, images, or any other visual or data-driven content restricted under IGI Global policy. All scholarly content, interpretations, and final editorial decisions reflect the independent academic judgment of the authors. All references were reviewed, verified, and cited in accordance with IGI Global and APA guidelines. This disclosure is provided to ensure transparency and compliance with IGI Global's standards for responsible AI use.

ACKNOWLEDGMENTS

This chapter would not have come to fruition without the mentorship and steadfast support of Llewellyn Dawn Smith, whose guidance extended from inception through completion. I am deeply grateful for her continued encouragement, professional insight, and confidence in the scholarly direction of this work.

I extend sincere appreciation to colleagues, collaborators, and members of the American Cannabis Nurses Association whose collective leadership, scholarship, and service continue to advance nurse-led, evidence-based cannabis care nationwide. Your dedication has strengthened this emerging specialty and contributed meaningfully to the professional infrastructure supporting cannabis nursing.

I also acknowledge the nursing students. particularly one student whose experience with cannabis during nursing school profoundly shaped my advocacy and reinforced my commitment to equitable, compassionate, and patient-centered care. I further recognize current and future nursing students who will lead the advancement of cannabis nursing education and practice, ensuring safe, ethical, and evidence-based care for healthcare consumers.

My deepest gratitude goes to my adult children, Jonathan, Serena, and Jason, and their friends, Reilly, Eman, David, and Alanna; whose curiosity, thoughtful discussions, and diverse perspectives have continually motivated me and enriched my understanding of the cannabis space. Your shared reflections have offered new viewpoints and continue to inspire my work.

REFERENCES

American Association of Colleges of Nursing. (2021). *The Essentials: Core competencies for professional nursing education.* Retrieved January 30, 2026, from American Association of Colleges of Nursing: https://www.aacnnursing.org/Portals/0/PDFs/Publications/Essentials-2021.pdf

American Cannabis Nurses Association & American Nurses Association. (2024). *Cannabis nursing: Scope and standards of practice*. American Nurses Association.

American Nurses Association. (2023). *ANA Enterprise impact report 2023; Imagining the Enterprise into 2040.* Silver Springs, MD: American Nurse Enterprise. Retrieved from https://www.nursingworld.org/ana/about-ana/annual-reports/

American Nurses Association. (2025). Code of ethics for nurses. In A. N. Association.

American Nurses Association. (2025). *Code of ethics for nurses with interpretive statements: Provisions 1-9.* ANA.

American Society for Quality. (n.d.). Retrieved February 4, 2026, from What is Six Sigma?: https://asq.org/quality-resources/six-sigma

Balneaves, L. G. (2018). Medical cannabis education: The Canadian experience. *Journal of Nursing Regulation*, *9*(2), 22–29.

Bass, B. M. (2006). *Transformational leadership*. Psychology Press. DOI: 10.4324/9781410617095

Braun, I. M.-J. (2023). Medical cannabis use in oncology: A review of clincal care models and patient-centered approaches. *Journal of Clinical Oncology*, *41*(2), 123–130. PMID: 38048518

Cawthorn, A. (2024, November 19). *The role of technology in modern nursing: From telehealth to AI.* Retrieved January 30, 2026, from Healthcare: https://www.indwes.edu/articles/2024/11/the-role-of-technology-in-modern-nursing-from-telehealth-to-ai

Centers for Disease Control and Prevention (CDC). (2025, March 7). *Cannabis and public health.* Retrieved January 30th, 2026, from Centers for Disease Control and Prevention: https://www.cdc.gov/cannabis/about/what-cdc-is-doing.html

Clark, C. (2021). The nurses's role: Providing cannabis care. In Clark, C. F., & Clark, C. (Eds.), *Cannabis: A handbook for nurses* (1st ed., p. 272). Wolters Kluwer.

Clark, C. M. (2019). *Fostering civility in nursing education* (2nd ed.). Sigma Theta Tau International.

Doody, O. D., & Doody, C. M. (2012). Transformational leadership in nursing practice. *British Journal of Nursing (Mark Allen Publishing)*, *21*(20), 1212–1218. DOI: 10.12968/bjon.2012.21.20.1212 PMID: 23132001

Gallagher, A. T. (2010). Educating for ethical leadership. *Nursing Ethics*, *17*(4), 421–432. PMID: 20610575

Gallup Poll. (2026, January 12). *Nurses continue to lead in honesty and ethics ratings.* Retrieved January 30th, 2026, from Gallup: https://news.gallup.com/poll/700736/nurses-continue-lead-honesty-ethics-ratings.aspx

Giddens, J. (2018). Transformational leadership: What every nursing dean should know. *Journal of Professional Nursing*, *117-121*(2), 117–121. Advance online publication. DOI: 10.1016/j.profnurs.2017.10.004 PMID: 29703313

Health Canada. (2018). *Cannabis legalization and regulation.* Government of Canada.

Hoch, E. H., Hall, W., & Feingold, D. (2025, February 14). Cannabis use in Europe. *European Archives of Psychiatry and Clinical Neuroscience*, *277-279*(2), 277–279. Advance online publication. DOI: 10.1007/s00406-025-01972-7 PMID: 39951121

International Council of Nurses. (n.d.). *The global voice of nursing.* Retrieved February 4, 2026, from ICN: https://www.icn.ch/

King, D. D., Gill, C. J., Cadieux, C. S., & Singh, N. (2024). The role of stigma in cannabis use disclosure: An exploratory study. *Harm Reduction Journal*, *21*(21), 1–13. DOI: 10.1186/s12954-024-00929-8 PMID: 38273362

Meiri, D. e. (2021). Cannabis clinical trials in Israel: A regulatory and scientific overview. *The Israel Medical Association Journal.*

National Academies of Sciences, Engineering, and Medicine. (2017). *The health effects of cannabis and cannabinoids: The current state of evidence and recommendations for research.* Washington, DC: National Academies Press. DOI: 10.17226/24625

NCSBN. (2018). The NCSBN National Nursing Guidelines for Medical Marijuana. *Journal of Nursing Regulation: Advancing Nursing Excellence for Public Protection*, S 3-S 58.

Parmelee, R. (2025). Nurse educators' experiences with medical cannabis education. Walden University, College of Nursing. Walden University., Retrieved December 15, 2025, from.

Parmelee, R. A., & Clark, C. S. (2022). Nursing students knowledge, skills, and attitudes regarding medicinal cannabis care. *Journal of Nursing Regulation*, *13*(3), 13–23. DOI: 10.1016/S2155-8256(22)00082-5

Parmelee, R. C. (2021). Cannabis pharmacology: From the whole plant to pharmaceutical applications. In Clark, C. (Ed.), *Cannabis: A handbook for nurses* (pp. 115–160). Wolters Kluwer.

QSEN Institute. (2020). *Quality and safety education for nurses: Competencies*. Retrieved January 30, 2026, from Quality and Safety Education for Nurses: https://www.qsen.org/competencies-pre-licensure-ksas

Russo, E. B. (2016). *Cannabis and Cannabinoids: Pharmacology, Toxicology, and Therapeutic Potential*. Routledge.

Senge, P. M. (2006). *The fifth discipline: The art and practice of learning the organization.* (Rev., Ed.) Doubleday.

Shepherd, J. M. (2024). Advancing nursing practice through artificial intelligence: Unlocking its transformative impact. *Online Journal of Issues in Nursing*, *29*(1). Advance online publication. DOI: 10.3912/OJIN.Vol29No01PPT77

Sherman, R. O. (2010). Growing future nurse leaders to build and sustain health work environments. *Nursing Administration Quarterly*, *34*(4), 346–358. PMID: 20838181

Shirey, M. R. (2013). Lewin's theory of planned change as a strategic resource. *The Journal of Nursing Administration*, *43*(2), 69–72. DOI: 10.1097/NNA.0b013e31827f20a9 PMID: 23343723

Sommers, D. M. (2023). Cannabis nursing scope and standards of practice: Panel Presentation. *ACNA National Conference* May 20-22, 2023 Denver, Colorado, (pp. 1-21). Denver.

Spears, L. (2010). Character and servant leadership: Ten characteristics of effective caring leaders. *The Journal of Virtues and Leadership*, *1*(1), 25–30.

Spector, C. B. (2018). Medical marijuana: A national survey of nursing education and practice. *Journal of Nursing Regulation*, *9*(2), 36–43.

Zolotov, Y. V. (2021). Medical cannabis education for health professionals: A systemic review. *Complementary Therapies in Medicine*, *56*, 102616.

KEY TERMS AND DEFINITIONS

Advocacy: Promoting patient rights, safety, and equitable access while supporting evidence-based cannabis care and reducing stigma.

Cannabis Nursing: A nursing specialty that applies evidence-based cannabinoid science to assess, educate, and support patients using cannabis safely.

Education: Building the knowledge and skills nurses need to practice safely, including cannabinoid science, legal issues, and patient teaching.

Ethics: The principles that guide safe, just, patient-centered decisions, including informed consent, autonomy, and professional responsibility.

Nursing Leadership: Guiding teams and systems through evidence-based decisions, advocacy, and strategic direction to improve care and advance the profession.

Policy: The rules and standards that shape how healthcare—and cannabis care—is delivered, documented, and regulated.

APPENDIX

Learning Application: NCLEX-Style Questions

1. A nurse leader is developing a hospital policy for cannabis healthcare consumer self-administration of medical cannabis. Which initial action best reflects evidence-based and ethical leadership?
   a. Review the institution's liability coverage and federal funding contracts.
   b. Conduct staff training before finalizing policy language.
   c. Implement the policy in selected units for pilot testing.
   d. Seeking board approval after state legislation changes.

Correct Answer: A

Rationale: Reviewing institutional liability and federal funding ensures legal compliance before policy development. Ethical leadership anticipates risk while protecting cannabis healthcare consumer and organizational integrity.

2. In preparing faculty to teach cannabis pharmacology, which strategy should an academic dean prioritize?
   a. Assign faculty to conduct independent literature reviews.
   b. Develop a comprehensive faculty development plan with ACNA resources.
   c. Hire adjunct instructors with clinical cannabis experience.
   d. Introduce elective courses rather than required modules.

Correct Answer: B

Rationale: Faculty development ensures knowledge consistency, aligns with national standards, and fosters institutional readiness for sustainable curriculum integration.

3. A nurse executive collaborates with policymakers to include cannabis content on the NCLEX. Which leadership competency is being demonstrated?
   a. Servant leadership
   b. Transformational leadership
   c. Transactional leadership
   d. Autocratic leadership

Correct Answer: B

Rationale: Transformational leadership inspires systemic change through advocacy, vision, and collaboration—qualities evident in national licensure reform efforts.

4. A nurse researcher is leading a study on cannabis use in palliative care. To uphold ethical standards, which principle should guide participant recruitment?
   a. Convenience sampling for rapid data collection.
   b. Inclusion of only cannabis healthcare consumers currently using cannabis.
   c. Recruitment that ensures diversity and equitable representation.

d. Exclusion of vulnerable populations to avoid risk.

Correct Answer: C

Rationale: Ethical research demands inclusivity and equity to produce valid, generalizable results and to address historical disparities in cannabis policy and access.

5. Which leadership action best aligns with the ANA 2040 Vision?
   a. Establishing separate cannabis care units in hospitals.
   b. Using artificial intelligence to predict cannabis treatment outcomes while maintaining cannabis healthcare consumer privacy.
   c. Limiting cannabis nursing education to graduate programs.
   d. Avoiding global collaborations to maintain national standards.

Correct Answer: B

Rationale: The ANA 2040 Vision emphasizes technologically advanced, cannabis healthcare consumer-centered, and equitable care; ethical use of AI to improve outcomes reflects these priorities.

Chapter 4
Developing Clinical Competence and Capability in Medical Cannabis Nursing

Hasan H. Alsararatee
http://orcid.org/0000-0003-4252-8201
Northampton General Hospital NHS Trust, UK

ABSTRACT

This chapter establishes an evidence-informed framework for clinical competence in medical cannabis nursing, integrating assessment, dosing, monitoring, patient education, ethical reasoning, and professional identity formation. Drawing on the current research, regulatory guidance, and theoretical models such as the biopsychosocial approach and therapeutic stewardship, the chapter outlines the clinical and ethical complexities associated with cannabinoid-based care. It explores variability in product pharmacology, the need for structured risk stratification, the importance of shared decision-making, and the challenges posed by stigma, misinformation, and regulatory inconsistencies. By synthesising empirical findings, ethical principles, and professional standards, the chapter delineates the knowledge, skills, and reflective capabilities required to ensure safe, accountable, and context-sensitive nursing practice within an evolving therapeutic landscape.

CHAPTER AIM

The aim of this chapter is to establish a comprehensive, evidence informed framework for clinical competence in medical cannabis nursing, integrating assessment, dosing, monitoring, patient education, ethical reasoning, legal accountability, and professional identity formation so that nurses can deliver safe, consistent, and accountable care within an evolving therapeutic landscape.

CHAPTER OBJECTIVES

By the end of this chapter, readers will be able to:

DOI: 10.4018/979-8-3373-7287-7.ch004

1. Critically evaluate the scientific, clinical, and regulatory evidence underpinning the therapeutic use of cannabis and its implications for nursing practice.
2. Apply a biopsychosocial and ethically grounded approach to the assessment of patients who may benefit from cannabinoid therapeutics, including risk stratification, symptom evaluation, and psychosocial appraisal.
3. Demonstrate competence in dosing and monitoring, including safe titration, recognition of adverse effects, management of drug interactions, and care of at risk populations.
4. Deliver effective patient education using shared decision making, transparent communication, and evidence informed counselling to correct misinformation and support safe use.
5. Analyse ethical and legal responsibilities associated with cannabis nursing, including consent, documentation standards, equity, governance, and role boundaries.
6. Understand and contribute to the development of professional identity within the emerging specialty of cannabis nursing, including collaboration with interdisciplinary teams and engagement with organisational policy.

INTRODUCTION

Cannabis-based medicines have transitioned from limited clinical use to greater clinical visibility as regulatory reform and emerging evidence have progressed (Ntais et al., 2025). Prescribing trends across several health systems indicate that cannabinoids are now encountered more frequently in the management of chronic pain, neurological spasticity, refractory epilepsies, and palliative care presentations (Johnson et al., 2010). These developments require nurses and clinicians to apply rigorous clinical judgement, evidence appraisal, and safe monitoring when supporting patients who use cannabinoid therapies (Sinclair et al., 2024).

The therapeutic application of cannabis has expanded rapidly as research, legislation, and patient interest have converged (Hossain and Chae, 2024). International data indicate a significant rise in the use of cannabinoid-based medicines for chronic pain, multiple sclerosis related spasticity, epilepsy, and palliative symptoms (Whiting et al., 2015). In parallel, patients increasingly use cannabis autonomously, often without clinical oversight. Studies show that up to 45 percent of patients who use medical cannabis do so without formal consultation and frequently underestimate potential interactions and adverse effects (Boehnke et al., 2019). These trends position nurses as critical figures in correcting misinformation and supporting safe practice. One of the most authoritative analyses of cannabis evidence is the extensive review published by the National Academies of Sciences, Engineering, and Medicine. Their committee found substantial evidence supporting efficacy for chronic pain, chemotherapy-induced nausea and vomiting, and multiple sclerosis related spasticity, but noted limited or insufficient evidence for many other frequently publicised uses (National Academies of Sciences, Engineering, and Medicine, 2017). This disparity between validated therapeutic outcomes and public belief underscores the need for nurses to apply critical, evidence informed reasoning in patient assessment and education.

Nurses frequently encounter patients who have initiated cannabis use independently, a phenomenon reflected in a UK-based qualitative study in which registered nurses reported feeling under-prepared to support patients using medicinal cannabis (McIntosh et al., 2024). This reflects a broader challenge: cannabis products vary widely in cannabinoid composition, terpenoid content, and bioavailability, and these differences influence therapeutic effect and risk (Vázquez et al, 2021). Nurses must therefore recognise product variability as a core element of clinical assessment and patient counselling. Despite the increasing presence of cannabis in healthcare, research demonstrates that nurses often feel underprepared. Crowell and colleagues conducted a national survey which found considerable gaps in nurses' knowledge of cannabis pharmacology, endocannabinoid function, adverse effects, and safety considerations (Crowell et al., 2021). Participants frequently expressed uncertainty when advising patients or interpreting claims about efficacy. These findings align with a scoping review by Zolotov et al (2021) which found that formal cannabis education is significantly limited across nursing curricula internationally.

In response to evolving clinical demands, the American Nurses Association formally recognised cannabis nursing as a specialty in 2023 (American Nurses Association, 2023). This recognition signifies a transition from informal, interest driven participation towards formalised, accountable, and standardised practice. Other regions have undertaken similar initiatives. For example, the College of Nurses of Ontario produced practice guidance for nurses involved in cannabis care, emphasising documentation, competence, and legal responsibilities (College of Nurses of Ontario, 2018). Structured educational programmes for nurses have been developed within the Israeli medical cannabis service to ensure consistent and safe clinical practice (Lewis et al., 2015). These developments demonstrate emerging international consensus around the need for specialised competencies. However, organisational infrastructures often lag behind clinical needs. Research by Philpot et al. found that many healthcare institutions lack clear policies on monitoring, documenting, or integrating medical cannabis into care pathways (Philpot et al., 2019). Without structured frameworks, nurses face uncertainty regarding scope of practice, liability, and interprofessional responsibilities. This chapter aims to address these gaps by articulating a comprehensive, evidence informed model of competence in cannabis nursing.

The conceptual foundation of the chapter is the biopsychosocial model, originally proposed by Engel (1977), which recognises that health outcomes arise from biological, psychological, and social influences. Cannabinoid therapeutics intersect with each of these domains through neurobiological mechanisms, psychological effects, and sociocultural factors such as stigma or patient belief systems. Within this model, the concept of therapeutic stewardship is used to describe the nurse's responsibility to ensure the safe, proportionate, and evidence informed use of cannabinoid therapies. Clinical prudence is introduced to signify reflective, cautious, and ethically grounded decision making in contexts where uncertainty is common. Shared decision making, supported by the work of Elwyn and colleagues, provides a framework for transparent communication, informed consent, and patient empowerment (Elwyn et al., 2012).

This chapter therefore situates cannabis nursing within a broader theoretical, empirical, and professional context. It synthesises evidence from clinical trials, observational studies, qualitative research, and regulatory guidance to support the development of a robust competency framework. It also examines the emergence of professional identity in cannabis nursing and discusses the implications for curriculum development, governance, and organisational policy.

CONTEXT AND THEORETICAL FOUNDATIONS FOR MEDICAL CANNABIS NURSING

Medical cannabis has received more clinical and scientific attention in recent years, partly because the endocannabinoid system was discovered in the 1990s (Nabil et al., 2024). This system, comprising endogenous ligands, receptors, and metabolic enzymes, regulates numerous physiological processes, including mood, appetite, pain perception, immune activity, and memory (Di Marzo, 2018). Understanding these mechanisms has contributed to increased interest in therapeutic cannabinoid modulation. Clinical research demonstrates potential benefits but also significant heterogeneity. A systematic review by Whiting et al. (2015) found moderate quality evidence supporting cannabis for chronic pain, but low-quality evidence for other conditions, owing to methodological limitations. Similarly, Bennett et al., (2012) note that while cannabinoids may produce analgesia, their effect sizes are often modest compared with patient expectations. These findings highlight the essential role of critical appraisal in nursing practice.

In addition to variation in efficacy, cannabis carries known risks. Acute adverse effects include anxiety, cognitive impairment, tachycardia, and dizziness (Hall & Degenhardt, 2014). Long term risks may include dependence in susceptible individuals, or induction of psychosis in those with a predisposition (Murray et al., 2017). Furthermore, cannabinoids interact with the cytochrome P450 system, creating potential interactions with warfarin, antiepileptic medicines, and sedatives (Brown et al., 2020). Nurses must incorporate such considerations into assessment and monitoring. Patient expectations often diverge from scientific evidence. Qualitative studies demonstrate that individuals frequently turn to cannabis to address symptoms such as anxiety or insomnia despite limited empirical support (Carliner et al., 2017). These expectations are shaped by cultural beliefs, personal narratives, and commercial marketing. Nurses must therefore be equipped to provide balanced, evidence informed counselling.

Legal frameworks further complicate clinical practice by creating variability in patient access, prescriber authority and nursing responsibilities within cannabinoid-based care pathways. In Australia, in-depth interviews with clinicians revealed that complex special access schemes and inconsistent regulatory guidance generate uncertainty in documentation and delay patient treatment initiation (Hallinan et al., 2021). In Israel, longitudinal data confirm that rapid expansion of licenced medical cannabis products outpaced the development of clinical protocols and nurse training frameworks, contributing to ambiguity around professional accountability in cannabis clinics (Bar-Lev Schleider et al., 2022). Understanding the legal context is essential for safe and accountable practice, particularly as the clinical use of cannabis-based medicines continue to expand across several therapeutic areas. In palliative care, recent evaluations indicate that cannabinoids are prescribed to address complex symptom clusters such as pain, nausea, and appetite disturbance, although benefits remain inconsistent and require careful monitoring (Hardy et al., 2023; Hardy et al., 2025). In neurology, cannabidiol retains robust evidence for severe childhood epilepsies, with sustained seizure reduction confirmed in longer term follow up studies (Bonanni et al., 2023). These developments underscore the necessity for nurses to hold specialist knowledge, critical appraisal capability, and confidence in navigating evolving clinical and regulatory expectations. This chapter therefore establishes the conceptual and evidence informed grounding required to support safe and effective nursing practice within this developing field.

SYNTHESIS OF THE EVIDENCE BASE FOR MEDICAL CANNABIS

The evidence base for medical cannabis continues to expand, yet remains characterised by variable methodological quality, modest effect sizes, and areas of sustained uncertainty. This reinforces the need for nurses to adopt evidence informed, critically appraised approach when supporting patients who use cannabinoid-based therapies. Foundational evidence was established by the National Academies of Sciences, Engineering, and Medicine (2017), which identified substantial evidence for cannabinoids in chronic pain, chemotherapy induced nausea and vomiting, and spasticity in multiple sclerosis, forming the basis of many contemporary clinical guidelines. More recent analyses refine and often temper these conclusions. The living systematic review produced by Chou et al. (2025) demonstrates that cannabinoids for subacute and chronic pain yield small improvements in pain intensity, usually less than one point on a 10-point scale, with increased adverse events and limited certainty regarding long term benefit. These findings are consistent with Schweiger et al. (2025), who report that although analgesic effects in randomised trials often achieve statistical significance, the absolute improvements frequently fall below clinically important thresholds, with somnolence and dizziness among the most common adverse effects. Observational evidence provides a related but distinct picture. O'Brien et al. (2023) found that real world patients reported small to moderate reductions in pain intensity and interference over a three-month period, alongside improvements in sleep and quality of life, although the absence of a comparator group and high attrition restrict the reliability of these findings.

The evidence for cancer related pain and palliative symptom management remains inconsistent. Earlier work by Bennett et al. (2012) identified only modest improvements in chronic cancer pain that often fell short of expectations. Subsequent trial data have not resolved this uncertainty. In the MedCan1 study, Hardy et al. (2023) showed that cannabidiol oil offered no meaningful improvement in total symptom distress compared with placebo in patients with advanced cancer. The later trial by Hardy et al. (2025), which evaluated a balanced tetrahydrocannabinol and cannabidiol oral oil, again demonstrated no difference in primary symptom burden, although a small improvement in pain scores occurred at the cost of higher psychotomimetic toxicity and treatment discontinuation. Narrative evidence from Bimonte et al. (2024) reinforces this pattern, concluding that while some studies report benefits, results across trials of cannabis-based medicines in cancer pain are inconsistent, and central nervous system adverse effects remain prevalent. Johnson et al. (2010) similarly observe that high quality cancer pain trials often fail to meet primary endpoints and that current evidence offers little support for an opioid sparing effect. These findings underline the responsibility of nurses to set realistic expectations and to monitor patients closely for both therapeutic response and adverse outcomes.

In neurology, cannabidiol represents one of the few indications supported by robust trial evidence. Devinsky et al. (2017) showed significant reductions in seizure frequency in Dravet and Lennox Gastaut syndromes, though adverse effects such as somnolence, diarrhoea, and elevated transaminases necessitate close supervision. Bonanni et al. (2023) extend this evidence by reporting sustained seizure reductions over longer periods, although liver toxicity remains a concern, particularly when valproate is co administered.

Mental health remains an area of considerable uncertainty. Black et al. (2019) identified insufficient evidence for cannabinoids in depressive disorders, anxiety, psychosis, or attention deficit disorders. This has been strengthened by De Bode et al. (2025), who synthesised 22 systematic reviews and found that evidence for mental health conditions is weak, heterogeneous, and often contradictory, with small improvements in some subgroups offset by potential worsening in others. The situation is similar in younger populations. Köck et al. (2024), in an analysis of randomised controlled trials in children, adolescents, and young adults, identified only modest benefits (Hedges g around 0.31), with most improvements observed in autism spectrum disorder. The authors emphasised insufficient evidence for routine use due to short follow up periods and incomplete safety profiles. Rice et al. (2024) also concluded that cannabinoid research in neurodevelopmental and neuropsychiatric disorders is underdeveloped, often uncontrolled, and unable to support confident recommendations. Together, these findings necessitate careful, evidence-based dialogue with patients who seek cannabinoids for psychological distress.

Safety considerations are central to nursing practice. Acute adverse events, including cognitive impairment, dizziness, anxiety, and somnolence, remain well documented across multiple trials. Long term risks are similarly important. Zeraatkar et al. (2022), in a systematic review involving 12 143 adults, reported that approximately 26 per cent experienced adverse events and 13.5 per cent experienced psychiatric events, with serious harms, dependence, cognitive impairment, and accidents occurring in fewer than 5 per cent, though certainty was low due to confounding. Experimental and observational data reviewed by Borrego-Ruiz & Borrego (2025) highlight potential immunomodulatory effects, pro inflammatory cytokine responses, and the association between heavy cannabis use and cognitive or mood disturbances. Complementary evidence from Sorkhou et al. (2021) shows that frequent or high potency cannabis use increases risks of psychotic like experiences, anxiety symptoms, and deficits in attention and memory, with younger users particularly vulnerable.

Drug interactions represent a further dimension of clinical risk. Lopera et al. (2022) identified nineteen clinically significant interactions, including high risk interactions with warfarin, where markedly elevated international normalised ratio values and bleeding events were reported, as well as interactions with buprenorphine and tacrolimus. Ho et al. (2024) identified interactions involving twenty drug classes, particularly antiepileptics, anticoagulants, and immunosuppressants, recommending therapeutic drug monitoring and cautious dose adjustment. These findings have direct implications for nursing responsibilities related to medicines reconciliation and interdisciplinary communication.

A persistent theme across the literature is the divergence between patient perceptions and trial evidence. Qualitative studies indicate that many patients believe cannabis is beneficial for anxiety, stress reduction, or sleep (Das et al., 2024; Ghelani, 2021; Hurn, 2023). Olson et al. (2022) found that patients with advanced cancer often consider cannabis safer than opioids and capable of providing substantial symptom relief, influencing both trial participation and treatment persistence despite minimal objective gains. Zeng et al. (2021) further report that individuals with chronic pain frequently hold high expectations regarding symptom relief and accept substantial risks of non-serious adverse events, while differing widely in their concerns about cognitive or psychiatric harm.

These studies demonstrate that cannabis has legitimate but limited therapeutic value across specific conditions, with modest effect sizes, heterogeneous evidence quality, and notable safety considerations. Nurses play a critical role in interpreting this complex evidence base, supporting patients through informed discussions, monitoring for adverse effects, and ensuring safe integration of cannabinoid products within wider clinical care.

THEORETICAL FOUNDATIONS FOR COMPETENCE IN CANNABIS NURSING

In order to develop a coherent professional framework for cannabis nursing, it is necessary to situate practice within appropriate theoretical perspectives. These foundations support competent clinical reasoning, ethical decision making, and effective communication.

The Biopsychosocial Model

The biopsychosocial model, first articulated by Engel, continues to underpin contemporary nursing practice by positioning health and illness within the dynamic interaction of biological, psychological, and social determinants rather than within a solely biomedical framework (Engel, 1977). Subsequent scholarship has reinforced its value: Borrell-Carrió et al. (2004) emphasise that the biopsychosocial model enhances clinical reasoning and supports more nuanced therapeutic relationships, while Wade and Halligan (2017) argue that it provides the most coherent framework for conditions characterised by complexity, multimorbidity, and subjectively mediated symptom burden. This theoretical foundation is particularly pertinent to cannabis nursing, where patient responses to cannabinoid therapeutics are shaped not only by pharmacological processes but also by cognitive, emotional, cultural, and contextual influences.

The biological dimension encompasses pharmacokinetics, pharmacodynamics, variability in product composition, and the potential for interactions with medicines metabolised through cytochrome P450 pathways. These factors demand precise assessment, ongoing monitoring, and an understanding of how biological vulnerability may heighten risks such as cognitive impairment or psychiatric instability (Zeraatkar et al., 2022). The psychological dimension draws attention to patient expectations, coping styles, symptom interpretation, and prior experiences with cannabis, all of which can influence perceived efficacy and adherence. Psychological factors also shape susceptibility to anxiety, perceptual changes, or cognitive effects associated with cannabinoid exposure (Sorkhou et al., 2021). The social dimension integrates the influence of cultural narratives, socioeconomic constraints, legal status, and persistent stigma. These factors affect patterns of disclosure, access to regulated products, and engagement with professional advice, with qualitative evidence showing that many patients navigate cannabis use outside formal healthcare channels due to perceived or actual stigma (Olson et al., 2022). By synthesising these domains, the biopsychosocial perspective provides a structured means of conducting holistic assessment and making context sensitive clinical decisions. It enables nurses to evaluate how biological mechanisms intersect with psychological meaning and social environment, thereby supporting safer and more person-centred use of cannabinoid-based therapies. This framework also aligns with contemporary nursing standards that emphasise personalised care, shared decision making, and professional accountability in emerging therapeutic areas.

Therapeutic Stewardship

Therapeutic stewardship reflects the nurse's responsibility to promote proportionate, evidence informed, and ethically defensible use of cannabinoid-based medicines. The concept aligns with established stewardship frameworks in antimicrobial and opioid management, where inappropriate or excessive use poses significant risks to individual and population health (Charani and Holmes, 2013; Dowell et al., 2022). Within the context of cannabis nursing, stewardship requires nurses to appraise indications with rigour, evaluate the strength and limitations of available evidence, and communicate transparently with patients regarding expected benefits, uncertainties, and potential harms. It further necessitates systematic monitoring for adverse events, including cognitive change, mood instability, and drug interactions, particularly given the variable quality and pharmacological complexity of cannabis products (Zeraatkar et al., 2022). Effective stewardship also relies on meticulous documentation, clear rationale for therapeutic decisions, and close collaboration with prescribers to ensure coherent, safe, and accountable care.

CLINICAL PRUDENCE

Clinical prudence, grounded in Aristotelian notions of phronesis or practical wisdom, has been advanced in contemporary nursing ethics as a cornerstone of reflective, context dependent clinical judgement (Gastmans, 2013). It denotes a mode of reasoning in which empirical evidence is integrated with professional experience, patient preferences, moral sensitivity, and an appreciation of situational nuance. Modern scholarship emphasises that prudence enables clinicians to navigate areas of uncertainty, particularly where evidence is incomplete, heterogeneous, or evolving, by drawing on a balanced and ethically attuned deliberative process (Begley, 2006; Sellman, 2024). In the context of cannabinoid therapeutics, clinical prudence is indispensable because the evidence base contains gaps, variable effect sizes, and condition specific limitations. It requires nurses to interpret research findings critically, to distinguish between well supported indications and speculative use, and to recognise when risks may outweigh benefits. Prudence also involves the capacity to identify when cannabis is unsuitable, when heightened vigilance is required due to comorbidities or polypharmacy, and when alternative interventions may offer safer or more effective outcomes. By fostering this mode of reasoning, nurses are better equipped to act responsibly, maintain patient safety, and uphold professional accountability within an emerging and ethically complex field.

Shared Decision Making

Shared decision making offers a structured and ethically grounded framework for collaborative communication between clinicians and patients. Elwyn et al. (2012) describe it as a deliberative process in which clinically appropriate options are outlined, the potential benefits and harms are conveyed with transparency, and patient values, goals, and preferences are integrated into the final decision. Evidence from decision science demonstrates that shared decision making improves patient knowledge, enhances accuracy of risk perception, and increases satisfaction with care, particularly in situations where evidence is uncertain or outcomes vary between individuals (Stacey et al., 2017).

Its importance within cannabis nursing is considerable, as patient expectations are frequently shaped by personal experience, cultural narratives, and commercial messaging that may not correspond with validated clinical evidence. Structured dialogue enables nurses to explore these expectations, clarify misconceptions, and support patients in weighing therapeutic possibility against potential risk. This approach strengthens informed consent, fosters trust, and ensures that decisions regarding cannabinoid-based therapies are both evidences informed and aligned with what matters most to the individual patient.

Professional Identity Formation

Professional identity constitutes a core element of advanced nursing practice, shaping how practitioners understand their roles, responsibilities, and contributions within the wider health system. The emergence of cannabis nursing as a recognised area of practice requires nurses to construct an identity grounded in clinical competence, ethical accountability, and robust engagement with evidence. Scholarship on advanced practice identity demonstrates that professional formation is influenced by education, role clarity, organisational culture, and opportunities for reflective practice, each of which contributes to confidence, authority, and effective role enactment (Pursio et al., 2021).

Within cannabis focused care, identity work is particularly salient because practitioners must navigate persistent stigma, challenge misconceptions about cannabis use, and articulate the clinical legitimacy of their role in a field where public discourse and evidence do not always align. Falk-Rafael (2005) points out that nurses who develop a coherent and theoretically informed identity demonstrate stronger role integration, greater resilience, and enhanced interprofessional credibility, especially in emerging or contested areas of practice. As cannabis nursing continues to evolve, the cultivation of such an identity is essential for ensuring that practitioners can advocate effectively for patients, uphold professional standards, and contribute meaningfully to safe and accountable clinical pathways.

CLINICAL USES, RISKS AND REGULATORY CONTEXT

Clinical Assessment

Clinical assessment forms the foundation of safe and effective cannabis nursing practice. Unlike conventional pharmacotherapy, cannabis products vary substantially in cannabinoid composition, potency, pharmacokinetics, and route of administration, which creates unique clinical challenges. Nurses must therefore conduct a comprehensive assessment that accounts for biological, psychological, and social dimensions of the patient's health, consistent with Engel's biopsychosocial model (Engel, 1977). The complexity of cannabinoid therapeutics requires nurses to use advanced clinical reasoning and awareness of the current evidence base, recognising that although cannabis has demonstrated efficacy for certain conditions, substantial uncertainty remains across many others (National Academies of Sciences, Engineering, and Medicine, 2017). The increasing prevalence of self-directed cannabis use adds further complexity. Boehnke and colleagues found that many patients obtain cannabis without clinical oversight and frequently use unregulated products characterised by unpredictable potency and contamination risk (Boehnke et al., 2019). Such patterns heighten the need for structured assessment, therapeutic stewardship, and shared decision making. Nursing assessment must therefore be more comprehensive than in traditional medicine management, integrating symptom evaluation, cannabis-specific history taking, polypharmacy review, mental health assessment, and legal considerations.

Clinical assessment determines whether a patient is a suitable candidate for cannabinoid therapy, identifies risks that require mitigation, supports safe dosing and monitoring, and provides the basis for ongoing evaluation. The following sections provide a detailed, evidence-based framework for cannabis assessment in nursing practice.

Comprehensive History-Taking

A holistic and structured history is essential for understanding the patient's therapeutic needs, expectations, prior experiences, and associated risks. Many patients who present for guidance with cannabis have already experimented with products purchased from informal markets, online sellers, or unregulated dispensaries. In a survey of authorised medical cannabis users, Lucas and Walsh (2017) found that patients often self-adjust doses or transition rapidly between products without understanding differences in cannabinoid ratios or potency. Nurses therefore require a cannabis-specific history that establishes:

1. Product type including THC and CBD content, whole-plant extracts, synthetic cannabinoids, or unregulated oils.
2. Route of administration such as inhaled vapour, oral oils, capsules, edibles, topicals, or tinctures, which have markedly different absorption profiles (Vázquez et al, 2021).
3. Frequency and timing of use, recognising that dose titration is influenced by tolerance, metabolism, and co-medication.

4. Perceived benefits and motivations, which often extend beyond evidence-supported indications (Carliner et al., 2017).
5. Adverse effects experienced, including anxiety, cognitive impairment, tachycardia, or sedation (Hall and Degenhardt, 2014).
6. Legal acquisition sources to identify potential contamination or unregulated product risks.

Eliciting this detail helps nurses identify discrepancies between patient expectations and the evidence base, correct harmful misconceptions, and construct an informed therapeutic plan.

Accurately establishing the patient's symptomatology is essential, particularly because cannabis is frequently used for conditions where evidence is limited. The systematic review conducted by the National Academies underscores that while there is substantial evidence for chronic pain, spasticity in multiple sclerosis, and chemotherapy-induced nausea and vomiting, the evidence for anxiety disorders, insomnia, or neurodegenerative conditions remains inadequate or insufficient (National Academies of Sciences, Engineering, and Medicine, 2017).

Clinical assessment should therefore document:

- ✓ Severity, frequency, and duration of symptoms.
- ✓ Impact on functioning, mobility, sleep, mood, and quality of life.
- ✓ Previous treatments attempted and reasons for discontinuation.
- ✓ Contraindications to first line or alternative therapies.

For instance, in chronic pain, cannabinoids may produce modest analgesia relative to patient expectations (Bennett et al., 2012). Without structured assessment, patients may mistakenly assume cannabis offers strong or immediate relief.

Treatment Goals and Patient Expectations

Patient beliefs about cannabis can shape expectations in ways that influence therapeutic adherence and satisfaction. Studies show that many individuals believe cannabis to be safer or more natural than conventional medicines, sometimes equating natural origin with reduced risk (Carliner et al., 2017). Nurses must therefore explore expectations and correct misconceptions using shared decision making (Elwyn et al., 2012). Goals should be realistic, measurable, and aligned with what current evidence supports.

Risk Stratification

Risk stratification ensures that clinicians identify individuals for whom cannabis may be unsuitable or require enhanced monitoring.

MENTAL HEALTH RISK ASSESSMENT

Cannabis has well documented psychotropic effects, which may exacerbate underlying mental health conditions. High-potency THC is associated with an increased risk of psychosis, particularly in genetically or clinically vulnerable individuals (Murray et al., 2017). Acute anxiety, panic, and paranoia are also common adverse effects associated with THC exposure (Hall and Degenhardt, 2014). Nurses should therefore assess:

- Personal or family history of psychosis.
- Previous cannabis-related psychiatric events.
- Current mood state, including depression or severe anxiety.
- Trauma history or severe stressors.
- Concurrent use of psychiatric medicines such as benzodiazepines or antidepressants.

Evidence suggests that CBD dominant preparations may present a lower psychiatric risk, yet robust evidence remains limited. Nurses must therefore exercise clinical prudence when supporting patients with complex mental health needs.

Assessment of Substance Use

Cannabis may pose risks for individuals with a history of substance dependency. Although cannabis dependence is less common than dependence on opioids or stimulants, it affects a subset of regular users, particularly those exposed to high potency THC (Murray et al., 2017). Assessment should cover:

- Past dependence or attempts at detoxification.
- Current alcohol, nicotine, or illicit substance use.
- Pattern of cannabis consumption, including compulsive use or withdrawal.
- Social context of use and peer influences.

Identifying problematic patterns is essential to support harm reduction and to determine whether cannabinoid therapy is clinically appropriate.

Polypharmacy and Drug Interactions

Cannabinoids interact with medicines metabolised by cytochrome P450 enzymes, including warfarin, antiepileptic medicines, benzodiazepines, and certain antidepressants (Brown and Winterstein, 2020). Nurses must conduct a detailed medication review, considering:

- Potential for raised INR in patients on warfarin.
- Altered serum levels of antiepileptics.
- Compounded sedative effects with benzodiazepines.
- CYP interactions affecting antidepressants, immunosuppressants, or cardiovascular drugs

Monitoring for interactions is essential, particularly in older adults or individuals with multiple comorbidities.

Physical Assessment

Physical assessment provides critical insight into potential contraindications and helps establish baseline physiological parameters, such as cardiovascular status, neurological function, respiratory patterns, mental state, and indicators of hepatic or renal impairment. These findings assist nurses in identifying vulnerabilities that may heighten the risks of cannabinoid exposure and in determining whether additional investigation or specialist review is indicated.

Neurological and Cognitive Assessment

Cannabinoids, particularly those containing THC, can impair short term memory, divided attention, reaction time, and executive functioning, and these effects are more pronounced in older adults (Hall and Degenhardt, 2014; Volkow et al., 2017). Chronic exposure is associated with disruptions across multiple memory systems, including encoding, storage, manipulation, and retrieval. Meta analyses show consistent deficits in verbal and visual memory among long term users, with reduced performance on established clinical assessments such as the Rey Auditory Verbal Learning Test, Deese Roediger McDermott paradigm, and N back tasks (Broyd et al., 2016; Figueiredo et al., 2020). Evidence also demonstrates heightened susceptibility to false memories, with regular users more likely to endorse incorrect information in both laboratory and immersive tasks, even after short periods of abstinence (Riba et al., 2015; Kloft et al., 2020). These findings have implications for safety, clinical reporting, and medicolegal contexts. Although some deficits may improve with sustained abstinence, residual impairments often persist beyond acute intoxication. Studies of supervised abstinence show partial recovery in verbal and visual memory after four weeks, yet not all domains return to baseline, suggesting that a subset of impairments may reflect longer term neuroadaptation (Schuster et al., 2018). Working memory deficits, particularly visual working memory, appear to be among the most robust and enduring effects of THC exposure, with randomised trials confirming acute impairments in task accuracy and attentional control (Adam et al., 2020). Neuroimaging studies also report altered hippocampal and prefrontal activation in chronic users, supporting a neurobiological basis for the observed functional changes (Batalla et al., 2013).

By contrast, language appears relatively preserved. Early and contemporary studies show no consistent evidence of chronic language impairment, with some cohorts demonstrating comparable or even enhanced verbal fluency compared with non-users (Roten et al., 2015; Becker et al., 2014). However, the evidence base remains limited, with methodological variability and a lack of recent studies employing rigorous linguistic testing. It is plausible that language, as a crystallised cognitive ability, is less vulnerable to cannabis related disruption compared with domains dependent on rapid processing and working memory. Motor coordination and psychomotor control are more reliably affected. Acute exposure impairs reaction time, vigilance, and fine motor performance, and these deficits can persist into the residual phase even after subjective intoxication has resolved (Ramaekers et al., 2006; Weinstein et al., 2008). Driving simulation studies indicate that experienced users may develop partial tolerance to subjective effects yet remain at increased risk of errors during tasks requiring sustained attention and rapid visuomotor responses (Hartley et al., 2019). Evidence of dose dependence further highlights the relevance of product potency, with higher THC concentrations linked to greater impairment (Hunault et al., 2009). These impairments are clinically relevant because subtle decrements in coordination can elevate risk of falls, collisions, and errors in activities requiring precision.

Given this evidence, cognitive screening in cannabis assessment should evaluate:

- Memory encoding, recall, and retention.
- Orientation, attention, and processing speed.
- Speech fluency and communicative coherence.
- Working memory capacity and ability to follow multi step instructions.
- Falls risk and fine motor coordination affecting daily living.

Neurological evaluation is essential because even mild deficits may compromise safety, particularly among older adults, those operating machinery, those who drive, or those managing complex treatment regimens. Integrating cognitive findings with psychosocial and biomedical assessment allows nurses to identify individuals at heightened risk, tailor harm reduction strategies, and ensure that cannabis is used within a framework of safe, evidence informed practice.

Cardiovascular and Respiratory Assessment

Cannabis can increase heart rate, alter blood pressure, and in some cases precipitate atrial and ventricular arrhythmias, with higher risk in younger males and in those with structural heart disease or channelopathies (Paulraj et al., 2025). Cardiovascular assessment should therefore include:

- Baseline heart rate and rhythm at rest, with repeat measurements after postural change.
- Blood pressure lying and standing to identify postural hypotension or labile hypertension.
- Focused cardiovascular history, including coronary artery disease, heart failure, prior myocardial infarction, congenital or structural heart disease, and any history of palpitations, syncope, or documented arrhythmia.
- Review of concomitant cardiovascular medicines, particularly beta blockers, calcium channel blockers, antiarrhythmic agents, and drugs that prolong the QT interval.
- Physical examination for signs of heart failure or structural disease, including peripheral oedema, raised jugular venous pressure, displaced apex beat, and cardiomegaly.
- Careful auscultation for added heart sounds and murmurs, especially evidence of valvular disease or hypertrophic cardiomyopathy, which may increase susceptibility to cannabis related arrhythmias.
- Baseline electrocardiogram where indicated, to detect conduction abnormalities, prolonged QT interval, or patterns suggestive of channelopathies.

Respiratory assessment is required for patients considering inhaled cannabis, as smoked or vapourised preparations may exacerbate existing respiratory disease even when exposure to combustion products is reduced. Assessment should include:

- Detailed respiratory history, including asthma, chronic obstructive pulmonary disease, interstitial lung disease, sleep apnoea, and tobacco or vaping history.
- Observation of respiratory rate, work of breathing, and oxygen saturation at rest and, where appropriate, on exertion.
- Chest auscultation for wheeze, crackles, or reduced breath sounds, which may indicate airway hyperreactivity or parenchymal disease.

- Consideration of baseline spirometry in patients with known or suspected chronic lung disease before initiating inhaled cannabis products.

Such structured cardiovascular and respiratory assessment enables nurses to identify patients at heightened risk of cannabis related haemodynamic instability or arrhythmia and those in whom non inhaled routes or alternative therapies may represent a safer option.

Falls Risk in Older Adults

Older adults constitute an expanding demographic within medical cannabis use, and emerging epidemiological evidence underscores the clinical relevance of falls risk. In the national cohort study by Pravosud et al. (2025) involving 4503 Veterans Health Administration patients aged 65 to 84 years, 34.4 percent reported at least one fall in the previous year, and deficits in activities of daily living significantly increased the odds of both current cannabis use and cannabis use disorder. The study also identified that more than one in ten older adults used cannabis within the preceding 30 days, with over half engaging in frequent use, patterns that may amplify falls risk through cognitive impairment, delayed reaction time, and orthostatic instability.

Given these findings, falls assessment must extend beyond routine mobility checks to include structured evaluation of orthostatic blood pressure, gait stability, and dual task performance, each of which may deteriorate with THC exposure. Cognitive screening is particularly important, as Pravosud et al. (2025) linked anxiety symptoms and functional impairment with elevated odds of cannabis use disorder, conditions that may interact with cannabis effects to compromise safe ambulation. Environmental assessment, including identification of home hazards and footwear safety, remains a core responsibility for nurses supporting older cannabis users. A comprehensive falls risk appraisal therefore forms a fundamental component of safe cannabis care in later life, ensuring that therapeutic intentions do not inadvertently heighten vulnerability to injury.

Assessing Psychosocial Context

Cannabis use in older adults and in those with chronic symptoms is shaped by far more than pharmacology alone. It is embedded within values, expectations, social roles, and cultural narratives. In a qualitative study of people living with chronic pain, Individuals' Values and Preferences Regarding Medical Cannabis for Chronic Pain: A Descriptive Qualitative Study (Cummings et al., 2024) found that participants emphasised improving sleep, reducing reliance on other medications, and enhancing daily functioning as key motivators for cannabis use; yet they also reported substantial experimentation, variable dosing, and frequent reliance on non-clinical information sources (Cummings et al., 2024). A comprehensive mixed-methods systematic review, Values and preferences towards medical cannabis among people living with chronic pain: a mixed-methods systematic review (Zeng et al., 2021) showed that patients' decisions to use medical cannabis were strongly influenced by social facilitators (such as family support) and barriers (such as stigma), and that many users accepted minor adverse effects (e.g., memory issues, fatigue) in exchange for perceived benefit.

Older adults present particular psychosocial issues when using cannabis. The study Cannabis Use Among Older Adults (Pravosud et al., 2025) found that in a sample of older veterans (aged 65–84), over one in ten reported past 30-day cannabis use and more than one-third of these met criteria for a cannabis use disorder; importantly, those with deficits in activities of daily living, anxiety symptoms, or social and functional vulnerabilities were at higher risk. In addition, a survey on older adults' attitudes, Older Adults' Use of Cannabis and Attitudes Around Disclosure and Use (Abu Baker et al., 2024) highlighted that many older adults using cannabis do so under the radar of formal healthcare, due to concerns about judgement or lack of clinician knowledge.

Given this evidence, a robust psychosocial assessment by nurses and clinicians must attend to several domains:

- Understanding motivation and goals: Explore the reasons the patient is using cannabis—are they motivated by pain relief, sleep improvement, medication reduction, coping with mood or isolation? Clarify whether expectations align with evidence and identify potential unrealistic beliefs (e.g., "cannabis will fix everything").
- Beliefs and information sources: Ask about the patient's beliefs regarding cannabis ("natural", "safe", "better than opioids") and their information sources. Many older adults rely on peers, online forums, or dispensary advice rather than clinical guidance (Cummings et al., 2024; Zeng et al., 2021).
- Social and cultural context: Assess stigma, disclosure behaviours, family attitudes and living arrangements. Older users may fear professional judgement, leading to non-disclosure and unsupervised use (Abu Baker et al., 2024).
- Functional and psychological vulnerabilities: Screen for anxiety, depression, cognitive concerns, deficits in daily living, frailty or isolation—these factors both drive cannabis use and increase risk of adverse effects (Pravosud et al., 2025).
- Support environment and adherence: Evaluate social support, caregiving responsibilities, financial constraints, housing stability and health literacy. These social determinants affect the ability to adhere to safer regimens and monitor for harm (Zeng et al., 2021).

By integrating these psychosocial domains alongside the usual biomedical assessment, nurses can better understand *why* an older adult is using cannabis, tailor interventions accordingly, set realistic expectations, ensure safe monitoring, and promote shared decision making. This holistic approach supports safer and more person-centred care in the context of cannabinoid use.

Stigma and Communication Barriers

Stigma surrounding cannabis use continues to influence clinical encounters, shaping how patients interpret their symptoms, disclose their behaviours, and engage with professional advice. Qualitative research demonstrates that individuals frequently minimise or conceal cannabis use because of anticipated judgement from clinicians, fear of being labelled as irresponsible, or concerns that disclosure may negatively affect their care (Baumbusch and Yip, 2022). Evidence from older adults further shows that stigma interacts with generational attitudes and cultural norms, leading to selective disclosure, fragmented self-management, and reliance on informal rather than clinical guidance (Abu Baker et al., 2024). In a clinical setting, such concealment may obscure important information about drug interactions, mental health vulnerability, and safety risks, thereby complicating accurate assessment and shared decision making.

For nurses, mitigating these barriers requires the deliberate creation of a communicative environment characterised by psychological safety, neutrality, and respect. Nyblade ey al. (2019) highlights that stigma reduction in healthcare emphasises that the clinician's tone, language, and assumptions strongly influence willingness to disclose sensitive information. Adopting open questioning techniques, validating patient experiences, and explicitly inviting disclosure about cannabis use reduce the likelihood of omission and improve therapeutic alliance. A non-judgemental stance is therefore essential not only to gather accurate clinical information but also to uphold ethical principles of dignity, autonomy, and person-centred care.

Social Support and Caregiving

Cannabis therapy often requires monitoring, especially during dose titration. The presence of a supportive caregiver enhances safety. Assessment should consider:

- Whether the patient has support for dosing, monitoring, and follow-up.
- Understanding of adverse effect recognition.
- The ability of the carer to provide practical or emotional support

In palliative care, where cannabinoids are frequently used for symptom management, carer involvement is particularly important (Johnson et al., 2010).

Socioeconomic Factors and Access to Regulated Products

Cannabis products from legal channels can be costly, which may influence patients to seek cheaper unregulated alternatives. Philpot et al. (2019) report that cost and access are among the most common barriers to safe cannabis use. Nurses must therefore incorporate socioeconomic assessment into care planning and signpost patients towards regulated, affordable pathways where possible.

Legal and Regulatory Assessment

Given the variation in cannabis legislation across jurisdictions, nurses must ensure that clinical recommendations comply with current regulations. Fischer et al. (2017) highlights that regulatory inconsistency creates uncertainty about documentation, clinical responsibility, and professional liability.

Assessment must therefore include:

- Whether cannabis is legally prescribed or recommended.
- Whether the nurse's involvement is permitted within local scope of practice.
- Documentation standards required by governing bodies.
- Patient understanding of legal restrictions, such as driving regulations.
- Institutional policies governing storage, administration, and monitoring

Clarity regarding legal boundaries protects both patient safety and professional integrity.

THE IMPORTANCE OF DOCUMENTATION

Documentation provides an auditable record of clinical reasoning, supports continuity of care, and protects against legal challenge. The College of Nurses of Ontario (2018) emphasises that documentation should capture:

1. Rationale for cannabis use.
2. Risk and benefit discussion.
3. Titration plan.
4. Monitoring plan.
5. Observed adverse reactions.
6. Patient understanding and consent

Comprehensive documentation ensures transparency and supports governance frameworks essential to emerging practice areas such as cannabis nursing.

Clinical Case Study 1: Managing spasticity in multiple sclerosis

A 42-year-old patient living with multiple sclerosis reports progressive spasticity despite physiotherapy and optimisation of first-line pharmacological therapies including baclofen. The patient has read online accounts of improvement with cannabis-based treatments and requests professional guidance. Comprehensive assessment identifies no history of psychosis, unstable mood disorder, or cardiovascular disease. Alcohol intake is low, illicit drug use is absent, and the patient benefits from strong domestic support. The patient expresses a wish to reduce reliance on sedating antispasmodic medicines that impair daily functioning.

Evidence from controlled trials demonstrates that nabiximols can produce modest but clinically meaningful reductions in spasticity severity in multiple sclerosis, although adverse effects such as dizziness, somnolence, and dry mouth are frequently reported (Whiting et al., 2015). The National Academies review concludes that there is *substantial* evidence supporting cannabinoid-based treatment for spasticity related to multiple sclerosis, while emphasising the need for careful monitoring because individual responses vary significantly (National Academies of Sciences, Engineering, and Medicine, 2017). These findings support a cautious, structured, and ethically grounded approach to cannabis initiation.

Drawing on this evidence, the nurse:

- Conducts a cannabis-specific assessment, including prior exposure, expectations, functional goals, potential contraindications, co-morbidities, and concomitant medicines.
- Provides balanced education about potential benefits, limitations, and uncertainties, drawing explicitly on findings from the National Academies and recent randomised trials.
- Assesses risks related to sedation, concentration, and driving, highlighting that nabiximols commonly impairs reaction time and that legal driving restrictions may apply.
- Develops an individualised titration and monitoring plan, focusing on symptom relief, tolerability, and functional outcomes, with agreed monitoring intervals.
- Collaborates closely with the prescriber to ensure the product is regulated, dose-standardised, and introduced under a shared governance framework.

- Uses structured shared decision making, ensuring that therapeutic choice aligns with the patient's priorities, such as reducing sedation while improving mobility.

This case illustrates how rigorous clinical assessment, ethical reasoning, and evidence informed dialogue form the foundation of safe and accountable cannabis nursing. It also demonstrates the importance of integrating patient goals with systematically appraised evidence to support proportionate and person-centred care.

DOSING, MONITORING, AND PATIENT EDUCATION IN CANNABIS NURSING

Dosing, monitoring, and education constitute the core competencies required for safe and effective cannabis nursing. Cannabinoid pharmacology is characterised by considerable inter-individual variability, complex pharmacokinetics, and dose dependent adverse effects, which necessitate cautious titration and structured surveillance (Vázquez et al, 2021). Evidence demonstrates that inappropriate initiation, lack of monitoring, or insufficient patient instruction can increase the likelihood of adverse events such as sedation, cognitive impairment, anxiety, falls, and drug interactions (Hall and Degenhardt, 2014; Brown and Winterstein, 2020).

Nurses therefore play a pivotal role in guiding patients through therapeutic initiation, identifying early signs of harm, correcting misinformation, and ensuring that treatments remain aligned with evidence informed practice and ethical guidance. This section outlines a comprehensive set of principles for dosing, monitoring, and education in cannabis nursing, supported by contemporary evidence and clinical guidelines.

Principles of Dosing in Cannabis Nursing

Start Low and Go Slow

The most consistently supported principle in cannabis dosing is the "start low and go slow" approach. This method reflects the unpredictable absorption profiles of cannabinoids, the interaction between THC and CBD, and the risk of dose related adverse effects (Lucas and Walsh, 2017). Nurses should initiate therapy with the lowest clinically appropriate dose and incrementally increase dosage only when symptoms remain insufficiently controlled and the patient demonstrates tolerability. The National Academies review supports gradual titration to mitigate risks such as dizziness, cognitive impairment, tachycardia, and anxiety, particularly in individuals using formulations containing THC (National Academies of Sciences, Engineering, and Medicine, 2017). Slow titration is especially important in older adults, who are more susceptible to delirium, falls, and cardiovascular instability (Philpot et al., 2019).

Understanding Cannabinoid Ratios

Cannabinoid formulations vary widely, and the proportions of THC and CBD significantly influence both therapeutic effect and risk.

- THC contributes to analgesic, antiemetic, and antispastic effects but also produces intoxication, anxiety, impaired memory, psychomotor slowing, and psychosis in vulnerable individuals (Murray et al., 2017).
- CBD demonstrates anticonvulsant, anxiolytic, and anti-inflammatory properties and may attenuate some adverse effects of THC (Devinsky et al., 2017).

Clinical selection of cannabinoid ratios must therefore reflect symptom profile, psychiatric history, age, and safety considerations. Evidence suggests that CBD dominant preparations are better tolerated and carry lower psychiatric and cognitive risks, and are often recommended for individuals with mood disorders, older adults, or those with no previous cannabis exposure (Whiting et al., 2015). Routes of administration shape how cannabinoids are absorbed, how quickly effects begin, how long they persist, and the overall safety profile of treatment. These differences are well documented in pharmacokinetic studies and must be considered carefully in nursing practice to prevent avoidable harm or therapeutic failure (Chayasirisobhon, 2021). The rout of administration attached in Table 1.

Monitoring in Cannabis Nursing

Monitoring is critical to ensure effectiveness, detect adverse effects, and recognise drug interactions.

Monitoring Therapeutic Response

Monitoring therapeutic response requires structured, longitudinal evaluation that prioritises functional improvement rather than isolated reductions in pain intensity. High-quality evidence demonstrates that cannabinoids offer only small reductions in chronic pain, typically below thresholds considered clinically important, which reinforces the need to monitor sleep, daily functioning, and participation in meaningful activities. A comprehensive meta-analysis of randomised trials by Wang et al. (2021) found that cannabinoids produced modest analgesic effects but were frequently accompanied by adverse events, highlighting the necessity for careful clinical review and titration. Existing real-world evidence from the Australian QUEST cohort study indicates that some patients experience improvements in health-related quality of life and sleep when initiating medicinal cannabis, though pain reductions remain moderate and outcomes vary widely across individuals (Tait et al., 2023). In this context, nurses should apply validated measures such as the Brief Pain Inventory or EQ-5D, document changes in medicine use including opioid reduction, and assess how symptoms affect mobility, self-care, mood, and social engagement.

Monitoring Adverse Effects

Cannabinoids can cause a wide range of dose dependent adverse effects. Common effects include:

- Dizziness, sedation, dry mouth
- Short-term memory impairment
- Tachycardia, hypotension
- Anxiety or panic

More serious risks include:

- Psychosis in susceptible individuals (Murray et al., 2017)
- Falls in older adults (Philpot et al., 2019)
- Interaction induced toxicity (Brown and Winterstein, 2020)

Nurses must routinely assess:

- Vital signs
- Cognitive status
- Mood and anxiety
- Motor coordination and gait
- Signs of intoxication
- Effects on sleep and appetite

Structured monitoring protects vulnerable populations and ensures early detection of harm.

Monitoring Drug Interactions

Cannabinoids interact with medicines metabolised by CYP450 enzymes. Identified interactions include:

- Increased INR with warfarin
- Reduced seizure control with antiepileptics
- Enhanced sedation with benzodiazepines
- Potential interactions with SSRIs, immunosuppressants, and cardiovascular medicines

These interactions are documented in previous literature (Damkier et al., 2019; Lopera et al., 2022; Balachandran et al., 2021; Srinivasana and Shukla, 2024). Nurses must conduct regular medication reviews and coordinate with prescribers and pharmacists.

Monitoring At-Risk Populations

Certain groups require enhanced surveillance.

Older Adults

Older adults require careful clinical monitoring because age-related physiological changes increase the pharmacodynamic and pharmacokinetic effects of cannabinoids. Slower hepatic metabolism, increased body fat, polypharmacy, and reduced physiological reserve heighten susceptibility to sedation, cognitive impairment, orthostatic hypotension, and falls. Evidence from observational studies demonstrates that older adults report higher rates of dizziness, impaired balance, and confusion when initiating cannabinoid therapies, particularly with THC dominant preparations (Abuhasira et al., 2018). Survey data further indicate that many older individuals use unregulated or informally sourced cannabis products because of cost, limited access to specialist prescribing, or uncertainty about legal pathways, which increases exposure to variable potency and inconsistent dosing (Philpot et al., 2019). These factors underscore the need for nurses to conduct structured monitoring focusing on cognition, gait stability, cardiovascular parameters, and medicine interactions, ensuring that risk is mitigated while supporting therapeutic goals.

Individuals With Mental Health Conditions

Those with a personal or family history of psychosis should avoid high-THC products due to increased psychiatric risk (Murray et al., 2017).

Patients With Cardiovascular Disease

Cannabis can precipitate tachycardia, orthostatic hypotension, and rarely arrhythmias, requiring close monitoring (Paulraj et al., 2025).

Patient Education in Cannabis Nursing

Patient education is essential for safety, informed consent, and adherence.

Correcting Misinformation

Studies indicate that patients frequently rely on informal sources such as the internet, peers, or commercial dispensaries rather than clinical evidence (Carliner et al., 2017). Nurses must therefore:

- Challenge inaccurate beliefs about safety.
- Clarify indications supported by evidence.
- Explain the variable quality of unregulated products
- Provide transparent information about risks.

Shared Decision Making

Shared decision making improves autonomy, adherence, and satisfaction. Elwyn et al. (2012) recommend a structured approach involving:

- Presentation of all clinically reasonable options.
- Discussion of risks and benefits.
- Exploration of patient preferences.
- Agreement on next steps.

This approach is especially important given the uncertainties in cannabis therapeutics.

Teaching Safe Dosing and Use

Education must include:

- Stepwise titration guidance

- Early signs of adverse effects
- Matching dosing to daily activities
- Avoiding poly-substance use with alcohol, sedatives, or opioids
- Safe storage away from children or vulnerable adults

Guidance on Regulated Versus Unregulated Products

Patients must be advised that unregulated products may contain contaminants or inaccurate cannabinoid concentrations. Philpot et al. (2019) highlight significant variability in unregulated supply chains.

Nurses should guide patients towards:

- Regulated, lab-tested products
- Trusted dispensaries or authorised pharmacies
- Products with clear labelling

Case Study 2: Integrating Dosing, Monitoring, and Education

A 58-year-old patient with chemotherapy-induced nausea is prescribed a balanced THC-CBD oromucosal spray. No psychiatric or cardiovascular risk factors are identified.

The nurse:

- Explains evidence supporting cannabinoids for chemotherapy-induced nausea (National Academies of Sciences, Engineering, and Medicine, 2017)
- Initiates low-dose titration
- Monitors sedation, appetite, mood, and functional status
- Provides education on driving restrictions and safe storage

The patient reports improved symptoms with minimal adverse effects, demonstrating the value of structured dosing, monitoring, and education.

ETHICAL, LEGAL, AND PROFESSIONAL RESPONSIBILITIES IN CANNABIS NURSING

Ethical, legal, and professional considerations form a crucial component of cannabis nursing practice. Nurses must uphold patient safety, respect autonomy, maintain legal compliance, and embody professional integrity within a complex and evolving therapeutic landscape. The evidence base for medical cannabis contains uncertainties, and clinical practice is shaped by regulatory variation, cultural sensitivity, and societal tensions. As a result, cannabis nursing demands rigorous ethical reflexivity, clear professional accountability, and careful engagement with legal requirements (Fischer et al., 2017).

This section examines the ethical foundations of practice, legal constraints, professional duties, and the emerging identity of cannabis nursing within contemporary health care.

Ethical Responsibilities in Cannabis Nursing

Supporting Autonomy While Safeguarding Wellbeing

Respect for autonomy is a core principle of health care ethics. Nurses must ensure that patients make informed decisions grounded in accurate knowledge rather than misinformation or commercial promotion. Evidence indicates that many individuals form beliefs about cannabis from non-clinical sources that may not reflect scientific findings (Carliner et al., 2017). Ethical practice requires nurses to provide balanced information, facilitate understanding, and support voluntary choice.

At the same time, beneficence and non-maleficence require the prevention of foreseeable harm. High potency THC carries known risks for anxiety, cognitive impairment, cardiovascular disturbance, and psychosis in vulnerable individuals (Murray et al., 2017). Nurses must therefore recognise tensions between patient preference and clinical safety, making cautious recommendations consistent with evidence informed therapeutic stewardship.

Ethical Communication and the Duty of Transparency

Ethical communication requires honesty about therapeutic limitations. The National Academies review identified substantial evidence for a small number of indications, alongside insufficient evidence for many others (National Academies of Sciences, Engineering, and Medicine, 2017). Nurses have a duty to ensure that patients are not misled regarding potential benefits or the certainty of outcomes.

Shared decision making provides a structured means of ethical communication. Elwyn and colleagues highlight that patients benefit from transparent discussion of risks and uncertainties and are more likely to adhere to treatment when decision making is collaborative (Elwyn et al., 2012). Cannabis nursing must therefore integrate shared decision making as a standard approach.

Equity and Access

Equitable access to safe, regulated cannabis products is an ethical concern. Philpot and colleagues report that socioeconomic constraints often lead patients to resort to unregulated products due to cost or availability (Philpot et al., 2019). These products carry risks of contamination and inaccurate labelling. Nurses must advocate for equitable access, support harm reduction, and provide guidance to vulnerable patients who may otherwise be exposed to unsafe products.

Legal Responsibilities

Working Within Jurisdictional Regulations

Cannabis laws vary widely across regions. Nurses must remain informed about:

- Which professionals can prescribe cannabis
- Approved indications
- Restrictions on administration within clinical facilities
- Requirements for documentation and consent

- Statutory reporting obligations

Regulatory uncertainty can compromise care and increase professional vulnerability (Fischer et al., 2017). Ethical practice therefore requires awareness of legal frameworks and the implementation of organisational policies that align with statutory expectations.

Documentation and Legal Accountability

Accurate documentation is essential for legal protection and continuity of care. Guidance from the College of Nurses of Ontario emphasises that documentation must include clinical rationale, discussion of risks and benefits, monitoring plans, adverse effects, and patient consent (College of Nurses of Ontario, 2018). In the context of cannabis, where risk profiles are variable and evidence is still evolving, comprehensive documentation is a critical safeguard against future disputes or allegations.

Fitness to Practise Considerations

Cannabis nursing requires clinicians to maintain professional competence. Failure to understand cannabis pharmacology, contraindications, or legal boundaries can compromise patient safety and bring professional sanction. Nurses engaged in cannabis related care must therefore pursue appropriate education, engage with current evidence, and recognise limits to their scope of practice.

Professional Responsibilities

The Emerging Identity of the Cannabis Nurse

The formal recognition of cannabis nursing as a specialty by the American Nurses Association marks an important milestone in professional evolution (American Nurses Association, 2023). This recognition emphasises that cannabis nursing requires a sophisticated body of knowledge, autonomous judgement, and ethical competence. Professional identity formation is essential for confidence, legitimacy, and interprofessional collaboration (Pursio et al., 2021).

Nurses working within this field must develop:

- Clinical expertise in cannabinoid therapeutics.
- Ethical literacy and sensitivity to contested values.
- Legal knowledge relevant to practice scope.
- Communication skills for managing stigma and misinformation.
- Commitment to reflective practice

These components support the consolidation of cannabis nursing as a credible and accountable domain of advanced practice.

Interprofessional Collaboration

Cannabis care is inherently interdisciplinary. Evidence indicates that optimal outcomes occur when nurses collaborate with prescribers, pharmacists, mental health specialists, and social care partners (Whiting et al., 2015). Interprofessional collaboration is vital for:

- Managing complex polypharmacy
- Conducting joint risk assessments
- Ensuring coherent therapeutic plans
- Responding to mental health concerns
- Coordinating palliative or supportive care

Nurses are often the practitioners who spend the most time with patients, placing them in a central position to identify emerging risks, support adherence, and coordinate care across disciplines.

Professional Boundaries and Role Clarity

Nurses must maintain boundaries consistent with their legal scope of practice. In some jurisdictions, nurses may administer but not prescribe cannabis. In others, they may support assessment and monitoring but not provide explicit therapeutic recommendations. Clear role boundaries prevent ethical conflicts and protect practitioners from liability while ensuring that patients receive appropriate, consistent guidance (Canadian Nurses Association, 2017; Russell et al., 2018).

CONCLUSION

Nursing practice involving cannabis-based medicinal products is an emerging area of care that requires clinical competence, ethical judgement, legal awareness, and a clear understanding of professional responsibilities. This chapter has demonstrated that safe and effective cannabis care depends upon rigorous assessment, evidence informed dosing, structured monitoring, and comprehensive patient education. The evidence base, as summarised by major reviews such as the National Academies of Sciences, Engineering, and Medicine (2017), identifies that cannabis offers potential therapeutic benefit for a limited number of conditions, while significant uncertainties remain across many others. Nurses therefore play a crucial role in applying clinical prudence, correcting misinformation, and safeguarding patients from avoidable harm.

The ethical and legal responsibilities of cannabis nursing extend beyond technical skill. Nurses must cultivate an environment that supports autonomy, transparency, shared decision making, and equitable access to regulated products. They must adhere to jurisdictional regulations, maintain accurate documentation, and remain aware of their professional scope and accountability. As the field matures, professional identity formation will become central to the consolidation of cannabis nursing as a recognised specialist practice. The future of cannabis nursing will depend on continued research, curriculum development, organisational governance, and interprofessional collaboration. By adopting a biopsychosocial perspective, embracing therapeutic stewardship, and committing to ongoing reflective practice, nurses can contribute to a responsible, ethically grounded, and evidence informed integration of cannabinoid therapeutics within contemporary health care. This chapter offers a foundation upon which education providers, health organisations, and policy makers can build as they prepare for the inevitable expansion and formalisation of cannabis nursing in the years ahead.

REFERENCES

Abu Baker, D., Cruz Rivera, P. N., Narasimhan, R., Nguyen, N., Tibiriçá, L., Kepner, W. E., O'Malley, P., Nguyen, A. L., & Moore, A. A. (2024). Older adults' use of cannabis and attitudes around disclosing medical cannabis use to their healthcare providers in California: A mixed methods study. *Drugs - Real World Outcomes*, *11*(4), 647–658. DOI: 10.1007/s40801-024-00451-0 PMID: 39294485

Abuhasira, R., Shbiro, L., & Landschaft, Y. (2018). Medical use of cannabis and cannabinoids containing products: Regulations in Europe and North America. *European Journal of Internal Medicine*, *49*, 2–6. DOI: 10.1016/j.ejim.2018.01.001 PMID: 29329891

Adam, K. C. S., Doss, M. K., Pabon, E., Vogel, E. K., & de Wit, H. (2020). Δ9-Tetrahydrocannabinol (THC) impairs visual working memory performance: A randomized crossover trial. *Neuropsychopharmacology : Official Publication of the American College of Neuropsychopharmacology*, *45*(11), 1807–1816. DOI: 10.1038/s41386-020-0690-3 PMID: 32386395

American Nurses Association. (2023, September 27). *ANA officially recognises cannabis nursing as a specialty nursing practice*. https://www.nursingworld.org/news/news-releases/2023/ana-officially-recognizes-cannabis-nursing-as-a-specialty-nursing-practice/

Balachandran, P., Elsohly, M., & Hill, K. P. (2021). Cannabidiol interactions with medications, illicit substances, and alcohol: A comprehensive review. *Journal of General Internal Medicine*, *36*(7), 2074–2084. DOI: 10.1007/s11606-020-06504-8 PMID: 33515191

Bar-Lev Schleider, L., Mechoulam, R., Sikorin, I., Naftali, T., & Novack, V. (2022). Adherence, safety, and effectiveness of medical cannabis and epidemiological characteristics of the patient population: A prospective study. *Frontiers in Medicine*, *9*, 827849. DOI: 10.3389/fmed.2022.827849 PMID: 35223923

Batalla, A., Bhattacharyya, S., Yücel, M., Fusar-Poli, P., Crippa, J. A., Nogué, S., Torrens, M., Pujol, J., Farré, M., & Martin-Santos, R. (2013). Structural and functional imaging studies in chronic cannabis users: A systematic review of adolescent and adult findings. *PLoS One*, *8*(2), e55821. DOI: 10.1371/journal.pone.0055821 PMID: 23390554

Baumbusch, J., & Yip, I. S. (2022). Older adults' experiences of using recreational cannabis for medicinal purposes following legalization. *The International Journal on Drug Policy*, *108*, 103812. DOI: 10.1016/j.drugpo.2022.103812 PMID: 35930902

Becker, M. P., Collins, P. F., & Luciana, M. (2014). Neurocognition in college-aged daily marijuana users. *Journal of Clinical and Experimental Neuropsychology*, *36*(4), 379–398. DOI: 10.1080/13803395.2014.893996 PMID: 24620756

Begley, A. M. (2006). Facilitating the development of moral insight in practice: Teaching ethics and teaching virtue. *Nursing Philosophy*, *7*(4), 257–265. DOI: 10.1111/j.1466-769X.2006.00284.x PMID: 16965307

Bennett, M. I., Rayment, C., Hjermstad, M., Aass, N., Caraceni, A., & Kaasa, S. (2012). Prevalence and aetiology of neuropathic pain in cancer patients: A systematic review. *Pain*, *153*(2), 359–365. DOI: 10.1016/j.pain.2011.10.028 PMID: 22115921

Bimonte, S., Nocerino, D., Schiavo, D., Crisci, M., Cascella, M., & Cuomo, A. (2024). Cannabinoids for cancer-related pain management: An update on therapeutic applications and future perspectives. *Anticancer Research*, *44*(3), 895–900. DOI: 10.21873/anticanres.16883 PMID: 38423660

Black, N., Stockings, E., Campbell, G., Tran, L. T., Zagic, D., Hall, W. D., & Farrell, M. (2019). Cannabinoids for the treatment of mental health disorders: A systematic review and meta-analysis. *The Lancet. Psychiatry*, *6*, 995–1010. DOI: 10.1016/S2215-0366(19)30401-8 PMID: 31672337

Boehnke, K. F., Scott, J. R., Litinas, E., & Clauw, D. J. (2019). Cannabis use for medical conditions: Patterns and outcomes. *Journal of Psychoactive Drugs*, *51*, 425–435.

Bonanni, P., Ragona, F., Fusco, C., Gambardella, A., Operto, F. F., Parmeggiani, L., Sartori, S., & Specchio, N. (2023). Cannabidiol use in patients with Dravet syndrome and Lennox–Gastaut syndrome: Experts' opinions using a nominal group technique approach. *Expert Opinion on Pharmacotherapy*, *24*(5), 655–663. DOI: 10.1080/14656566.2023.2187697 PMID: 37021712

Borrego-Ruiz, A., & Borrego, J. J. (2025). A holistic review of cannabis and its potential risks and benefits in mental health. *Psychiatry International*, *6*(3), 92. DOI: 10.3390/psychiatryint6030092

Borrell-Carrió, F., Suchman, A. L., & Epstein, R. M. (2004). The biopsychosocial model 25 years later: Principles, practice, and scientific inquiry. *Annals of Family Medicine*, *2*(6), 576–582. DOI: 10.1370/afm.245 PMID: 15576544

Brown, J. D., & Winterstein, A. G. (2020). Potential adverse drug events and drug–drug interactions with medical cannabis. *Journal of Clinical Medicine*, *9*, 989. DOI: 10.3390/jcm9040919

Broyd, S. J., van Hell, H. H., Beale, C., Yücel, M., & Solowij, N. (2016). Acute and chronic effects of cannabinoids on human cognition: A systematic review. *Biological Psychiatry*, *79*(7), 557–567. DOI: 10.1016/j.biopsych.2015.12.002 PMID: 26858214

Canadian Nurses Association. (2017). Cannabis for medical purposes: Legal implications for nurses. *The Canadian Nurse*, *113*(1), 16–18. PMID: 29236416

Carliner, H., Mauro, P. M., Brown, Q. L., Shmulewitz, D., Rahim-Juwel, R., Sarvet, A. L., Wall, M. M., & Hasin, D. S. (2017). The widening gender gap in marijuana use prevalence in the United States during a period of economic change. *JAMA Psychiatry*, *74*, 567–575.

Charani, E., & Holmes, A. H. (2013). Antimicrobial stewardship programmes: The need for wider engagement. *BMJ Quality & Safety*, *22*(11), 885–887. DOI: 10.1136/bmjqs-2013-002444 PMID: 24046440

Chayasirisobhon, S. (2021). Mechanisms of action and pharmacokinetics of cannabis. *The Permanente Journal*, *25*, 19–200. PMID: 33635755

Chou, R., Ahmed, A. Y., Dana, T., Morasco, B. J., Bougatsos, C., Fu, R., & Williams, L. (2025). *Living systematic review on cannabis and other plant-based treatments for chronic pain: 2025 update*. Agency for Healthcare Research and Quality. DOI: 10.23970/AHRQEPCCER250UPDATE2025

College of Nurses of Ontario. (2018). *Practice standard: Medical cannabis*. https://www.cno.org/en/learn-about-standards-guidelines/educational-tools/ask-practice/medical-marijuana/

Crowell, B., Seamon, M., Buckley, T., & Gildner, J. (2021). Nurses' knowledge, perceptions and clinical experiences with medical cannabis. *Journal of Clinical Nursing*, *30*, 3530–3540.

Cummings, H., Ul Haq, M. Z., Dargham, A., Shakeel, N., Busse, J. W., Darzi, A. J., & Alvarez, E. (2024). Individuals' values and preferences regarding medical cannabis for chronic pain: A descriptive qualitative study. *Journal of Pain Research*, *17*, 21–34. DOI: 10.2147/JPR.S432823 PMID: 38192366

Damkier, P., Lassen, D., Christensen, M. M. H., Madsen, K. G., Hellfritzsch, M., & Pottegård, A. (2019). Interaction between warfarin and cannabis. *Basic & Clinical Pharmacology & Toxicology*, *124*(1), 28–31. DOI: 10.1111/bcpt.13152 PMID: 30326170

Das, A., Hendershot, C. S., Husain, M. I., Knyahnytska, Y., Elsaid, S., Le Foll, B., & Kloiber, S. (2024). Perceptions, experiences and patterns of cannabis use in individuals with mood and anxiety disorders in the context of cannabis legalization and medical cannabis programme in Canada: A qualitative study. *Pharmacopsychiatry*, *57*(3), 141–151. DOI: 10.1055/a-2264-1047 PMID: 38467156

de Bode, N., Kroon, E., Sznitman, S. R., & Cousijn, J. (2025). The differential effects of medicinal cannabis on mental health: A systematic review. *Clinical Psychology Review*, *118*, 102581. DOI: 10.1016/j.cpr.2025.102581 PMID: 40186931

Devinsky, O., Cross, H., Laux, L., Marsh, E., Miller, I., Nabbout, R., Scheffer, I., Thiele, E., & Wright, S.Cannabidiol Study Group. (2017). Trial of cannabidiol for drug-resistant seizures in the Dravet syndrome. *The New England Journal of Medicine*, *376*(21), 2011–2020. DOI: 10.1056/NEJMoa1611618 PMID: 28538134

Di Marzo, V. (2018). New approaches and challenges to targeting the endocannabinoid system. *Nature Reviews. Neuroscience*, *19*, 723–738. PMID: 30116049

Dowell, D., Ragan, K. R., Jones, C. M., Baldwin, G. T., & Chou, R. (2022). CDC clinical practice guideline for prescribing opioids for pain—United States, 2022. *MMWR. Recommendations and Reports*, *71*(3), 1–95. DOI: 10.15585/mmwr.rr7103a1 PMID: 36327391

Elwyn, G., Frosch, D., Thomson, R., Joseph-Williams, N., Lloyd, A., Kinnersley, P., Coulter, A., Barry, M., Eden, A., & Rollnick, S. (2012). Shared decision making: A model for clinical practice. *Journal of General Internal Medicine*, *27*(10), 1361–1367. DOI: 10.1007/s11606-012-2077-6 PMID: 22618581

Engel, G. L. (1977). The need for a new medical model: A challenge for biomedicine. *Science*, *196*(4286), 129–136. DOI: 10.1126/science.847460 PMID: 847460

Falk-Rafael, A. (2005). Advancing nursing theory through theory-guided practice: The emergence of a critical caring perspective. *Advances in Nursing Science*, *28*(1), 38–49. DOI: 10.1097/00012272-200501000-00005 PMID: 15718937

Figueiredo, P. R., Tolomeo, S., Steele, J. D., & Baldacchino, A. (2020). Neurocognitive consequences of chronic cannabis use: A systematic review and meta-analysis. *Neuroscience and Biobehavioral Reviews*, *108*, 358–369. DOI: 10.1016/j.neubiorev.2019.10.014 PMID: 31715191

Fischer, B., Russell, C., Sabioni, P., Van den Brink, W., Le Foll, B., Hall, W., Rehm, J., & Room, R. (2017). Lower-risk cannabis use guidelines: A comprehensive update of evidence and recommendations. *American Journal of Public Health, 107*(8), e1–e12. DOI: 10.2105/AJPH.2017.303818 PMID: 28644037

Gastmans, C. (2013). Dignity-enhancing nursing care: A foundational ethical framework. *Nursing Ethics, 20*(2), 142–149. DOI: 10.1177/0969733012473772 PMID: 23466947

Ghelani, A. (2021). Cannabis use among mental health professionals: A qualitative study of cannabis-related risk perceptions. *Journal of Drug Issues, 51*(4), 679–689. DOI: 10.1177/00220426211032558 PMID: 34511638

Hall, W., & Degenhardt, L. (2014). The adverse health effects of chronic cannabis use. *Drug Testing and Analysis, 6*(1–2), 39–45. DOI: 10.1002/dta.1506 PMID: 23836598

Hallinan, C. M., Gunn, J. M., & Bonomo, Y. A. (2021). Implementation of medicinal cannabis in Australia: Innovation or upheaval? *BMJ Open, 11*(10), e054044. DOI: 10.1136/bmjopen-2021-054044 PMID: 34686558

Hardy, J., Greer, R., Huggett, G., Kearney, A., Gurgenci, T., & Good, P. (2023). Phase IIb randomised, placebo-controlled, dose-escalating, double-blind study of cannabidiol oil for symptom relief in advanced cancer (MedCan1-CBD). *Journal of Clinical Oncology, 41*(7), 1444–1452. DOI: 10.1200/JCO.22.01632 PMID: 36409969

Hardy, J. R., Greer, R. M., Pelecanos, A. M., Huggett, G. E., Kearney, A. M., Gurgenci, T. H., & Good, P. D. (2025). Medicinal cannabis for symptom control in advanced cancer: A double-blind, placebo-controlled, randomised clinical trial of 1:1 tetrahydrocannabinol and cannabidiol. *Supportive Care in Cancer, 33*(8), 1–12. DOI: 10.1007/s00520-025-09763-5 PMID: 40705150

Hartley, S., Simon, N., Larabi, A., Vaugier, I., Barbot, F., Quera-Salva, M. A., & Alvarez, J. C. (2019). Effect of smoked cannabis on vigilance and accident risk using simulated driving in occasional and chronic users and the pharmacokinetic–pharmacodynamic relationship. *Clinical Chemistry, 65*(5), 684–693. DOI: 10.1373/clinchem.2018.299727 PMID: 30872375

Ho, J. J. Y., Goh, C., Leong, C. S. A., Ng, K. Y., & Bakhtiar, A. (2024). Evaluation of potential drug–drug interactions with medical cannabis. *Clinical and Translational Science, 17*(5), e13812. DOI: 10.1111/cts.13812 PMID: 38720531

Hossain, M. K., & Chae, H. J. (2024). Medical cannabis: From research breakthroughs to shifting public perceptions and ensuring safe use. *Integrative Medicine Research, 13*(4), 101094. DOI: 10.1016/j.imr.2024.101094 PMID: 39640076

Hunault, C. C., Mensinga, T. T., Böcker, K. B. E., Schipper, C. M. A., Kruidenier, M., Leenders, M. E., de Vries, I., & Meulenbelt, J. (2009). Cognitive and psychomotor effects in males after smoking a combination of tobacco and cannabis containing up to 69 mg delta-9-tetrahydrocannabinol (THC). *Psychopharmacology, 204*(1), 85–94. DOI: 10.1007/s00213-008-1440-0 PMID: 19099294

Hurn, S. (2023). An individual's lived experiences of taking cannabis-based medicinal products to treat anxiety. *International Journal of Environmental Research and Public Health, 20*(18), 6776. DOI: 10.3390/ijerph20186776 PMID: 37754635

Johnson, J. R., Burnell-Nugent, M., Lossignol, D., Ganae-Motan, E. D., Potts, R., & Fallon, M. T. (2010). Multicentre, double-blind, randomised, placebo-controlled study of nabiximols in patients with opioid-refractory cancer pain. *Journal of Pain and Symptom Management*, *39*, 167–179. DOI: 10.1016/j.jpainsymman.2009.06.008 PMID: 19896326

Kloft, L., Otgaar, H., Blokland, A., Monds, L. A., Toennes, S. W., Loftus, E. F., & Ramaekers, J. G. (2020). Cannabis increases susceptibility to false memory. *Proceedings of the National Academy of Sciences of the United States of America*, *117*(9), 4585–4589. DOI: 10.1073/pnas.1920162117 PMID: 32041881

Köck, P., Badek, A., Meyer, M., Klaassen, A. L., Walter, M., & Kindler, J. (2024). Cannabinoids for treating psychiatric disorders in youth: A systematic review of randomised controlled trials. *Child and Adolescent Psychiatry and Mental Health*, *18*(1), 158. DOI: 10.1186/s13034-024-00846-5 PMID: 39696457

Lewis, N., Broitman, D., & Sznitman, S. R. (2015). Medical cannabis: A framing analysis of Israeli newspaper coverage. *Science Communication*, *37*(6), 675–702. DOI: 10.1177/1075547015608507

Lopera, V., Rodríguez, A., & Amariles, P. (2022). Clinical relevance of drug interactions with cannabis: A systematic review. *Journal of Clinical Medicine*, *11*(5), 1154. DOI: 10.3390/jcm11051154 PMID: 35268245

Lucas, P., & Walsh, Z. (2017). Medical cannabis access, use, and substitution for prescription opioids and other substances: A survey of authorised medical cannabis patients. *Harm Reduction Journal*, *14*, 58. DOI: 10.1186/s12954-017-0183-9 PMID: 28821296

McIntosh, N., Wilson, N. J., Povalej, P., Hunt, L., & Lewis, P. (2024). An exploration of registered nurses' experiences caring for patients taking medicinal cannabis. *Nursing Open*, *11*(10), e70063. DOI: 10.1002/nop2.70063 PMID: 39455290

Murray, R. M., Quigley, H., Quattrone, D., Englund, A., & Di Forti, M. (2017). Traditional marijuana, high-potency cannabis, and synthetic cannabinoids: Increasing risk for psychosis. *The Lancet. Psychiatry*, *4*, 643–653.

Nabil, E. L., Metouekel, A., Serondo, H. U., El Koufi, C., El Amri, H., El Fahime, E., & El Kazzouli, S. (2024). Cannabis unveiled: From history to innovation, exploring the world of cannabis strains, chemistry, industry and economic impact. *Chemical Review and Letters*, *7*(5), 827–845.

National Academies of Sciences, Engineering, and Medicine. (2017). *The health effects of cannabis and cannabinoids: The current state of evidence and recommendations for research*. National Academies Press.

Ntais, C., Kontodimopoulos, N., & Melanthiou, Y. (2025). Marketing management and policymaking for medical cannabis: Overcoming barriers and shaping strategies. *Cannabis (Research Society on Marijuana)*. Advance online publication. DOI: 10.26828/cannabis/2025/000316 PMID: 40909146

Nyblade, L., Stockton, M. A., Giger, K., Bond, V., Ekstrand, M. L., Lean, R. M., Mitchell, E. M., Nelson, L. R. E., Sapag, J. C., Siraprapasiri, T., Turan, J., & Wouters, E. (2019). Stigma in health facilities: Why it matters and how we can change it. *BMC Medicine*, *17*(1), 25. DOI: 10.1186/s12916-019-1256-2 PMID: 30764806

O'Brien, K., Beilby, J., Frans, M., Lynskey, M., Barnes, M., Jayasuriya, M., Athanasiou-Fragkouli, A., Blair, P., & Nutt, D. (2023). Medicinal cannabis for pain: Real-world data on three-month changes in symptoms and quality of life. *Drug Science, Policy and Law*, *9*, 20503245231172535. DOI: 10.1177/20503245231172535

Olson, R. E., Smith, A., Huggett, G., Good, P., Dudley, M., & Hardy, J. (2022). Using a qualitative sub-study to inform the design and delivery of randomised controlled trials on medicinal cannabis for symptom relief in patients with advanced cancer. *Trials*, *23*(1), 752. DOI: 10.1186/s13063-022-06691-1 PMID: 36064621

Paulraj, S., Upreti, P., Tamirisa, K., & Batnyam, U. (2025). Arrhythmias and cannabis use: A comprehensive overview. *Heart Rhythm O2*, *6*(1), 78–85. DOI: 10.1016/j.hroo.2024.10.020 PMID: 40224259

Philpot, L. M., Ebbert, J. O., & Hurt, R. T. (2019). A survey of the attitudes, beliefs, and knowledge about medical cannabis among primary care providers. *BMC Family Practice*, *20*(1), 17. DOI: 10.1186/s12875-019-0906-y PMID: 30669979

Pravosud, V., Lum, E., Vali, M., Cohen, B. E., Hoggatt, K. J., Byers, A. L., Austin, P. C., Walter, L. C., Hasin, D., Zaman, T., & Keyhani, S. (2025). Cannabis use among older adults. *JAMA Network Open*, *8*(5), e2510173. DOI: 10.1001/jamanetworkopen.2025.10173 PMID: 40366653

Pursio, K., Kankkunen, P., Sanner-Stiehr, E., & Kvist, T. (2021). Professional autonomy in nursing: An integrative review. *Journal of Nursing Management*, *29*(6), 1565–1577. DOI: 10.1111/jonm.13282 PMID: 33548098

Ramaekers, J. G., Kauert, G., van Ruitenbeek, P., Theunissen, E. L., Schneider, E., & Moeller, M. R. (2006). High-potency marijuana impairs executive function and inhibitory motor control. *Neuropsychopharmacology : Official Publication of the American College of Neuropsychopharmacology*, *31*(10), 2296–2303. DOI: 10.1038/sj.npp.1301068 PMID: 16572123

Riba, J., Valle, M., Sampedro, F., Rodríguez-Pujadas, A., Martínez-Horta, S., Kulisevsky, J., & Rodríguez-Fornells, A. (2015). Telling true from false: Cannabis users show increased susceptibility to false memories. *Molecular Psychiatry*, *20*(6), 772–777. DOI: 10.1038/mp.2015.36 PMID: 25824306

Rice, L. J., Cannon, L., Dadlani, N., Cheung, M. M. Y., Einfeld, S. L., Efron, D., Dossetor, D. R., & Elliott, E. J. (2024). Efficacy of cannabinoids in neurodevelopmental and neuropsychiatric disorders among children and adolescents: A systematic review. *European Child & Adolescent Psychiatry*, *33*(2), 505–526. DOI: 10.1007/s00787-023-02169-w PMID: 36864363

Roten, A., Baker, N. L., & Gray, K. M. (2015). Cognitive performance in a placebo-controlled pharmacotherapy trial for youth with marijuana dependence. *Addictive Behaviors*, *45*, 119–123. DOI: 10.1016/j.addbeh.2015.01.013 PMID: 25661990

Russell, K., Cahill, M., Gowen, K., Cronquist, R., Smith, V., & Borris-Hale, C. (2018). Nursing care of the patient using medical marijuana. *Journal of Nursing Regulation*, *9*(2), S23–S27. DOI: 10.1016/S2155-8256(18)30094-2

Schuster, R. M., Gilman, J., Schoenfeld, D., Evenden, J., Hareli, M., Ulysse, C., Nip, E., Hanly, A., Zhang, H., & Evins, A. E. (2018). One month of cannabis abstinence in adolescents and young adults is associated with improved memory. *The Journal of Clinical Psychiatry, 79*(6), 18m12138.

Schweiger, V., Ganz, B., Martini, A., Sarzi-Puttini, P., Bazzichi, L., Bonora, E., Vendramin, P., Nizzero, M., Zamboni, L., Polati, L., Lugoboni, F., Raniero, D., Polati, E., & Del Balzo, G. (2025). Medical cannabis for chronic pain management: Questions and answers between clinical and medico-legal issues. *Clinical and Experimental Rheumatology*. Advance online publication. DOI: 10.55563/clinexprheumatol/o23y55 PMID: 40556619

Sellman, D. (2024). Virtue ethics and nursing practice. In *Key Concepts and Issues in Nursing Ethics* (pp. 135–146). Springer Nature Switzerland. DOI: 10.1007/978-3-031-54108-7_9

Sinclair, J., Parker, M., & Armour, M. (2024). Cultivating understanding: Navigating the complexities associated with medicinal cannabis and implications for nursing practice. *The Australian Journal of Advanced Nursing*, *41*(3), 1–5.

Sorkhou, M., Bedder, R. H., & George, T. P. (2021). The behavioural sequelae of cannabis use in healthy people: A systematic review. *Frontiers in Psychiatry*, *12*, 630247. DOI: 10.3389/fpsyt.2021.630247 PMID: 33664685

Srinivasana, G., & Shukla, D. (2024). Cannabis-derived pharmaceutical products: Therapeutic, pharmacokinetic and clinical implications – A comprehensive review. *Indian Drugs, 61*(10).

Stacey, D., Légaré, F., Lewis, K., Barry, M. J., Bennett, C. L., Eden, K. B., Holmes-Rovner, M., Llewellyn-Thomas, H., Lyddiatt, A., Thomson, R., & Trevena, L. (2017). Decision aids for people facing health treatment or screening decisions. *Cochrane Database of Systematic Reviews*, *4*(4), CD001431. DOI: 10.1002/14651858.CD001431.pub5 PMID: 28402085

Tait, M. A., Costa, D. S., Campbell, R., Norman, R., Warne, L. N., Schug, S., & Rutherford, C. (2023). Health-related quality of life in patients accessing medicinal cannabis in Australia: The QUEST initiative results of a 3-month follow-up observational study. *PLoS One*, *18*(9), e0290549. DOI: 10.1371/journal.pone.0290549 PMID: 37672515

Vázquez, M., García-Carnelli, C., Maldonado, C., & Fagiolino, P. (2021). Clinical pharmacokinetics of cannabinoids and potential drug–drug interactions. In *Cannabinoids and sleep: Molecular, functional and clinical aspects* (pp. 27–42). Springer International Publishing. DOI: 10.1007/978-3-030-61663-2_3

Volkow, N. D., Hampson, A. J., & Baler, R. D. (2017). Don't worry, be happy: Endocannabinoids and cannabis at the intersection of stress and reward. *Annual Review of Pharmacology and Toxicology*, *57*(1), 285–308. DOI: 10.1146/annurev-pharmtox-010716-104615 PMID: 27618739

Wade, D. T., & Halligan, P. W. (2017). The biopsychosocial model of illness: A model whose time has come. *Clinical Rehabilitation*, *31*(8), 995–1004. DOI: 10.1177/0269215517709890 PMID: 28730890

Wang, L., Hong, P. J., May, C., Rehman, Y., Oparin, Y., Hong, C. J., Hong, B. Y., AminiLari, M., Gallo, L., Kaushal, A., Craigie, S., Couban, R. J., Kum, E., Shanthanna, H., Price, I., Upadhye, S., Ware, M. A., Campbell, F., Buchbinder, R., & Busse, J. W. (2021). Medical cannabis or cannabinoids for chronic non-cancer and cancer-related pain: A systematic review and meta-analysis of randomised clinical trials. *BMJ (Clinical Research Ed.)*, *374*(1034), n1034. DOI: 10.1136/bmj.n1034 PMID: 34497047

Weinstein, A., Brickner, O., Lerman, H., Greemland, M., Bloch, M., Lester, H., Chisin, R., Sarne, Y., Mechoulam, R., Bar-Hamburger, R., Freedman, N., & Even-Sapir, E. (2008). A study investigating the acute dose–response effects of 13 mg and 17 mg Δ9-tetrahydrocannabinol on cognitive-motor skills, subjective and autonomic measures in regular users of marijuana. *Journal of Psychopharmacology (Oxford, England)*, *22*(4), 441–451. DOI: 10.1177/0269881108088194 PMID: 18635724

Whiting, P. F., Wolff, R. F., Deshpande, S., Di Nisio, M., Duffy, S., Hernández, A. V., Keurentjes, J. C., Lang, S., Misso, K., Ryder, S., Schmidlkofer, S., Westwood, M., & Kleijnen, J. (2015). Cannabinoids for medical use: A systematic review and meta-analysis. *Journal of the American Medical Association*, *313*(24), 2456–2473. DOI: 10.1001/jama.2015.6358 PMID: 26103030

Zeng, L., Lytvyn, L., Wang, X., Kithulegoda, N., Agterberg, S., Shergill, Y., Esfahani, M. A., Heen, A. F., Agoritsas, T., Guyatt, G. H., & Busse, J. W. (2021). Values and preferences toward medical cannabis among people living with chronic pain: A mixed-methods systematic review. *BMJ Open*, *11*(9), e050831. DOI: 10.1136/bmjopen-2021-050831 PMID: 34493521

Zeraatkar, D., Cooper, M. A., Agarwal, A., Vernooij, R. W., Leung, G., Loniewski, K., Dookie, J. E., Ahmed, M. M., Hong, B. Y., Hong, C., Hong, P., Couban, R., Agoritsas, T., & Busse, J. W. (2022). Long-term and serious harms of medical cannabis and cannabinoids for chronic pain: A systematic review of non-randomised studies. *BMJ Open*, *12*(8), e054282. DOI: 10.1136/bmjopen-2021-054282 PMID: 35926992

Zolotov, Y., Metri, S., Calabria, E., & Kogan, M. (2021). Medical cannabis education among healthcare trainees: A scoping review. *Complementary Therapies in Medicine*, *58*, 102675. DOI: 10.1016/j.ctim.2021.102675 PMID: 33539943

KEY TERMS AND DEFINITIONS

Adverse effects: Unintended and harmful effects associated with treatment, such as dizziness, sedation, anxiety, tachycardia, or cognitive impairment.

Biopsychosocial model: A framework for assessment and care that considers biological, psychological, and social influences on health and illness.

Cannabidiol (CBD): A non-intoxicating cannabinoid that has recognised therapeutic uses, particularly in some seizure disorders, and is generally associated with a lower risk of psychotropic adverse effects than THC.

Cannabinoids: Active chemical compounds found in cannabis, such as tetrahydrocannabinol and cannabidiol, which produce physiological and clinical effects.

Cannabis nursing: An emerging field of nursing practice focused on the assessment, monitoring, education, and safe management of patients using cannabis-based medicines.

Clinical competence: The integrated knowledge, skills, judgement, and professional behaviour required to deliver safe, effective, and accountable care.

Clinical governance: The systems and processes through which healthcare organisations maintain standards of safety, quality, and accountability.

Clinical prudence: Careful and ethically informed professional judgement used when making decisions in situations where evidence is limited, evolving, or uncertain.

Drug interactions: Changes in the effect of one medicine caused by the presence of another substance, including cannabis-derived products.

Endocannabinoid system: A biological regulatory system made up of receptors, endogenous cannabinoids, and enzymes that influences pain, mood, appetite, memory, and immune responses.

Informed consent: A patient's voluntary agreement to treatment after receiving sufficient information about benefits, risks, alternatives, and uncertainties.

Interprofessional collaboration: Joint working between nurses and other healthcare professionals to ensure coordinated, safe, and effective patient care.

Medical cannabis: The therapeutic use of cannabis-derived products for symptom management or treatment within a clinical context.

Patient education: The process of providing clear, balanced, and evidence-based information to help patients understand treatment, risks, and safe use.

Polypharmacy: The use of multiple medicines by one patient, increasing the risk of drug interactions and adverse effects.

Professional accountability: The duty of nurses to justify their actions and decisions in relation to professional, ethical, and legal standards.

Professional identity formation: The development of a clear sense of role, values, responsibilities, and professional purpose within a specialist area of practice.

Risk stratification: The process of identifying factors that may increase a patient's likelihood of harm or poor outcomes from cannabis use, such as mental illness, cardiovascular disease, or polypharmacy.

Shared decision making: A collaborative process in which clinicians and patients discuss options, risks, benefits, and personal preferences before agreeing on a treatment plan.

Stigma: Negative social attitudes or judgements that may discourage patients from disclosing cannabis use or seeking professional support.

Tetrahydrocannabinol (THC): The principal psychoactive cannabinoid in cannabis, associated with symptom relief in some conditions but also with intoxication, anxiety, and cognitive impairment.

Therapeutic stewardship: The professional responsibility to ensure that cannabis-based therapies are used cautiously, proportionately, ethically, and on the basis of the best available evidence.

Titration: The careful adjustment of dose over time in order to achieve therapeutic benefit while minimising harm.

Chapter 5
Comprehensive Nursing Approaches to Cannabis Nursing:
The Cannabis Nurse Navigator®

Nique Pichette
http://orcid.org/0009-0008-0017-7427
Olin Neuropsychiatry Research Center, USA

Ariana Caruso
http://orcid.org/0009-0004-0845-8494
Olin Neuropsychiatry Research Center, USA

Cole Arnold
http://orcid.org/0009-0008-5755-7201
Olin Neuropsychiatry Research Center, USA

Lisa Capitani
Olin Neuropsychiatry Research Center, USA

Jodi Chapin
http://orcid.org/0009-0004-4271-4340
Olin Neuropsychiatry Research Center, USA

Susan Rosen
Olin Neuropsychiatry Research Center, USA

ABSTRACT

The Cannabis Nurse Navigator is a registered nurse with specialized training in cannabis science, clinical assessment, and patient education. Functioning at the intersection of nursing care, clinical research, and patient advocacy, the Cannabis Nurse Navigator serves as a guide and liaison between patients, providers, and healthcare systems. This integrative approach allows nurses to address patient needs that often fall outside traditional care models, needs shaped by stigma, inconsistent regulation, and rapidly emerging evidence. The Cannabis Nurse Navigator does not recommend specific products, direct patients to commercial vendors, or engage in prescribing; rather, the role focuses on assessment, education, harm reduction, and systems navigation within the nursing scope of practice.

CHAPTER OBJECTIVES

At the conclusion of this chapter, the reader will be able to:

DOI: 10.4018/979-8-3373-7287-7.ch005

1. define the cannabis nurse navigator role as a competency based, systems level nursing role grounded in professional standards, with a focus on reducing barriers to safe, coordinated care across the healthcare continuum;
2. differentiate the cannabis nurse navigator role from prescriptive, advisory, commercial and direct care cannabis roles, with clear delineation of scope of practice and professional boundaries;
3. apply core principles of nurse navigation, including assessment, care coordination, education, advocacy, and systems literacy, to cannabis-related care across healthcare systems;
4. examine the current evidence base supporting the need for structured nursing roles in cannabis-related care, including implications for safety, quality, and patient outcomes;
5. analyze implementation considerations for integrating the cannabis nurse navigator within healthcare systems, including organizational barriers, resource allocation, ethical safeguards, and interdisciplinary coordination; and
6. describe the scope and boundaries of navigation, including when and how cannabis nurse navigator involvement is initiated, operationalized, and transitioned within the continuum of care.

KEY ARGUMENT

Cannabis integration is not solely a pharmacologic or policy issue but a nursing problem of navigation, education, care coordination, case management, and safety. The cannabis nurse navigator is proposed as a systems-level nursing response designed to reduce fragmentation, improve communication, and support safe, evidence-informed cannabis-related care within healthcare systems.

CONCEPTUAL MODEL AND ROLE DEFINITION

Nurse navigation has been extensively studied in oncology and chronic care settings. Oncology nurse navigators coordinate appointments, facilitate referrals, educate patients and families, and provide psychosocial support. The oncology nurse navigator model has demonstrated improved patient outcomes, increased treatment adherence, and reduced system inefficiencies.

Core principles of nurse navigation include assessment, care coordination, education, advocacy, and systems literacy. Together, these competencies enable nurses to guide patients through complex healthcare systems and support informed decision-making. This holistic mindset moves beyond isolated patient events to see the underlying structures while fostering awareness that individual actions ripple through larger networks, crucial for tackling global challenges, such as sustainability. These principles of the Cannabis Nurse Navigator are directly transferable to cannabis care, where similar challenges exist. The Cannabis Nurse Navigator, therefore, occupies a critical intersection between clinical expertise, organizational systems, and patient-centered advocacy (Katerenchuk & Salas, 2023).

The Cannabis Nurse Navigator is responsible for integrating cannabis-related care into existing healthcare systems. Functioning at the intersection of nursing leadership, clinical research, and patient advocacy, the cannabis nurse navigator serves as a guide and liaison between patients, providers, and healthcare systems (Pruitt & Sportsman, 2013). This integrative approach allows nurses to address patient needs that often fall outside traditional care models, particularly those shaped by stigma, inconsistent regulation, and rapidly emerging evidence. The Cannabis Nurse Navigator does not recommend specific products, direct patients to commercial vendors, or engage in prescribing; rather, the role focuses on system oversight, protocol development, care coordination, education, harm reduction, and systems navigation within the nursing scope of practice. Modeled on proven navigation roles in oncology and chronic care, the Cannabis Nurse Navigator's primary focus is system navigation and care integration, without direct prescribing.

The Cannabis Nurse Navigator acts as the essential bridge between the patient, their clinical team, and the complex legal, regulatory, and clinical landscape of medical cannabis. The role emphasizes coordination, policy alignment, and organizational leadership, rather than direct bedside care. The Cannabis Nurse Navigator does this by leading the development of evidence-based educational frameworks, staff training, and patient education pathways to ensure access to accurate cannabis-related educational resources across the healthcare system.

Transitioning from theory to practice, the Cannabis Nurse Navigator fulfills five core functions that define its professional scope:

1. Assessment: Develops, standardizes, and supports implementation of cannabis-related assessment pathways across care settings; may oversee or coordinate specialty assessment processes performed by the cannabis nurse or other qualified clinicians.
2. Education: Leads development of evidence-based educational frameworks, staff training, and patient education pathways; ensures access to accurate cannabis-related educational resources across the healthcare system.
3. Care coordination: Facilitates communication among the interdisciplinary healthcare team, ensuring cannabis-related patient information is documented and integrated into overall care planning.
4. Advocacy: Promotes destigmatization and equitable access for patients who use medical cannabis, with particular attention to marginalized or underserved populations.
5. Harm reduction and safety monitoring: Establishes screening and referral workflows for identifying misuse, dependence risk, cannabis use disorder (CUD), cannabis hyperemesis syndrome (CHS), and other cannabis-related safety concerns within interdisciplinary care systems.

The primary responsibilities of the Cannabis Nurse Navigator include:

- coordinating cannabis-related care across interdisciplinary teams;
- developing referral pathways and structured care protocols;
- integrating cannabis-related documentation into electronic health records;
- aligning institutional policies with evolving legal and regulatory frameworks;
- leading interprofessional education and simulation exercises; and
- supporting healthcare teams in complex cannabis-related clinical decision making.

Through these activities, the Cannabis Nurse Navigator helps healthcare organizations move beyond fragmented or informal approaches to cannabis use, replacing them with structured and evidence-informed systems of care. The Cannabis Nurse Navigator's patient interaction is typically indirect, occurring through guidance of care teams, development of care pathways, and coordination of interdisciplinary services. The ultimate impact of the role is reflected at the organizational level, including improvements in care continuity, patient safety oversight, and equitable access to cannabis-related healthcare services.

As previously defined, the Cannabis Nurse Navigator model is grounded in a standardized set of core nursing competencies, its application is inherently adaptable to clinical specialties and practice settings. Oncology, hospice and palliative care, psychiatry, primary care, and chronic disease management each present distinct patient needs, symptom targets, risk profiles, and regulatory considerations related to cannabis use. Accordingly, the Cannabis Nurse Navigator applies a common framework of system oversight, protocol development, coordination, and escalation, while integrating specialty-specific clinical knowledge, population-based risk assessment, and interdisciplinary collaboration (American Cannabis Nurses Association, 2024; Freeman & Rodriguez, 2011; Pruitt & Sportsman, 2013).

As federal and state policies continue to evolve, cannabis-related conditions, such as CUD and CHS, become widely recognized and diagnosed, the need for systemic screening and management of cannabis use is increasingly clear (Patel, 2022; Russo et al., 2022). The Cannabis Nurse Navigator will address this gap by providing specialized knowledge and care coordination, which may otherwise be lacking in general healthcare systems (Carter et al., 2018; Kokorelias et al., 2022; Kokorelias et al., 2021; Zibrik et al., 2016).

Evidence provided by Chan et al.'s 2023 systematic review of research on the oncology nurse navigator role suggests that the implementation of this role has positive effects on patients' quality of life, satisfaction with care, and hospital use, and can suggest cost-effectiveness of navigator programs within oncology. The rise in cannabis use for both medical and nonmedical purposes, coupled with the medical community's lack of knowledge regarding the endocannabinoid system and cannabinoid therapeutics, raises the question of whether a Cannabis Nurse Navigator can similarly enhance patient outcomes. Studies have shown that physicians and nurses may be able to influence patients' cannabis use through education and health strategies, but the lack of provider training in cannabis-related healthcare limits their ability to provide effective care (Rice et al., 2022; Szaflarski et al., 2020).

To ensure consistency, safety, and professional accountability, the Cannabis Nurse Navigator role aligns with existing nursing standards and regulatory systems. The model builds upon established principles of nurse navigation as defined by the ANA Nursing Scope and Standards of Practice. It further integrates the competencies outlined in Clinical Research Nursing: Scope and Standards of Practice (International Association of Clinical Research Nurses, 2024) and Cannabis Nursing: Scope and Standards of Practice (American Cannabis Nurses Association, 2024). Together, these systems provide a foundation for an evidence-based nursing role that promotes ethical, compassionate, and patient-centered navigation for individuals utilizing cannabinoid therapeutics. Additionally, the Cannabis Nurse Navigator incorporates guidelines from the National Council of State Boards of Nursing for medical cannabis nursing (Russell et al., 2018). According to these guidelines, nurses in this role are expected to:

1. possess a clear understanding of the current legal landscape surrounding cannabis, concise knowledge of medical cannabis programs, and patient rights;
2. maintain expertise in the endocannabinoid system and cannabinoid pharmacology;
3. safely and effectively manage patient care related to cannabis use, including, but not limited to, patient education and harm reduction strategies; and
4. approach patients without bias regarding their treatment choices, including cannabis use.

While the Cannabis Nurse Navigator model is grounded in a standardized set of core nursing competencies, its application is inherently adaptable to clinical specialties and practice settings. For example, while an oncology focused cannabis nurse may support symptom palliation, patient education regarding potential drug–drug interactions, and continuity of care, the hospice and palliative cannabis nurse emphasizes comfort, quality of life, and caregiver education within established plans of care; the psychiatric-focused cannabis nurse prioritizes risk identification, screening for CUD and psychosis risk, patient education, and harm-reduction strategies which are consistent with cannabis nursing scope of practice and public protection mandates (National Academies of Sciences, Engineering, and Medicine, 2017; National Consensus Project for Quality Palliative Care, 2018; Russell et al., 2018; Szaflarski et al., 2020).

While these professional frameworks establish the ethical and clinical parameters of practice, ongoing research continues to expand the empirical foundation for cannabis-related nursing care. The Cannabis Nurse Navigator role positions the nurse as a central agent in bridging the research-to-practice gap, herein referred to as the "cannabis care gap." Through this model, cannabis nurses are equipped to identify risk, monitor patterns of use, and implement evidence-based interventions within real-world healthcare environments. Building on these theoretical foundations, early research has begun to explore how cannabis-related care is understood and managed within clinical systems. Initial findings from the pilot study of Pichette et al. (2025) informed the ongoing expansion of the research into *Exploring Cannabis Patient Care: Hartford HealthCare Staff Experience and Knowledge*, which examines a broader institutional knowledge, perception, and practices surrounding medical cannabis use across diverse care settings. In parallel, the completed study *Evaluating Individual Criteria to Support Cannabis Use Disorder: A Provider Review* (Pichette, 2024) provides critical insight differentiating between therapeutic use and problematic consumption patterns. Collectively, these studies underscore the need for a structured, evidence-based nursing framework to guide assessment and intervention in the context of cannabinoid therapeutics. Furthermore, the forthcoming Cannabis Assessment Reliability and Validity Evaluation tool aims to establish a standardized measure to support clinical decision-making, promote diagnostic clarity, and reinforce the integration of cannabis care within the nursing practice (Pichette, 2024).

The cannabis nurse navigator model is grounded in the legacy of Dr. Harold Freeman's pioneering Patient Navigation framework (Freeman & Rodriguez, 2011), which redefined health equity through guided access, advocacy, and culturally competent care. Aligned with nursing's ethical, scientific, and social mission of advancing holistic, equitable healthcare for all populations (Natale-Pereira et al., 2011; Russell et al., 2018), this model expands those principles into an emerging field that demands both compassion and clinical precision within the healthcare systems.

The Cannabis Nurse Navigator embodies the profession's core values of compassion, advocacy, and evidence-based practice while ensuring that no patient is left outside the reach of informed, stigma-free care within the healthcare system. By operationalizing the principles of education, ethics, and integrative science, nurses are well positioned to shape emerging models of healthcare through empathy, innovation, and evidence (Melnyk & Raderstorf, 2024). A future in cannabis care reflects not only controversy but also competence and compassion. The Cannabis Nurse Navigator operationalizes this role by leading the development of evidence-based educational frameworks, staff training initiatives, and patient education pathways that support accurate cannabis-related information across the healthcare system.

Importantly, the Cannabis Nurse Navigator should be distinguished from the role of the cannabis nurse, as defined in the ACNA Cannabis Nursing: Scope and Standards of Practice (2024). While both roles operate within the domain of cannabis-related healthcare, they function at different levels of practice and address different aspects of care delivery. The Cannabis Nurse Navigator operates primarily at the systems level, focusing on care coordination, policy integration, documentation structures, and interdisciplinary communication within healthcare organizations. In contrast, the cannabis nurse provides direct clinical care to patients, including assessment of cannabis use, patient education, harm reduction strategies, symptom monitoring, and motivational interviewing. Together, these complementary roles form a dual-level framework in which system-level coordination and direct patient care operate in alignment to support safe, evidence-informed cannabis integration within healthcare environments. To support the clinical relevance of this role, it is essential to examine the current evidence base.

EVIDENCE BASE FOR CANNABIS THERAPEUTICS

The increasing use of cannabis across clinical and community settings requires a balanced appraisal of both potential therapeutic benefit and known safety concerns. Although patient interest and use continue to expand, the evidence base remains heterogeneous, and many healthcare professionals report insufficient education regarding cannabinoid therapeutics, dosing, risk, and appropriate monitoring (National Academies of Sciences, Engineering, and Medicine, 2017; Szaflarski et al., 2020). This gap between patient use and provider preparedness reinforces the need for structured nursing leadership in cannabis-related care.

Current evidence suggests that cannabis and cannabinoids may offer therapeutic benefit in selected clinical contexts, but the strength of evidence varies by indication. The NASEM (2017) concluded that there is substantial evidence supporting the effectiveness of cannabis or cannabinoids for chronic pain in adults and for chemotherapy-induced nausea and vomiting. Evidence for improving sleep associated with chronic illness is more modest, and the literature remains limited by variability in product composition, routes of administration, dosing strategies, and study design. These methodological inconsistencies complicate translation into clinical practice and underscore the importance of careful assessment, patient education, and interdisciplinary oversight.

In oncology and palliative care, patients commonly report using cannabis to manage pain, nausea, appetite loss, insomnia, and anxiety. Emerging literature suggests that cannabinoids may help alleviate symptom clusters in some patients, particularly when conventional treatments are insufficient or poorly tolerated (Johnson et al., 2023; National Academies of Sciences, Engineering, and Medicine, 2017). However, the overall quality of evidence in these populations remains mixed, and rigorous randomized controlled trials are still limited. As a result, cannabis should not be framed as universally effective or risk free but, rather, as a therapeutic consideration requiring individualized evaluation within the broader plan of care.

Psychiatric and behavioral health considerations require particular caution. While some patients report perceived benefits for anxiety or sleep, evidence remains mixed, especially for tetrahydrocannabinol-dominant products. Cannabis exposure may exacerbate anxiety, impair cognition, and in vulnerable individuals contribute to psychosis risk or functional decline (National Academies of Sciences, Engineering, and Medicine, 2017). In addition, long-term or high-frequency use may be associated with problematic patterns of consumption, including CUD, and clinicians must remain alert to increasingly recognized complications, such as CHS. These concerns are especially relevant in psychiatric nursing, adolescent populations, and patients with co-occurring substance use or mental health disorders (Kansagara et al., 2026).

The evidence surrounding cannabis as an opioid-sparing intervention also remains inconclusive. Some observational literature suggests potential benefit in reducing opioid reliance or improving symptom burden, yet findings are not uniform and should be interpreted cautiously (Vyas et al., 2017). For nursing practice, this means cannabis should not be approached through ideology, but through evidence-informed clinical reasoning, harm reduction, and patient-centered communication.

Taken together, the literature supports neither uncritical endorsement nor categorical dismissal of cannabis therapeutics. Instead, it supports the need for structured nursing roles that can interpret evolving evidence, identify risk, coordinate referrals, and promote safe, stigma-free communication within healthcare systems. This is precisely where the Cannabis Nurse Navigator offers value, not by prescribing or promoting cannabis but by ensuring that cannabis-related care is approached with the same rigor, coordination, and ethical accountability expected of all complex clinical issues. The distinctions between these roles are summarized in Table 1.

Table 1. Comparative overview of the Cannabis Nurse Navigator and the cannabis nurse (King, 2024)

Domain	Cannabis Nurse Navigator	Cannabis Nurse
Level of practice	System/organization	Patient/clinical
Primary focus	Navigation, integration, policy alignment	Direct patient care and interaction
Core functions	Care coordination, referral pathways, documentation systems, and team leadership	Assessment, education, harm reduction, symptom monitoring
Interprofessional role	Leads or facilitates interdisciplinary planning	Supports care teams as a cannabis subject expert
Organizational impact	Improves system efficiency and equitable access	Improves patient knowledge, safety, and symptom management
Patient interaction	Indirect	Direct
Leadership role	Often serves as program lead or patient care navigator	Clinical expert within care teams

Note. Qualitative findings from Institutional Review Board-approved pilot study by Pichette et al. (2025).

BACKGROUND

The National Council of State Boards of Nursing has already developed guidelines for medical cannabis nursing,[1] which can serve as the foundation for this role. Nurses in this role would need to:

1. understand the legal landscape surrounding cannabis use;
2. be knowledgeable about medical cannabis programs and patient rights;
3. have expertise in the endocannabinoid system and cannabinoid pharmacology;
    2. safely and effectively manage patient care related to cannabis use, including patient education and harm reduction strategies; and
    3. approach patients without bias regarding their treatment choices, including cannabis use.[1]

The scope of practice for the Cannabis Nurse Navigator would extend beyond the general nursing scope defined by the ANA,[2,3] to include competencies specific to cannabis care. This specialized role could bridge the gap between healthcare providers' limited knowledge and the growing patient need for cannabis-related care, thereby enhancing overall patient outcomes.

Research Gaps and Proposed Study

Despite the potential for nurse navigators to improve care in cannabis-related healthcare, little research has been done on this specific role. The literature lacks comprehensive studies on the integration of Cannabis Nurse Navigators into interdisciplinary healthcare teams.

PURPOSE

To address the experience, knowledge and perceptions of healthcare staff at the Institute of Living (IOL) regarding the care of patients who use medical cannabis. The study aims to determine whether implementing a Cannabis Nurse Navigator, based on the opinions of participating IOL staff, might improve care coordination, patient education, and health outcomes.

METHODS

This exploratory study used a survey distributed via REDCap to IOL staff which included a 13-item balanced Likert scale and two open-ended questions assessing staff knowledge of cannabis use and care, attitudes toward cannabis patients, and willingness to collaborate with a cannabis nurse navigator. Specific items measured knowledge of cannabis pharmacology, the endocannabinoid system, patient safety, and organizational policies.

Responses from 23 participants were analyzed. The 13-item Likert-scale total score (range: 13–65; Q12 reverse-coded, ideal max = 61) was summarized with minimum, maximum, and median/IQR.

Qualitative data from two open-ended questions were analyzed thematically using Microsoft Word (Version 2019) or NVivo (Version 1.4, 2023).

RESULTS

Using Braun and Clarke's (2006) thematic analysis, the following themes were generated and determined:

1. would provide and/or improve education: participants emphasized the educational value a Cannabis Nurse Navigator could offer to both patients and providers;
2. would improve and/or assist with patient care: the role was viewed as a potential enhancer of care coordination;
3. lack of knowledge: staff acknowledged limited knowledge around cannabis therapeutics
4. too few patients: some felt patient volume may not justify the role, highlighting institutional hesitation; and
5. lack of staff, acceptance, and money: concerns around resource allocation and stigma were noted as barriers.

Figure 1 illustrates possession of working knowledge of the current state of cannabis legislation; Figure 2 provides confidence of assessing signs and symptoms of cannabis adverse effects, routes of administration, medical cannabis dosage, purpose for use, and relief; Figure 3 shows possession of general knowledge to assess and document a patient's medical cannabis use; and Figure 4 demonstrates willingness to refer a patient to a cannabis nurse navigator.

Figure 1. Possession of working knowledge of the current state of cannabis legislation

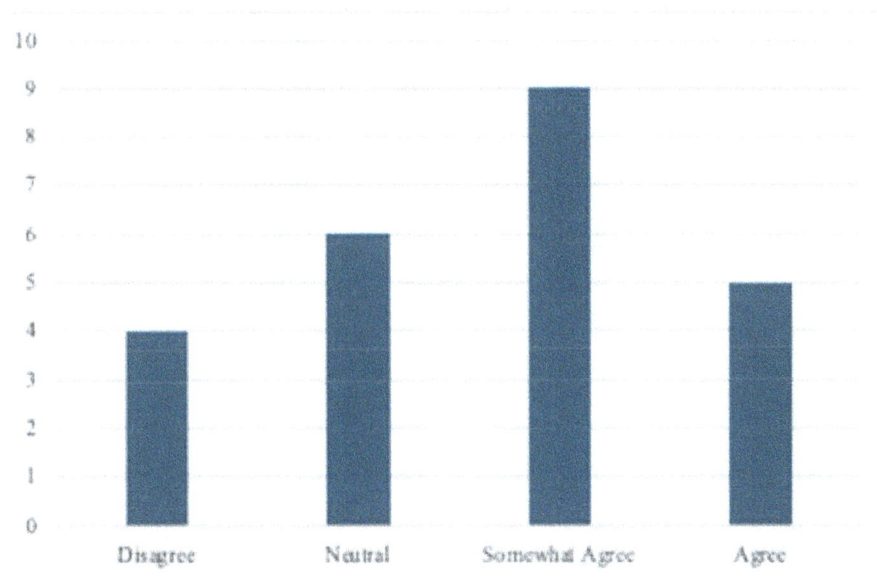

Figure 2. Confidence of assessing signs and symptoms of cannabis adverse effects, routes of administration, medical cannabis dosage, purpose for use, and relief

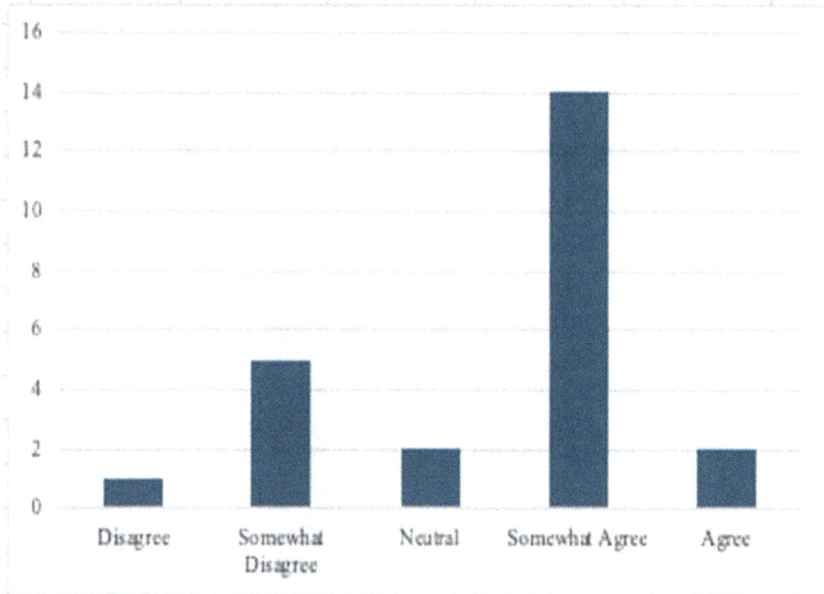

Figure 3. Possession of general knowledge to assess and document a patient's medical cannabis use

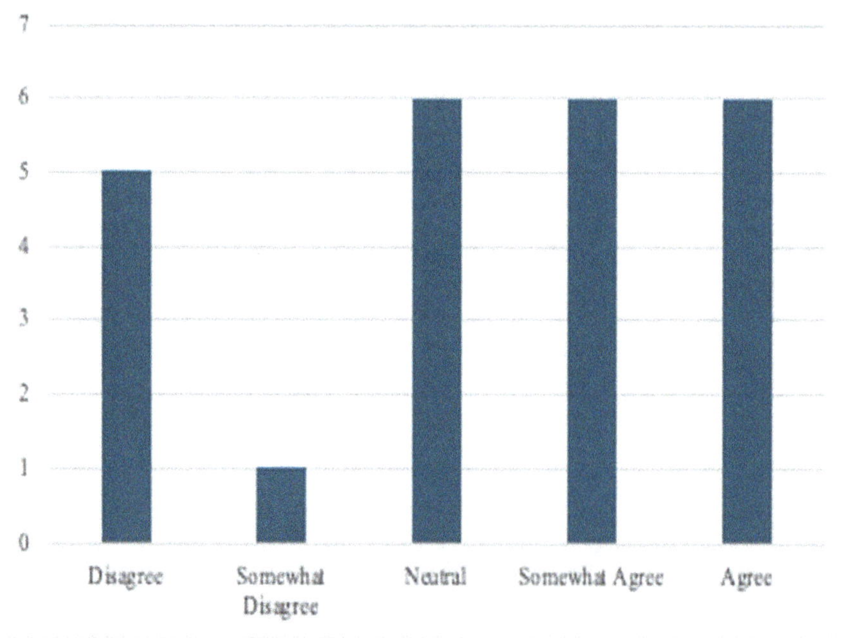

Figure 4. Willingness to refer a patient to a Cannabis Nurse Navigator

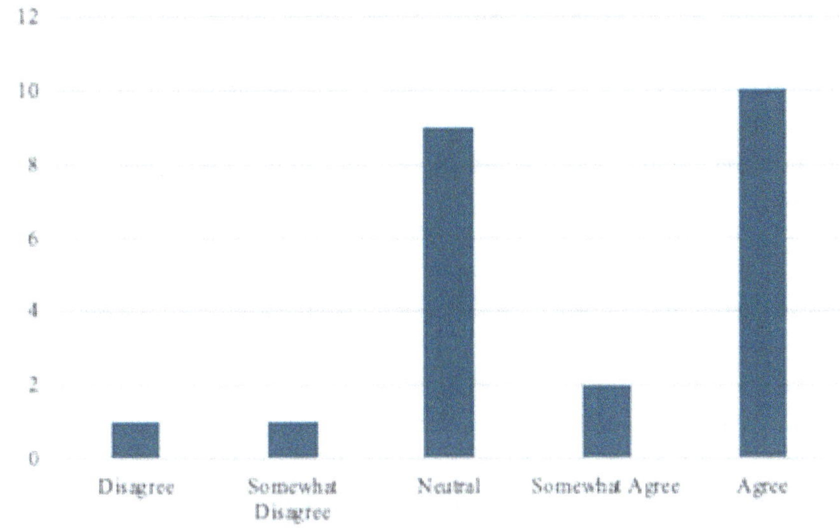

Perceived Benefits of a Cannabis Nurse Navigator

The Institutional Review Board approved pilot study provided critical exploration and hypothesis-generating insight into nursing perceptions regarding the potential integration of a role within a health-care system. Using Braun and Clarke's (2006) thematic analysis framework, both perceived benefits and perceived implementation considerations were identified. Together, these findings offer a balanced understanding of how frontline nursing staff conceptualize cannabis-related care, professional preparedness, and organizational feasibility rather than definitive outcome measurements.

1. The Cannabis Nurse Navigator will provide and/or improve education: The most common reported benefit was having access to a nurse with detailed, factual, evidence-based knowledge of medical cannabis. Participants in the study consistently described themselves as lacking the time, training, or confidence to investigate cannabis-related resources, pharmacology, safety considerations, and regulatory constraints. The Cannabis Nurse Navigator was viewed as a resource capable of translating complex and evolving evidence into clinically meaningful guidance. This theme emphasizes that the demand is not for advocacy or promotion of cannabis but for clinical accuracy, risk awareness, and informed decision-making.
2. The Cannabis Nurse Navigator will improve and/or assist with patient care: The Cannabis Nurse Navigator would support symptom management in pain, anxiety, hospice, palliative care, digestive health, and neurology through guidance on safe and effective alternative or adjunct therapies for complex and chronic conditions. The navigator would also identify and mitigate drug-drug interactions, dosing concerns, and adverse effects. Participants in the study referenced specialty-specific concerns, such as stroke patients and breastfeeding. This reinforces the need for a role grounded in evidence and clinical refinement, rather than generalized advice.

3. The Cannabis Nurse Navigator eliminates barriers: Participants in the study repeatedly emphasized the importance of a judgment-free, stigma-reducing space for patients. The Cannabis Nurse Navigator is viewed as fulfilling a core ethical nursing function described as advocacy for patient dignity, autonomy, and informed choice. The education this position provides is described as bidirectional in that it supports both patients and healthcare staff. This highlights the Cannabis Nurse Navigator role in counteracting misinformation and bias within the healthcare system itself. The navigator's alignment is with foundational nursing principles, including beneficence, nonmaleficence, and respect for people.

In addition to perceived benefits, participants identified several system-level considerations that may influence implementation. These themes are best understood not as a rejection of the role but as indicators of organizational readiness.

- Too few patients: Some respondents expressed uncertainty regarding whether sufficient patient volume existed to justify a dedicated navigation role. This perception may reflect the current lack of integration of cannabis-related care within formal clinical workflow. Cannabis use is frequently underreported, documented inconsistently or not at all, or addressed outside structured assessments, which may obscure actual demand for cannabis care. This phenomenon has been widely documented in early-stage development of nurse navigation, such as the oncology nurse navigator, where patient needs often became more apparent only after a standardized referral pathway was established. Therefore, perceived low volume of patient care may represent a limitation of current infrastructure rather than the absence of clinical need.
- Lack of staff, acceptance, and resources: Participants in the study raised concerns regarding staffing availability, interdisciplinary acceptance, and funding sustainability. The responses from the pilot study reflect realistic concerns common to the introduction of any new specialty role within complex healthcare systems. The uncertainty regarding the scope of practice, referral mechanisms, and role differentiation may contribute to hesitancy during early implementation phases. Questions regarding financial justification and resource allocation emphasize the importance of aligning new roles with organizational priorities, value-based care metrics, and measurable outcomes.

INTERPRETATION OF PILOT STUDY RESULTS

Within the nursing realm, the ANA Scope and Standards of Practice (American Nurses Association, 2015) helps frame the perspective from which nursing innovation takes place: Nursing is the protection, promotion, and optimization of health and abilities, prevention of illness and injury, facilitation of healing, alleviation of suffering through the diagnosis and treatment of human response, and advocacy in the care of individuals, families, groups, communities, and populations (p. 1). The ANA scope and standards of practice document call for all nurses to be leaders within the profession, working to influence policies and encourage innovation (American Nurses Association, 2015).

The findings of this pilot study reflect a classic early-stage implementation profile. A strong identification of perceived clinical value, paired with concerns related to readiness and sustainability, is consistent with the implementation of scientific literature examining the adoption of innovative nursing roles. As an early-stage implementation study, these findings are intended to inform future research, program design, and scalability outcomes across healthcare settings.

The themes of the pilot study suggest that successful development of a Cannabis Nurse Navigator model requires attention to:

1. clearly defined scope and competencies;
2. education aligned with established nursing standards;
3. standardized referral and documentation pathways;
4. necessity of culture change supported by nursing and organizational leadership; and
5. outcome measurement demonstrating safety, quality, and efficiency.

SCHOLARLY IMPLICATIONS FOR ROLE DEVELOPMENT

The findings provide a realistic foundation for future research, program design, and scalability. The Cannabis Nurse Navigator role's success depends on thoughtful integration within nursing structures, institutional policy, and healthcare system priorities. The pilot study contributes in a meaningful way to the emerging global discourse on cannabis nursing by shifting the conversation from ideological debates toward disciplined role development grounded in evidence, ethics, and innovative systems thinking.

THE CANNABIS NURSE NAVIGATOR: SYSTEM LEVEL INTEGRATION AND COORDINATION

The Cannabis Nurse Navigator is responsible for integrating cannabis-related care into existing healthcare systems. Rather than providing direct bedside care, the navigator focuses on care coordination, policy alignment, and organizational leadership to ensure that patients who use cannabis receive safe, consistent, and equitable care across clinical settings. The primary responsibilities of the Cannabis Nurse Navigator include:

- coordinating cannabis-related care across interdisciplinary teams;
- developing referral pathways and structured care protocols;
- integrating cannabis-related documentation into electronic health records;
- aligning institutional policies with evolving legal and regulatory frameworks;
- leading interprofessional education and simulation exercises; and
- supporting healthcare teams in complex cannabis-related clinical decision making.

Through these activities, the Cannabis Nurse Navigator helps healthcare organizations move beyond fragmented or informed approaches to cannabis use, replacing them with structures and evidence-informed systems of care. The navigator's patient interaction is typically indirect, occurring through guidance of care teams, development of care pathways, and coordination of interdisciplinary services. The ultimate impact of the role is reflected at the organizational level, including improvements in continuity of care, harm reduction, and equitable access to cannabis-related healthcare services.

THE CANNABIS NURSE: DIRECT CARE AND PATIENT SUPPORT

The cannabis nurse operates primarily at the patient care level, providing direct clinical support for individuals who use cannabis therapeutically or nonmedically. The cannabis nurse focuses on patient assessment, education, and symptom monitoring within the context of individualized care. The cannabis nurse's core responsibilities are:

- conducting comprehensive cannabis use assessments;
- educating patients on dosing principles, routes of administration, and safety considerations;
- providing harm reduction strategies to minimize adverse effects or misuse;
- monitoring symptoms, therapeutic outcomes, and potential side effects;
- supporting motivational interviewing and behavioral change strategies; and
- delivering culturally sensitive patient education related to cannabis use.

The cannabis nurse interacts directly with the patients and families, helping individuals understand the potential benefits and risks associated with cannabis use while promoting safe and informed decision-making. Within the interdisciplinary teams, the cannabis nurse often functions as a subject matter expert in cannabinoid therapeutics, providing clinical insights that support team-based care planning (Clark, 2021).

The Cannabis Nurse Navigator and the cannabis nurse are designed to be complementary rather than hierarchical. The Cannabis Nurse Navigator focuses on system integration, coordination, and leadership, while the cannabis nurse focuses on clinical implementation and patient support. Together, these roles create a structured approach to cannabis-related healthcare that addresses both organizational systems of care and individual patient needs.

The Cannabis Nurse Navigator develops the infrastructure necessary for safe and equitable cannabis integration within healthcare systems, while the cannabis nurse operationalizes the framework through direct patient engagement. This dual-level model allows healthcare organizations to move beyond provisional cannabis guidance and toward coordinated, evidence-informed cannabis care across clinical environments.

OPERATIONALIZING THE CANNABIS NURSE NAVIGATOR WITHIN HEALTHCARE SYSTEMS

While the conceptual framework of the Cannabis Nurse Navigator establishes the philosophical and professional foundation of the role, successful integration within healthcare systems requires a structural implementation strategy. Implementing the Cannabis Nurse Navigator would involve aligning clinical practice, institutional policy, interdisciplinary communication, and regulatory compliance into a coordinated system of care. As cannabis use continues to expand in both medical and recreational platforms, healthcare institutions are increasingly encountering patients whose cannabis use intersects with conventional medical treatment. Without structured guidance, this intersection often results in fragmented communication, undocumented cannabis use, and inconsistent patient education. The Cannabis Nurse Navigator addresses these gaps by creating standardized pathways for assessment, documentation, and care coordination.

The illustrative workflow for the cannabis nurse navigator is given in Figure 5.

Figure 5. Illustrative workflow for the Cannabis Nurse Navigator

Patient disclosure or identification of cannabis use

↓↓↓

Clinical Team consults Cannabis Nurse Navigator™

↓↓↓

Navigator evaluates clinical context and institutional policies

↓↓↓

Referral to Cannabis Nurse or appropriate specialist

↓↓↓

Interdisciplinary care coordination and documentation

↓↓↓

Ongoing monitoring and evaluation of patient outcomes

This workflow allows healthcare teams to respond to cannabis-related issues in a systematic manner that prioritizes patient safety, informed decision-making, and coordinated care.

PHASE ONE: INSTITUTIONAL NEEDS ASSESSMENT

The first step in implementing a Cannabis Nurse Navigator program is a comprehensive evaluation of the institutional needs. This assessment identifies gaps in cannabis-related knowledge among staff and providers, evaluates existing documentation practices, and assesses the current level of coordination within the healthcare system. Key areas of the assessment include:

- prevalence of patient-reported cannabis use;

- provider knowledge and comfort discussing cannabis;
- documentation practices within electronic health records;
- legal and regulatory considerations within the institution's jurisdiction; and
- existing patient navigation or care coordination structures.

Needs assessments may incorporate provider surveys, patient intake data, and institutional policy reviews. Preliminary findings from the pilot study Pichette et al. (2025) indicate that many healthcare providers report limited formal education on cannabis therapeutics, highlighting the need for structured support within clinical teams.

PHASE TWO: ROLE INTEGRATION AND SCOPE ALIGNMENT

Following the needs assessment, healthcare organizations must define how the Cannabis Nurse Navigator will integrate into existing care structures. The navigator already operates primarily at the systems level; therefore, the role typically intersects with departments that already manage complex care coordination. Common integration points include:

- oncology services;
- pain management programs;
- psychiatry and behavioral health services;
- palliative care teams; and
- primary care coordinated programs.

During this phase, healthcare systems establish clear reporting structures, referral pathways, and documentation procedures to ensure that cannabis-related care is integrated within the broader patient care framework.

PHASE THREE: DEVELOPMENT OF CLINICAL PATHWAYS AND REFERRAL SYSTEMS

A central function of the Cannabis Nurse Navigator is the creation of structured clinical pathways that guide healthcare providers when cannabis use impacts clinical care. These pathways help standardize how cannabis-related discussions, assessments, and referrals occur within the healthcare system. Clinical pathway components include:

- standardized screening questions for cannabis use;
- referral mechanisms to cannabis nurses or other specialists;
- interdisciplinary consultation protocols; and
- integration of cannabis documentation into electronic health records.

By developing these structured pathways, the Cannabis Nurse Navigator ensures that cannabis use is addressed consistently across clinical settings rather than through provisional conversations or undocumented patient disclosures.

PHASE FOUR: INTERPROFESSIONAL EDUCATION AND TEAM DEVELOPMENT

Healthcare providers frequently report limited training in cannabinoid pharmacology, dosing principles, and harm reduction strategies (Kruger et al., 2022; Worster et al., 2023). The Cannabis Nurse Navigator plays a critical leadership role in addressing this educational gap by facilitating interdisciplinary learning opportunities. These educational initiatives may include:

- clinical workshops on the endocannabinoid system;
- continuing education sessions on cannabinoid pharmacology;
- simulation exercises addressing complex cannabis-related patient scenarios; and
- guidance on legal and regulatory considerations.

Through these initiatives, the Cannabis Nurse Navigator strengthens provider competence and reduces stigma surrounding cannabis discussions in clinical practice.

PHASE FIVE: POLICY DEVELOPMENT AND REGULATORY ALIGNMENT

Cannabis regulation varies widely across jurisdictions and continues to evolve as new legislation emerges. Healthcare institutions must maintain policies that reflect current legal requirements while supporting patient-centered care. The Cannabis Nurse Navigator contributes to policy development by:

- reviewing institutional policies related to cannabis use;
- aligning documentation procedures with regulatory standards;
- supporting compliance with state and federal laws; and
- assisting leadership teams in interpreting emerging legislation.

This policy level involvement ensures that cannabis-related care is delivered within ethically and legally appropriate frameworks. Efforts to address institutional barriers to medical cannabis use at the end of life have gained traction through legislation, such as Ryan's Law in California. Enacted as the *Compassionate Access to Medical Cannabis Act* (SB 311/SB 988), Ryan's Law permits terminally ill patients to use state-authorized medical cannabis within specified healthcare facilities under regulated conditions. The law was inspired by the experience of Ryan Bartell, a patient with advanced pancreatic cancer whose access to cannabis was restricted during hospitalization, necessitating reliance on high-dose opioids. This regimen reduced pain but limited alertness and meaningful interaction with loved ones. Following transfer to a facility that permitted cannabis use, Ryan experienced improved symptom control while remaining more communicative and present, highlighting cannabis's potential role in supporting both comfort and connection at the end of life (Sobel, 2023).

Since its implementation, healthcare institutions in California have operationalized compassionate access through structured protocols, including secure storage of patient-supplied products, documentation in the medical record, administration oversight, and prohibitions on smoking or vaping while allowing oral or other noncombustible forms (McKaig et al., 2025). These frameworks demonstrate that cannabis integration can occur safely within existing regulatory structures without requiring facilities to prescribe or dispense cannabis directly.

Despite these advances, gaps persist between state-level legalization and real-world access within healthcare systems. Connecticut's proposed legislation (H.B. 5242, 2026), introduced in March 2026, seeks to require hospitals, nursing homes, hospice inpatient facilities, and short-term hospital special hospices to allow terminally ill qualifying patients to continue using medical cannabis during inpatient care. Modeled in part after Ryan's Law, the proposal preserves institutional oversight while preventing abrupt discontinuation of a therapy that may already be effectively managing symptoms (Capitani, 2026). At the time of writing, there are 13 states considering bills similar to Ryan's Law (Jaeger, 2026). As states pass such bills, there will be a need for systems to integrate policies and procedures for cannabis use in healthcare facilities, underscoring the need for professionals, such as the Cannabis Nurse Navigator, to coordinate such policies in a legal and ethical manner.

Clinical testimony supporting such legislation underscores the implications of current restrictions. Patients achieving symptom relief with medical cannabis in outpatient settings are often required to discontinue its use upon admission, necessitating higher opioid doses and other sedatives. The trade-offs can include reduced alertness, impaired communication, and diminished quality of life (Capitani, 2026).

From a palliative care perspective, these policy-driven treatment shifts raise important ethical and clinical considerations. While opioids remain essential for many patients, the inability to continue cannabis therapy may exacerbate symptoms and limit engagement with family and participation in end-of-life decisions. Emerging evidence suggests that cannabinoids may alleviate symptom clusters, including pain, nausea, appetite loss, insomnia, and anxiety, though the overall quality of evidence is still developing and heterogeneous (Johnson et al., 2023; National Academies of Sciences, Engineering, and Medicine, 2017).

As recently as February 2026, the Washington State House of Representatives passed legislation modeled on Ryan's Law, restoring compassionate access for terminally ill patients and emphasizing dignity at the end of life (Washington State House of Representatives, 2026). These examples reflect a growing national trend to align end-of-life care policies with patient-centered and legally authorized therapies.

From a nursing perspective, compassionate access addresses not only symptom relief but also the ability of patients to remain awake, interactive, and engaged with family and caregivers. Evidence indicates that cannabis may improve symptom clusters in palliative populations, though standardized dosing, long-term safety, and integration with conventional pharmacotherapy remain areas of uncertainty (Johnson et al., 2023). This highlights the need for clinician education, institutional policy development, and interdisciplinary roles, such as the cannabis nurse navigator, to support safe, ethical, and evidence-informed integration of cannabis into palliative and hospice care (Kansagara et al., 2020).

Despite positive observational evidence and implementation experience, rigorous randomized controlled trials and systematic evaluations in hospice and palliative care populations are limited. Further research is needed to inform clinical guidelines, dosing standards, and integration strategies (Johnson et al., 2023).

PHASE SIX: PROGRAM EVALUATION AND CONTINUOUS QUALITY IMPROVEMENT

The Cannabis Nurse Navigator role requires ongoing evaluation to measure their impact on patient care and system efficiency. Evaluation frameworks should incorporate both patient-level outcomes and organizational metrics. Potential evaluation indicators include patient safety metrics, care coordination metrics, patient experience metrics, and organizational outcomes.

Patient safety metrics evaluate documentation of cannabis use in clinical records and monitoring of adverse events related to cannabinoid therapeutics. Care coordination metrics evaluate referral completion rates and interdisciplinary outcomes. Patient experience metrics evaluate patient satisfaction with cannabis-related education and support, as well as perceived stigma reduction within healthcare interactions. Organizational outcomes evaluate provider knowledge improvement following educational initiatives, as well as improved integration of cannabis-related information within care planning. Continuous quality improvement processes allow healthcare organizations to refine the Cannabis Nurse Navigator positions as clinical evidence and regulatory environments evolve.

SUPPORTING SAFE AND COORDINATED CANNABIS CARE

The combined efforts of the Cannabis Nurse Navigator and the cannabis nurse create a dual level framework for cannabis-related healthcare. The Cannabis Nurse Navigator provides the organizational infrastructure that supports coordinated care while the cannabis nurse ensures that individual patients receive informed clinical guidance. Together, these roles allow healthcare systems to improve communication among healthcare providers regarding cannabis use, reduce stigma surrounding cannabis-related discussions in clinical practice, enhance patient safety through structured assessment and monitoring, and ensure that cannabis-related care is integrated into interdisciplinary treatment planning.

By clearly defining the complementary responsibilities of these roles, healthcare organizations can move beyond fragmented or informal approaches to cannabis guidance and instead develop a coordinated care system that supports both clinical care and organizational oversight.

COORDINATED CANNABIS CARE IN PRACTICE

A 45-year-old patient receiving chemotherapy for metastatic breast cancer reports using cannabis products purchased from a local dispensary to manage nausea, insomnia, and anxiety related to treatment. During a routine oncology visit, the patient discloses using edible cannabis products several times per week but expresses uncertainty about appropriate dosing and potential interactions with prescribed medications. The oncology provider acknowledges limited knowledge with cannabinoid therapeutics and requests a consultation through the institution's Cannabis Nurse Navigator program.

Upon receiving the referral, the Cannabis Nurse Navigator reviews the patient's clinical information including the current treatment plan, medication profile, and institutional policies regarding cannabis-related documentation and care coordination. The Cannabis Nurse Navigator then facilitates a referral to the cannabis nurse, ensuring that the patient receives a comprehensive clinical assessment, while also coordinating communication among the oncology team and other relevant providers. The Cannabis Nurse

Navigator then integrates these findings into the broader care plan by ensuring appropriate documentation within the electronic health record, coordinating interdisciplinary communication, and confirming that the patient's cannabis use is considered in ongoing symptom management discussions.

EVIDENCE BASE FOR CANNABIS THERAPEUTICS AND CLINICAL CONSIDERATIONS

The expanding use of cannabis for both medical and nonmedical purposes has prompted increasing attention to the scientific evidence surrounding cannabinoid therapeutics. Patients frequently report using cannabis for symptom management related to chronic pain, oncology treatment, sleep disturbance, anxiety, and other conditions. However, the clinical evidence supporting these applications varies in strength, and healthcare providers often report limited training in interpreting cannabis-related research. Therefore, a critical synthesis of the literature is necessary to inform nursing practice and guide safe patient care (McIntosh et al., 2024).

One of the most comprehensive evaluations of cannabis therapeutics was conducted by the National Academies of Sciences, Engineering, and Medicine (2017). This report reviewed more than 10,000 scientific abstracts and concluded that there is substantial evidence supporting the use of cannabis or cannabinoids for chronic pain in adults, particularly neuropathic pain. Cannabinoid therapies have also demonstrated strong evidence for reducing chemotherapy-induced nausea and vomiting, as well as moderate evidence for improving sleep disturbances associated with chronic illness.

Subsequent systematic reviews and meta-analyses have further explored these findings. Studies examining chronic pain management suggest that cannabinoids may offer modest analgesic effects, particularly in cases of neuropathic pain where conventional therapies may provide limited relief. However, the clinical effectiveness of cannabinoid therapies remains variable due to heterogeneity in study design, dosing regimens, cannabinoid composition, and routes of administration. These variations make it difficult to establish standardized treatment guidelines, highlighting the need for healthcare professionals who can interpret emerging evidence and guide patients safely.

In oncology settings, cannabis use is commonly reported among patients seeking relief from treatment-related symptoms, including nausea, appetite loss, anxiety, and insomnia (Valente et al., 2024). Cannabinoid-based medications, such as dronabinol and nabilone, have demonstrated antiemetic properties in patients undergoing chemotherapy, and observational studies suggest that some patients report improved appetite and overall quality of life when using cannabis products. Nevertheless, high-quality randomized controlled trials examining cannabis in oncology symptom management remain limited, and further research is needed to clarify optimal dosing, formulation, and long-term safety.

Mental health outcomes associated with cannabis use present a more complex and sometimes contradictory evidence base. Some patients report reductions in anxiety and improvements in sleep when using cannabis, particularly products containing cannabidiol. However, evidence regarding psychiatric outcomes remains mixed. High concentrations of tetrahydrocannabinol have been associated with increased risk of anxiety, paranoia, and, in vulnerable populations, psychotic symptoms (Kansagara et al., 2026). Epidemiological research has also identified associations between heavy cannabis use and increased risk of psychosis in individuals with underlying genetic or psychiatric vulnerabilities. These findings underscore the importance of careful clinical assessment and patient education when cannabis is used in the context of mental health conditions.

Another area of growing interest involves the potential relationship between cannabis use and opioid utilization. Early ecological studies suggested that states with medical cannabis programs experienced reductions in opioid prescribing and opioid-related mortality. However, more recent analyses have produced mixed results, with some studies failing to replicate these associations. As a result, the role of cannabis as a substitute or adjunct to opioid therapy remains an area of ongoing scientific debate (Mok et al., 2023).

Alongside potential therapeutic applications, cannabis use also presents clinical risks that must be carefully considered within healthcare settings. Adverse effects associated with cannabis include cognitive impairment, dizziness, anxiety, and, in some cases, dependence or problematic use. The diagnostic framework for CUD highlights patterns of problematic cannabis consumption that may interfere with social, occupational, or health functioning. In addition, emerging clinical conditions, such as CHS, have been increasingly recognized in patients with chronic cannabis exposure.

Therefore, healthcare providers face the challenge of balancing patient-reported benefits with potential safety concerns and scientific uncertainty. Despite the increasing prevalence of cannabis use among patients, surveys consistently demonstrate that many physicians, nurses, and pharmacists report limited formal education regarding cannabinoid pharmacology and cannabis therapeutics. This gap between patient behavior and provider knowledge contributes to inconsistent clinical guidance and may leave patients navigating cannabis-related decisions without reliable medical support.

Within this context, nurses are uniquely positioned to contribute to safe and evidence-informed cannabis care. Nursing practice emphasizes holistic assessment, patient education, harm reduction, and care coordination and principles that are particularly relevant in addressing complex and evolving therapeutic landscapes (Theisen & Konieczny, 2019). The Cannabis Nurse Navigator model builds upon these foundations by creating a structured system through which healthcare teams can interpret emerging cannabis evidence, coordinate interdisciplinary care, and ensure that patient cannabis use is addressed transparently within clinical decision-making.

Rather than promoting or discouraging cannabis use categorically, the Cannabis Nurse Navigator framework supports an evidence-informed and patient-centered approach. By integrating scientific evidence, clinical assessment, and interdisciplinary communication, nurses can help ensure that cannabis-related care is approached with the same rigor, safety considerations, and ethical accountability that guide other therapeutic interventions within modern healthcare systems.

GLOBAL LANDSCAPE OF MEDICAL CANNABIS

The Cannabis Nurse Navigator model is a bridge between theoretical systems thinking and applied social practice by demonstrating its applicability in diverse healthcare systems and legal frameworks. The Cannabis Nurse Navigator model also outlines a phased implementation framework and provides guidance for nurse leaders, administrators, and policymakers on adopting, scaling, or evaluating the role. The chapter highlights the unique contribution of a doctorate-prepared nurse in designing, implementing, and assessing the Cannabis Nurse Navigator role, positioning nursing as the central driver of safe and effective cannabis care integration.

The global landscape of cannabis therapeutics is slowly evolving. Countries across North America, Europe, Latin America, and parts of Asia and Africa are adopting medical cannabis programs, while recreational legalization continues to expand access. With these advances, healthcare systems face critical challenges in safety in integrating cannabis into patient care. Providers often report insufficient education, fragmented information, and inconsistent legal frameworks. Nurses are on the frontlines and are uniquely positioned to bridge these gaps. Nursing practice encompasses assessment, patient advocacy, education, and care coordination with skills directly aligned to the needs posed by medical cannabis integration. However, traditional nursing curricula often do not include cannabis therapeutics, the endocannabinoid system, or regulatory knowledge, leaving practitioners ill-prepared to navigate patient questions and coordinate care across complex systems.

THE NEED FOR A NURSE-LED SOLUTION

Nursing personnel are uniquely qualified to lead the Cannabis Nurse Navigator role. Their foundational education and scope of practice emphasize holistic, patient-centered care, therapeutic communication, advocacy, patient and family education, and seamless coordination across the entire care continuum. These competencies enable nurses to simultaneously address clinical, psychosocial, regulatory, and systemic dimensions of cannabis use functions that pharmacists (whose expertise centers on pharmacological safety and drug interactions) or internal medicine specialists (whose focus is primarily diagnostic and prescriptive) are not positioned to integrate as comprehensively or relationally.

Evidence from multiple healthcare systems shows that patients who use cannabis encounter substantial barriers, including stigma, lack of evidence-based guidance, and fragmented care (Breuning et al., 2026). To address these systemic challenges, the Cannabis Nurse Navigator role was developed as a health-system and policy-level intervention. Modeled after successful navigator programs in oncology, chronic care management, and other chronic disease settings, this role does not provide medical authorization, prescribing guidance, diagnosis, or direct bedside care. Instead, the Cannabis Nurse Navigator functions as a systems-level coordinator, educator, and advocate who translates complex clinical, institutional, and regulatory information into clear, actionable guidance for both patients and clinical teams, driving organizational change and policy integration.

The Cannabis Nurse Navigator specifically addresses three critical gaps in patient care:

1. knowledge gaps among patients and healthcare staff;
2. fragmented care and lack of coordination; and
3. stigma and patient mistrust of the healthcare system.

By establishing the Cannabis Nurse Navigator as an evidence-based, nurse-led intervention, healthcare organizations can enhance patient safety, optimize symptom management, and reduce reliance on opioids while remaining fully compliant with legal and institutional policies (Vyas et al., 2017). Clear delineation of roles is essential to prevent duplication of effort, confusion, or scope-of-practice conflicts. The Cannabis Nurse Navigator role complements but does not replace other professionals, as follows:

- **Primary care providers**: Prescribe medications, manage overall health, and integrate the cannabis nurse navigator's recommendations into the patient's care plan.
- **Pharmacists**: Provide medication safety oversight, identify potential interactions, and advise on cannabinoid formulations.

- **Behavioral health clinicians**: Address psychiatric comorbidities, substance use disorders, and psychosocial interventions.
- **Cannabis nurses**: Provide direct bedside assessment, diagnosis (where authorized), prescribing (within scope of practice), hands-on care, and patient education.
- **Other specialties**: Collaborate as needed for complex medical or neurological conditions.

Importantly, the Cannabis Nurse Navigator operates distinctly at the health-system and policy level as a coordinator and change agent, whereas cannabis nurses deliver direct clinical care at the bedside. By clarifying these responsibilities, the Cannabis Nurse Navigator ensures cohesive, patient-centered care and facilitates the seamless integration of cannabis-related expertise into traditional healthcare structures.

The Cannabis Nurse Navigator represents an innovative evolution of evidence-based nursing practice grounded in advocacy, holistic care, and science. As cannabis use and societal acceptance continue to grow worldwide, this role offers a structured, professional model that bridges gaps in safety, communication, and interdisciplinary collaboration. Ultimately, it improves patient outcomes, reduces stigma, and advances the global field of cannabis nursing.

CONCLUSION

The Cannabis Nurse Navigator represents a transformative evolution in nursing practice, bridging the gap between emerging cannabis science and patient-centered clinical care. By integrating assessment, education, care coordination, advocacy, and harm reduction, Cannabis Nurse Navigators ensure that medical cannabis patients will receive safe, effective, and stigma-free guidance within the healthcare system when they seek care.

This role was developed from the foundation of the legacy of patient navigation, nursing theory, and interdisciplinary collaboration while responding to the unique challenges of cannabis care, including legal variability, social stigma, and rapidly evolving pharmacology. The Cannabis Nurse Navigator promotes equity and evidence-based practice, empowering patients to make informed decisions and supporting healthcare teams in delivering coordinated, high-quality care.

As cannabis use continues to expand globally, the Cannabis Nurse Navigator is positioned to lead in advancing clinical knowledge, shaping policy, and contributing to research that informs best practice. By operationalizing the principles of compassion, ethics, education, and science (Sitzman & Watson, 2018), the Cannabis Nurse Navigator embodies nursing's commitment to holistic, person-centered care, while simultaneously addressing systemic gaps and advancing health equity. The Cannabis Nurse Navigator exemplifies the capacity of nursing to innovate within emerging therapeutic landscapes while strengthening patient safety, interprofessional collaboration, and health system responsiveness.

REFERENCES

American Cannabis Nurses Association. (2024). *Cannabis nursing: Scope and standards of practice*. American Nurses Association.

American Nurses Association. (2015). *Nursing: Scope and standards of practice* (3rd ed.).

Braun, V., & Clarke, V. (2006, January 1). Using Thematic Analysis in Psychology. *Qualitative Research in Psychology*, *3*(2), 77–101. DOI: 10.1191/1478088706qp063oa

Breuning, M., Nie, J., Schlesinger, M., Smith, L., Lavie-Ajayi, M., Babinski, S., & Law, S. (2026). The persistence of stigma and other challenges experienced by medical cannabis users: A thematic synthesis of qualitative studies. *Medical Cannabis and Cannabinoids*, •••, 1–36. DOI: 10.1159/000551584

Capitani, L. (2026, February 20). *Supporting terminally ill patients in Connecticut health care facilities to use cannabis (HB 5242)* [Testimony]. Connecticut General Assembly Public Health Committee. https://www.d4dpr.org/post/expert-testimony-terminally-ill-cannabis-use-hb-5242

Carter, N., Valaitis, R. K., Lam, A., Feather, J., Nicholl, J., & Cleghorn, L. (2018). Navigation delivery models and roles of navigators in primary care: A scoping literature review. *BMC Health Services Research*, *18*(1), 96. Advance online publication. DOI: 10.1186/s12913-018-2889-0 PMID: 29422057

Clark, C. (2021). *Cannabis: A handbook for nurses* (1st, North American ed.). Lippincott Williams & Wilkins.

Freeman, H. P., & Rodriguez, R. L. (2011). History and principles of patient navigation. *Cancer*, *117*(S15), 3537–3540. DOI: 10.1002/cncr.26262 PMID: 21780088

International Association of Clinical Research Nurses. (2024). *Clinical research nursing: Scope and standards of practice* (2nd ed.). American Nurses Association.

Jaeger, K. (2026, February 3). Lawmakers in multiple states push to allow medical marijuana use in hospitals by qualifying patients. *Marijuana Moment*. https://www.marijuanamoment.net/lawmakers-in-multiple-states-push-to-allow-medical-marijuana-use-in-hospitals-by-qualifying-patients/

Johnson, E. C., Colbert, S. M., Jeffries, P. W., Tillman, R., Bigdeli, T. B., Karcher, N. R., Chan, G., Kuperman, S., Meyers, J. L., Nurnberger, J. I., Plawecki, M. H., Degenhardt, L., Martin, N. G., Kamarajan, C., Schuckit, M. A., Murray, R. M., Dick, D. M., Edenberg, H. J., D'Souza, D. C., & Agrawal, A. (2023). Associations between cannabis use, polygenic liability for schizophrenia, and cannabis-related experiences in a sample of cannabis users. *Schizophrenia Bulletin*, *49*(3), 778–787. DOI: 10.1093/schbul/sbac196 PMID: 36545904

Kansagara, D., Morasco, B. J., Iacocca, M. O., Bair, M. J., Hooker, E. R., & Becker, W. C. (2020). Clinician knowledge, attitudes, and practice regarding cannabis: Results from a National Veterans Health Administration survey. *Pain Medicine*, *21*(11), 3180–3186. DOI: 10.1093/pm/pnz322 PMID: 31909803

Kansagara, D., Terry, G. E., Ayers, C. K., & D'Souza, D. C. (2026). Cannabis and mental health: A review. *JAMA Internal Medicine*, *186*(5), 618. Advance online publication. DOI: 10.1001/jamainternmed.2025.8215 PMID: 41801216

Katerenchuk, J., & Salas, A. S. (2023). An integrative review on the oncology nurse navigator role in the Canadian context. *Canadian Oncology Nursing Journal = Revue Canadienne de Nursing Oncologique*, *33*(4), 385–399. DOI: 10.5737/23688076334385 PMID: 38919590

King, K. (2024). Cannabis nursing. *AJN. The American Journal of Nursing*, *124*(5), 31. DOI: 10.1097/01.NAJ.0001016368.03202.a8 PMID: 38661699

Kokorelias, K. M., DasGupta, T., & Hitzig, S. L. (2022). Designing the ideal patient navigation program for older adults with complex needs: A qualitative exploration of the preferences of key informants. *Journal of Applied Gerontology*, *41*(4), 1002–1010. DOI: 10.1177/07334648211059056 PMID: 34905440

Kokorelias, K. M., Shiers-Hanley, J. E., Rios, J., Knoepfli, A., & Hitzig, S. L. (2021). Factors influencing the implementation of patient navigation programs for adults with complex needs: A scoping review of the literature. *Health Services Insights*, *14*, 11786329211033267. Advance online publication. DOI: 10.1177/11786329211033267 PMID: 34349519

Kruger, D. J., Mokbel, M. A., Clauw, D. J., & Boehnke, K. F. (2022). Assessing health care providers' knowledge of medical cannabis. *Cannabis and Cannabinoid Research*, *7*(4), 501–507. DOI: 10.1089/can.2021.0032 PMID: 34463161

McIntosh, N., Wilson, N., Povalej, P., Hunt, L., & Lewis, P. (2024). An exploration of registered nurses' experiences caring for patients taking medicinal cannabis. *Nursing Open*, *11*(10), e70063. Advance online publication. DOI: 10.1002/nop2.70063 PMID: 39455290

McKaig, A., Varilla Ridad, A. R., Bell, A., McParlane, R., & Quirch, M. (2025). Implementing Ryan's Law on an inpatient medical oncology unit. *Clinical Journal of Oncology Nursing*, *29*(1), 86–90. DOI: 10.1188/25.CJON.86-90 PMID: 39933092

Melnyk, B. M., & Raderstorf, T. (Eds.). (2024). *Evidence-based leadership, innovation, and entrepreneurship in nursing and healthcare: A practical guide for success* (2nd ed.). Springer Publishing Company. DOI: 10.1891/9780826160720

Mok, J., Milloy, M. J., Grant, C., Lake, S., DeBeck, K., Hayashi, K., Kerr, T., & Socías, M. E. (2023). Use of cannabis as a harm reduction strategy among people who use drugs: A cohort study. *Cannabis and Cannabinoid Research*, *8*(4), 670–678. DOI: 10.1089/can.2021.0229 PMID: 35647886

Natale-Pereira, A., Enard, K. R., Nevarez, L., & Jones, L. A. (2011). The role of patient navigators in eliminating health disparities. *Cancer*, *117*(S15), 3543–3552. DOI: 10.1002/cncr.26264 PMID: 21780089

National Academies of Sciences, Engineering, and Medicine. (2017). *The health effects of cannabis and cannabinoids: The current state of evidence and recommendations for research.* National Academies Press. DOI: 10.17226/24625

Patel, D. (2022). Cannabis use disorder. In Avery, J. D., & Hankins, D. (Eds.), *Addiction medicine: A case and evidence-based guide.*, DOI: 10.1007/978-3-030-86430-9_4

Pichette, N. (2024). *Provider review: Evaluating individual criteria to support cannabis use disorder* (Publication No. 1816) [Doctoral dissertation, Salve Regina University]. Sigma Repository. https://www.sigmarepository.org/dissertations/1816

Pichette, N., O'Sullivan, D., Caruso, A., Blair, E., & Pearlson, G. (2025, November 13). *Exploring cannabis patient care: Institute of Living staff experience and knowledge* [Poster presentation]. Trinity Health of New England Annual Research Day, Hartford, CT, United States. https://www.trinityhealthofne.org/sites/default/files/Education%20and%20Research/Research%20Day%202025/34-Exploring-Cannabis-Patient_Care.pdf

Pruitt, Z., & Sportsman, S. (2013). The presence and roles of nurse navigators in acute care hospitals. *The Journal of Nursing Administration, 43*(11), 592–596. DOI: 10.1097/01.NNA.0000434510.74373.40 PMID: 24153201

Rice, J., Hildebrand, A., Waslo, C. S., Cameron, M. H., & Jones, K. D. (2022). Cannabis for medical purposes: A cross-sectional analysis of health care professionals' knowledge. *Journal of the American Association of Nurse Practitioners, 34*(1), 100–106. DOI: 10.1097/JXX.0000000000000590 PMID: 33767121

Russell, K., Cahill, M., Gowen, K., Cronquist, R., Smith, V., Borris-Hale, C., Fischer, H., Heywood, D., Johnston, J., & Sutton-Johnson, S. (2018). The National Council of State Boards of Nursing national nursing guidelines for medical marijuana. *Journal of Nursing Regulation, 9*(2), S1–S60. https://www.ncsbn.org/public-files/The_NCSBN_National_Nursing_Guidelines_for_Medical_Marijuana_JNR_July_2018.pdf

Russo, E. B., Spooner, C., May, L., Leslie, R., & Whiteley, V. L. (2022). Cannabinoid hyperemesis syndrome survey and genomic investigation. *Cannabis and Cannabinoid Research, 7*(3), 336–344. DOI: 10.1089/can.2021.0046 PMID: 34227878

Sitzman, K., & Watson, J. (2018). *Caring science, mindful practice: Implementing Watson's human caring theory* (2nd ed.). Springer Publishing Company. DOI: 10.1891/9780826135568

Sobel, K. (2023). *Testimony of Ken Sobel, Esq. Exhibit SHHS1069AC submitted to the Nevada Senate Committee on Health and Human Services, 82nd Nevada Legislative Session*. Nevada Legislature. https://archive.leg.state.nv.us/Session/82nd2023/Exhibits/Senate/HHS/SHHS1069AC.pdf

Szaflarski, M., McGoldrick, P., Currens, L., Blodgett, D., Land, H., Szaflarski, J. P., & Segal, E. (2020). Attitudes and knowledge about cannabis and cannabis-based therapies among US neurologists, nurses, and pharmacists. *Epilepsy & Behavior, 109*, 107102. Advance online publication. DOI: 10.1016/j.yebeh.2020.107102 PMID: 32442891

Theisen, E., & Konieczny, E. (2019). Medical cannabis: What nurses need to know. *American Nurse Today, 14*(11), 6–11. https://www.myamericannurse.com/medical-cannabis-what-nurses-need-to-know/

Valente, A. C., Lopes, L. P. N., & Matheus, M. E. (2024). Medical cannabis use in oncology and associated outcomes: A scoping review. *Journal of Oncology Pharmacy Practice, 30*(4), 737–751. DOI: 10.1177/10781552241239006 PMID: 38477532

Vyas, M. B., LeBaron, V. T., & Gilson, A. M. (2017). The use of cannabis in response to the opioid crisis: A review of the literature. *Nursing Outlook, 66*(1), 56–65. DOI: 10.1016/j.outlook.2017.08.012 PMID: 28993073

Washington State House of Representatives. (2026, February 12). *House passes "Ryan's Law," restoring compassion and dignity to end-of-life care.* https://housedemocrats.wa.gov/blog/2026/02/12/house-passes-ryans-law-restoring-compassion-and-dignity-to-end-of-life-care/#:~:text=OLYMPIA%20%E2%80%94%20In%20the%20final%20chapter%20of,hospice%20facilities%20can%20access%20medical%20cannabis%20as

Worster, B., Ashare, R. L., Hajjar, E., Garber, G., Smith, K., & Kelly, E. L. (2023). Clinician attitudes, training, and beliefs about cannabis: An interprofessional assessment. *Cannabis and Cannabinoid Research, 8*(3), 547–556. DOI: 10.1089/can.2021.0022 PMID: 34978882

Zibrik, K., Laskin, J., & Ho, C. (2016). Integration of a nurse navigator into the triage process for patients with non-small-cell lung cancer: Creating systematic improvements in patient care. *Current Oncology (Toronto, Ont.), 23*(3), 280–283. DOI: 10.3747/co.23.2954 PMID: 27330366

KEY TERMS AND DEFINITIONS

Cannabinoid Hyperemesis Syndrome (CHS): A clinical syndrome involving cyclical, severe nausea and vomiting associated with chronic, heavy cannabis use. Recognition and appropriate referral pathways for CHS are key safety functions within the navigator role.

Cannabis Nurse Navigator™: A standardized, systems-level advanced nursing role focused on organizational leadership and infrastructure. The Cannabis Nurse Navigator develops and implements protocols, referral pathways, documentation standards, staff education, policy alignment, interdisciplinary coordination, and harm-reduction systems to integrate cannabis-related care safely and equitably into healthcare organizations. This role operates primarily at the system/organizational level rather than through direct bedside care.

Cannabis Nurse: A direct, patient-level clinical nursing role that provides hands-on assessment, education, symptom monitoring, harm reduction, motivational interviewing, and individualized care for patients using medical cannabis. This role complements the Cannabis Nurse Navigator within a dual-level model.

Cannabis Use Disorder (CUD): A diagnosable condition characterized by problematic, continued cannabis use despite clinically significant impairment or distress. The Cannabis Nurse Navigator supports system-wide screening and referral pathways for CUD.

Care Coordination: The deliberate organization of patient care activities between different participants (providers, settings, and services) to facilitate appropriate, timely, and safe delivery of healthcare, including integration of cannabis-related information into the overall care plan.

Dual-Level Cannabis Nursing Model: A complementary framework in which the Cannabis Nurse Navigator functions at the systems/organizational level (coordination, policy, education infrastructure) while the Cannabis Nurse provides direct clinical care at the patient level. Together, these roles create structured, safe integration of cannabis-related care.

Endocannabinoid System (ECS): The complex biological system composed of endocannabinoids, receptors (CB1 and CB2), and enzymes that helps regulate pain, mood, appetite, sleep, immune function, and inflammation. Proficiency in the ECS is foundational to cannabis nursing practice.

Harm Reduction: Evidence-based strategies aimed at minimizing negative health, social, and legal consequences associated with cannabis use without necessarily requiring cessation. In cannabis nursing, this includes screening for Cannabis Use Disorder, education on safe dosing and routes of administration, and management of risks such as drug interactions.

Patient Navigation: A established nursing model, originally developed in oncology and chronic illness care, that emphasizes assessment, care coordination, education, advocacy, and systems literacy to help patients overcome barriers and move effectively through complex healthcare systems.

Systems-Level Nursing Role: A nursing practice focused on organizational infrastructure, policy development, staff education, and care system redesign rather than direct individual patient care. The Cannabis Nurse Navigator exemplifies this level of practice.

Chapter 6
A Framework for Health-Focused Medical Cannabis Care:
Using a Structured, Process-Based Approach

David Gordon
http://orcid.org/0009-0004-2008-8131
Community College of Denver, USA

ABSTRACT

Medical cannabis consumption is expanding rapidly in the United States, yet increased access has not been accompanied by consistent clinical processes. This has created a "clinical vacuum" for patients in which cannabis is often used in unstructured settings with inconsistent outcomes. This chapter argues that these challenges reflect a failure of care delivery rather than a limitation of the cannabis plant itself. It proposes a health-focused definition of medical cannabis centered on intentionality, monitoring, and evidence-based decision-making. To operationalize this definition, a five-step clinical framework is presented: Intention, Education, Implementation, Assessment, and Adjustment. The chapter also highlights the essential role of nurses in facilitating this framework, while also recognizing that this process can be applied in self-directed use when core elements are maintained. Emphasis is placed on future research evaluating process-based cannabis care using longitudinal, patient-centered outcomes across diverse care contexts.

INTRODUCTION

Medical Cannabis Access ≠ Medical Cannabis Care

Beth brings her medical cannabis certification to a local dispensary, excited to try a therapy that might help her. She has lived with chronic pain for over 20 years, with comorbid diagnoses of insomnia and depression. However, she received little guidance during her certification visit, and even less at the dispensary. She leaves with a bag of products, feeling overwhelmed; two days later, she is recovering

DOI: 10.4018/979-8-3373-7287-7.ch006

from hours of anxiety and marked impairment. Experiences such as Beth's are common and reflect not a failure of cannabis as a medicine, but shortcomings in the clinical process that surrounds its use.

Cannabis consumption for medicinal purposes in the United States (U.S.) has grown rapidly (Boehnke et al., 2024), accompanied by increased availability for most Americans (Schauer, 2024). However, access is not synonymous with effective medical cannabis care, and in the U.S., access is often prioritized over care. Medical care fundamentally requires a process of guidance, monitoring, and outcome assessment. These core elements are frequently absent from the medical cannabis experience, leaving patients in a clinical vacuum. The Association of Cannabinoid Specialists reinforces this concern, characterizing current state-based medical cannabis programs as a failure of healthcare infrastructure due to their emphasis on access rather than care (Tishler, n.d.).

The objective of this chapter is to propose a health-focused, process-based definition of medical cannabis, alongside a five-step framework that operationalizes it. Together, these emphasize a patient-centered approach applicable across diverse clinical contexts. In doing so, this chapter reviews the current landscape of medical cannabis care and identifies key clinical and systemic shortcomings that a process-based approach can address. It further highlights the essential role of nurses in helping patients implement this framework to support safe, effective, and sustainable medical cannabis use.

BACKGROUND

Cannabis Resurgence in a Chronic Disease Era

Interest in the medicinal use of cannabis has entered a renewed era (Boehnke et al., 2024), reaching a level of attention not seen since William Brooke O'Shaughnessy reintroduced the plant to the European medical community in the mid-19th century (Russo, 2017). This resurgence has unfolded alongside widespread regulatory change in the U.S. over the past three decades (Schauer, 2024) and against the backdrop of an accelerating chronic disease burden, in which declining quality of life has become increasingly common for millions of Americans (Olfson et al., 2018; Garmany & Terzic, 2024).

More than three-quarters of U.S. adults live with at least one chronic condition, and over 10% manage five or more (Benavidez et al., 2024). Beyond the human toll, the economic impact is substantial, with approximately 90% of nearly $5 trillion in annual U.S. healthcare expenditures now directed toward the management of chronic health conditions (Benavidez et al., 2024).

Chronic Disease, Homeostasis, and Systems Dysregulation

While chronic health conditions often arise from multifactorial drivers, a unifying feature across many diagnoses is disruption of the body's homeostatic regulatory capacity (Muth et al, 2019). This dysregulation commonly manifests as a persistent imbalance within the autonomic nervous system (ANS), characterized by chronic sympathetic dominance and reduced parasympathetic activity (Mancia & Grassi, 2014; Malpas, 2010). Because the nervous and immune systems are intrinsically interconnected, sustained sympathetic activation contributes directly to immune dysregulation. The downstream consequence—chronic inflammation—underlies many of the leading causes of global morbidity and mortality and is estimated to contribute to more than half of all deaths worldwide (Furman et al., 2019; GBD 2017 Causes of Death Collaborators, 2018).

Why Patients Turn to Medical Cannabis

Many of the conditions for which cannabis is most commonly sought, such as chronic pain, insomnia, emotional health challenges, autism, and cancer-related symptoms, exemplify the pattern of high healthcare utilization paired with suboptimal outcomes (Geurts et al., 2017; Cashin et al., 2025; McIntyre et al., 2023; Benca et al., 2023; Holdman et al., 2022). Patients navigating these complex conditions often find themselves within a healthcare system optimized for acute, episodic care (Institute of Medicine [IOM], 2001), rather than the integrated, whole-person approaches required to manage multiple, interacting chronic conditions. This misalignment has facilitated a "satisfaction gap," with many patients reporting that their needs are not adequately addressed by standard models of care (Rimmelzwaan et al., 2020; Christidis et al., 2025). For many individuals, conventional pharmaceuticals provide incomplete relief or are accompanied by adverse effects that further diminish daily functioning and quality of life (Boehnke et al., 2024). As a result, an increasing number of patients are turning to medical cannabis to address concerns that remain insufficiently managed by existing treatments (Bruce et al., 2018; Martin et al., 2021; Mercurio et al., 2019; Garcia-Romeu et al., 2022; Boehnke et al., 2024).

This growing interest has translated into approximately four million certified medical cannabis patients in the U.S. (Marijuana Policy Project, 2024), with millions more estimated to be using cannabis for medical purposes without formal certification (Compton et al., 2016). However, this expansion has occurred within a fragmented regulatory and academic landscape, contributing to the absence of a clear, consistently applied definition of "medical cannabis."

Medical Cannabis in the U.S.: Access Pathways and Definitions

Think back to Beth. After arbitrarily selecting one of the gummies she purchased and taking one nightly before bed, is she now a medical cannabis patient?

Some would argue that medical treatment requires a formal physician prescription for a Food and Drug Administration (FDA)–approved product (U.S. Congress, 1938; FDA, 2023). In the U.S., defining medical cannabis in this manner restricts treatment to a narrow set of options, including cannabidiol (Epidiolex) for rare seizure disorders and synthetic Δ-9-tetrahydrocannabinol (THC) formulations for chemotherapy-induced nausea and vomiting (FDA, 2023). Others apply a broader definition, extending medical cannabis status to individuals holding state-issued certifications, or more expansively, to anyone who self-identifies a health condition and consumes cannabis for therapeutic purposes (Graham et al., 2025).

This definitional ambiguity is further complicated by cannabis's evolving federal regulatory status. In the U.S., most cannabis remains classified as a Schedule I substance under the Controlled Substances Act (Controlled Substances Act, 1970). In contrast, low-THC varieties, commonly referred to as "hemp," are regulated separately under federal law (Agriculture Improvement Act of 2018). Legal status also remains in flux. A December 2025 executive order directed the Attorney General to expedite cannabis's transition to Schedule III, a designation reserved for substances with a "currently accepted medical use" under federal law (The White House, 2025), although no definitive timeline has been established. Additionally, legislation enacted in November 2025 amended the federal definition of "hemp," with changes taking effect in November 2026 and potentially altering product availability for patients absent further revision (Congressional Research Service, 2025). Regardless of cannabis's administrative classification as a controlled substance, the absence of a standardized clinical process for care remains the primary barrier to its integration into mainstream medical practice (National Academies of Sciences, Engineering, and Medicine, 2017).

Patients also face substantial challenges accessing guidance through conventional healthcare infrastructure (Boehnke et al., 2019). Most healthcare professionals receive little formal education in cannabis therapeutics (Evanoff et al., 2017) and frequently report low confidence in counseling patients on its use (Ronne et al., 2021). Estimates further suggest that fewer than 2% of licensed U.S. physicians actively participate in state registries as authorizing clinicians (Boehnke et al., 2024). When combined with anticipated stigma that discourages patients from disclosing cannabis use to their primary care providers (King et al., 2024), the result is a fragmented landscape in which patients often bypass their established medical teams. Instead, many rely on cannabis-only clinics or obtain products through adult-use markets or informal channels (Romero et al., 2025; Salter et al., 2022; Reed et al., 2020).

Nurse Leadership in Cannabis

Nurses have already shown leadership in attempting to help patients navigate this complex arena. The growth of the American Cannabis Nurses Association (American Cannabis Nurses Association, n.d.), the development of Cannabis as a nursing specialty (American Nurses Association, 2023), and the creation of Nursing Competencies in cannabis care (American Cannabis Nurses Association, 2021) all highlight the important roles nurses are already playing in improving health outcomes with cannabis consumption. This has led to nurses already working in varied spaces within the medical cannabis arena (American Nurses Association, 2023; Moore, 2024), some of which are highlighted below:

- working in cannabis dispensaries offering education and guidance to patients who qualify for medical cannabis
- serving as cannabis navigators that guide patients and help connect them to quality resources to facilitate informed decision-making
- directing treatment as a primary cannabis practitioner, a role that is open to nurse practitioners in some states
- supporting cannabis research in academic and private settings through education, recruitment, outcome measurement, and research design

MAIN FOCUS OF THE CHAPTER

Issues, Controversies, Problems

Definitional Ambiguity and Clinical Confusion

The absence of a shared, operational definition of "medical cannabis" in the U.S. has contributed to a fragmented and often clinically incoherent landscape, resulting in confusion among both patients and clinicians. Notably, the lack of a "common or agreed-upon definition" (European Monitoring Centre for

Drugs and Drug Addiction, 2018) represents an additional barrier to clinical integration, as state-level cannabis laws vary substantially in how they define permissible medical use (Ryan et al., 2021).

Medical cannabis is frequently discussed as though it were a single therapeutic entity, analogous to conventional pharmaceuticals; however, cannabis encompasses a wide range of potential "medications." It is not a single medicine, but a plant containing multiple active constituents (Russo, 2011) that interact with numerous receptor systems (Pertwee et al., 2010) and can be administered through diverse routes (National Academies of Sciences, Engineering, and Medicine, 2017). As a result, clinical effects vary substantially across individuals and clinical contexts (National Academies of Sciences, Engineering, and Medicine, 2017).

Although isolated compounds are more readily studied and more likely to gain regulatory approval, restricting the definition of medical cannabis to these options excludes a broader array of products that demonstrate promise in both clinical research and patient experience. Conversely, expanding the definition to include anyone with state certification, or even individuals with self-reported health conditions consuming cannabis, substantially enlarges the medical cannabis patient population (Graham et al., 2025). Yet clinical encounters limited to certification alone—without education, guidance, or monitoring—or unstructured self-treatment do not meet accepted standards of medical care (Dowell et al., 2022).

Access Without Care: Structural Gaps in Support

As a result, most patients who use cannabis for medicinal purposes do so without support from cannabis-trained professionals, and as many as 78% rely on self-directed learning or non-medical dispensary staff for therapeutic guidance (Clobes et al., 2025). Some patients turn to "cannabis-only" clinics; however, these settings are often high-volume access models that prioritize certification over clinical guidance and provide limited follow-up care (Boehnke et al., 2024). Others depend on point-of-sale recommendations, even though dispensary employees generally lack formal medical training (Haug et al., 2016) and may base guidance on non-clinical considerations (Merlin et al., 2021).

Nurses report "overwhelming support" for medical cannabis while looking to overcome cannabis stereotypes and provide the education and advocacy patients require (Kurtzman et al., 2022). However, nurses report insufficient education on cannabis science and therapeutics (Paiva et al., 2024; Balneaves et al., 2023; King, 2024). Because of this, nurses must often facilitate their own self-education to gain the necessary knowledge to be an effective cannabis nurse (King, 2024). Nurses already caring for medical cannabis patients report looking for "predictable processes" while noting "there is a lot to learn" and having "one conundrum after another" (McIntosh et al., 2024).

Safety and Efficacy in Unmonitored Use

The absence of a coherent system for medical cannabis care has important implications for both safety and efficacy, particularly among a relatively small subgroup of higher-risk consumers (Fischer et al., 2022). In unmonitored settings, cannabis use may be associated with the development of cannabis use disorder (CUD) and related adverse outcomes (National Academies of Sciences, Engineering, and Medicine, 2017). Emerging evidence suggests that an access-over-care approach in the U.S. may contribute to higher-risk use patterns, including associations between earlier medical cannabis certification and behaviors consistent with CUD (Schuster et al., 2022), as well as higher rates of CUD among medical cannabis cardholders compared with recreational consumers (Han et al., 2023).

Efficacy may also be compromised in the absence of structured clinical guidance. In a cohort of patients who received access-only medical cannabis for musculoskeletal pain, 58% discontinued treatment within one year, with nearly half discontinuing within the first three months (Khak et al., 2025). Discontinuation was most common among older adults, with a mean age of 71.5 years, raising concerns about the adequacy of unstructured, dispensary-based care for populations that often require more precise dosing, closer monitoring, and professional support (Khak et al., 2025). These findings are particularly relevant given that older adults represent the fastest-growing demographic of cannabis consumers in the U.S. (Han et al., 2025).

Limits of Disease-Centric Models for Cannabis Care

As patient interest in medical cannabis continues to grow, substantial challenges remain in ensuring access to appropriate guidance and clinical support (Clobes et al., 2025). Even when cannabis is incorporated into care, it is frequently introduced into existing disease- and symptom-centric models of medicine (Institute of Medicine, 2001; Tinetti et al., 2012). These models are poorly suited to the management of complex chronic conditions, where addressing individual symptoms or diagnoses in isolation often contributes to polypharmacy and escalating adverse effects (Institute of Medicine, 2001; Rimmelzwaan et al., 2020; Khezrian et al., 2020). This downstream focus also fails to address upstream drivers of chronic disease, including systemic inflammation and regulatory imbalance (Furman et al., 2019).

Within this context, clinical discussions of cannabis often center on questions such as whether it is effective for a specific diagnosis or symptom, with legitimacy typically conferred one condition at a time. State medical cannabis programs reinforce this framing by requiring certification for specific qualifying diagnoses, which vary considerably across jurisdictions (Ryan et al., 2021). However, this approach does not adequately account for the pharmacologic complexity of cannabis, including its multiple bioactive constituents, varied formulations, and diverse routes of administration.

As a result, nearly two centuries after O'Shaughnessy reintroduced cannabis to Western medicine, discussion continues to focus on the wrong questions, emphasizing safety and efficacy in isolation rather than the processes that govern real-world use. Framed in this way, medical cannabis is reduced to a product–diagnosis pairing that mirrors the limitations of conventional disease-centric care models. Accumulating evidence suggests that this framing is poorly aligned with the realities of chronic, multisystem disease (Muth et al., 2019). This disconnect underscores the need for a more clinically useful framework for integrating cannabis into medical care.

SOLUTIONS AND RECOMMENDATIONS

A Health-Focused Definition of Medical Cannabis

To address this mismatch, medical cannabis must be defined not by a product, a certification, or a diagnosis-specific treatment, but as a structured clinical process. This chapter proposes the following definition of medical cannabis: "the intentional and monitored use of the cannabis plant, or its constituents, to improve health, as guided by evidence-based medicine (EBM)."

This definition, illustrated in Figure 1, is intentionally broad yet demanding. It places improvement in health at the center of care, requiring outcomes to be evaluated holistically across physical, emotional, social, and cognitive domains. It accommodates the diversity of cannabis products that patients already access and use, while simultaneously insisting on core principles of medical care: intention, monitoring, and the application of EBM. Framed in this way, medical cannabis becomes generalizable, prioritizing process over product, monitoring over certification, and health over diagnoses.

Figure 1. A health-focused definition of medical cannabis

Medical Cannabis is...

the **intentional** and **monitored** use of the cannabis plant, or its constituents to **improve health**, as guided by **evidence-based medicine**

Figure 1. A Health-Focused Definition of Medical Cannabis.
This definition reframes medical cannabis as a clinical process rather than a product or access designation. It establishes intention, monitoring, and alignment with evidence-based medicine as necessary conditions for medical use, with health improvement serving as the primary criterion for evaluating effectiveness.

Intention anchors medical cannabis in patient-centered care, guiding both the decision to incorporate cannabis and the goals that shape individualized dosing strategies. Monitoring ensures ongoing assessment and adjustment, which are core components of medical care.

Health is intentionally aligned with the World Health Organization's (WHO) description as "a state of complete physical, mental, and social well-being and not merely the absence of disease or infirmity" (World Health Organization, 1948). The definition centers medical cannabis use on the goal of improving health, rather than treating isolated symptoms or diagnoses. This framing emphasizes lived experience across multiple domains and highlights well-being as a core construct, often described as an internal sense of judging life positively and feeling good (Centers for Disease Control [CDC], n.d.; Diener et al., 2018).

Accordingly, this approach prioritizes quality of life, function, and resilience, moving beyond a narrow focus on symptoms or diagnoses alone. Such multidimensional assessment should be familiar to nurses, for whom person-centered evaluation across physical, psychological, and social domains is foundational to professional practice (McCance & McCormack, 2025).

A Definition Applicable Across Clinical Contexts

Medical cannabis is ideally used with guidance and support from a cannabis-trained professional. Such clinicians can help patients clarify intentions, monitor benefits and adverse effects, interpret the evolving evidence base, and translate that knowledge into practical recommendations. This guidance may include product selection, safe consumption practices, and individualized dosing strategies.

At the same time, this definition accommodates self-directed cannabis use, provided that the core elements of intention, monitoring, and evidence-based decision-making are actively maintained. When patients work independently, this requires deliberate self-education, self-regulation, and careful observation over time to ensure that use remains intentional and health-focused.

A Practical Framework to Operationalize the Definition

Throughout this chapter, Beth has served as an illustrative example of a patient living with multiple chronic conditions who is interested in using medical cannabis to improve her health. Despite having access, she struggles to determine how and what to consume, and how to replicate the benefits observed in clinical trials and other structured care environments. These challenges underscore the need for a clear, structured framework to ensure that the core elements of this chapter's definition of medical cannabis—intention, monitoring, and the use of EBM—are consistently present.

This framework, illustrated in Figure 2, consists of five core steps, each essential for translating the definition of medical cannabis into a practical, usable process for improving health:

- **Intention**: defines purpose and direction
- **Education**: aligns action with evidence and values
- **Implementation**: translates knowledge into a workable regimen
- **Assessment**: determines whether intentions are being met
- **Adjustment**: refines therapy based on feedback and new information

Figure 2. A health-focused framework for medical cannabis use

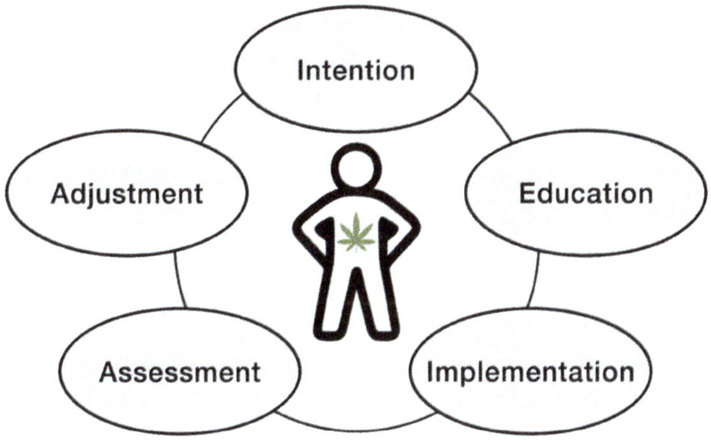

Figure 2. A Health-Focused Framework for Medical Cannabis Use.
This framework illustrates five interdependent components—intention, education, implementation, assessment, and adjustment—that operationalize a health-focused approach to medical cannabis use. Intention serves as the conceptual cornerstone of the framework and the starting point for defining medical cannabis use, while the circular structure emphasizes that care is not linear. Ongoing assessment and adjustment allow earlier components, including intention and education, to be revisited and refined over time in response to individual needs and outcomes.

At every stage, the framework places the patient at the center of the process, ensuring care remains personalized while grounded in EBM. It is applicable across a wide range of symptoms, intentions, diagnoses, and clinical contexts, and can be used by both cannabis-naïve individuals and long-term consumers. Although presented sequentially, effective use of the framework is inherently iterative, with continual reassessment and refinement as treatment evolves.

The framework is intentionally pragmatic. It does not depend on a specific disease model, biologic theory, or therapeutic philosophy. Whether cannabis is used to manage discrete symptoms, as an adjunct to other treatments, or in pursuit of broader health goals, the same core process applies.

Regardless of whether cannabis use is self-directed or supported by a cannabis-trained professional, the process begins in the same place: clarifying intention. Intention establishes the foundation that guides all subsequent decisions and ensures that medical cannabis is approached in a patient-centered manner, oriented not only toward symptom relief but toward whole-person, health-focused care.

Intention

Intention is the cornerstone of health-focused cannabis therapy and the essential starting point of this chapter's proposed definition of medical cannabis. While Beth presents with multiple diagnoses, these do not fully capture her goals or the intentions she brings to her care. She may be seeking better sleep, improved work productivity, or a greater sense of acceptance and emotional balance in daily life.

Philosophical scholarship defines intention as a purposeful, goal-directed focus that shapes action (Anscombe, 1963; Bratman, 1987). In this framing, intention is not a passive statement of desire, but an active process requiring patient participation. Importantly, intention is not merely a philosophical construct. It is one of the strongest predictors of follow-through in health-related behaviors (Ajzen, 1991) and has been shown to influence physical activity (McEachan et al., 2011), medication adherence (Lin et al., 2016), and broader health-related outcomes (Tabaei-Aghdaei et al., 2023).

Because cannabis can support multiple, and sometimes opposing, experiences, clarity of intention is particularly important in cannabis therapeutics. The following considerations may be helpful when working with patients to establish clear and realistic intentions:

- Is treatment intended to focus on specific symptoms, and if so, which are prioritized? Alternatively, is the patient seeking to address upstream drivers such as inflammation, stress physiology, or trauma?
- Is treatment intended to support engagement with daily life and relationships, or to provide brief periods of disconnection from chronic challenges?
- What types of activities will the patient engage in while using cannabis? Do these activities require cognitive focus, coordination, or physical movement, or do they benefit more from spontaneity and creativity?
- Is the goal to enhance efficiency and task completion, or to allow for more open, less goal-directed thought?

These considerations are not exhaustive, but they highlight why defining intentions is essential as the framework progresses. To assess whether intention-setting has been effective, clinicians and educators can reflect on the following questions with patients:

- Can the patient clearly articulate what they want to be different in their day-to-day life?
- Are they thinking beyond a list of symptoms and diagnoses?
- Have they distinguished between overarching intentions for cannabis therapy and specific intentions for individual dosing sessions?
- Do their non-cannabis behaviors align with their stated intentions?

Clarifying intention also helps guide adjunctive, non-cannabis interventions. For example, when improving sleep quality is identified as a priority, this naturally leads to education on sleep hygiene and the incorporation of supportive behavioral strategies into the care plan.

Although patients can engage in this process independently, intention-setting is often more effective when supported by a care team. Many patients manage multiple concerns and conditions, making it easy to become overwhelmed by symptom-by-symptom approaches. Nurses are well positioned to help patients define and prioritize intentions (McCance & McCormack, 2025) and play a critical role in supporting subsequent steps in this framework.

Clear intentions alone, however, do not provide a roadmap for action. Patients frequently encounter uncertainty around products, dosing, routes of administration, timing, and risk. Without appropriate education, even well-defined intentions may devolve into ineffective or unsafe trial-and-error. For this reason, education is the logical next step in the framework, translating intention into informed action aligned with EBM.

Education

Beth hopes cannabis can be an effective tool and wants to use it medically, yet she has already encountered significant challenges. She has clarified her intentions—improving sleep and becoming more proactive about healthy behaviors—while also hoping for broader symptom relief. After navigating these early hurdles, she recognizes that better information is essential for making informed decisions about her treatment.

Education is critical because confusion surrounding cannabis remains widespread among patients, clinicians, and industry professionals alike. Cannabis is inherently complex, encompassing a wide range of products, dosing strategies, and routes of administration (National Academies of Sciences, Engineering, and Medicine, 2017). As a result, education serves as the bridge between intention and action, translating evidence into a reliable foundation from which patients can begin treatment. Education is also essential for reinforcing a core pillar of this chapter's definition of medical cannabis: that use is guided by EBM.

In 1996, Sackett and colleagues outlined the foundational principles of EBM. They described three essential components: best available scientific evidence, clinical expertise, and patient values, emphasizing that effective care requires integration of all three (Sackett et al., 1996). This model remains highly relevant to medical cannabis and provides a practical structure for education and decision-making.

Best Available Scientific Evidence

Sackett emphasized that EBM is not limited to randomized controlled trials (RCTs) and meta-analyses, but involves identifying the best external evidence available to answer clinical questions (Sackett et al., 1996). In cannabis therapeutics, this includes RCTs alongside real-world evidence derived from non-interventional studies, patient registries, electronic health records, and insurance datasets (Banerjee et al., 2022; Schlag et al., 2022). This broader evidence base is particularly important given the inherent limitations of RCTs (Ahuja, 2019; Ioannidis, 2005), and the impracticality of studying every possible formulation, route of administration, dose range, and clinical indication in controlled trials.

Clinical Expertise

Clinical expertise is already embedded within mainstream medical decision-making alongside formal research evidence. For example, approximately half of recommendations issued by the American College of Cardiology/American Heart Association and the European Society of Cardiology rely primarily on expert consensus (Level 3 evidence), while fewer than 10% are based on Level 1 evidence such as RCTs and systematic reviews (Fanaroff et al., 2019).

In cannabis care, a growing number of clinicians work directly with patients to guide therapeutic use (Boehnke et al., 2024). Contemporary practice also draws upon thousands of years of historical medicinal cannabis use (Russo, 2007), as well as shared insights exchanged through professional societies, conferences, and collaborative clinical communities. Within Sackett's framework, this clinical expertise is essential for translating evidence into individualized, practical starting points for treatment.

Patient Values

Scientific evidence and clinical expertise represent only two components of EBM; the third is patient values. These include beliefs, preferences, lived experience, goals, risk tolerance, priorities, and cultural or moral frameworks. As discussed in the prior section, intention-setting plays a central role in identifying and incorporating these values into evidence-based decision-making.

Putting it all Together

A complete EBM approach aligns particularly well with cannabis therapeutics, given both the wide range of conditions cannabis may affect (Pacher & Kunos, 2013) and the diversity of available treatment options (National Academies of Sciences, Engineering, and Medicine, 2017). Education is therefore necessary to translate evidence into actionable care. Effective medical cannabis education is reflected by several key indicators:

- Patients express confidence using medical cannabis
- Patients remain open to adjustment and personalization
- Patients can identify benefits without requiring marked impairment
- Patients remain consistent with their treatment plans
- Patients can make small, informed adjustments independently

Education functions as more than information delivery; it is a central mechanism for risk mitigation. By translating evidence into practical guidance, education reduces risks associated with unguided use. This is particularly important for vulnerable populations, including older adults, individuals with emotional health concerns, and those with cognitive impairment. In these groups, risks may include interactions with existing polypharmacy, destabilization of sleep or emotional health, or increased caregiver burden.

While physician education and engagement remain important areas for growth, many other healthcare professionals play essential roles in delivering cannabis education and bridging the gap between intention and implementation. Nurses have emerged as leaders in this space with one example being LEAF411, a nonprofit organization that provides nurse-led education and directional support to the public regarding the safe use of legal cannabis.

This model is especially relevant for older adults, the fastest-growing demographic of cannabis consumers in the U.S. (Han et al., 2025). Given higher rates of multimorbidity and polypharmacy, this population has distinct educational needs and can benefit substantially from accessible, nurse-led guidance. Figure 3 summarizes age demographics and engagement patterns among individuals contacting the LEAF411 nurse-led cannabis education helpline between October 2019 and January 2026. This example illustrates how education can function as a first-line risk mitigation strategy, complementing the recommendations of treating clinicians.

Figure 3. Nurse-led cannabis education: Client age distribution and primary concerns

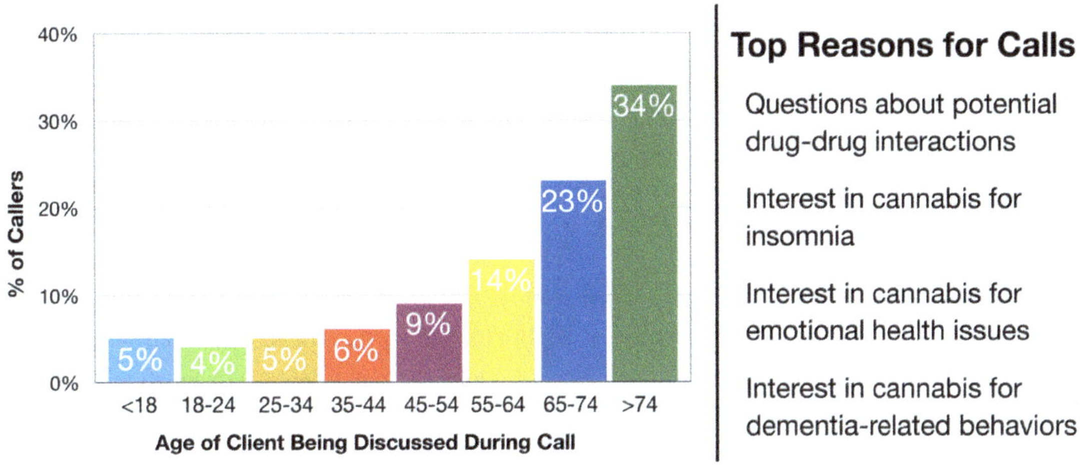

Figure 3. Nurse-Led Cannabis Education: Client Age Distribution and Primary Concerns

Client age distribution and primary reasons for engagement with the nurse-led cannabis education helpline operated by LEAF411 between October 2019 and January 2026. Data are derived from internal organizational records shared via personal communication with Katherine Golden, CEO of LEAF411. These data illustrate how nurse-led cannabis education supports evidence-informed decision making, personalization of care, and assessment of readiness for implementation within a health-focused cannabis framework.

Whether a patient is supported by nurses, another cannabis-trained professional, or managing use independently, education plays a critical role in determining readiness for implementation. Although guidance from a cannabis-trained professional is ideal, many patients now have access to high-quality educational resources developed by clinicians, researchers, and educators actively engaged in both evidence appraisal and patient care. These tools allow some individuals to use cannabis in accordance with this chapter's definition without a formal practitioner relationship.

By serving as the bridge between intention and action, education prepares patients to enter the next stage of this framework. When grounded in EBM, it enables cannabis therapy to begin thoughtfully, safely, and with clear direction. The next step—implementation—translates this preparation into practice.

Implementation

Beth has spent time with a cannabis educator and understands the differences between THC- and CBD-dominant products, as well as the advantages and limitations of various routes of administration. She drives to work and, at this stage, wants to avoid impairment during the workday. She begins taking a CBD-dominant oil infusion (commonly labeled as a tincture) orally in the morning and early afternoon. After dinner, she uses a different product containing 2.5 mg of each CBD and THC, also taken orally. The regimen is easy to follow and fits well with her daily routines and priorities.

Implementation translates the preceding steps into a personalized, evidence-based cannabis regimen. Importantly, this represents a starting point—not a fixed endpoint—designed to fit the patient's life and align with their intentions, rather than applying a standardized approach to a specific symptom or diagnosis. For example, two patients with fibromyalgia may share similar symptoms yet require different recommendations based on their goals, daily responsibilities, and clinical context. An effective implementation plan should be accessible, understandable, and manageable, while clearly specifying key elements such as constituents, dose, frequency, and route of administration.

Appropriate dosing and titration are central to identifying a patient's therapeutic window—the range in which benefit occurs with minimal adverse effects. A thoughtful implementation strategy can also reduce higher-risk use patterns, including regular combustion (smoking), frequent use of high-concentration THC products, and rapid tolerance development (Fischer et al., 2022). For patients already using cannabis in ineffective or higher-risk ways, implementation should emphasize gradual transitions rather than abrupt changes. When done well, implementation reduces the risk of overwhelm, over-treatment, abandonment, and harm.

EBM provides general operating principles that apply across conditions and populations. In addition, published protocols and clinical guidelines are available to inform therapeutic use (Bell et al., 2024; Bhaskar et al., 2021; MacCallum & Russo, 2018). The following themes, while not exhaustive, align with both the literature and clinical expertise and help identify effective starting points for implementation.

Dosing Considerations

"Start low, go slow" remains a foundational principle in cannabis therapeutics (MacCallum & Russo, 2018), particularly when initiating Type 1 (THC-dominant) products. This approach minimizes adverse effects, which are consistently dose-dependent (Fischer et al., 2022), while also allowing identification of efficacy. Notably, the effective dose range for cannabis often begins much lower than patients expect. Many assume impairment is required for benefit, although meaningful improvements may occur at THC doses that do not produce such effects (Wallace et al., 2015). Clinical guidance typically defines a low starting THC dose as 0.5–2.5 mg and rarely recommends exceeding this range in cannabis-naïve patients (MacCallum & Russo, 2018).

CBD has a substantially wider therapeutic window than THC and has been studied at doses up to 1,500 mg per day (Iffland & Grotenhermen, 2017). In clinical practice, however, many patients report benefit at considerably lower doses (Shannon et al., 2019). Initial CBD dosing commonly ranges from 10–30 mg per dose, with pediatric dosing adjusted by weight.

Ratio Selection

Cannabis products are often categorized by CBD-to-THC ratio: Type 1 products are THC-dominant, Type 2 products contain relatively balanced amounts of CBD and THC, and Type 3 products are CBD-dominant. While no universal thresholds exist, ratios between approximately 3:1 and 1:3 CBD:THC serve as practical guides for Type 2 products.

Beginning with a 1:1 CBD:THC whole-plant preparation is a simple and evidence-supported approach. Sativex (nabiximols)—a sublingually administered spray that is an approved pharmaceutical in more than 25 countries—delivers approximately 2.5 mg each of THC and CBD per spray and has been extensively studied, demonstrating positive safety and efficacy (Prieto González & Vila Silván, 2021a; Prieto González & Vila Silván, 2021b). Although not optimal for all patients, 1:1 products with similar constituent profiles are widely available in retail markets and well supported by clinical evidence, making them practical starting points.

Higher CBD:THC ratios may be preferable when limiting impairment is a priority. Although CBD is psychoactive (Iffland & Grotenhermen, 2017), it does not produce the classic impairment associated with THC. Increasing the relative CBD content using Type 3 products may enhance tolerability and acceptance, particularly early in treatment.

Route of Administration

Ingestion and inhalation remain the most common routes of cannabis administration, though sublingual, transdermal, and rectal routes are also used (National Academies of Sciences, Engineering, and Medicine, 2017). Inhalation produces rapid onset, often within minutes, and the shortest duration, typically under four hours (Huestis, 2007). Oral ingestion is more variable due to gastrointestinal absorption and first-pass hepatic metabolism, but generally produces slower onset (1–2 hours) and longer duration (6–12 hours) (Huestis, 2007). Newer ingestible formulations with more predictable and rapid onset are increasingly available (Reddy et al., 2023).

Sublingual administration is often described as intermediate in onset and duration; however, in practice it frequently resembles oral ingestion (Lefebvre et al., 2024). Transdermal formulations provide slower onset and longer duration up to 12 hours, but offer less flexibility and higher cost, particularly at therapeutic doses (Lefebvre et al., 2024).

Aligning patient intentions with expected pharmacokinetics is a key component of implementation and increases patient confidence. Familiarity with these parameters also supports accurate post-dosing assessment, discussed in the next section.

Temporal Patterns: Maintenance vs. Rapid Relief

Onset and duration are central to aligning cannabis use with patient intentions. For example, rapid-onset options such as inhalation or fast-acting ingestibles may benefit patients seeking appetite stimulation or acute nausea relief. Inhalation may be used for intermittent or breakthrough symptoms, or when minimizing the duration of impairment is a primary goal.

For persistent symptoms, longer-acting maintenance strategies are often preferable. These allow cannabinoids to reach a steady state, supporting homeostatic regulation of nervous and immune system activity while providing consistent symptom relief. In this way, cannabis therapy may address upstream contributors to illness while also managing symptoms.

With adequate education and confidence, many patients use more than one product or route to support different intentions. For example, a non-impairing oral product may be used two to three times daily for baseline support, while inhaled THC is reserved for breakthrough symptoms or brief, intentional periods of euphoria.

Harm Reduction Strategies

Implementation should incorporate harm-reduction strategies that minimize risk while supporting intentional cannabis use. When monitored and intentional, cannabis use is not typically associated with severe adverse outcomes (Fischer et al., 2022), and deliberate implementation choices can further enhance safety.

For patients who require inhalation, dry-herb vaporizers are preferred. These devices heat ground flower without combustion, substantially reducing exposure to toxic byproducts associated with smoking (Fischer et al., 2022). Compared with vaporizer pens or concentrates, dry-herb vaporizers allow more precise dose control and generally carry lower risk of excessive THC exposure or contaminants.

Evidence regarding CBD's mitigation of THC-related adverse effects is mixed; however, clinical experience and selected data support an entourage effect in which CBD may widen THC's therapeutic window (Russo, 2011; Englund et al., 2013). Accordingly, incorporating CBD alongside THC should be routinely considered, with product selection guided by patient intentions and tolerance.

Cannabinoids can interact with the liver's cytochrome P450 enzymes and cause clinically significant drug-drug interactions. These interactions are most common with higher dosages of CBD (>100 mg daily) but warrant consideration in any cannabis treatment plan, particularly for patients taking immunosuppressants, anti-epileptics, anticoagulants, antifungals, or other central nervous system depressants (Nachnani et al., 2024). Additional consideration is warranted when cannabis is used alongside immune checkpoint inhibitor immunotherapy, as the immunomodulatory properties of cannabinoids may interact with treatment response in ways that remain incompletely understood (Behling-Hess et al., 2025).

A comprehensive harm-reduction approach also includes non-cannabis behavioral and lifestyle strategies. Recommendations often focus on nutrition, movement, stress regulation, and social connection, all of which independently improve health outcomes and reduce reliance on cannabis as a sole therapeutic tool.

Many patients are already using cannabis when they seek guidance, though not in ways that align with this framework. In these cases, meeting patients where they are and prioritizing gradual, achievable changes is essential. Completing intention-setting and education before modifying a regimen fosters engagement. Simple adjustments, such as switching from smoking to dry-herb vaporization or adding a daily Type 3 maintenance product, are often effective first steps toward healthier use patterns.

Collaboration and Patient Success

Successful implementation depends not only on the regimen itself, but also on the surrounding systems of support, collaboration, and readiness.

Nurses play a critical role during this stage. In collaboration with physicians, they help translate recommendations into daily routines, address access and affordability, assist with product labeling, and identify barriers to adherence. Nurses excel in nonjudgmental harm reduction and behavior change support, both for cannabis use and complementary lifestyle interventions. In many states, nurse practitioners may serve as an authorizing provider for medical certification and direct a comprehensive treatment plan.

Clinical experience and emerging evidence indicate that nurse involvement improves patient satisfaction, adherence, and outcomes. Meta-analyses demonstrate that structured nurse-led programs enhance medication adherence and clinical outcomes across chronic conditions (Rehman et al., 2025; Ruksakulpiwat et al., 2025). In medical cannabis specifically, specialized nursing consultations have been identified as a key factor in improving adherence and symptom management (Bassi et al., 2025).

As implementation marks the beginning of a patient's cannabis journey, success is ultimately evaluated during the next step: assessment. However, as regimens are established, several practical questions help identify readiness and effectiveness of the implementation strategy:

- Can the patient clearly articulate what, when, how, and how much to consume?
- Do they have reliable access to recommended products, and can they afford them?
- Does the regimen align with daily responsibilities, such as driving or safety-sensitive work?
- Do they understand which products may cause impairment or have narrower therapeutic windows?
- Are they prepared to incorporate non-cannabis recommendations alongside treatment?

Implementation establishes a plan that is accessible, tolerable, safe, and aligned with patient intentions. Given the diversity and complexity of cannabis, ongoing personalization is expected. Implementation is the starting point; assessment determines how well the plan is working and how it should evolve.

Assessment

Beth has been following her regimen for several weeks. Her partner asks whether it is helping. How does she know? She might respond globally, "yes, I feel better." Others may notice changes before she does, commenting that she seems happier or that she complains less about abdominal symptoms. In research or clinical settings, she would likely complete questionnaires pre- and post-treatment. Beth has multiple ways to assess whether cannabis therapy is helping, and learning how to use them is central to success.

Monitoring is a core pillar of this chapter's definition of medical cannabis because it reveals what is working, what is not, and provides the feedback needed to guide future adjustments. Assessment should be an active process with meaningful patient engagement; feedback from multiple perspectives is particularly valuable and may include a cannabis-trained professional, the patient themselves, and individuals close to them. Within this framework, assessment serves several essential functions in the pursuit of improved health:

- Prevents treatment without feedback
- Optimizes dosing to limit unwanted cognitive effects, sedation, and functional impairment
- Promotes multi-domain appraisal of health
- Guards against reductionism and symptom chasing
- Incorporates multiple perspectives

Within cannabis treatment, both assessment after individual dosing sessions and longitudinally are important, as each provides distinct and complementary information.

Dosing Session Assessment

A brief clinical example highlights the importance of real-time assessment. Mary used cannabis after work to manage anxiety that they accumulated throughout the day. By the time they arrived home, they felt overstimulated and disconnected, often skipping dinner and struggling to engage with their partner. While cannabis provided some relief, they frequently felt overly impaired and sedated, most often after smoking a full joint shortly after arriving home. Their intention was present, but they were not assessing whether their consumption was actually achieving it.

Rather than continuing this pattern, Mary was instructed to take a single puff, assess after 10 minutes, and then decide whether re-dosing was necessary. Within a short period, they discovered that two puffs were sufficient to calm their nervous system, restore their appetite, and allow them to be present with their partner, without unwanted sedation or impairment. Post-dosing assessment helped transform cannabis from an unstructured tool into a targeted, medical intervention.

Even when patients are using consistent, maintenance regimens, it's important to assess after dosing, particularly early in treatment. Chronic conditions still fluctuate moment to moment, and immediate effects can provide valuable guidance. This is especially relevant when THC is involved, as its effects tend to be more acute and dose-sensitive. By reassessing after each dose, patients can determine whether their current dose and cannabinoid ratio are appropriate for their needs.

Several tools can support this type of session-level assessment, depending on patient preference. Figure 4 highlights Dr. Dustin Sulak's Inner Inventory, a brief four-question framework that prompts patients to check in with their breath, body, mind, and symptoms before and after dosing (Sulak, n.d.). There are also apps that allow patients to track individualized goals, document subjective effects, and link outcomes to specific products and doses (Giangregorio et al., 2024). In practice, some patients prefer simple 0–10 symptom ratings or reflective journaling.

Figure 4. Session-level assessment using Dr. Dustin Sulak's inner inventory

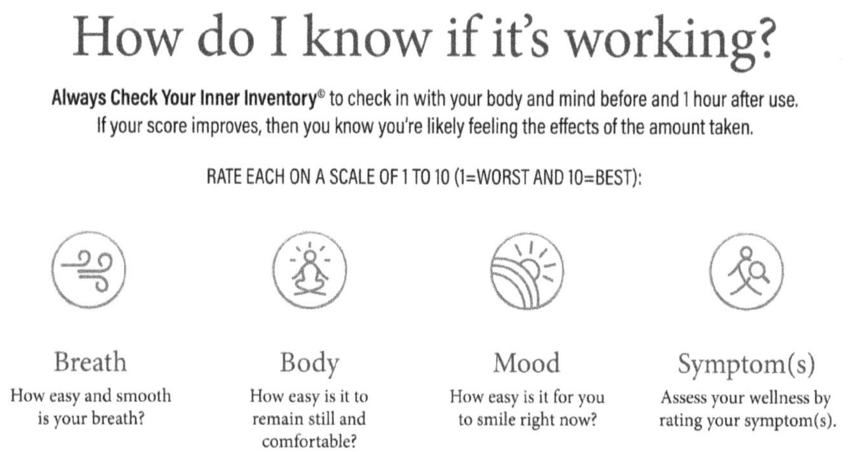

Figure 4. Session-Level Assessment Using Dr. Dustin Sulak's Inner Inventory.
Assessment at the level of individual dosing sessions provides actionable information for guiding cannabis therapy. Dr. Dustin Sulak's Inner Inventory is a brief, four-item self-assessment that prompts patients to rate breath, body, mood, and symptom burden before and after dosing, supporting patient awareness and informed dose titration through structured, self-evaluation (Sulak, n.d.).

Longitudinal Assessment

Monitoring over time is equally critical. Longitudinal assessment allows patients and clinicians to evaluate whether therapy is contributing to the central goal of this chapter's definition of medical cannabis: improving health. This intentionally broad outcome helps avoid an overly reductionist focus on isolated symptoms and instead emphasizes the whole person, including physical, emotional, social, and cognitive domains.

For example, a patient may begin using an oral cannabis product for sleep and find that they are sleeping more deeply than ever before. However, if this improvement is accompanied by prolonged morning grogginess or impaired work performance, overall health may not be improved despite better sleep. Longitudinal assessment makes these trade-offs visible and creates opportunities for adjustment. As such, assessment must extend beyond symptom severity to include function, confidence, well-being, and quality of life.

A range of validated tools can support assessment over time, provided they are used consistently and interpreted in context. PROMs and HRQoL instruments are widely used across chronic disease management (Black, 2013) and have also been incorporated into the cannabis literature (Arkell et al., 2023; Tait et al., 2025). Although primarily developed for research settings, many are practical and accessible for clinical use.

Patient Global Impression of Change (PGIC)

The PGIC is a widely used PROM that captures a patient's global perception of treatment effectiveness using a single question (Hurst & Bolton, 2004). Responses are recorded on a symmetrical 7-point scale ranging from "Very Much Improved" to "Very Much Worse," with "No Change" at the midpoint. For cannabis therapy, a representative question might be: "Since beginning this cannabis treatment regimen, how would you describe the change (if any) in your overall health?" Its simplicity makes the PGIC particularly useful for capturing overall treatment impact while remaining adaptable to specific symptoms or domains.

PROMIS Global Health-10 (PROMIS GH-10)

The PROMIS GH-10 expands assessment across ten items evaluating overall health, quality of life, physical function, pain, fatigue, emotional distress, and social health (Hays et al., 2009). This brief instrument has been validated against longer tools such as the Short Form (36) Health Survey (SF-36) and offers a practical balance between depth and feasibility (Kasturi et al., 2018).

The PROMIS Toolbox

PROMIS GH-10 is part of the broader PROMIS toolbox, which includes validated modules assessing multiple domains (Cella et al., 2010). Clinicians and patients may combine the GH-10 with selected short-form modules—such as Pain Interference, Sleep Disturbance, or Anxiety—to create a tailored yet manageable assessment battery.

These instruments are only a subset of available options. The specific tool matters less than the presence of consistent, interpretable feedback to guide decision-making and ongoing optimization.

Regardless of whether a patient is working with a practitioner or self-managing their care, monitoring remains essential. Assessment tells a story, both in the moment and over time, about whether intentions are being met and whether overall health is improving. That story directly informs the next step in the framework: adjustment, where treatment is refined to keep the patient moving toward improved health.

Adjustment

Beth returns after a month on her new treatment regimen, which is evidence-based and personalized to her intentions. Ongoing education gave her confidence in implementing the regimen. Regular self-assessment then guided action, leading to micro-adjustments in both her daytime and evening regimen. During follow-up, she reports a positive global impression of treatment, along with improvements in quality of life and sleep. However, she continues to experience daytime pain that interferes with her work. Beth also notes that her current daytime product has become cost-prohibitive at her present dosing. Taken together, this information supports a change to a more cost-effective daytime product, with an adjusted cannabinoid ratio designed to improve pain while minimizing impairment.

Adjustment naturally follows assessment and provides the opportunity to optimize a patient's cannabis regimen to better align with their intentions. In guided care, it is uncommon for patients to discontinue treatment shortly after initiation (Tait et al., 2023), though it remains important to evaluate whether continued use is appropriate. Cost, stigma, adverse effects, and regimen complexity are just some of the potential reasons for cessation (Khak et al., 2025). Patients who struggle during this stage may benefit from working with a cannabis-trained professional, who can offer clinical and educational guidance and introduce products or strategies a patient may not otherwise consider. Once the decision is made to continue therapy, the adjustment stage allows for targeted changes in dose, constituents, ratios, routes of administration, and specific products or brands.

For example, if a patient continues to have difficulty with sleep onset despite using an ingested product dosed a few hours before bedtime, an appropriate adjustment may be to trial a more rapidly absorbed option, such as inhalation or a rapid-acting ingestible formulation. Alternatively, if sleep maintenance remains the primary issue, shifting the original ingested product closer to bedtime may better align pharmacokinetics with the patient's needs.

Adjustment often requires behavioral and logistical support, not just pharmacologic change. Working with cannabis-trained nurses can be valuable during this stage. They can assist by:

- Helping patients interpret assessment data
- Supporting behavior change during regimen shifts
- Addressing barriers related to cost, access, and adherence
- Reinforcing harm-reduction strategies during transitions
- Helping patients avoid premature abandonment of therapy

Variability is expected in cannabis treatment, and adjustment is the critical step in this framework where therapy becomes truly personalized. This process ensures that care is optimized rather than constrained by rigid, disease-centric regimens. The importance of adjustment is highlighted by data from Siani-Rose and colleagues, who evaluated ten patients in a metabolomics study under good disease control on stable cannabis regimens (Siani-Rose et al., 2023). Table 1 illustrates the substantial diversity of these regimens, even within a single clinical condition, underscoring the need for continual adjustment.

Table 1. Diversity of cannabis regimens among patients with autism under good disease control

	Cannabinoid content (mg) per treatment						
Age	**Method of Administration**	**THC**	**CBD**	**CBG**	**CBN**	**THCA**	**CBDA**
6	Edible	1				17	
7	Tincture	10	30		30		
7	Edible	10		20			
8	Tincture	1		20		15	
8	Tincture	10	35				
9	Edible	5	100	20			
10	Tincture	50					75
10	Tincture	3	50				
11	Edible		60	50			
11	Edible		85	25			
11	Edible	10	100				
11	Tincture		200				
12	Edible	15	7.5				
12	Tincture	4.5	10		3		
12	Tincture	0.05				5	12

Source: Siani-Rose et al. (2023)

As adjustments are considered, all prior stages of the framework are revisited. Information gathered during assessment—both in real time during dosing sessions and longitudinally—is integrated alongside any changes in patient intentions or emerging evidence that may inform care. In this way, the five steps of the framework are not strictly linear but iterative and continuously applied. Patients can engage in this process independently; however, working with cannabis-trained professionals across multiple stages of the framework adds meaningful value and supports more consistent, successful application in practice.

A Process-Based Definition and Framework Fits Cannabis Biology

This chapter proposes a holistic, process-based definition and corresponding framework for medical cannabis in lieu of a disease- or symptom-centric approach. This strategy also aligns with cannabis biology. Cannabinoids work through the endocannabinoid system (ECS), an evolutionarily conserved regulatory system (Elphick, 2012) that helps maintain homeostasis, regulates physiological parameters such as sleep, appetite, mood and pain, and plays a central role in modulating both nervous and immune system activity (de Roon-Cassini et al., 2020). By addressing these upstream, root causes of chronic disease, medical cannabis could have broad relevance across a range of chronic conditions (Pacher & Kunos, 2013).

This is reflected in evidence from structured care environments—such as randomized controlled trials (RCTs), open-label extension studies, prospective observational research, and national medical cannabis registries—where process is prioritized over access. In real-world environments, multiple different cannabinoid formulations and methods of administration are used for an extensive array of clinical indications. Despite the heterogeneity in products and indications, data supports both the efficacy and safety of medical cannabis (Mick & Douek, 2024), and consistently suggests improvements in clinical outcomes, well-being, and quality-of-life measures (Bar-Lev Schleider et al., 2022; Tait et al., 2025; Erridge et al., 2026). Taken together, these patterns suggest that outcomes depend less on a specific cannabis product or the underlying diagnoses, and more on the care environment in which it is used, further underscoring the need for a clear process-based definition and clinical framework.

The Framework in Practice

The following examples illustrate how this framework functions in practice and contributes to effective medical cannabis treatment as defined in this chapter. The first is a case from this author's clinical practice; the second is a published intervention in a Veterans clinic that independently operationalized a similar framework.

Bob presented for a consultation after several years of medical cannabis certification and use for a range of conditions and symptoms, including headaches, depression, anxiety, insomnia, irritable bowel syndrome, and attention deficit disorder. His use consisted of repeated daily inhalation via combustion or dabbing (rapid vaporization and inhalation of concentrate cannabis extracts). Although he reported short-term symptom relief immediately after consumption, he also described escalation of many chronic symptoms over time and a generally poor quality of life. His use patterns were consistent with CUD and were likely contributing to poorer overall health, thus inconsistent with this chapter's definition of medical cannabis.

Guided by this definition, the proposed framework was used to help Bob transition to a cannabis regimen that was intentional, monitored, and guided by EBM. First, Bob was guided to clarify his intentions. He identified symptom relief and improved ability to engage in activities he enjoyed as primary goals. Another important intention was avoiding pharmaceutical treatments which, despite multiple trials, had historically been ineffective for him.

Education followed. Foundational aspects of medical cannabis were reviewed, including differences between THC, CBD, and other cannabinoids, as well as the relative advantages and disadvantages of various routes of administration. He learned how tolerance, particularly to THC, can affect therapeutic response, and gained insight on behavioral strategies that might support his goals.

With this foundation, a new strategy was implemented. He started a daytime maintenance regimen using a Type 3, CBD-dominant ingestible product. To optimize THC use, he separately began a low-dose ingested THC maintenance regimen alongside the Type 3 product. He was given guidance on the role of inhalation for short-term symptom relief with the priority that any inhaled use should be guided by structured self-monitoring rather than habitual escalation.

Early reassessments demonstrated reduced overall cannabis use; however, improvements on the PGIC were minimal, and other PROMs continued to show disruption across several domains. Guided by this assessment data, his regimen was adjusted by increasing the ingested THC dose while maintaining other components. Follow-up also provided opportunities to revisit education topics, including sleep hygiene, breathing techniques for anxiety, and the benefits of dry-herb vaporization compared to smoking or dabbing.

Over subsequent reassessments, Bob reported progressive improvement, which was reflected in his assessment tools. Daytime inhalation became minimal and, when used, involved a Type 2 (1:1 CBD:THC) flower variety that he found more effective than the THC-dominant products he had previously used.

Six months into his revised treatment approach, Bob reported being "very much improved" on the PGIC. Notably, cannabis had become only one component of a broader health strategy, as he had also made meaningful changes in behavioral domains. While he continued to report multiple symptoms, they were milder. Their impact on his social, cognitive, physical, and emotional functioning was substantially reduced. This case demonstrates the application of the framework within a structured clinician–patient relationship, though the framework itself is intentionally designed to extend beyond physician-led care.

In parallel, published evidence supports the effectiveness of a structured, process-based approach to medical cannabis care in other settings. In January 2025, researchers at the University of Michigan reported on a Veteran-focused coaching intervention designed to optimize cannabis use for chronic pain management. Although developed independently, the program closely mirrored this framework, operationalizing core elements such as intention setting, individualized implementation, and ongoing assessment and adjustment (Boehnke et al., 2025).

The intervention emphasized patient-centered goal setting, education regarding cannabis constituents and routes of administration, and iterative reassessment guided by patient-reported outcomes. Outcomes were favorable, with high patient satisfaction and significant improvements across multiple patient-reported measures, including global impression of change and pain-related quality-of-life (Boehnke et al., 2025).

Together, this Veteran-focused pilot and the clinical case example presented earlier illustrate how structured, intentional, and monitored cannabis care contrasts with the largely unstructured consumption patterns that remain common in the U.S. When applied as a process rather than a product-driven intervention, medical cannabis can be consistently operationalized in alignment with the definition proposed in this chapter.

Implications for Nursing Practice and Clinical Care

This health-focused framework functions as a clinical analogue of the Nursing Process—Assessment, Diagnosis, Planning, Implementation, and Evaluation (ANA, 2021)—adapted for the unique pharmacodynamics and regulatory landscape of cannabinoid therapeutics.

Nurses can play an essential role at every stage of this framework, and Table 2 summarizes key nursing functions associated with each step. This framework is not aspirational; it is immediately implementable, using existing nursing competencies and care models.

Table 2. Nursing contributions in the application of this chapter's proposed framework

Framework Step	Primary Purpose	Key Nursing Contributions in Practice
Intention	Define the purpose and direction of cannabis therapy	• Facilitate patient-centered goal clarification beyond diagnoses • Help patients prioritize intentions (e.g., sleep, function, emotional regulation) • Translate vague symptom goals into actionable, health-focused intentions • Support alignment between cannabis use and non-cannabis behaviors
Education	Align treatment decisions with evidence, values, and safety	• Provide evidence-based education on cannabinoids, ratios, dosing, and routes of administration • Address misconceptions and normalize uncertainty • Integrate patient values, risk tolerance, and lived experience into decision-making • Deliver accessible education through scalable models (e.g., nurse-led helplines, coaching)
Implementation	Translate knowledge into a workable, personalized regimen	• Assist patients in operationalizing treatment plans within daily routines • Support harm-reduction strategies (e.g., safer routes, lower-risk products) • Help patients interpret product labels and dosing instructions • Identify and mitigate barriers related to cost, access, and adherence
Assessment	Determine whether intentions and health goals are being met	• Guide patients in session-level and longitudinal self-monitoring • Administer and interpret PROMs • Encourage holistic assessment beyond symptom severity (e.g., function, well-being) • Incorporate feedback from patients and caregivers
Adjustment	Refine therapy based on feedback and evolving needs	• Help patients interpret assessment data to guide changes • Support gradual, safe adjustments in dose, product, or method • Reinforce harm-reduction principles during regimen changes • Reduce premature discontinuation by addressing concerns and setbacks

Source: Author's own work

FUTURE RESEARCH DIRECTIONS

This chapter's proposed holistic, process-based definition of medical cannabis and the five-step framework used to operationalize it are both testable and scalable, yet remain understudied. To date, most cannabis research has focused on discrete outcome measures rather than the clinical processes that govern real-world use. Future research should emphasize implementation science approaches that examine how cannabis can be integrated into structured care models that support sustained benefit, minimize harm, and promote long-term, responsible use.

The University of Michigan Veteran coaching study may be viewed as an early feasibility model for structured, health-focused cannabis care. The intervention incorporated multiple elements of the framework proposed in this chapter, including intention setting, patient education, ongoing assessment using patient-reported outcomes, and individualized adjustment over time (Boehnke et al., 2025). Developed using available scientific literature, clinical expertise from cannabis-trained professionals, and collaboration with Veteran-focused advocacy groups, the intervention involved four coaching sessions over a 14-week period. During sessions coaches emphasized education regarding cannabis constituents and routes of administration, methodical "start low, go slow" dosing, and safety considerations.

Outcomes from this pilot provide early support for the feasibility of structured cannabis care. Patient satisfaction was high, with 87.5% of participants reporting they were very or completely satisfied with the intervention and 81.3% rating coaching as very or extremely helpful. Clinically, 63% of participants reported much or very much improvement on the PGIC, while the remaining participants reported mild improvement. Statistically significant improvements were also observed in PROMs of social satisfaction, pain interference, and pain intensity (Boehnke et al., 2025).

While encouraging, this pilot was not designed to compare structured cannabis care with the access-only certification models that predominate in most U.S. jurisdictions. Future research should build on this work by directly evaluating whether framework-based care improves outcomes relative to unstructured access pathways. One proposed approach is a tiered study design in which patients seeking medical cannabis certification are randomized to one of three arms: (1) access-only medical cannabis certification; (2) access plus self-guided framework education (e.g., a handbook or digital tool); or (3) access plus nurse-led framework implementation. After a follow-up period of approximately three to six months, primary outcomes could include:

- patient-reported quality of life
- goal attainment and intention alignment
- adverse effects and treatment discontinuation
- patterns of use over time, such as escalation versus stabilization

In addition to comparative care models, another important future direction is the development and validation of instruments designed to assess use of this chapter's proposed framework. These Health-focused Cannabis Process Measures (HFCPMs) could examine participation across each framework component—intention, education, implementation, assessment, and adjustment. Each component could be measured using a small set of items capturing domains such as intention clarity, evidence comprehension, consistency of implementation, monitoring behaviors, and willingness to adjust treatment. When used alongside validated PROMs, these tools could help determine whether greater engagement with specific framework components correlates with improved safety, quality of life, or long-term sustainability of cannabis use.

Finally, future work should examine how nurse-led cannabis care models can be integrated into existing healthcare systems. Key considerations include training standards, scope-of-practice, reimbursement pathways, and operational feasibility. Addressing these factors will be critical for determining whether structured, health-focused cannabis care models can be implemented and sustained at scale.

CONCLUSION

Medical cannabis access has expanded substantially in the U.S., yet medical cannabis care has not. This imbalance has created a gap between access and clinical support, leaving safety, efficacy, and health outcomes often unclear or unmeasured. The central barrier to effective medical cannabis, therefore, lies less in the plant itself and more in how care is accessed, structured, and delivered.

This chapter proposes a health-focused definition of medical cannabis as the intentional and monitored use of the cannabis plant, or its constituents, to improve health, as guided by EBM. This definition prioritizes process and whole-person outcomes over specific products, diagnoses, or symptom-based algorithms. To operationalize this definition in a manner that is practical and adaptable across diverse clinical contexts, the chapter introduces a five-step, iterative framework:

- **Intention**: defines patient values, goals, and direction for care
- **Education**: aligns treatment decisions with EBM and supports patient competency
- **Implementation**: translates intention and education into a manageable starting regimen
- **Assessment**: measures outcomes holistically, both longitudinally and at the level of individual dosing sessions
- **Adjustment**: personalizes ongoing treatment based on feedback, alongside continued education and intention setting

Together, the definition and framework support effective medical cannabis use across a wide range of clinical and real-world settings. While guidance from a cannabis-trained professional is ideal, the framework is intentionally designed to support both clinician-guided and self-directed use, provided that intention, monitoring, and evidence-based decision-making are actively maintained.

Cannabis is a uniquely diverse therapeutic modality, characterized by wide variability in products, routes of administration, dosing strategies, constituent ratios, and pharmacodynamic effects. As a result, optimal outcomes depend less on disease- or symptom-centric algorithms and more on a personalized clinical process grounded in intentional use, monitoring, and iterative refinement. This relationship is reflected in both research and real-world data, where meaningful clinical benefits and favorable safety profiles are observed despite substantial heterogeneity in cannabis regimens.

Nurses are already leaders in cannabis education and patient guidance and are essential to implementing this framework at scale. Their roles span every stage of the process, including clarifying patient goals and translating intentions into actionable plans; delivering evidence-based education and risk counseling; supporting implementation logistics such as routines, labeling, and harm-reduction strategies; facilitating monitoring through patient-reported outcome measures and structured check-ins; and coaching safe adjustment over time to optimize outcomes and reduce premature discontinuation.

Looking ahead, priorities must extend beyond cannabis access to include comparative evaluation of access-only versus framework-based models; development and validation of HFCPMs alongside PROMs and HRQoL instruments; and the creation of training, reimbursement, and integration pathways for nurse-led, process-based cannabis care.

Ultimately, improved patient health and well-being must remain the central aim of medical cannabis use. Ensuring that cannabis remains truly "medical" requires repeatable clinical processes, consistent and validated measurement, and scalable guidance and support. When these elements are in place, medical cannabis is better positioned to deliver the safety, efficacy, and holistic health benefits it has the potential to provide.

ACKNOWLEDGEMENTS

This research received no specific grant from any funding agency in the public, commercial, or not-for-profit sectors. The author thanks Katherine Golden, RN (CEO, Executive Director, and Founder of LEAF411) and Whitney Wacker, RN, staff nurse at LEAF411, for collating and providing data from LEAF411's nurse-led helpline.

Generative artificial intelligence and large language models were used solely for proofreading, grammar, and readability improvements. All content, concepts, and structure were developed by the author.

REFERENCES

Act, C. S. 21 U.S.C. §§ 801–971 (1970). https://www.govinfo.gov/content/pkg/USCODE-2023-title21/pdf/USCODE-2023-title21-chap13.pdf

Agriculture Improvement Act of 2018, Pub. L. No. 115-334, 132 Stat. 4490 (2018). https://www.congress.gov/115/plaws/publ334/PLAW-115publ334.pdf

Ahuja, A. S. (2019). Should RCTs be used as the gold standard for evidence-based medicine? *Integrative Medicine Research*, *8*(1), 31–32. DOI: 10.1016/j.imr.2019.01.001 PMID: 30805294

Ajzen, I. (1991). The theory of planned behavior. *Organizational Behavior and Human Decision Processes*, *50*(2), 179–211. DOI: 10.1016/0749-5978(91)90020-T

American Cannabis Nurses Association. (2021). *About ACNA*. https://cannabisnurses.org/about-the-acna

American Nurses Association. (2021). *Nursing: Scope and standards of practice* (4th ed.). American Nurses Association.

American Nurses Association. (2023, July 10). *ANA officially recognizes cannabis nursing as a specialty nursing practice*. https://www.nursingworld.org/news/news-releases/2023/ana-officially-recognizes-cannabis-nursing-as-a-specialty-nursing-practice/

American Nurses Association. (2023). *Cannabis nursing: Scope and standards of practice*. American Nurses Association. https://www.nursingworld.org/nurses-books/cannabis-nursing-scope-and-standards-of-practice/

Anscombe, G. E. M. (1963). *Intention* (2nd ed.). Basil Blackwell. (Original work published 1957)

Arkell, T. R., Downey, L. A., Hayley, A. C., & Roth, S. (2023). Assessment of medical cannabis and health-related quality of life. *JAMA Network Open*, *6*(5), e2312522. DOI: 10.1001/jamanetworkopen.2023.12522 PMID: 37159196

Balneaves, L. G., Watling, C. Z., Strus, J. A., Boscow, M., Davis, L., Graveline, K., Harrigan, T., Henriquez, N., Mitchell, K., & Thompson, G. (2023). Baccalaureate nursing students' knowledge, attitudes, educational needs, and use of medical and non-medical cannabis at five institutions in Manitoba, Canada: A cross-sectional analysis. *Nurse Education Today*, *130*, 105955. Advance online publication. DOI: 10.1016/j.nedt.2023.105955 PMID: 37677985

Banerjee, R., Erridge, S., Salazar, O., Mangal, N., Couch, D., Pacchetti, B., & Sodergren, M. H. (2022). Real-world evidence in medical cannabis research. *Therapeutic Innovation & Regulatory Science, 56*(1), 8–14. DOI: 10.1007/s43441-021-00346-0 PMID: 34748204

Bar-Lev Schleider, L., Mechoulam, R., Sikorin, I., Naftali, T., & Novack, V. (2022). Adherence, safety, and effectiveness of medical cannabis and epidemiological characteristics of the patient population: A prospective study. *Frontiers in Medicine, 9*, 827849. DOI: 10.3389/fmed.2022.827849 PMID: 35223923

Bassi, G. M., Giorgi, V., Lazzarin, M., Meanti, R., Omeljaniuk, R. J., Sarzi-Puttini, P., & Torsello, A. (2025). Symptom management, adherence to therapy, and filling the gaps of medical cannabis therapy: A qualitative study on the importance of nursing consultations for fibromyalgia patients. *Journal of Cannabis Research, 7*(1), 84. Advance online publication. DOI: 10.1186/s42238-025-00346-z PMID: 41163201

Behling-Hess, C., Simonson, G., Salz, T., Feuerstein, N., & Zullig, L. L. (2025). The impact of cannabis on immune checkpoint inhibitor therapy: A systematic review of immunomodulatory effects of cannabis in patients with and without cancer. *Supportive Care in Cancer, 33*(3), 166. Advance online publication. DOI: 10.1007/s00520-025-09218-x PMID: 39921765

Bell, A. D., MacCallum, C. A., Margolese, S., Walsh, Z., Wright, P., Daeninck, P. J., Mandarino, E., Lacasse, G., Deol, J. K., de Freitas, L., St. Pierre, M., Belle-Isle, L., Gagnon, M., Bevan, S., Sanchez, T., Arlt, S., Monahan-Ellison, M., O'Hara, J., Boivin, M., & Costiniuk, C. (2024). Clinical practice guidelines for cannabis and cannabinoid-based medicines in the management of chronic pain and co-occurring conditions. *Cannabis and Cannabinoid Research, 9*(2), 669–687. DOI: 10.1089/can.2021.0156 PMID: 36971587

Benca, R. M., Bertisch, S. M., Ahuja, A., Mandelbaum, R., & Krystal, A. D. (2023). Wake up America: National survey of patients' and physicians' views and attitudes on insomnia care. *Journal of Clinical Medicine, 12*(7), 2498. Advance online publication. DOI: 10.3390/jcm12072498 PMID: 37048582

Bhaskar, A., Bell, A., Boivin, M., Briques, W., Brown, M., Clarke, H., Cyr, C., Eisenberg, E., de Oliveira Silva, R. F., Frohlich, E., Georgius, P., Hogg, M., Horsted, T. I., MacCallum, C. A., Müller-Vahl, K. R., O'Connell, C., Sealey, R., Seibolt, M., Sihota, A., & Moulin, D. E. (2021). Consensus recommendations on dosing and administration of medical cannabis to treat chronic pain: Results of a modified Delphi process. *Journal of Cannabis Research, 3*(1), 22. DOI: 10.1186/s42238-021-00073-1 PMID: 34215346

Black, N. (2013). Patient-reported outcome measures could help transform healthcare. *BMJ (Clinical Research Ed.), 346*(jan28 1), f167. DOI: 10.1136/bmj.f167 PMID: 23358487

Boehnke, K. F., Bowyer, G., McAfee, J., Smith, T., Klida, C., Kurtz, V., Litinas, E., Purohit, P., Arewasikporn, A., Horowitz, D., Thomas, L., Eckersley, J., Railing, M., Williams, D. A., Clauw, D. J., Kidwell, K. M., Bohnert, A. S. B., & Bergmans, R. S. (2025). Feasibility pilot of a novel coaching intervention to optimize cannabis use for chronic pain management among veterans. *Journal of Cannabis Research, 7*(1), 7. Advance online publication. DOI: 10.1186/s42238-025-00265-z PMID: 39856785

Boehnke, K. F., Scott, J. R., Litinas, E., Sisley, S., Clauw, D. J., Goesling, J., & Williams, D. A. (2019). Cannabis use preferences and decision-making among medical cannabis patients with chronic pain. *The Journal of Pain, 20*(11), 1362–1372. DOI: 10.1016/j.jpain.2019.05.009 PMID: 31132510

Boehnke, K. F., Scott, J. R., Martel, M. O., Smith, T., Bergmans, R. S., Kruger, D. J., Williams, D. A., & Fitzcharles, M. A. (2024). Substituting medical cannabis for medications among patients with rheumatic conditions in the United States and Canada. *ACR Open Rheumatology*, *6*(12), 826–835. DOI: 10.1002/acr2.11717 PMID: 39236308

Bratman, M. E. (1987). *Intention, plans, and practical reason*. Harvard University Press.

Bruce, D., Brady, J. P., Foster, E., & Shattell, M. (2018). Preferences for medical marijuana over prescription medications among persons living with chronic conditions. *Journal of Alternative and Complementary Medicine (New York, N.Y.)*, *24*(2), 146–153. DOI: 10.1089/acm.2017.0184 PMID: 28945457

Cashin, A. G., Furlong, B. M., Kamper, S. J., De Carvalho, D., Machado, L. A. C., Davidson, S. R. E., Bursey, K. K., Abdel Shaheed, C., & Hall, A. M. (2025). Analgesic effects of non-surgical and non-interventional treatments for low back pain: A systematic review and meta-analysis of placebo-controlled randomized trials. *BMJ Evidence-Based Medicine*, bmjebm-2024-112974. Advance online publication. DOI: 10.1136/bmjebm-2024-112974 PMID: 40101974

Cella, D., Riley, W., Stone, A., Rothrock, N., Reeve, B., Yount, S., Amtmann, D., Bode, R., Buysse, D., Choi, S., Cook, K., DeVellis, R., DeWalt, D., Fries, J. F., Gershon, R., Hahn, E. A., Lai, J.-S., Pilkonis, P., Revicki, D., & Hays, R. (2010). The Patient-Reported Outcomes Measurement Information System (PROMIS): Development and testing of adult self-reported health outcome item banks, 2005–2008. *Journal of Clinical Epidemiology*, *63*(11), 1179–1194. DOI: 10.1016/j.jclinepi.2010.04.011 PMID: 20685078

Centers for Disease Control and Prevention. (n.d.). *Well-being concepts*. https://archive.cdc.gov/www_cdc_gov/hrqol/wellbeing.htm

Christidis, M., Al-Moraissi, E. A., Miah, T., Mihasi, L., Razavian, A., Christidis, N., & De la Torre Canales, G. (2025). Living with pain: A systematic review on patients' subjective experiences. *Systematic Reviews*, *14*(1), 188. Advance online publication. DOI: 10.1186/s13643-025-02953-6 PMID: 41053837

Clobes, T. A., Mee, M. M., Jimenez, J. M., Maldonado, J., & Song, J. R. (2025). Impact of healthcare provider awareness and guidance on the medical cannabis experience. *Medical Cannabis and Cannabinoids*, *8*(1), 47–57. DOI: 10.1159/000544125 PMID: 40104431

Compton, W. M., Han, B., Jones, C. M., Blanco, C., & Hughes, A. (2016). Marijuana use and use disorders in adults in the USA, 2002–14: Analysis of annual cross-sectional surveys. *The Lancet. Psychiatry*, *3*(10), 954–964. DOI: 10.1016/S2215-0366(16)30208-5 PMID: 27592339

Congressional Research Service. (2025, December 3). *Change to federal definition of hemp and implications for federal enforcement* (CRS Insight No. IN12620). https://www.congress.gov/crs-product/IN12620

de Roon-Cassini, T. A., Stollenwerk, T. M., Beatka, M., & Hillard, C. J. (2020). Meet your stress management professionals: The endocannabinoids. *Trends in Molecular Medicine*, *26*(10), 953–968. DOI: 10.1016/j.molmed.2020.07.002 PMID: 32868170

Diener, E., Oishi, S., & Tay, L. (2018). Advances in subjective well-being research. *Nature Human Behaviour*, *2*(4), 253–260. DOI: 10.1038/s41562-018-0307-6 PMID: 30936533

Dowell, D., Ragan, K. R., Jones, C. M., Baldwin, G. T., & Chou, R. (2022). CDC clinical practice guideline for prescribing opioids for pain—United States, 2022. *MMWR. Recommendations and Reports*, *71*(3, RR-3), 1–95. DOI: 10.15585/mmwr.rr7103a1 PMID: 36327391

Elphick, M. R. (2012). The evolution and comparative neurobiology of endocannabinoid signalling. *Philosophical Transactions of the Royal Society of London. Series B, Biological Sciences*, *367*(1607), 3201–3215. DOI: 10.1098/rstb.2011.0394 PMID: 23108540

Englund, A., Morrison, P. D., Nottage, J., Hague, D., Kane, F., Bonaccorso, S., Stone, J. M., Reichenberg, A., Brenneisen, R., Holt, D., Feilding, A., Walker, L., Murray, R. M., & Kapur, S. (2013). Cannabidiol inhibits THC-elicited paranoid symptoms and hippocampal-dependent memory impairment. *Journal of Psychopharmacology (Oxford, England)*, *27*(1), 19–27. DOI: 10.1177/0269881112460109 PMID: 23042808

Erridge, S., Clarke, E., McLachlan, K., Coomber, R., Beri, S., Khan, S., Weatherall, M. W., Platt, M. W., Rucker, J. J., Mediano, P. A. M., & Sodergren, M. H. (2026). Clinical outcomes and patient profiles in the UK medical cannabis registry: A k-means clustering analysis. *Journal of Clinical Pharmacology*, *66*(1), e70151. Advance online publication. DOI: 10.1002/jcph.70151 PMID: 41510842

European Monitoring Centre for Drugs and Drug Addiction. (2018). *Medical use of cannabis and cannabinoids: Questions and answers for policymaking*. https://doi.org/DOI: 10.2810/979004

Evanoff, A. B., Quan, T., Dufault, C., Awad, M., & Bierut, L. J. (2017). Physicians-in-training are not prepared to prescribe medical marijuana. *Drug and Alcohol Dependence*, *180*, 151–155. DOI: 10.1016/j.drugalcdep.2017.08.010 PMID: 28892720

Fanaroff, A. C., Califf, R. M., Windecker, S., Smith, S. C.Jr, & Lopes, R. D. (2019). Levels of evidence supporting American College of Cardiology/American Heart Association and European Society of Cardiology guidelines, 2008–2018. *Journal of the American Medical Association*, *321*(11), 1069–1080. DOI: 10.1001/jama.2019.1122 PMID: 30874755

Fischer, B., Robinson, T., Bullen, C., Curran, V., Jutras-Aswad, D., Medina-Mora, M. E., Pacula, R. L., Rehm, J., Room, R., Brink, W., & Hall, W. (2022). Lower-risk cannabis use guidelines for reducing health harms from non-medical cannabis use: A comprehensive evidence and recommendations update. *The International Journal on Drug Policy*, *99*, 103381. DOI: 10.1016/j.drugpo.2021.103381 PMID: 34465496

Furman, D., Campisi, J., Verdin, E., Carrera-Bastos, P., Targ, S., Franceschi, C., Ferrucci, L., Gilroy, D. W., Fasano, A., Miller, G. W., Miller, A. H., Mantovani, A., Weyand, C. M., Barzilai, N., Goronzy, J. J., Rando, T. A., Effros, R. B., Lucia, A., Kleinstreuer, N., & Slavich, G. M. (2019). Chronic inflammation in the etiology of disease across the life span. *Nature Medicine*, *25*(12), 1822–1832. DOI: 10.1038/s41591-019-0675-0 PMID: 31806905

Garcia-Romeu, A., Elmore, J., Mayhugh, R. E., Schlienz, N. J., Martin, E. L., Strickland, J. C., Bonn-Miller, M., Jackson, H., & Vandrey, R. (2022). Online survey of medicinal cannabis users: Qualitative analysis of patient-level data. *Frontiers in Pharmacology*, *13*, 965535. Advance online publication. DOI: 10.3389/fphar.2022.965535 PMID: 36147312

Garmany, A., & Terzic, A. (2024). Global healthspan–lifespan gaps among 183 World Health Organization member states. *JAMA Network Open*, *7*(12), e2450241. Advance online publication. DOI: 10.1001/jamanetworkopen.2024.50241 PMID: 39661386

GBD 2017 Causes of Death Collaborators. (2018). Global, regional, and national age-sex-specific mortality for 282 causes of death in 195 countries and territories, 1980–2017: A systematic analysis for the Global Burden of Disease Study 2017. *The Lancet, 392*(10159), 1736–1788. https://doi.org/DOI: 10.1016/S0140-6736(18)32203-7

Geurts, J. W., Willems, P. C., Lockwood, C., van Kleef, M., Kleijnen, J., & Dirksen, C. (2017). Patient expectations for management of chronic non-cancer pain: A systematic review. *Health Expectations*, *20*(6), 1201–1217. DOI: 10.1111/hex.12527 PMID: 28009082

Giangregorio, A., Wang, L., Sprague, S., Arbus, M., & Busse, J. W. (2024). Predictors of response to medical cannabis for chronic pain: A retrospective review of real-time observational data. *Cannabis (Research Society on Marijuana)*, *7*(3), 167–176. DOI: 10.26828/cannabis/2024/000259 PMID: 39781554

Graham, M., Pacula, R. L., Pessar, S. C., Ge, Y., Kritikos, A. F., Hall, W., & Hammond, D. (2025). Understanding medical cannabis use internationally: Why definitions and context matter. *Addiction (Abingdon, England)*, *120*(10), 2141–2146. DOI: 10.1111/add.70117 PMID: 40590488

Han, B. H., Compton, W. M., Blanco, C., & Jones, C. M. (2023). Trends in cannabis use disorder prevalence among medical and nonmedical cannabis users in the United States. *JAMA Network Open*, *6*(1), e2251621. Advance online publication. DOI: 10.1001/jamanetworkopen.2022.51621 PMID: 36701154

Han, B. H., Yang, K. H., Cleland, C. M., & Palamar, J. J. (2025). Trends in past-month cannabis use among older adults. *JAMA Internal Medicine*, *185*(7), 881–883. DOI: 10.1001/jamainternmed.2025.1156 PMID: 40455425

Haug, N. A., Kieschnick, D., Sottile, J. E., Babson, K. A., Vandrey, R., & Bonn-Miller, M. O. (2016). Training and practices of cannabis dispensary staff. *Cannabis and Cannabinoid Research*, *1*(1), 244–251. DOI: 10.1089/can.2016.0024 PMID: 28861496

Hays, R. D., Bjorner, J. B., Revicki, D. A., Spritzer, K. L., & Cella, D. (2009). Development of physical and mental health summary scores from the PROMIS global items. *Quality of Life Research: An International Journal of Quality of Life Aspects of Treatment, Care and Rehabilitation*, *18*(7), 873–880. DOI: 10.1007/s11136-009-9496-9 PMID: 19543809

Holdman, R., Vigil, D., Robinson, K., Shah, P., & Contreras, A. E. (2022). Safety and efficacy of medical cannabis in autism spectrum disorder compared with commonly used medications. *Cannabis and Cannabinoid Research*, *7*(4), 451–463. DOI: 10.1089/can.2020.0154 PMID: 34432543

Huestis, M. A. (2007). Human cannabinoid pharmacokinetics. *Chemistry & Biodiversity*, *4*(8), 1770–1804. DOI: 10.1002/cbdv.200790152 PMID: 17712819

Hurst, H., & Bolton, J. (2004). Assessing the clinical significance of change scores recorded on subjective outcome measures. *Journal of Manipulative and Physiological Therapeutics*, *27*(1), 26–35. DOI: 10.1016/j.jmpt.2003.11.003 PMID: 14739871

Iffland, K., & Grotenhermen, F. (2017). An update on safety and side effects of cannabidiol: A review of clinical data and relevant animal studies. *Cannabis and Cannabinoid Research*, *2*(1), 139–154. DOI: 10.1089/can.2016.0034 PMID: 28861514

Institute of Medicine. (2001). *Crossing the quality chasm: A new health system for the 21st century*. National Academies Press., DOI: 10.17226/10027

Ioannidis, J. P. A. (2005). Why most published research findings are false. *PLoS Medicine*, *2*(8), e124. Advance online publication. DOI: 10.1371/journal.pmed.0020124 PMID: 16060722

Kasturi, S., Szymonifka, J., Burket, J. C., Berman, J. R., Kirou, K. A., Levine, A. B., & Mandl, L. A. (2018). Feasibility, validity, and reliability of the 10-item PROMIS Global Health Short Form in outpatients with systemic lupus erythematosus. *The Journal of Rheumatology*, *45*(3), 397–404. DOI: 10.3899/jrheum.170590 PMID: 29419473

Khak, M., Ramtin, S., Chung, J., Ilyas, A. M., & Greis, A. (2025). Discontinuation rates and predictors of medical cannabis cessation for chronic musculoskeletal pain. *PLoS One*, *20*(8), e0329897. Advance online publication. DOI: 10.1371/journal.pone.0329897 PMID: 40773423

Khezrian, M., McNeil, C. J., Murray, A. D., & Myint, P. K. (2020). An overview of prevalence, determinants, and health outcomes of polypharmacy. *Therapeutic Advances in Drug Safety*, *11*, 2042098620933741. Advance online publication. DOI: 10.1177/2042098620933741 PMID: 32587680

King, D. D., Gill, C. J., Cadieux, C. S., & Singh, N. (2024). The role of stigma in cannabis use disclosure: An exploratory study. *Harm Reduction Journal*, *21*(1), 21. Advance online publication. DOI: 10.1186/s12954-024-00929-8 PMID: 38273362

King, K. (2024). Cannabis nursing. AJN. *The American Journal of Nursing*, *124*(5), 31. DOI: 10.1097/01.NAJ.0001016368.03202.a8 PMID: 38661699

Kurtzman, E. T., Greene, J., Begley, R., & Drenkard, K. N. (2022). "We want what's best for patients." Nurse leaders' attitudes about medical cannabis: A qualitative study. *International Journal of Nursing Studies Advances*, *4*, 100065. Advance online publication. DOI: 10.1016/j.ijnsa.2022.100065 PMID: 38745605

Lefebvre, È., Tawil, N., & Yahia, L. (2024). Transdermal delivery of cannabidiol for the management of acute inflammatory pain: A comprehensive review of the literature. *International Journal of Molecular Sciences*, *25*(11), 5858. Advance online publication. DOI: 10.3390/ijms25115858 PMID: 38892047

Lin, C.-Y., Updegraff, J. A., & Pakpour, A. H. (2016). The relationship between the theory of planned behavior and medication adherence in patients with epilepsy. *Epilepsy & Behavior*, *61*, 231–236. DOI: 10.1016/j.yebeh.2016.05.030 PMID: 27390026

MacCallum, C. A., & Russo, E. B. (2018). Practical considerations in medical cannabis administration and dosing. *European Journal of Internal Medicine*, *49*, 12–19. DOI: 10.1016/j.ejim.2018.01.004 PMID: 29307505

Malpas, S. C. (2010). Sympathetic nervous system overactivity and its role in the development of cardiovascular disease. *Physiological Reviews*, *90*(2), 513–557. DOI: 10.1152/physrev.00007.2009 PMID: 20393193

Mancia, G., & Grassi, G. (2014). The autonomic nervous system and hypertension. *Circulation Research*, *114*(11), 1804–1814. DOI: 10.1161/CIRCRESAHA.114.302524 PMID: 24855203

Marijuana Policy Project. (2024). *Medical marijuana patient numbers*. https://www.mpp.org/issues/medical-marijuana/state-by-state-medical-marijuana-laws/medical-marijuana-patient-numbers/

Martin, E. L., Strickland, J. C., Schlienz, N. J., Munson, J., Bonsu, H., Mueller, A. S., & Vandrey, R. (2021). Antidepressant and anxiolytic effects of medicinal cannabis use in an observational subset of patients with anxiety and depression. *Frontiers in Psychiatry*, *12*, 729800. Advance online publication. DOI: 10.3389/fpsyt.2021.729800 PMID: 34566726

McCance, T., & McCormack, B. (2025). The person-centred nursing framework: A mid-range theory for nursing practice. *Journal of Research in Nursing : JRN*, *30*(1), 47–60. DOI: 10.1177/17449871241281428 PMID: 40093819

McEachan, R. R. C., Conner, M., Taylor, N. J., & Lawton, R. J. (2011). Prospective prediction of health-related behaviours with the theory of planned behaviour: A meta-analysis. *Health Psychology Review*, *5*(2), 97–144. DOI: 10.1080/17437199.2010.521684

McIntosh, N., Wilson, N. J., Povalej, P., Hunt, L., & Lewis, P. (2024). An exploration of registered nurses' experiences caring for patients taking medicinal cannabis. *Nursing Open*, *11*(10), e70063. Advance online publication. DOI: 10.1002/nop2.70063 PMID: 39455290

McIntyre, R. S., Alsuwaidan, M., Baune, B. T., Berk, M., Demyttenaere, K., Goldberg, J. F., Gorwood, P., Ho, R., Kasper, S., Kennedy, S. H., Ly-Uson, J., Mansur, R. B., McAllister-Williams, R. H., Murrough, J. W., Nemeroff, C. B., Nierenberg, A. A., Rosenblat, J. D., Sanacora, G., Schatzberg, A. F., & Maj, M. (2023). Treatment-resistant depression: Definition, prevalence, detection, management, and investigational interventions. *World Psychiatry; Official Journal of the World Psychiatric Association (WPA)*, *22*(3), 394–412. DOI: 10.1002/wps.21120 PMID: 37713549

Mercurio, A., Aston, E. R., Claborn, K. R., Waye, K., & Rosen, R. K. (2019). Marijuana as a substitute for prescription medications: A qualitative study. *Substance Use & Misuse*, *54*(11), 1894–1902. DOI: 10.1080/10826084.2019.1618336 PMID: 31179810

Merlin, J. S., Merlin, J. S., Althouse, A., Feldman, R., Arnsten, J. H., Bulls, H. W., Liebschutz, J. M., Nugent, S. M., Orris, S. R., Rohac, R., Starrels, J. L., Morasco, B. J., & Kansagara, D. (2021). Analysis of state cannabis laws and dispensary staff recommendations to adults purchasing medical cannabis. *JAMA Network Open*, *4*(9), e2124511. DOI: 10.1001/jamanetworkopen.2021.24511 PMID: 34524435

Mick, G., & Douek, P. (2024). Clinical benefits and safety of medical cannabis products: A narrative review on natural extracts. *Pain and Therapy*, *13*(5), 1063–1094. DOI: 10.1007/s40122-024-00643-0 PMID: 39096481

Moore, E. (2024). Connecting the dots with cannabis care. *American Nurse Journal*, *19*(7), 30–32. DOI: 10.51256/ANJ072430

Muth, C., Blom, J. W., Smith, S. M., Johnell, K., Gonzalez-Gonzalez, A. I., Nguyen, T. S., Brueckle, M. S., Cesari, M., Tinetti, M. E., & Valderas, J. M. (2019). Evidence supporting the best clinical management of patients with multimorbidity and polypharmacy: A systematic guideline review and expert consensus. *Journal of Internal Medicine*, *285*(3), 272–288. DOI: 10.1111/joim.12842 PMID: 30357955

Nachnani, R., Knehans, A., Neighbors, J. D., Kocis, P. T., Lee, T., Tegeler, K., Trite, T., Raup-Konsavage, W. M., & Vrana, K. E. (2024). Systematic review of drug-drug interactions of delta-9-tetrahydrocannabinol, cannabidiol, and cannabis. *Frontiers in Pharmacology*, *15*, 1282831. Advance online publication. DOI: 10.3389/fphar.2024.1282831 PMID: 38868665

National Academies of Sciences, Engineering, and Medicine. (2017). The health effects of cannabis and cannabinoids: The current state of evidence and recommendations for research. *National Academies Press*. https://doi.org/DOI: 10.17226/24625

Olfson, M., Wall, M., Liu, S.-M., Schoenbaum, M., & Blanco, C. (2018). Declining health-related quality of life in the United States. *American Journal of Preventive Medicine*, *54*(3), 325–333. DOI: 10.1016/j.amepre.2017.11.012 PMID: 29338955

Order, E. Increasing medical marijuana and cannabidiol research. (2025, December 18). The White House. https://www.whitehouse.gov/presidential-actions/2025/12/increasing-medical-marijuana-and-cannabidiol-research/

Pacher, P., & Kunos, G. (2013). Modulating the endocannabinoid system in human health and disease: Successes and failures. *The FEBS Journal*, *280*(9), 1918–1943. DOI: 10.1111/febs.12260 PMID: 23551849

Paiva, C., Santos, T., Cunha-Oliveira, A., Rosendo, I., & Pita, J. R. (2024). Knowledge, opinions and experiences of nurses and nursing students in Portugal regarding the use of medical cannabis. *BMC Nursing*, *23*(1), 788. Advance online publication. DOI: 10.1186/s12912-024-02443-5 PMID: 39468501

Pertwee, R. G., Howlett, A. C., Abood, M. E., Alexander, S. P. H., Di Marzo, V., Elphick, M. R., Greasley, P. J., Hansen, H. S., Kunos, G., Mackie, K., Mechoulam, R., & Ross, R. A. (2010). Cannabinoid receptors and their ligands: Beyond CB1 and CB2. *Pharmacological Reviews*, *62*(4), 588–631. DOI: 10.1124/pr.110.003004 PMID: 21079038

Prieto González, J. M., & Vila Silván, C. (2021a). Safety and tolerability of nabiximols oromucosal spray: A review of more than 15 years of accumulated evidence from clinical trials. *Expert Review of Neurotherapeutics*, *21*(7), 755–778. DOI: 10.1080/14737175.2021.1935879 PMID: 34092180

Prieto González, J. M., & Vila Silván, C. (2021b). Safety and tolerability of nabiximols oromucosal spray: A review of real-world experience in observational studies, registries, and case reports. *Expert Review of Neurotherapeutics*, *21*(5), 547–558. DOI: 10.1080/14737175.2021.1904896 PMID: 33749480

Reddy, T. S., Zomer, R., & Mantri, N. (2023). Nanoformulations as a strategy to overcome the delivery limitations of cannabinoids. *Phytotherapy Research*, *37*(4), 1526–1538. DOI: 10.1002/ptr.7742 PMID: 36748949

Reed, M., McCartney, D., & Guttmannova, K. (2020). Marijuana sources in a medical marijuana environment: Dynamics in access and use among a cohort of young adults in Los Angeles, California. *Drugs: Education Prevention & Policy*, *27*(1), 69–78. DOI: 10.1080/09687637.2018.1557595 PMID: 31949332

Rehman, A., Naz, Z., Ali, A., Naz, F., & Siddique, F. (2025). Meta-analysis of nurse-led interventions on medication adherence and clinical outcomes in patients with chronic illnesses. *Insights: Journal of Health and Rehabilitation*, *3*(10), 38–47. DOI: 10.71000/w46qy993

Rimmelzwaan, L. M., Bogerd, M. J. L., Schumacher, B. M. A., Slottje, P., van Hout, H. P. J., & Reinders, M. E. (2020). Multimorbidity in general practice: Unmet care needs from a patient perspective. *Frontiers in Medicine*, *7*, 530085. Advance online publication. DOI: 10.3389/fmed.2020.530085 PMID: 33415113

Romero, D., Mendez, D., Fowler, L. A., Morales, J., & Glantz, S. A. (2025). Medical cannabis utilization across U.S. states with varying legal status. *Preventive Medicine Reports*, *39*, 102582. Advance online publication. DOI: 10.1016/j.pmedr.2025.102582

Ronne, S. T., Rosenbaek, F., Pedersen, L. B., Waldorff, F. B., Nielsen, J. B., Riisgaard, H., & Søndergaard, J. (2021). Physicians' experiences, attitudes, and beliefs toward medical cannabis: A systematic literature review. *BMC Family Practice*, *22*(1), 212. Advance online publication. DOI: 10.1186/s12875-021-01559-w PMID: 34674661

Ruksakulpiwat, S., Pongsuwun, K., Junphongsri, P., Preeprem, C., Nguantad, S., & Samart, B. (2025). Nurse-led interventions to improve health, adherence, and functional outcomes in adults and older adults with multimorbidity: A systematic review of randomized and quasiexperimental studies. *Journal of Nursing Management*, *2025*(1), 6252049. Advance online publication. DOI: 10.1155/jonm/6252049 PMID: 41019866

Russo, E. B. (2007). History of cannabis and its preparations in saga, science, and sobriquet. *Chemistry & Biodiversity*, *4*(8), 1614–1648. DOI: 10.1002/cbdv.200790144 PMID: 17712811

Russo, E. B. (2011). Taming THC: Potential cannabis synergy and phytocannabinoid–terpenoid entourage effects. *British Journal of Pharmacology*, *163*(7), 1344–1364. DOI: 10.1111/j.1476-5381.2011.01238.x PMID: 21749363

Russo, E. B. (2017). History of cannabis as medicine: Nineteenth-century Irish physicians and correlations of their observations to modern research. In Collen, L., & Robson, P. (Eds.), *Cannabinoids in neurologic and mental disease* (pp. 3–20). Academic Press.

Ryan, J. E., McCabe, S. E., & Boyd, C. J. (2021). Medicinal cannabis: Policy, patients, and providers. *Policy, Politics & Nursing Practice*, *22*(2), 126–133. DOI: 10.1177/1527154421989609 PMID: 33567970

Sackett, D. L., Rosenberg, W. M. C., Gray, J. A. M., Haynes, R. B., & Richardson, W. S. (1996). Evidence-based medicine: What it is and what it isn't. *BMJ (Clinical Research Ed.)*, *312*(7023), 71–72. DOI: 10.1136/bmj.312.7023.71 PMID: 8555924

Salter, A. R., Cutter, G. R., Tyry, T., Marrie, R. A., & Fox, R. J. (2022). Sources of cannabis information and medical guidance among people with multiple sclerosis. *Neurology. Clinical Practice*, *12*(1), 52–60. DOI: 10.1212/CPJ.0000000000001081 PMID: 35733947

Schauer, G. L. (2024). Improving cannabis policy research at a pivotal time for policy development. *American Journal of Public Health*, *114*(S8, Suppl. 8), S635–S638. DOI: 10.2105/AJPH.2024.307799 PMID: 39442025

Schlag, A. K., Zafar, R. R., Lynskey, M. T., Athanasiou-Fragkouli, A., Phillips, L. D., & Nutt, D. J. (2022). The value of real-world evidence: The case of medical cannabis. *Frontiers in Psychiatry, 13*, 1027159. Advance online publication. DOI: 10.3389/fpsyt.2022.1027159 PMID: 36405915

Schuster, R. M., Mermelstein, R., & Gonzalez, R. (2022). Early onset of cannabis use is associated with greater risk of cannabis use disorder in adulthood. *Drug and Alcohol Dependence, 231*, 109245. Advance online publication. DOI: 10.1016/j.drugalcdep.2021.109245

Shannon, S., Lewis, N., Lee, H., & Hughes, S. (2019). Cannabidiol in anxiety and sleep: A large case series. *The Permanente Journal, 23*(1), 18–041. DOI: 10.7812/TPP/18-041 PMID: 30624194

Siani-Rose, M., Cox, S., Goldstein, B., Abrams, D., Taylor, M., & Kurek, I. (2023). Cannabis-responsive biomarkers: A pharmacometabolomics-based application to evaluate the impact of medical cannabis treatment on children with autism spectrum disorder. *Cannabis and Cannabinoid Research, 8*(1), 126–137. DOI: 10.1089/can.2021.0129 PMID: 34874191

Sulak, D. (n.d.). *The inner inventory: A method for finding your optimal cannabis dose*. Healer. https://healer.com/programs/the-inner-inventory/

Tabaei-Aghdaei, Z., McColl-Kennedy, J. R., & Coote, L. V. (2023). Goal setting and health-related outcomes in chronic diseases: A systematic review and meta-analysis of the literature from 2000 to 2020. *Medical Care Research and Review : MCRR, 80*(2), 145–164. DOI: 10.1177/10775587221113228 PMID: 35904147

Tait, M. A., Costa, D. S. J., Campbell, R., Norman, R., Warne, L. N., Schug, S., & Rutherford, C. (2023). Health-related quality of life in patients accessing medicinal cannabis in Australia: The QUEST initiative results of a 3-month follow-up observational study. *PLoS One, 18*(9), e0290549. Advance online publication. DOI: 10.1371/journal.pone.0290549 PMID: 37672515

Tait, M. A., Costa, D. S. J., Campbell, R., Warne, L. N., Norman, R., Schug, S., & Rutherford, C. (2025). Improvements in health-related quality of life are maintained long-term in patients prescribed medicinal cannabis in Australia: The QUEST initiative 12-month follow-up observational study. *PLoS One, 20*(4), e0320756. Advance online publication. DOI: 10.1371/journal.pone.0320756 PMID: 40173146

Tinetti, M. E., Fried, T. R., & Boyd, C. M. (2012). Designing health care for the most common chronic condition: Multimorbidity. *Journal of the American Medical Association, 307*(23), 2493–2494. DOI: 10.1001/jama.2012.5265 PMID: 22797447

Tishler, J. (n.d.). *Many patients using cannabis yet medical cannabis systems failing*. Association of Cannabinoid Specialists. https://www.cannaspecialists.org/medical_cannabis_systems_are_failing

U.S. Congress. (1938). *Federal Food, Drug, and Cosmetic Act*, 21 U.S.C. § 301 et seq. https://www.govinfo.gov/content/pkg/USCODE-2023-title21/pdf/USCODE-2023-title21-chap9.pdf

U.S. Food and Drug Administration. (2023). *FDA and cannabis: Research and drug approval process*. https://www.fda.gov/news-events/public-health-focus/fda-and-cannabis-research-and-drug-approval-process

Wallace, M. S., Marcotte, T. D., Umlauf, A., Gouaux, B., & Atkinson, J. H. (2015). Efficacy of inhaled cannabis on painful diabetic neuropathy. *The Journal of Pain*, *16*(7), 616–627. DOI: 10.1016/j.jpain.2015.03.008 PMID: 25843054

World Health Organization. (1948). *Constitution of the World Health Organization*. https://www.who.int/about/governance/constitution

KEY TERMS AND DEFINITIONS

Cannabis-trained professional: A healthcare professional with formal and/or experiential training in cannabis science, pharmacology, therapeutic application, and harm reduction.

Clinical Vacuum: A gap in structured care where access to treatment exists without consistent education, monitoring, outcome measurement, or longitudinal guidance.

Evidence-based medicine (EBM): The integration of the best available research evidence with clinical expertise and patient values to guide healthcare decisions.

Harm Reduction: An approach that prioritizes reducing potential harms associated with a behavior rather than requiring abstinence or cessation, with the goal of improving safety, function, and overall well-being.

Health: A state of physical, emotional, and social well-being and resilience, not defined solely by the absence of disease or formal medical diagnoses.

Holistic: An approach that considers the whole person, including physical, emotional, social, cognitive, and functional domains, rather than focusing solely on isolated symptoms or diagnoses.

Homeostasis: The ability of biological systems to maintain internal stability and balance despite changing internal or external conditions.

Intentional Use: Purposeful use of cannabis aligned with clearly defined health goals, values, and expectations rather than reactive or habitual consumption.

Iterative Care: A care model in which treatment is continuously refined through reassessment, feedback, and adjustment over time.

Monitoring: The systematic tracking of subjective and objective outcomes over time to assess effectiveness, tolerability, and unintended effects.

Patient-reported outcome measures (PROMs): Validated tools used to capture patient-reported symptoms, function, and quality of life across multiple health domains.

Therapeutic window: The dose range of a compound or product in which clinical benefits are achieved with adverse effects that are limited and tolerable.

Chapter 7
The Cannabis Nurse: A New Paradigm for Patient and Community Care

Elisabeth Mack
http://orcid.org/0009-0008-1418-6201
Holistic Caring, USA

ABSTRACT

As cannabis nursing develops, it meets the growing demand for expert support among patients using cannabis therapeutically. This chapter outlines the Cannabis Nurse's role and practical strategies for integrating it into healthcare and communities. It covers six core knowledge areas, essential skills, workflows, and quality metrics from the National Council of State Boards of Nursing. Real-world examples highlight its impact in oncology, geriatrics, palliative care, mental health, and pain management. The chapter also discusses entrepreneurial, administrative and business opportunities, offering resources for administrators and nurse leaders, and clear pathways for nurses' education and leadership in value-based care.

INTRODUCTION: FROM RECOGNITION TO PRACTICE

The formal recognition of cannabis nursing as a specialty by the American Nurses Association in 2023 marks an important development in contemporary nursing practice (American Nurses Association, 2023). Patients across the lifespan are increasingly using cannabis therapeutically for conditions including chronic pain, sleep disturbance, anxiety, and symptom management in serious illness. Yet clinical guidance, standardized workflows, and clearly defined nursing roles have not evolved at the same pace as patient use. As a result, gaps remain in patient education, safety monitoring, and care coordination across healthcare settings.

National epidemiologic data illustrate the growing relevance of these conversations in clinical practice. Recent surveillance from the Centers for Disease Control and Prevention indicates that nearly one in five adults in the United States report cannabis use within the past year, with increasing prevalence among older adults (Centers for Disease Control and Prevention, 2025). Among adults aged 65 and older, past-year cannabis use has risen substantially in recent years, reflecting broader societal changes in legalization, perceived therapeutic benefit, and accessibility of cannabis products. These trends have

DOI: 10.4018/979-8-3373-7287-7.ch007

important implications for healthcare systems, particularly as patients increasingly initiate discussions about cannabinoid therapies with clinicians managing chronic disease, cancer care, and palliative needs.

Despite this shift in patient behavior, most nursing and medical education programs provide limited formal instruction on the endocannabinoid system (ECS), cannabinoid pharmacology, dosing considerations, or potential drug interactions (National Council of State Boards of Nursing [NCSBN], 2018; Zolotov, 2025). Consequently, clinicians may feel unprepared to address patient questions or to guide safe therapeutic decision-making.

Oncology and palliative care clinicians have noted that conversations about cannabis frequently arise in clinical encounters, yet providers often lack structured frameworks for responding to these discussions (DiGirolamo, 2026). In parallel, studies examining real-world cannabis guidance have identified significant variability in recommendations provided by non-clinical retail staff, highlighting inconsistencies in dosing, product selection, and safety counseling (Mee, et al., 2026). Together, these gaps underscore the need for clinically trained professionals, including nurses, to support safe and evidence-informed cannabis use.

This chapter addresses that gap by translating policy recognition of cannabis nursing into practical implementation and situates cannabis nursing within the broader transformation of healthcare delivery toward patient-centered, integrative, and value-based models. Drawing on national nursing guidance, emerging clinical research, and frontline nursing experience, the chapter defines the role and scope of the professional Cannabis Nurse across healthcare and community settings. Particular attention is given to how nurses collaborate within interdisciplinary teams, conduct risk screening and patient education, and monitor outcomes associated with cannabinoid use.

Cannabinoid therapeutics remain an evolving area of clinical research. Evidence supporting therapeutic applications varies across conditions, and important limitations persist, including heterogeneity in product composition, variability in dosing approaches, and regulatory barriers to large, randomized trials (Chou et al., 2025; National Academies of Sciences, Engineering, and Medicine, 2017). For this reason, cannabis nursing emphasizes careful assessment, patient education, and harm-reduction strategies rather than prescriptive treatment models.

The chapter also examines cannabis nursing through the lens of healthcare administration and workforce development. As healthcare systems, insurers, and employers explore cannabinoid-based approaches within disease management and population health initiatives, nurses may play an important role in translating emerging evidence into safe clinical practice. By outlining competencies, practice pathways, and future workforce needs, this chapter positions cannabis nursing not as an alternative discipline but as a developing component of modern, patient-centered care.

The objectives of this chapter are to:

- Define the role, scope, and core competencies of the Cannabis Nurse across clinical, community, and emerging healthcare settings
- Apply structured clinical workflows for cannabis nursing practice, including assessment, risk screening, patient education, dosing guidance, and ongoing monitoring
- Evaluate safety considerations, ethical responsibilities, and interprofessional collaboration strategies in the use of cannabinoid therapeutics
- Examine the integration of cannabis nursing within healthcare systems, population health, and value-based care models, including emerging opportunities in policy, reimbursement, and nurse-led innovation

BACKGROUND: ROLE AND SCOPE OF THE CANNABIS NURSE

The Cannabis Nurse is a licensed nurse who applies evidence-informed cannabinoid science, clinical assessment skills, and patient education principles to support the safe and appropriate therapeutic use of cannabis. As an emerging specialty, cannabis nursing integrates foundational nursing competencies with focused knowledge of the endocannabinoid system (ECS), cannabis pharmacology, safety considerations, and evolving regulatory frameworks. The role does not replace medical prescribing authority; rather, it strengthens the clinical care surrounding it through assessment, education, monitoring, and coordination within interprofessional teams (National Council of State Boards of Nursing [NCSBN], 2018; American Cannabis Nurses Association & American Nurses Association [ACNA & ANA], 2024).

At its core, cannabis nursing is grounded in established nursing principles, including patient education, safety, therapeutic communication, ethical practice, and advocacy. The ECS provides a biologically relevant framework for understanding the potential role of cannabinoids in regulating homeostasis across multiple physiological systems, including pain modulation, inflammation, mood, sleep, and neuroprotection (Di Marzo, 2018; Russo, 2018). Clinical translation of ECS science into practice has been further described in cannabinoid-based therapeutic models that emphasize individualized dosing, route selection, and symptom-targeted care (Russo & MacCallum, 2016).

The role of the Cannabis Nurse is not to teach molecular biology in depth, but to translate these concepts into practical, patient-centered guidance. This includes helping patients understand routes of administration, dosing strategies, expected effects, and potential risks within the context of their overall health status and treatment goals. This work is grounded in therapeutic presence and recognition of the patient's lived experience, including the psychological, emotional, and spiritual dimensions of care. Recognizing that patient experiences are highly individualized, the goal of cannabis nursing is to support improvement across one or more domains of health—biological, mental, emotional, spiritual, or social—without creating unintended harm in others (Mack 2025; Clark, 2021).

While the ECS offers a compelling framework for therapeutic application, clinical outcomes associated with cannabinoid use remain variable. Differences in product composition, dosing strategies, and individual patient response contribute to inconsistent findings across studies. In addition, regulatory constraints have historically limited large-scale randomized controlled trials. As a result, current clinical guidance emphasizes cautious, individualized approaches informed by evolving evidence (Chou et al., 2025; Bell et al., 2023).

The Cannabis Nursing Scope and Standards of Practice are guided by state nurse practice acts, institutional policies, and national nursing guidance, including recommendations from the NCSBN and ACNA (ACNA & ANA, 2024; NCSBN, 2018). Within these parameters, Cannabis Nurses commonly conduct risk screening, review health history and medications, provide patient and caregiver education, support symptom tracking, and monitor for adverse events. They also serve as liaisons between patients, prescribers, pharmacists, dispensary personnel, and caregivers, helping to ensure continuity and clarity across often fragmented care environments.

Competencies within cannabis nursing expand with experience and role setting. Frontline nurses may focus on education, safety screening, and documentation, while advanced practice nurses and nurse leaders may engage in protocol development, quality improvement initiatives, staff training, research collaboration, and policy development. Across all levels, maintaining clear role boundaries is essential. Cannabis Nurses do not diagnose conditions or prescribe cannabis; instead, they operate within a harm-reduction framework that prioritizes patient safety, informed decision-making, and alignment with professional nursing standards (ACNA & ANA, 2024; NCSBN, 2018).

Nurses require a range of core competencies that are applicable in various healthcare environments, with each level of practice determining the entry point into cannabis nursing. For example, frontline staff will emphasize patient education, assessment, and foundational knowledge of the endocannabinoid system within clinical settings, whereas advanced practice nurses will drive systems and policy development as this specialty becomes more established within the broader healthcare system. Entrepreneurial nurses may concentrate on education and coaching, often engaging in industry-related or business-focused activities. By explicitly outlining scope of practice, defining competencies, and establishing clear collaborative roles, cannabis nursing transitions from an informal advisory capacity to a well-defined clinical discipline. This framework underpins the creation of standardized workflows, enhances patient safety, and facilitates integration into comprehensive healthcare delivery and disease management models discussed in subsequent sections.

Table 1. Cannabis nursing competency matrix

Level	Core Functions	Skills	Settings
Frontline RN	Education, screening, safety	ECS basics, dosing awareness	Clinics, community
Specialist	Complex care coordination	Case management, protocols	Oncology, pain clinics
Advanced Practice	Leadership, program design	Policy, research, training	Health systems
Entrepreneur	Independent / industry roles	Business, education, consulting	Dispensaries, startups

Health Equity, Social Justice, and the Legacy of Cannabis Prohibition

Cannabis has been used as an herbal remedy for millennia; however, its prohibition in the 1930s resulted in its withdrawal from mainstream healthcare. The convergence of corporate interests, xenophobia, racism, and economic challenges during the Great Depression contributed to the implementation of prohibition. In 1941, cannabis was removed from the pharmacopeia, preventing physicians from recommending it for medical use. Furthermore, prohibition had considerable social consequences, disproportionately impacting Black and Brown communities due to policies enacted by white legislators (Martin-Willett et al., 2023).

The emergence of cannabis nursing occurs within this broader historical and social context shaped by decades of prohibition and unequal enforcement. Communities disproportionately impacted by the War on Drugs, particularly marginalized populations, continue to face barriers to access, economic participation, and trust in healthcare systems (National Academies, 2017; Martin-Willett, et al., 2023).

Despite legalization trends, disparities persist in:

- access to safe, regulated products, or the ability to grow their own plants
- affordability of care due to a lack of reimbursement
- inclusion in industry ownership due to steep investment needs
- representation in clinical research due to a majority white test pool

Cannabis Nurses have an ethical responsibility to address these inequities through:

- culturally responsive education on cannabis as a medicine for all people
- advocacy for equitable access regardless of demographics and economic status
- harm-reduction approaches for those who may be stereotyped
- community-based engagement to promote the reemergence of cannabis

Equity-focused cannabis care includes recognizing financial barriers, stigma, and historical mistrust, while ensuring patients receive nonjudgmental, evidence-informed support. As healthcare systems evolve, nurses will play a critical role in shaping models that prioritize access, inclusion, and justice, not just clinical outcomes.

Cannabis nursing has the potential to either reinforce or reduce existing disparities depending on how care models are designed and implemented. Intentional integration of equity-focused practices—such as inclusive education, community engagement, and advocacy for policy reform—will be essential to ensuring that the benefits of cannabinoid therapeutics are accessible across diverse populations. In this way, cannabis nursing extends beyond clinical care into a broader commitment to social accountability within healthcare systems.

MAIN FOCUS OF THE CHAPTER

Clinical Foundations of Cannabis Nursing Practice

Clinical cannabis nursing practice is grounded in the integration of cannabinoid science with core nursing processes, including assessment, clinical reasoning, patient education, and ongoing monitoring. As patient use of cannabis expands across medical and wellness contexts, nurses are increasingly called upon to interpret evolving evidence and translate it into safe, individualized care strategies. This requires a balance between emerging research, clinical judgment, and patient-centered communication within a rapidly changing regulatory environment (National Council of State Boards of Nursing [NCSBN], 2018; Bell et al., 2023).

Endocannabinoid System and Clinical Relevance

The endocannabinoid system (ECS) plays a central role in maintaining physiological homeostasis across multiple organ systems. It is composed of endogenous cannabinoids (endocannabinoids), cannabinoid receptors (primarily CB1 and CB2), and enzymes responsible for synthesis and degradation. This system influences a wide range of processes, including pain modulation, immune response, mood regulation, sleep, appetite, and neuroprotection (Di Marzo, 2018; Russo, 2018).

Phytocannabinoids such as delta-9-tetrahydrocannabinol (THC) and cannabidiol (CBD) interact with the ECS in distinct ways. THC acts as a partial agonist at CB1 receptors, contributing to its psychoactive and analgesic effects, while CBD exhibits more complex modulatory actions, including indirect effects on cannabinoid receptors and influence on non-cannabinoid pathways such as serotonin and transient receptor potential (TRP) channels (Russo & MacCallum, 2016; Bruni et al., 2018).

For the Cannabis Nurse, understanding the ECS provides a clinical framework rather than an end in itself. This knowledge supports the ability to explain why cannabinoids may influence multiple symptom domains and why patient responses can vary significantly. While ECS science offers biologic plausibility for therapeutic use, variability in product composition, dosing, and individual physiology contributes to inconsistent clinical outcomes, reinforcing the need for cautious, individualized care approaches (Chou et al., 2025; Bell et al., 2023).

Routes of Administration and Dosing Principles

Cannabis products can be administered through multiple routes, each with distinct pharmacokinetic profiles that influence onset, duration, and intensity of effects. Common routes include inhalation (smoked or vaporized), oral ingestion (oils, capsules, edibles), sublingual administration (tinctures), and topical or transdermal applications.

Inhaled cannabis typically produces rapid onset within minutes, with shorter duration of action, making it potentially useful for acute symptom relief. Oral formulations have delayed onset—often 1 to 3 hours—but longer duration, which may be beneficial for chronic symptom management. Sublingual products offer an intermediate profile, though absorption can be variable. Topical and transdermal formulations are generally used for localized effects or sustained systemic delivery, depending on formulation. Patients can be taught how to employ a short-acting, long-acting approach with a variety of cannabis products (Bruni et al., 2018).

Dosing in cannabis therapeutics remains highly individualized. A "start low and go slow" approach is widely recommended, particularly when introducing THC-containing products. Factors influencing dosing include patient age, prior cannabis exposure, comorbid conditions, concurrent medications, and treatment goals (Sulak, 2021). Nurses play a key role in helping patients titrate dosing safely, recognize therapeutic thresholds, and avoid adverse effects.

Cannabis Nurses reinforce that therapeutic cannabis use is not static; dosing and product selections may require adjustments over time based on response, tolerance, and changes in health status (Clark, 2021). Our bodies are always renewing, and dosing requirements change over time as the ECS is toned and balanced.

Safety, Drug Interactions, and Risk Mitigation

Safety is a central component of cannabis nursing practice. While cannabinoids are generally well tolerated, potential adverse effects include dizziness, sedation, cognitive impairment, anxiety, and, in some cases, paradoxical worsening of symptoms. THC-containing products carry additional risks related to psychoactive effects, particularly in vulnerable populations (NASEM, 2017).

Cannabinoids, particularly CBD, may interact with commonly prescribed medications through hepatic enzyme pathways, including cytochrome P450 isoenzymes. These interactions can alter serum concentrations of medications such as anticoagulants, antiepileptics, and certain psychotropic drugs, necessitating careful monitoring and collaboration with prescribing clinicians (Graham et al., 2022).

Risk mitigation strategies include comprehensive medication reconciliation, screening for contraindications, patient education on safe storage and use, and ongoing monitoring for adverse events. Special attention is required for populations such as older adults, individuals with cardiovascular or psychiatric conditions, pregnant or breastfeeding patients, and those with a history of substance use disorder (Graham et al., 2022).

Evidence Landscape and Clinical Interpretation

The evidence base for cannabis therapeutics continues to evolve, with a growing body of observational studies, systematic reviews, and meta-analyses supporting its use in select conditions, including chronic pain, chemotherapy-induced nausea and vomiting, and spasticity associated with multiple sclerosis (National Academies of Sciences, Engineering, and Medicine, 2017; Castle et al., 2025).

At the same time, limitations in study design, product standardization, and regulatory barriers contribute to variability in findings. Recent clinical guidelines emphasize the importance of cautious interpretation, shared decision-making, and individualized care planning (Bell et al., 2023; Chou et al., 2025).

In oncology and palliative care, emerging evidence suggests potential benefits in symptom management, including pain, appetite stimulation, sleep, and quality of life, though further high-quality trials are needed (Troyer & Tanco, 2024; National Cancer Institute, 2024). Similarly, ongoing research is exploring the role of cannabinoids in neurological conditions, mental health, and substance use disorders, highlighting both therapeutic promise and areas of uncertainty (Chye et al., 2019; Russo, 2018).

For nurses, the role is not to resolve these uncertainties, but to navigate them, responsibly translating available evidence into practical guidance while maintaining transparency about limitations. This requires strong communication skills, critical appraisal of emerging research, and a commitment to patient-centered care.

Integrating Clinical Knowledge into Practice

Clinical cannabis nursing practice is ultimately defined by the ability to translate complex and evolving information into safe, actionable care strategies. This includes helping patients set realistic expectations, identify therapeutic goals, and integrate cannabis use within broader care plans.

Importantly, many patients seeking cannabis guidance are doing so after experiencing limitations or dissatisfaction with conventional treatment approaches. As a result, cannabis nursing often intersects with holistic and integrative models of care that emphasize a harm-reduction approach for whole-person health, patient autonomy, and quality of life (Clark, 2021).

Within this context, nurses serve as both clinical guides and care coordinators—bridging gaps between traditional healthcare systems, emerging cannabinoid therapeutics, and patient-driven care pathways. This role requires not only clinical competence, but also adaptability, ethical awareness, and a commitment to ongoing learning as the evidence base continues to evolve.

CLINICAL WORKFLOWS, SAFETY, AND ETHICAL PRACTICE IN CANNABIS NURSING

Clinical cannabis nursing practice is defined not only by knowledge of cannabinoid science, but by the ability to implement structured, safe, and ethically grounded workflows across diverse care settings. As cannabis use expands within both medical and consumer-driven contexts, nurses play a critical role in establishing consistency, mitigating risk, and ensuring that patient care aligns with professional standards and evolving evidence.

Variability in cannabis guidance extends beyond clinical settings. Studies evaluating recommendations provided in retail environments have demonstrated substantial inconsistency in product selection, dosing advice, and safety considerations, particularly among non-clinical personnel (Mee et al., 2026). While dispensary staff play an important role in patient access and product navigation, the absence of standardized clinical training can contribute to gaps in patient education and risk mitigation. This reinforces the need for healthcare professionals, including nurses, to serve as trusted sources of evidence-informed guidance and to collaborate with dispensary teams to improve patient safety and continuity of care.

Table 2. Clinical workflow model

Intake → Assessment → Risk Screening →
Education → Product Selection Guidance → Titration →
Monitoring → Follow-Up

Assessment, Risk Screening, and Medication Review

The clinical encounter begins with a comprehensive assessment that mirrors traditional nursing practice while incorporating cannabis-specific considerations. This includes a detailed health history, current symptom burden, prior experience with cannabis, and patient-defined goals of care.

Medication reconciliation is a critical component of this process. Given the potential for cannabinoid interactions with commonly prescribed medications—particularly those metabolized through cytochrome P450 pathways—nurses must assess for risks related to polypharmacy, dose-dependent interactions, and therapeutic duplication (Graham et al., 2022).

Risk screening should also evaluate for contraindications and precautions, including a history of psychiatric conditions (e.g., psychosis), cardiovascular instability, pregnancy or breastfeeding status, and substance use disorders. Special attention is required for older adults, who may be more susceptible to sedation, falls, and drug interactions due to age-related physiological changes (NCSBN, 2018).

This assessment phase establishes the clinical foundation for safe and individualized cannabis use, ensuring that recommendations are aligned with both patient goals and safety considerations.

Care Planning, Education, and Dosing Implementation

Following assessment, nurses support the development of an individualized care plan that incorporates cannabis as one component of a broader therapeutic strategy. This includes selecting appropriate product types, routes of administration, and dosing approaches based on patient needs, preferences, and risk profile.

Patient education is central to this phase. Nurses translate complex information into practical guidance, including:

- differences between THC and CBD, and how to use them together

- expected onset and duration based on route for safer, predictable outcomes
- titration strategies ("start low and go slow"), especially with THC
- rotating routes and dosing to avoid tolerance buildup
- avoidance of concurrent use with other substances, i.e., alcohol
- recognizing therapeutic effects versus adverse reactions
- safe storage of cannabis products and use practices with ADLs

Importantly, this process emphasizes shared decision-making. Patients are active participants in care planning, and education is tailored to health literacy, cultural context, and prior experience (Clark, 2021).

Dosing implementation is iterative rather than prescriptive. Nurses guide patients through gradual titration, helping them identify effective doses while minimizing unwanted effects. This approach reflects both the variability of cannabinoid response and the current limitations of standardized dosing guidelines.

Monitoring, Documentation, and Outcome Tracking

Ongoing monitoring is essential to safe cannabis use. Nurses support patients in tracking symptom response, functional outcomes, and any adverse effects over time. This may include structured tools such as symptom logs, sleep tracking, pain scales, or quality-of-life assessments. Informal tools such as cannabis tracking apps may be useful to some patients.

Documentation practices should align with professional standards and institutional policies, capturing baseline symptoms and goals, and what product types and dosing strategies were introduced. This will provide a clear picture of the patient-reported outcomes, and any adverse events or safety concerns that were identified. Any adjustments made over time will be elucidated to see how the clinical picture changed with respect to cannabinoids, dosing, and use patterns.

This structured approach not only supports continuity of care but also contributes to emerging data on real-world cannabis use, which remains a critical gap in the evidence base. This iterative process reflects nursing's traditional role in symptom management and chronic disease support, adapted to an emerging therapeutic category (ACNA & ANA, 2024).

Clear communication pathways are integral to workflow integrity. Cannabis Nurses often serve as liaisons among patients, prescribers, pharmacists, dispensary staff, and caregivers, helping to align messaging and reduce conflicting guidance. Documentation supports continuity of care and provides a record of education, risk screening, monitoring, and escalation decisions, reinforcing accountability and professional standards (NCSBN, 2018).

Table 3. Safety & documentation checklist

Domain	Key Elements
Risk Screening	**Medications, contraindications**
Education	**Dosing, routes, expectations**
Monitoring	**Symptom tracking, adverse effects**
Documentation	**Patient goals, outcomes**
Follow-Up	**Adjustments, escalation**

Harm Reduction and Safety Across Populations

Safety considerations are central to cannabis nursing practice, particularly given variability in product composition, routes, potencies, patient sensitivity, and limited long-term outcome data. Cannabis Nurses apply nursing judgment, conservative dosing principles, and ongoing monitoring to reduce preventable adverse events and to support informed decision-making.

A harm-reduction framework is central to cannabis nursing practice. Rather than promoting or discouraging use, nurses provide balanced, evidence-informed guidance that prioritizes patient safety and informed choice (Clark, 2021).

Key safety considerations include:

- avoiding high-dose THC in naïve or vulnerable patients
- minimizing risks of impairment, particularly related to driving or operating machinery
- recognizing signs of overuse or cannabis use disorder
- educating patients on product variability and labeling limitations

Special populations require tailored approaches. Older adults, oncology patients, individuals with chronic disease, and those with mental health or substance use histories may have unique risks and therapeutic considerations. Older adults may experience increased sensitivity to psychoactive effects, orthostatic hypotension, and increased fall risk.

In pediatric populations, cannabis nursing involvement focuses primarily on caregiver education, developing brain concerns, risk–benefit discussions, and coordination with specialty providers. During pregnancy and lactation, nurses emphasize current evidence limitations and professional guidance discouraging use, while supporting nonjudgmental counseling and referral when appropriate (NCSBN, 2018; ANA, 2016). Nurses must adapt care plans accordingly while maintaining close monitoring and collaboration with other providers.

Ethical Practice and Professional Boundaries

Cannabis nursing practice exists within a complex ethical and regulatory landscape. Nurses must balance patient autonomy with professional responsibility, ensuring that care remains within legal and scope-of-practice boundaries.

Key ethical considerations include:

- maintaining transparency about the limits of current evidence
- avoiding conflicts of interest, particularly in retail or product-affiliated settings
- ensuring that patient recommendations are not influenced by financial incentives
- supporting informed consent and shared decision-making

In emerging care environments such as dispensaries, nurses may play a valuable role in patient education and safety. However, clear role delineation is essential to preserve professional integrity and public trust.

Meeting patients where they're at is an important first step in listening and recognizing alternative modalities. Cultural humility, stigma reduction, and respect for diverse beliefs about cannabis use are essential, particularly in populations historically affected by criminalization or healthcare inequities (ANA, 2016; NCSBN, 2018).

Interprofessional Collaboration and Care Coordination

Cannabis regulations are highly variable, and its use remains stigmatized, inconsistently integrated into healthcare systems, and often siloed outside traditional medical settings. Cannabis Nurses frequently function as clinical translators—bridging the gaps between patients, licensed prescribers, pharmacists, dispensary professionals, caregivers, and institutional policies. This integrative role is essential for ensuring safety, continuity of care, and ethical practice across fragmented environments (NCSBN, 2018; Clark, 2021). Because cannabis therapeutics is such a novel field, Cannabis Nurses offer a valuable differentiator for health systems in which they operate.

Effective collaboration includes communicating patient goals and responses to treatment, and identifying potential medication interactions or safety concerns. The Cannabis Nurse will be the bridge in supporting continuity of care across settings, and contributing to team-based decision-making for all to gain from and grow through.

As healthcare systems increasingly explore cannabinoid-based therapies, nurses are uniquely positioned to bridge knowledge gaps and support safe integration into clinical practice.

From Workflow to System Integration

Structured clinical workflows provide the foundation for broader system integration. By standardizing assessment, education, monitoring, and documentation practices, cannabis nursing can evolve from an informal, patient-driven activity into a recognized component of healthcare delivery.

These workflows support not only individual patient outcomes, but also larger efforts related to quality improvement, population health, and emerging models of care. As such, they serve as a critical bridge between clinical practice and the healthcare administration, policy, and business opportunities explored in the next section.

Clinical Case Vignettes Across Care Settings

Clinical vignettes illustrate how cannabis nursing principles translate into real-world care across diverse populations and settings. These examples reflect common clinical scenarios and highlight assessment, education, safety, and interdisciplinary coordination.

Oncology (Chemotherapy Support)

A 58-year-old patient undergoing chemotherapy presents with nausea, poor appetite, and insomnia. The Cannabis Nurse conducts a symptom assessment, reviews medications for potential interactions, and educates the patient on low-dose THC for appetite stimulation and CBD-dominant formulations for anxiety. Assistance with identification of medical products in various dose forms at nearby dispensaries via online menus may be provided to expedite effective choices. Coordination with oncology providers ensures alignment with treatment goals and safety monitoring.

Geriatrics / Dementia Care

An 82-year-old patient with dementia experiences agitation and disrupted sleep. Caregiver education focuses on low-dose THC, with CBD and the minor cannabinoids as the preferred strategies, non-inhaled routes, and fall risk mitigation. Emphasis is placed on gradual titration, behavioral observation, medication interactions, especially opioids, and caregiver support. Monitoring and availability for follow up care is essential to aid the family in understanding effects versus side effects, and making adjustments.

Chronic Pain & Opioid Reduction

A middle-aged patient with chronic pain seeks alternatives to long-term opioid therapy. The Cannabis Nurse supports a harm-reduction approach, introducing cannabinoids as an adjunct therapy while coordinating with a potential opioid dose reduction from the prescribing providers. Functional goals include mobility, sleep, and quality of life, and these are prioritized over pain elimination. Documentation of efficacy with cannabinoids and a reduction of opioids will be critical to demonstrate a safe and effective pathway for healthcare providers to adopt and insurance carriers to reimburse.

Mental Health & Sleep

A 32-year old patient with anxiety and insomnia explores cannabinoid use after limited success with conventional treatments. Education includes daytime CBD use and cautious nighttime THC introduction, alongside behavioral health strategies and monitoring for adverse effects. Patient teaching around various cannabinoids, routes, and tracking outcomes is important to support the more nuanced cannabinoid pathway versus the pharmaceutical model of care.

Substance Use Recovery

A 44-year-old patient in recovery from alcohol use disorder explores CBD as a supportive tool. The nurse provides education on craving modulation, safety considerations, and integration with existing recovery supports (Chye et al., 2019). Ensuring understanding of appropriate use of CBD and minor cannabinoids versus cannabis use disorder with high dose THC is key to maintaining support from providers, family, and even the patient in sensitive situations.

BUSINESS, HEALTH SYSTEMS, AND THE FUTURE OF CANNABIS NURSING

The integration of cannabis into healthcare systems represents both a clinical and economic inflection point. As patient demand continues to rise and policy frameworks evolve, healthcare organizations, insurers, and employers are increasingly compelled to examine cannabinoid-based therapies through the lens of cost, outcomes, and population health. Within this landscape, Cannabis Nurses are uniquely positioned to bridge gaps between emerging therapeutics, traditional care models, and real-world patient use.

Cannabis as a Cost-Containment and Value-Based Care Strategy

As healthcare systems shift toward value-based care, interest in cannabinoid therapies is increasingly framed through disease management and population health. Conditions such as chronic pain, sleep disorders, anxiety, neurodegenerative disease, and cancer-related symptoms represent areas where patients already use cannabis, often without guidance, and where coordinated, nurse-led support may improve outcomes (Stanford Medicine, 2025).

Chronic disease remains the primary driver of healthcare expenditures in the United States, accounting for the majority of costs across Medicare, Medicaid, and commercial health insurance plans. Conditions such as chronic pain, cancer, neurodegenerative disorders, autoimmune disease, and mental health conditions often require long-term pharmacologic management, frequently associated with high cost and significant side effect burden. Although medicine has made significant strides in recent years, most progress centers on treating acute issues, offering limited benefits for individuals dealing with chronic illnesses that demand ongoing care to improve their quality of life.

Emerging evidence suggests that cannabinoid-based therapies may offer a complementary or, in some cases, substitutive approach to traditional treatment pathways, particularly in the context of pain management and opioid reduction (Kvamme et al., 2021; Chou et al., 2025). Observational studies and patient-reported outcomes indicate potential reductions in opioid use, improved symptom control, and enhanced quality of life among certain patient populations (NASEM, 2017).

From a healthcare administration perspective, these findings raise important questions regarding cost-effectiveness. Compared to many pharmaceutical interventions, cannabinoid therapies, particularly hemp-derived CBD products, may offer lower-cost alternatives when used appropriately and under clinical guidance. As value-based care models continue to evolve, there is increasing interest in therapies that can improve outcomes while reducing total cost of care (Mack, 2020).

At the same time, variability in product quality, lack of standardized dosing, and limited insurance coverage present ongoing challenges. These factors underscore the need for structured clinical oversight, which Cannabis Nurses are well positioned to provide.

Insurance Coverage, Policy Shifts, and Emerging Reimbursement Models

Recent federal and state-level policy discussions have signaled a potential shift toward greater integration of cannabinoid therapies within formal healthcare systems. Proposed changes related to cannabis rescheduling and expanded coverage pathways, particularly for non-psychoactive cannabinoids such as CBD have prompted insurers and policymakers to reconsider how these therapies may fit within existing reimbursement frameworks, or to invent new mechanisms for coverage that are unique to the promise of cannabinoid care (JD Supra, 2025).

Organizations such as the American Council of Cannabis Medicine are actively exploring frameworks to integrate medically guided cannabis reimbursement programs into the broader healthcare delivery and financing models (Lange, 2025). At the federal level, evolving policy discussions around cannabidiol, rescheduling, and pilot coverage mechanisms suggest that cannabinoid-based therapies may increasingly intersect with payer systems, including employer-sponsored benefits, workers' compensation programs, and public insurance pathways administered by the Centers for Medicare & Medicaid Services (The White House, 2025).

Pilot programs, research initiatives, and advocacy efforts, including those led by organizations such as Realm of Caring, the Commonwealth Project, and academic registries are generating real-world data to inform these decisions. These efforts focus on outcomes related to chronic pain, epilepsy, cancer care, and palliative populations, with an emphasis on safety, efficacy, and cost-benefit analysis (The Commonwealth Project, 2025; Cannabis and Health Research Initiative, 2025).

For payers, the central question is not whether patients are using cannabis, but whether structured, clinically guided use can reduce downstream costs associated with unmanaged symptoms, polypharmacy, and avoidable healthcare utilization. As this shift unfolds, Cannabis Nurses may play a critical role in supporting documentation, outcomes tracking, and care coordination necessary for reimbursement models to develop.

Disease Management and Population Health Applications

Disease management represents one of the most promising and practical applications of cannabis nursing within payer-aligned systems. Cannabis nursing aligns naturally with disease management and population health strategies, particularly in conditions characterized by chronic symptom burden and complex medication regimens. Nurses trained in cannabinoid therapeutics can support targeted interventions across several key areas:

- chronic pain and opioid tapering
- oncology and management of chemotherapy-related side effects
- palliative and end-of-life care
- neurological and neurodegenerative conditions (e.g., multiple sclerosis, Parkinson's disease, dementia)
- autoimmune disorders and inflammatory conditions
- mental health and substance use recovery support

Chronic Pain and Opioid Weaning

Chronic pain remains one of the most costly and challenging conditions in healthcare. Opioid-centered approaches have contributed to dependency, adverse events, and escalating costs without reliably improving function. Cannabinoid-based strategies, when guided clinically, offer an alternative or adjunct pathway that may support pain reduction, improved sleep, and functional gains while reducing opioid exposure (NASEM, 2017). Clinical experience indicates that patients benefit from formulations containing both CBD and THC. The use of a combination of short-acting and long-acting administration methods, such as tinctures and capsules for regular dosing and inhalation for breakthrough pain, has proven effective in practice.

Cannabis Nurses working in pain management or case management roles can support opioid weaning by:

- Assessing pain patterns and functional goals
- Educating patients on non-intoxicating and low-dose options
- Monitoring withdrawal symptoms and safety concerns
- Coordinating with prescribers and behavioral health providers
- Providing lifestyle tips to complement cannabinoid-based therapies

This role aligns directly with payer priorities around risk mitigation, disability management, and return-to-function outcomes. For the Cannabis Industry, nurses may be key to adoption, optimization, and retention, as a new study confirmed that over 58% of older adults prescribed medical cannabis for chronic pain stopped taking it within one year. These numbers indicate that a more personalized, guided approach is necessary (Respiratory Therapy, 2025).

Cancer Care and Chemotherapy Support

In oncology settings, cannabinoids are commonly used for symptom management. Cannabinoids provide support for chronic pain, neuropathic pain, nausea, vomiting (especially chemo-induced), loss of appetite, insomnia, fear, anxiety, and depression. CB1 receptors modulate nausea, pain, and mood, while CB2 receptors are anti-inflammatory and may support immune defense. The CB1 and CB2 receptors, along with non-classical targets like TRPV1, TRPV2, PPAR-Alpha, and PPAR-Gamma, are actively being studied for their roles in regulating tumor growth, inflammation, angiogenesis, and immune modulation (NCI, 2025; CannaKeys, 2024). A 2025 meta-analysis revealed a significant consensus supporting the use of medical cannabis in the categories of health metrics, cancer treatments, and cancer dynamics. (Castle et al., 2025).

Although the National Cancer Institute has offered cautious recommendations regarding the incorporation of cannabinoids into cancer treatment plans, many oncologists remain hesitant to endorse cannabis use, resulting in patients often managing these therapies independently (NCI 2025; DiGirolamo, 2026). In such circumstances, cancer patients may seek advice from dispensary staff or online forums that advocate for unproven dosing strategies, such as the daily consumption of one gram of THC oil. While anecdotal evidence suggests occasional positive outcomes, Cannabis Nurses can facilitate safer integration by encouraging evidence-based dosing, monitoring potential drug interactions and titration, assessing functional tolerance, and promoting adherence to prescribed oncology care plans (Clark, 2021). For healthcare systems and insurers, enhanced symptom management may lead to reduced emergency department visits, improved compliance with treatments, fewer side effects, and higher quality-of-life metrics—results that are increasingly valued within contemporary, outcome-focused oncology models.

Palliative Care, Hospice, and Medicare Populations

Palliative and hospice populations represent a natural intersection between cannabinoid therapeutics and Medicare-funded care. Goals in these settings prioritize comfort, dignity, and quality of life rather than disease modification. Cannabis Nurses can help align cannabinoid use with these goals while addressing safety concerns such as cognition, fall risk, caregiver burden, and medication interactions. Limited evidence suggests that cannabis may relieve numerous symptoms in palliative care patients, however, cannabis is associated with several neuropsychiatric and systemic adverse effects and drug interactions warrant clinical oversight (Troyer & Tanco, 2024).

Older adults represent the fastest-growing group of cannabis users, frequently pursuing alternatives to sedatives, analgesics, and anxiolytics. Given their slower metabolic rates and prevalence of polypharmacy, it is essential that older adults receive guidance beyond retail recommendations, particularly regarding high-THC products. Initiating therapy with a high-CBD regimen, and introducing THC in a gradual, measured, and monitored manner, is advisable. Recent research emphasizes both the therapeutic possibilities and the necessity for clinically supervised, cautious use within this population, reinforcing the critical role of nursing oversight (Stanford Medicine, 2025).

Neurological, Autoimmune, and Neurodegenerative Conditions

Epilepsy is widely regarded as a challenging neurological disorder for both patients and their families. Cannabinoids have emerged as a promising avenue for addressing treatment-resistant epilepsy. The introduction of cannabidiol (CBD) in the United States initially focused on young individuals with Dravet Syndrome who experienced frequent seizures and showed positive responses to CBD oil therapy. In 2018, Epidiolex, a purified CBD oil, received FDA approval and has since had a significant impact on affected families globally (Epidiolex, n.d.).

Conditions such as multiple sclerosis, Parkinson's disease, neuropathy, and autoimmune disorders often involve overlapping symptoms—pain, spasticity, fatigue, sleep disruption, and mood changes. Cannabinoid therapeutics, through ECS modulation, may influence multiple pathways relevant to these conditions, offering a systems-oriented approach that resonates with holistic care models (Russo, 2018).

Cannabis Nurses support these populations by coordinating care across specialties, tracking functional outcomes, and ensuring that symptom relief does not come at the expense of cognition, mobility, or safety. Fear of falls, adverse effects, and worsening outcomes makes nursing care invaluable to the families as well, through cannabinoid education, reassurance, and ongoing support (Mack, 2020).

Mental Health and Substance Use Substitution

Anxiety and depression are prevalent issues among individuals using cannabis for symptom relief, despite limited clinical evidence supporting its efficacy and significant concerns regarding adverse effects and the potential exacerbation of symptoms. Given the biphasic effects of cannabinoids and the varying protocols used for episodic versus chronic conditions, clinical guidance is essential to optimize outcomes and improve the likelihood of therapeutic success (National Academies Press, 2017).

Although conventional psychiatry continues to exercise caution, especially with respect to THC, there is increasing interest in the potential applications of cannabidiol (CBD) and other non-intoxicating cannabinoids for harm reduction and substance substitution approaches. Current evidence indicates that CBD may play a beneficial role in mitigating cravings, anxiety, and stress responses associated with substance use disorders (Chye et al., 2019).

Although CBD is generally regarded as the preferred treatment option, a significant number of patients choose high-THC products for their rapid effects and immediate sense of well-being, despite the associated risks. Cannabis nurses engaged in behavioral health or recovery contexts work to prioritize structure, ongoing monitoring, and interdisciplinary collaboration with mental health professionals. Cannabinoid therapy is presented not as a substitute for conventional treatments, but as an adjunctive support within comprehensive recovery plans.

Within all of the above clinical contexts, cannabis is not positioned as a replacement for conventional care, but as an adjunctive tool that may improve symptom control, enhance quality of life, and support patient-centered care goals (Troyer & Tanco, 2024; Castle et al., 2025). The role of the nurse is to integrate these therapies thoughtfully within existing care plans, ensuring safety, coordination, and alignment with broader treatment strategies.

The Cannabis Nurse as Consultant and Systems Integrator

A significant barrier to the integration of cannabis into healthcare is the knowledge gap among clinicians, administrators, and policymakers. Despite increasing patient use, most healthcare professionals receive little formal education on cannabinoid science, dosing, or safety considerations (Zolotov, 2025).

Cannabis Nurses are uniquely positioned to serve as consultants within healthcare systems, health plans, and community-based organizations. In this role, they:

- educate clinical teams and leadership on cannabinoid therapeutics
- develop protocols and clinical workflows
- support policy development and compliance
- assist with program implementation and evaluation
- bridge communication between patients, providers, and ancillary services

This consultative function reflects a broader shift in nursing toward leadership in care innovation, quality improvement, and systems transformation.

Systems-Level Example: Integrating Cannabis Nursing into Value-Based Care

A regional healthcare system implementing value-based care for chronic pain has observed elevated utilization among patients with prolonged opioid use, frequent emergency department admissions, and suboptimal functional outcomes. To address these concerns, the system has established a nurse-led cannabis education and monitoring initiative, which is incorporated into existing nursing case management services. Located in the New York metropolitan area, this healthcare system benefits from legal access to cannabis products and serves a population with a significant proportion of individuals already choosing cannabinoid use, often without structured clinical guidance.

Cannabis Nurses conduct structured assessments, provide comprehensive education on cannabinoid therapeutics, including CBD, THC, and routes of administration with a focus on short-acting and long-acting stacking protocols, and support for the gradual integration alongside existing treatment plans. Patients are then monitored for symptom improvement, opioid reduction, sleep quality, and functional outcomes over time.

Over time, preliminary outcomes of cannabis care demonstrate:

- reduced reliance on opioid medications
- improved patient-reported quality of life
- fewer urgent care visits related to uncontrolled symptoms

For healthcare administrators, these findings highlight the potential for cannabis nursing to contribute to cost containment and improved outcomes within value-based care models. For nurses, this represents a scalable pathway to using their unique skillsets to make a difference within population health and care innovation roles.

Entrepreneurship and Emerging Practice Models

In addition to traditional healthcare roles, cannabis nursing has given rise to new models of nurse-led entrepreneurship. These models often emerge in response to gaps in the healthcare system, particularly where patients lack access to providers who are knowledgeable in cannabis therapeutics.

Common entrepreneurial pathways include:

- private cannabis care coaching and consultation practices
- educational programs for patients, clinicians, and industry professionals
- partnerships with dispensaries to provide patient education and safety guidance
- product development and advisory roles within cannabinoid companies
- participation in research initiatives and clinical trials

While these opportunities offer increased autonomy and innovation, they also require careful attention to ethical considerations, scope of practice, and potential conflicts of interest. Maintaining professional integrity and patient trust remains paramount.

Importantly, dispensaries represent a rapidly evolving practice environment. While traditionally viewed as retail settings, many are seeking to incorporate clinical expertise to improve patient experience and safety. Nurses working in these settings can elevate standards of care, provided that clear boundaries are maintained between education and product promotion (Mack, 2020; Clark, 2021).

Dispensaries have become a primary point of contact for patients seeking guidance, often in the absence of formal clinical support. This reality presents both ethical challenges and professional opportunities for nurses. While concerns about conflicts of interest and scope of practice are valid, the absence of clinically trained professionals in dispensary environments may pose greater risks to patient safety than thoughtfully structured nursing involvement.

There is a clear distinction between retail sales and clinical guidance. While dispensary staff tend to focus on desired effects, Cannabis Nurses focus on ensuring patient understanding of chemotypes, routes of administration, and safety. Cannabis Nurses do not function as retail staff; rather, they provide independent, evidence-informed clinical guidance that prioritizes patient care, ethical practice, and alignment with nursing standards for community-based care (ACNA & ANA, 2024).

Industry-adjacent roles may include personalized or small group education, clinical advisory positions, research coordination, or program development. There is a tremendous need for guidance and interpretation of evidence-based research on how cannabinoids may supplement the conventional care treatment plans. When nurses engage with dispensaries in ethically sound roles such as patient education, safety screening, referral coordination, or clinical program development, they can significantly improve the quality and consistency of information patients receive. Clear boundaries, transparency, and adherence to nursing standards are essential to protecting licensure and public trust (Clark, 2021; Mack, 2025).

Moreover, nurses with business acumen and access to capital may be uniquely suited to lead or own dispensary-based enterprises. Nurse-led dispensaries can be designed from inception with safety, education, documentation, and referral pathways embedded into operations. In such models, clinical integrity is not compromised; rather, it becomes a defining feature of the organization. These environments demonstrate how entrepreneurship, when grounded in nursing ethics and holistic care principles, can elevate standards and better serve patients navigating complex therapeutic choices (Mack, 2020).

Toward a New Model of Care: From Fragmentation to Integration

Many patients who seek cannabis as part of their care journey do so after experiencing adverse outcomes and limitations within conventional healthcare systems. Fragmentation, time constraints, and a focus on disease-specific interventions can leave patients feeling unsupported in managing complex, chronic conditions.

Cannabis nursing offers an opportunity to reintroduce a more integrative, patient-centered approach, one that considers the whole person and emphasizes function, quality of life, and individualized care. By incorporating cannabinoid therapeutics into this model, nurses can help bridge the gap between traditional medical care and holistic healing practices (Clark, 2021).

This shift does not reject conventional medicine, but rather expands the toolkit available to patients and providers. It reflects a broader evolution toward care models that are collaborative, flexible, and responsive to modern patient needs.

Workforce Development and the Future of the Profession

As cannabis policy and healthcare integration continue to evolve, the demand for trained Cannabis Nurses is expected to grow. This includes roles in clinical care, education, research, policy, and healthcare administration.

Workforce development efforts must focus on:

- standardized education and competency frameworks
- integration into nursing curricula and continuing education programs
- development of clinical guidelines and best practices
- research initiatives to strengthen the evidence base
- leadership pathways within healthcare systems and policy environments

Nurses are well positioned to lead this transformation due to their foundational role in patient care, education, and advocacy. By combining clinical expertise with emerging knowledge in cannabinoid therapeutics, Cannabis Nurses can help shape the future of healthcare in a way that is both innovative and grounded in professional values (ACNA & ANA, 2024; NCSBN, 2018).

As healthcare systems evolve, the emergence of cannabis nursing reflects a broader trend toward interdisciplinary, integrative, and patient-centered care models. Future workforce development is expected to encompass the implementation of formal credentialing processes, integration into academic curricula, and increased engagement in healthcare leadership and policy. Nurses specializing in cannabinoid therapeutics are poised to meet current patient needs and play a pivotal role in establishing future standards, frameworks, and policies within this specialty.

This burgeoning field offers diverse opportunities for nurses across various sectors. Clinical practice and private holistic coaching businesses present entrepreneurial avenues, while a systems-focused approach enhances health systems, payers, case management, and disease-oriented care. The industry sector includes roles in dispensary and retail education, on-site education and counseling, as well as positions related to product development, brand innovation, and design. With ongoing cannabis legalization, opportunities in research, clinical trials, observational studies, and FDA regulatory pathways will expand.

In addition, policy and advocacy work will foster meaningful careers focused on advancing legislative initiatives and change leadership.

Table 4. Cannabis nurse career pathways

Function Map	Focus	Settings
Entrepreneurial Oriented	Clinical Practice	Private Holistic Coaching Business
Systems Oriented	Health Systems / Payers	Case Management / Disease Focused
Industry Oriented	Dispensary & Retail Education	On-site Educator and Counselor
Industry Oriented	Product Development / Industry	Brand Innovation and Design
Research Oriented	Research & Clinical Trials	Observational & FDA Pathways
Policy Oriented	Policy & Advocacy	Legislative, Changemaking

HOLISTIC CARE, PATIENT CHOICE, AND THE FUTURE OF HEALING

Holistic care, patient choice, and the future of healing converge in the realm of cannabis nursing. This field bridges clinical science and holistic care, recognizing that cannabinoid therapeutics are increasingly studied within biomedical frameworks. However, patient use often reflects a broader quest for healing that transcends mere symptom management. Many individuals exploring cannabis as part of their care have encountered limitations within conventional healthcare systems and seek approaches that address the intricate tapestry of their health and lived experience.

The endocannabinoid system (ECS) emerges as a unifying biological framework that aligns with this integrative model of care. By simultaneously influencing multiple physiological systems, the ECS plays a pivotal role in regulating processes deeply interconnected, including pain, mood, sleep, immune function, and stress response (Di Marzo, 2018; Russo, 2018). This systems-based perspective underscores the notion that health cannot be fully addressed through isolated interventions alone.

Holistic nursing embraces a multidimensional view of health, encompassing biological, mental, emotional, spiritual, and social factors. Cannabis nursing aims to enhance function, resilience, meaning, and quality of life, often impacting several aspects concurrently, such as improving sleep while alleviating pain and anxiety (Clark, 2021; Mack, 2026). Effective care eschews the notion of cannabis as a singular solution or blindly following trends. Instead, it tailors doses, considers individual differences, and takes specific circumstances into account (Russo, 2011).

This approach holds immense value for individuals grappling with chronic illness or persistent pain. For them, cannabis is not a mere last resort but a means to restore a harmonious balance between mind, body, and spirit. Cannabis nurses play a crucial role in helping patients set goals across various domains, ensuring that improvements in one area do not inadvertently harm others.

Nurses may resonate with this holistic model, especially given the persistent high levels of stress and burnout, and have been leaving the workforce in droves. Over 138,000 U.S. nurses have left since 2022, primarily due to stress, burnout, workload, understaffing, and salary issues (NCSBN, 2025). In contrast, nurses working within various aspects of cannabis care often feel professionally rejuvenated by reconnecting with core values such as listening, advocacy, and relationship-centered care, which fuels their interest in pursuing cannabis nursing (Mack, 2025).

Importantly, this approach doesn't replace conventional medicine. Instead, it complements existing treatments by broadening the range of therapeutic options available to patients. Cannabis can serve as an adjunctive tool within broader care plans, providing symptom relief while also addressing aspects of health that are often overlooked in traditional models of care.

Patient choice is paramount in this framework. As access to cannabis expands, individuals are increasingly making independent decisions about its use, often without clinical guidance. Cannabis Nurses play a crucial role in ensuring that these decisions are informed, safe, and aligned with each patient's health goals. This involves providing clear, evidence-based education while acknowledging both the potential benefits and limitations of current research (Bell et al., 2023; Chou et al., 2025).

At the same time, this work necessitates a shift in how healthcare systems perceive healing. Moving from fragmented, condition-specific models to more integrative approaches require flexibility, collaboration, and openness to emerging evidence. It also demands clinicians who are willing to engage with patients as active participants in their care, rather than passive recipients of conventional treatment.

Cannabis nursing embodies this evolution. By combining clinical expertise with a whole-person perspective, nurses are contributing to the development of a model of care that is both scientifically grounded and deeply human. As research progresses and healthcare systems adapt, this approach has the potential to enhance not only clinical outcomes but also the overall experience of care.

CONCLUSION

Cannabis nursing represents a natural evolution of professional nursing practice in response to changing patient needs, emerging science, and shifting healthcare systems. As cannabis use becomes increasingly integrated into both medical and consumer health landscapes, the role of the nurse in ensuring safe, ethical, and evidence-informed care is more important than ever.

This chapter has outlined the foundational elements of cannabis nursing, including role definition, clinical workflows, safety considerations, and system-level applications. It has also highlighted the expanding opportunities for nurses to contribute across clinical care, education, research, policy, and healthcare innovation.

While challenges remain, including variability in evidence, regulatory complexity, and gaps in professional education, the trajectory of this field is clear. Patients are already using cannabis therapeutically, and healthcare systems are beginning to respond. Nurses are uniquely positioned to lead this integration in a way that prioritizes safety, equity, and patient-centered care. This collaboration and paradigm change may contribute to cost containment and improved outcomes for medical patients.

Looking ahead, Cannabis Nurses are poised to play an essential role in shaping the delivery, evaluation, and reimbursement of cannabinoid therapies. Whether practicing independently, within healthcare systems, serving as consultants for employers and payers, or pursuing entrepreneurial and future business roles, nurses possess unique qualifications to lead this evolving discipline with professionalism and integrity. Their contributions facilitate the reintroduction of cannabis into medical practice, emphasizing compassion, safety, and a commitment to comprehensive care.

By grounding their practice in scientific evidence and holistic principles, cannabis nursing sets a standard for the future of healthcare—one that is integrative, adaptable, and attuned to the diverse needs of human health.

REFERENCES

American Cannabis Nurses Association & American Nurses Association. (2024). Cannabis nursing: Scope and standards of practice (2nd ed.). American Nurses Association. https://www.nursingworld.org/nurses-books/cannabis-nursing-scope-and-standards-of-practice/

American Nurses Association. (2016). Therapeutic use of marijuana and related cannabinoids [Position statement]. American Nurses Association. https://www.nursingworld.org/~49a8c8/globalassets/practiceandpolicy/ethics/therapeutic-use-of-marijuana-and-related-cannabinoids-position-statement.pdf

American Nurses Association. (2023). ANA officially recognizes cannabis nursing as a specialty nursing practice [News release]. American Nurses Association. https://www.nursingworld.org/news/news-releases/2023/ana-officially-recognizes-cannabis-nursing-as-a-specialty-nursing-practice/

Bell, A. D., MacCallum, C., Margolese, S., Walsh, Z., Wright, P., Daeninck, P. J., Mandarino, E., Lacasse, G., Deol, J. K., De Freitas, L., St Pierre, M., Belle-Isle, L., Gagnon, M., Bevan, S., Sanchez, T., Arlt, S., Monahan-Ellison, M., O'Hara, J., Boivin, M., & Balneaves, L. (2023). Clinical practice guidelines for cannabis and cannabinoid-based medicines in the management of chronic pain and co-occurring conditions. *Cannabis and Cannabinoid Research*, *8*(1). Advance online publication. DOI: 10.1089/can.2021.0156 PMID: 36971587

Bruni, N., Della Pepa, C., Oliaro-Bosso, S., Pessione, E., Gastaldi, D., & Dosio, F. (2018). Cannabinoid delivery systems for pain and inflammation treatment. *Molecules (Basel, Switzerland)*, *23*(10), 2478. DOI: 10.3390/molecules23102478 PMID: 30262735

Cannabis and Health Research Initiative. (2025). The National Cannabis Study.

CannaKeys. (2024). Cannabis and cancer: Research summary. https://cannakeys.com/the-cbd-for-cancer/#top-dboard

Castle, R. D., Marzolf, J., Morris, M., & Bushell, W. C. (2025). Meta-analysis of medical cannabis outcomes and associations with cancer. *Frontiers in Oncology*, *15*, 1490621. Advance online publication. DOI: 10.3389/fonc.2025.1490621 PMID: 40303989

Center for Disease Control and Prevention. (2025). Cannabis and Public Health. CDC. https://www.cdc.gov/cannabis/data-research/facts-stats/index.html

Chou, R., Ahmed, A., Dana, T., Morasco, B., Bougatsos, C., Fu, R., & Williams, L. (2025). Living Systematic Review on Cannabis and Other Plant-Based Treatments for Chronic Pain. DOI: 10.23970/AHRQEPCCER250UPDATE2025

Chye, Y., Christensen, E., Solowij, N., & Yücel, M. (2019). The endocannabinoid system and cannabidiol's promise for the treatment of substance use disorder. *Frontiers in Psychiatry*, *10*, 63. DOI: 10.3389/fpsyt.2019.00063 PMID: 30837904

Clark, C. S. (2021). *Cannabis: A handbook for nurses*. Wolters Kluwer.

Commonwealth Project. (2025). Policy briefs on cannabinoid integration in value-based care. https://commonwealthproject.org

Di Marzo, V. (2018). New approaches and challenges to targeting the endocannabinoid system. *Nature Reviews. Drug Discovery*, *17*(9), 623–639. DOI: 10.1038/nrd.2018.115 PMID: 30116049

DiGirolamo, E. (2026). Approaching conversations about cannabis use with patients. *Oncology Times*, *48*(5), 17–18. https://journals.lww.com/oncology-times/fulltext/2026/03000/approaching_conversations_about_cannabis_use_with.11.aspx. DOI: 10.1097/01.COT.0000000000000330

EPIDIOLEX® (cannabidiol). (n.d.). EPIDIOLEX.com. https://www.epidiolex.com/

Graham, M., Martin, J. H., Lucas, C. J., Murnion, B., & Schneider, J. (2022). Cannabidiol drug interaction considerations for prescribers and pharmacists. *Expert Review of Clinical Pharmacology*, *15*(12), 1383–1397. DOI: 10.1080/17512433.2022.2142114 PMID: 36317739

Kvamme, S. L., Pedersen, M. M., Thomsen, K. R., & Thylstrup, B. (2021). Exploring the use of cannabis as a substitute for prescription drugs in a convenience sample. *Harm Reduction Journal*, *18*(1), 72. Advance online publication. DOI: 10.1186/s12954-021-00520-5 PMID: 34246279

Lange, T. (2025). American Council of Cannabis Medicine unveils major industry initiative to expand medical cannabis access. Cannabis Business Times. https://www.cannabisbusinesstimes.com/business-issues-benchmarks/medical-cannabis-access-and-pricing/news/15769892/american-council-of-cannabis-medicine-unveils-major-industry-initiative-to-expand-medical-cannabis-access

Mack, E. A. (2020). Cannabis for health: Become a coach. AuthorHouse. https://www.authorhouse.com/en/bookstore/bookdetails/812353-cannabis-for-health-become-a-coach

Mack, S. (2025). Cannabis nursing: the heart of holistic care. Holistic Caring. https://holisticcaring.com/cannabis-nursing-the-heart-of-holistic-care/

Mack, S. (2026). Coherence in cannabis care. Ask The Green Nurse. https://thegreennurse.substack.com/p/coherence-in-cannabis-care

Martin-Willett, R., Stanger, M., James, W., Bryan, A. D., & Bidwell, L. C. (2023). Effects of historical inequity and institutional power on cannabis research: Moving toward equity and inclusion. *PNAS Nexus*, *2*(12), pgad383. Advance online publication. DOI: 10.1093/pnasnexus/pgad383 PMID: 38089600

Mee, M., Maldonado, J., Jimenez, J., Villegas, M., & Clobes, T. (2026). Dispensary budtender guidance versus clinician consensus: A comparative study of medical cannabis advice. Clinical Therapeutics. https://www.sciencedirect.com/science/article/pii/S0149291826000470

National Academies of Sciences, Engineering, and Medicine. (2017). The health effects of cannabis and cannabinoids: The current state of evidence and recommendations for research. National Academies Press. DOI: 10.17226/24625

National Academies Press (US). (2017). Mental health. The Health Effects of Cannabis and Cannabinoids - NCBI Bookshelf. https://www.ncbi.nlm.nih.gov/books/NBK425748/

National Cancer Institute. (2025). Cannabis and cannabinoids (PDQ®)–Health professional version. https://www.cancer.gov/about-cancer/treatment/cam/hp/cannabis-pdq

National Council of State Boards of Nursing. (2018). The NCSBN national nursing guidelines for medical marijuana. *Journal of Nursing Regulation*, *9*(2), 19–26. DOI: 10.1016/S2155-8256(18)30094-2

Respiratory Therapy. (2025). Chronic pain patients stop medical cannabis within 1 year | RT. https://respiratory-therapy.com/public-health/healthcare-policy/general-healthcare/chronic-pain-medical-cannabis/

Russo, E. B. (2011). Taming THC: Potential cannabis synergy and phytocannabinoid-terpenoid entourage effects. *British Journal of Pharmacology*, *163*(7), 1344–1364. DOI: 10.1111/j.1476-5381.2011.01238.x PMID: 21749363

Russo, E. B. (2018). Cannabis therapeutics and the future of neurology. *Frontiers in Integrative Neuroscience*, *12*, 51. DOI: 10.3389/fnint.2018.00051 PMID: 30405366

Russo, E. B., & MacCallum, C. A. (2016). Practical considerations in medical cannabis administration and dosing. *European Journal of Internal Medicine*, *31*, 12–19. https://pubmed.ncbi.nlm.nih.gov/29307505/ PMID: 29307505

Stanford Medicine. (2025). Cannabis and older adults: Five things medical experts want you to know. News Center. https://med.stanford.edu/news/insights/2025/10/cannabis-marijuana-seniors-cautions.html

Sulak, D. (2021). Handbook of cannabis for clinicians: Principles and practice. https://wwnorton.com/books/9780393714180

Supra, J. D. (2025). Taking the LEAD: CMS unveils the new LEAD model, focused on Long-Term Primary Care success. https://www.jdsupra.com/legalnews/taking-the-lead-cms-unveils-the-new-6671061

The White House. (2025). INCREASING MEDICAL MARIJUANA AND CANNABIDIOL RESEARCH. https://www.whitehouse.gov/presidential-actions/2025/12/increasing-medical-marijuana-and-cannabidiol-research/

Troyer, J., & Tanco, K. (2024). Review of the use of medicinal cannabis products in palliative care. *Cancers (Basel)*, *16*(7), 1412. DOI: 10.3390/cancers16071412 PMID: 38611090

Zolotov, Y. (2025). Developing Medical Cannabis Competencies a consensus statement. JAMA Network. https://jamanetwork.com/journals/jamanetworkopen/fullarticle/2839750

KEY TERMS AND DEFINITIONS

Cannabis Nursing: A recognized nursing specialty that applies evidence-informed cannabinoid science, clinical assessment, patient education, and ethical practice to support the safe and appropriate therapeutic use of cannabis across healthcare and community settings.

Endocannabinoid System (ECS): A biological regulatory system involved in maintaining homeostasis across multiple physiological processes, including pain modulation, immune function, mood, sleep, appetite, and stress response.

Harm Reduction: A patient-centered clinical approach that prioritizes safety, education, and risk mitigation when individuals are using or considering cannabis, rather than insisting on abstinence or punitive responses.

Healthcare Innovation: The development and implementation of new care models, services, or workflows that improve patient outcomes, access, quality, or cost-effectiveness within evolving healthcare systems.

Holistic Care: A framework of care that addresses the interconnected biological, mental, emotional, spiritual, and social dimensions of health, recognizing the whole person rather than isolated symptoms or diagnoses.

Nurse Entrepreneurship: The application of nursing expertise to independent or nontraditional practice models, including private consultative services, education, product development, or leadership roles within emerging healthcare sectors.

Nursing Leadership: The ability of nurses to influence clinical practice, organizational culture, policy development, and system-level change through ethical decision-making, collaboration, and advocacy.

Routes of Administration: The methods by which cannabis is introduced into the body—such as oral, sublingual, inhaled, or topical—which influence onset, duration, intensity, and safety considerations.

Scope of Practice: The legally defined boundaries within which nurses may practice, guided by state nurse practice acts, institutional policies, and professional standards that govern cannabis-related nursing care.

Value-Based Care: A healthcare delivery model that emphasizes patient outcomes, safety, quality, and cost-effectiveness, aligning clinical decision-making with long-term health and economic value rather than volume of services.

Chapter 8
Forensic Nursing Perspectives in Cannabis-Related Clinical and Legal Contexts

Baljeet Yadav
http://orcid.org/0000-0003-0624-6784
K.R. Mangalam University, Gurugram, India

Mahima Choudhary
K.R. Mangalam University, Gurugram, India

Rakhi Sahrawat
http://orcid.org/0009-0002-8741-489X
K.R. Mangalam University, Gurugram, India

Mahipal Singh Sankhla
K.R. Mangalam University, Gurugram, India

Sameer Saharan
http://orcid.org/0000-0002-7487-6297
Mody University of Science and Technology, India

ABSTRACT

Cannabis use presents complex clinical, legal, and ethical challenges within forensic nursing practice. Containing psychoactive constituents such as THC and CBD, cannabis is regulated under varying legal frameworks, including the Controlled Substances Act in the United States and the Cannabis Act in Canada, while cannabis use disorder is recognized in the DSM-5. Forensic nurses manage acute intoxication, withdrawal, and Cannabinoid Hyperemesis Syndrome, particularly among vulnerable populations such as pregnant individuals, adolescents, older adults, and persons with serious mental illness. Toxicological detection through urine and oral fluid testing, along with strict chain-of-custody procedures, supports evidence integrity in legal contexts. However, biological markers do not reliably establish real-time impairment, creating interpretive challenges.It may be concluded that cannabis-focused forensic nursing demands the integration of clinical competence, ethical accountability, and legal awareness to ensure patient-centered care, maintain evidentiary & equitable policy development.

DOI: 10.4018/979-8-3373-7287-7.ch008

1. INTRODUCTION AND SCOPE

Cannabis is defined as the dried flower tops, leaves, stems, and seeds of Cannabis sativa L., Cannabis indica L., and Cannabis ruderalis Janisch. They contain phytocannabinoids such as Δ9-tetrahydrocannabinol (THC) and cannabidiol (CBD) (A. Klein & S. Clark, 2022) which are regulated as Schedule I controlled substances in Canada and USA. Cannabis, cannabis use disorder, and cannabis dependence are listed in the Diagnostic and Statistical Manual of Mental Disorders, Fifth Edition. It is administered by inhalation and ingestion (Carla Monti, 2022). The term 'forensic' is defined as 'relating to, used in, or suitable to courts of law or to public discussion and debate'. Forensic nursing integrates nursing science with criminology and forensic sciences to investigate trauma victims. Forensic nurses provide specialized care and collect legal evidence from patients who may be intoxicated, to enable legal proceedings and policy formulation. Cannabis use may adversely affect certain populations such as children and older adults. It can complicate other health conditions and substances, including tobacco, alcohol, stimulants, opioids, benzodiazepines, and sedative hypnotics.

In forensic nursing practice, cannabis-related findings may arise during trauma examinations, impaired driving investigations, workplace incidents, sexual assault assessments, and other medicolegal situations requiring objective clinical documentation and evidence-informed evaluation.

Cannabis focused forensic nursing which corresponds to three categories of the World Health Organization Framework for Action on Interprofessional Education and Collaborative Practice. In collaborative practice, forensic nurses address health, safety, and well-being needs, assist victims and facilitate early intervention and preventive measures for the legal, policy, and political domains. Forensic nurses also consider the decriminalisation of cannabis possession and use from the aspects of public health, safety, and health care to ensure effective enforcement of legislation. Cannabis focused on forensic nursing research faces methodological challenges arising from legislative discrepancies and limited availability of psychoactive substances for clinical studies. Forensic nurses must apply trauma-informed, rights-based, and non-stigmatizing approaches while assessing cannabis-related presentations, recognizing that cannabis use does not necessarily indicate impairment, criminality, or causation of injury.

The existing policy oriented practices include educational and training initiatives on the therapeutic use of cannabis, digital information sharing technologies, and palliative complementary therapies to enable timely data collection on the impact of cannabis management on patients.

1.1 Historical Background

Cannabis has complicated and lengthy history that links to geography, society, and medicine to each other. It used for pain treatment, digestive issues, and ritual practices is documented in early documents from China, India, and the Middle East. Indian traditions emphasize its importance in Ayurveda and Hindu festivities like Shivratri and Holi. (Karki, P., & Rangaswamy, M. 2023) The extracts of cannabis were first prescribed for neuralgia, migraines, and insomnia in Western pharmacopeias in the 19th century. But due to variation in plant strength, it challenged with dose standardization, and the emergence of synthetic medications and the use of cannabis in medicine decreased in the early 20th century (Kalant, H. 2001).

Charitos et al. (2021) also illustrated about how cannabis is spread throughout the world via trade and colonization which emphasizing out how marijuana adapted to various therapeutic and cultural situations on different continents. While Warf (2014) placed cannabis within a geographical framework, documenting its spread and the sociopolitical dynamics influencing its regulation. Wills

(1998) offered a more comprehensive historical perspective which highlighted its medical uses and patterns of abuse. When taken as a whole, these studies show that although cannabis's analgesic, anti-inflammatory, and psychedelic qualities have always been valued, its acceptance has varied due to shifting scientific data, societal norms, and legal constraints. Based on examinations of archaeological human remains, the study by Giordano et al. (2023) offered impressive forensic toxicological evidence of cannabis use in Milan, Italy during the 1600s. This study demonstrates how cannabis was both prevalent and actively used in early modern Europe, providing concrete evidence of its incorporation into daily life as well as potential medical or recreational uses. The results highlight the importance of archaeotoxicology in reconstructing past drug usage trends and connecting forensic science and cultural history. Despite its long history, there are still large gaps in systematic research, especially in places like India where cultural acceptability contrasts with few scientific studies and stringent restriction.

1.2. Definitions And Conceptual Framework

The expanded use of cannabis for recreational and medical purposes triggers the need for a careful consideration of the implications for patients, families, and communities. Forensic nursing perspectives engage in clinical contexts, including acute care and substance use withdrawal supportive services. Forensic nursing includes the psychological, physical, and social areas of a person under examination. Forensic psychology refers to the clinical service with legal and administrative connection. Forensic psychiatry and clinical forensic medicine examines the clinical aspects of crimes.

Clinical distinctions between forensic and general nursing care include evidence integrity, documentation processes, and policy implications. Evidence chain-of-custody verification derives from the forensics, law and legal psychology perspectives. Recent legal and policy decisions refresh forensic work and bring direct identity disturbance; the need for identification triggers psychological disorder during the neural substance use process. Policy changes allow cannabis smoking tenants and enhance community strain.

Contemporary forensic nursing frameworks emphasize trauma-informed, patient-centered, and rights-based approaches when addressing cannabis-related clinical and medicolegal situations. Cannabis use should be interpreted objectively within the context of patient presentation, toxicology findings, and legal circumstances.

1.3. Relevance To Forensic Nursing Practice

The relevance of cannabis to forensic nursing encompasses considerations pertaining to personal well-being, legal contexts, ethical obligations, and professional policy. Cannabis has demonstrated efficacy in alleviating certain medical conditions, yet healthcare providers may confront complex scenarios following cannabis use. Changes in legislation, evolving public attitudes, and market availability have further increased patient inquiries and the likelihood of legal involvement following cannabis-related incidents. The legislation also influences the nurse's duty to maintain documentation associated with cannabis use. Forensic nursing thus weaves together the various forces of cannabis-related personal, legal, and policy contexts.

A range of clinical, legal, and policy considerations surrounding forensic cannabis shape the orientations of practice and research. Understanding cannabis pharmacology is essential for interpreting toxicology findings, which in turn informs the differential diagnosis the conditions such as Cannabinoid Hyperemesis Syndrome and the management of vulnerable populations also exposed to opioids.

Documentation, policy, and ethical issues connect cannabis use to rights-based and practice-oriented procedures. Forensic nursing intertwines clinical and legal arenas guidance for interdisciplinary evidence collection and documentation therefore remains relevant alongside patient centred clinical, procedural, and rights-based approaches, directly linking to advocacy and collaborative efforts concerning cannabis use.

The intersection of cannabis and forensic nursing is multifaceted yet resource intensive to investigate. Emerging legislation and public attitudes are modernizing cannabis-related policy and practice.

Forensic nurses may encounter cannabis-related findings in sexual assault examinations, workplace incidents, impaired driving investigations, trauma care, and child protection settings. Accurate assessment and unbiased documentation are essential to preserve evidentiary integrity and patient rights.

2. CANNABIS PHARMACOLOGY, TOXICOLOGY, AND DETECTION

Cannabis is a plant of genus Cannabis, an herbaceous plant cultivated for drug, industrial and food purposes. At harvest, the plant contains over 500 discrete compounds of which over 100 are cannabinoids, psychoactive compounds that alter human cognitions. Dronabinol, which is chemically identical to the principal psychoactive constituent of Cannabis, is a Food and Drug Administration (FDA)-approved cannabis-based product in the United States for two indications. Cannabinoids are also the basis of a schedule-I classification of cannabis. Initial exposure to high dosages of cannabis is likely to produce signs and symptoms that correspond with overdose, but these effects do not occur consistently across individuals and with repeated low-dosage administrations. Storage of cannabis products should consider the possible concentration of contaminants. Oral fluid has been identified as the most preferred biological specimen to detect cannabinoids shortly after consumption since it enables on-site analysis and visual interaction for compliance (Trif et al., 2024). The amount of time needed to collect, test and produce results from an oral-fluid device is essential for on-site instant detection in line with proposed legislation. In conclusion, compounds found within cannabis continued to be under study for detection in body fluids other than urine. Cannabis and its constituent compounds likely remain topics of interest from pharmacological, toxicological and legislative perspectives.

Also the stability of natural and synthetic cannabinoids in biological matrices is significantly impacted by storage conditions. Djilali et al. (2022) noted that temperature, light exposure, and duration can change metabolite detectability, which in turn affects the accuracy of forensic toxicology analyses. Ashton (2001) gave a succinct summary of the effects of cannabis from a pharmacological point of view, highlighting the role of Δ9-tetrahydrocannabinol (THC) in producing psychoactive outcomes like euphoria, anxiety, and impaired cognition as well as the therapeutic potential in managing pain and nausea. Extending this, Adams and Martin (1996) provided a comparative study of cannabis pharmacology and toxicology in humans and animals, describing its dose-dependent effects on behavior, the cardiovascular system, and the central nervous system while emphasizing the dangers of dependence and cognitive impairment with long-term use. Amin and Ali (2019) looked at the pharmacology of medical cannabis, concentrating on cannabinoids like THC and cannabidiol (CBD), how they interact with the endocannabinoid system, and how they can be used therapeutically to treat conditions like multiple sclerosis, epilepsy, and chronic pain. However, they cautioned about the variability in efficacy and safety.

2.1. Pharmacokinetics And Pharmacodynamics

The pharmacokinetics and pharmacodynamics of cannabinoids encompass their absorption, distribution, metabolism, and elimination, influencing biological activity. Assessing these processes helps evaluate therapeutic effects and potential toxicity. In humans, the main cannabinoid delta-9-tetrahydrocannabinol (Δ9-THC) produces psychoactive effects through central cannabinoid receptor 1 (CB1) binding. Δ9-THC is commonly detected along with its metabolite 11-nor-delta-9-tetrahydrocannabinol-9-carboxylic acid (THCA-COOH) in cannabis-related evaluations; however, THCA-COOH is a prodrug that cannot penetrate the blood-brain barrier. Standard detection and pattern analysis are therefore considered inadequate to establish cannabis impairment. On the other hand, recent studies address the physiology of cannabidiol (CBD) and Δ9-THC metabolism and some of the implications for differentiation and analysis of tetrahydrocannabinol and cannabidiol consumption. Δ9-THC and CBD are metabolized through human cytochrome P450 (CYP) enzymes, which constitute an important pathway for drug metabolic clearance as well as crucial determinants of drug-drug interactions (Nasrin et al., 2021).

Understanding the pharmacokinetics of THC and CBD assists forensic nurses in interpreting clinical presentations and toxicological findings within medicolegal contexts. The effects of cannabis may vary depending on route of administration, frequency of use, and individual physiology.

Figure 1. Key stages in cannabinoid pharmacokinetics and pharmacodynamics

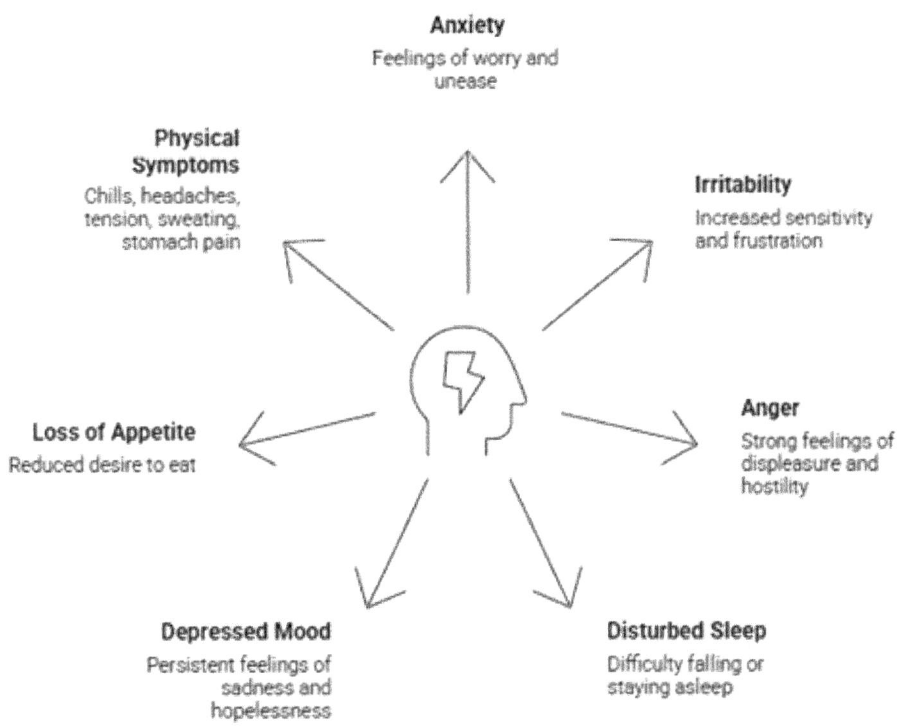

2.2. Toxicology Methods And Interpretation

Cannabis administration is a complex process that varies depending on the route and formulation. Neither acute pharmacokinetic nor pharmacodynamic data are easily applicable to long-term smokers. Cross-reference the section 'Definition' for generic drugs, and with the section 'Cannabis Use in Special Populations' for testimony limitatons with grandparents echoing impaired memory ("I had the goods on 'em and still do not recall what I have taken'"). Several cohorts (adolescents, psychotic patients, pregnant females, and grandparents) furnish apologies characteristic of cannabis intoxication.

Toxicological detection of cannabis does not always indicate active impairment or causation of an event. Forensic nurses should recognize the limitations of biological testing while correlating laboratory findings with clinical observations and case history.

Table 1. Representation of cannabis administration and effect

Characteristic	THC	11-OH-THC	THC-COOH
Psychoactive	Yes	Yes	No
Half-life	30 hours	105 hours	Weeks
Forensic marker	Limited	Limited	Useful
Detection time	Short	Short	Long

2.3. Limitations Of Current Testing And Window Of Detection

Cannabinoids, especially Δ9-tetrahydrocannabinol (THC), are primarily detected in urine and oral fluid specimens. Urinary detection is based on the presence of inactive THCCOOH, an inactive metabolite excreted in urine, while THC and 11-hydroxy-THC can be detected from oral fluid. Confirmation of a positive result is provided by measuring THCCOOH concentrations in biological fluids (Sharma et al., 2023). Testing methods depend on the specimen type. Urine drugs of abuse screening tests are used for initial laboratory screening, either instrumental or immunochemical methods, and only positive results are confirmed. Current cannabis testing methods may not accurately distinguish recent impairment from prior exposure, particularly among chronic users. These limitations highlight the importance of comprehensive forensic assessment and contextual interpretation.

Cannabinoids are lipophilic molecules stored in adipose tissues for a prolonged period also the THC window of detection in oral fluid is limited (R. Arkell et al., 2019). The combination of elevated body temperature, increased drive for fluids, and physiological anxiety caused by cannabinoid-induced psychoactive effects, along with the daily or multiple-times-a-day intake of cannabinoid-containing substances, can lead to Cannabinoid Hyperemesis Syndrome (CHS), characterized by bouts of uncontrollable vomiting, crampy abdominal pain, and compulsive hot showers. Few studies report an estimate on window of detection of cannabinoids in oral fluid, associated with cannabinoid rapid dissipation in these specimens. Appropriate oral-fluid sampling/witnessing devices and collection strategies must be strictly followed in order to obtain accurate indication of fresh intoxication following cannabis consumption.

Table 2. Representation of cannabinoid detection methods

Characteristic	Urine	Oral Fluid	Hair
Primary Analyte	THCCOOH	THC, 11-hydroxy-THC	Phytocannabinoids
Detection Basis	Presence of THCCOOH	Presence of THC	Presence of cannabinoids
Window of Detection	Longer	Shorter	Longer
Specificity	High	Moderate	Low
Advantages	Standard method	Rapid tests available	Long-term detection
Disadvantages	Invasive	Short detection window	Environmental contamination

3. CLINICAL MANIFESTATIONS AND CARE IMPLICATIONS

Acute intoxication may arise with any route after initiation or dose increases, and risk escalates when cannabis is consumed in combination with other sedating substances (Roberts, 2019). The effects typically commence within seconds to minutes for inhalation, by 30 minutes for edible or drinkable forms, and within 90 minutes for capsules, and persist from 1 hour to 4–12 hours, respectively. Cannabis withdrawal syndrome applies to regular users without recent exposure and can exceed 1 month. Symptoms, which begin within 1–3 days and persist up to 2 weeks after abstinence, include insomnia, irritability, anxiety, restlessness, depressed mood, decreased appetite, weight loss, nausea, vomiting, abdominal pain, and sweating.

Cannabinoid Hyperemesis Syndrome (CHS) is characterized by severe cyclic nausea and vomiting, along with abdominal pain and compulsive hot shower use. A diagnosis of CHS requires long-term cannabis use, 5 days or longer of increased dosage or frequency before symptom onset, and symptom resolution upon abstinence. An alternative explanation for nausea and vomiting should be excluded (Hasin,

2023). Use frequency among Colorado patients with CHS reaches 40% daily and 78% weekly or more; almost half started using cannabis by age 18. Chronic cannabis consumption is correspondingly prevalent among teenage presenters. Special populations, such as individuals with mental health concerns or co-occurring substance use, or patients undergoing polypharmacy, should also be considered. Substances compatible with cannabis use warrant assessment to enhance consideration of the therapeutic ratio, risk benefit balance, treatment response prediction, and legal classification when cannabis has been detected.

3.1. Acute Cannabis Intoxication And Withdrawal

Acute cannabis intoxication arises from the Cannabis sativa plant and its tetrahydrocannabinol (THC) compound. Cannabis withdrawal occurs after abrupt cessation or reduction in THC-containing cannabis products, especially in regular and heavy users (P. Connor et al., 2022). Symptoms typically begin within 24–48 hours and peak at days 2–6, lasting up to 2–3 weeks in heavy users. The prevalence varies, with about 47% of regular users experiencing withdrawal symptoms, higher in inpatient and outpatient settings. The severity and duration depend on prior cannabis consumption and co-occurring substance use. Cannabis withdrawal can potentially cause relapse, impacting personal relationships and work. Synthetic cannabinoids are more potent and may lead to more severe withdrawal than natural cannabis. Acute cannabis intoxication may present with altered cognition, anxiety, impaired coordination, or behavioral changes that require careful forensic assessment. Objective documentation of observed findings is important in medicolegal investigations.

Cannabis intoxication impairs reaction times and errors of omission, which are risk factors for impaired driving. Additional acute effects include sedation, euphoria, disconnection, cognitive impairment, and dizziness. Involved populations should be monitored following documented intoxication, for example, during police custody. Evidence indicates increased drivers under the influence of cannabis on the roads since legalization, although no estimates of the impact on traffic accidents are available. Suspected cannabis intoxication raises visual observation during traffic stops; the widely cited, optical A-B test outlines a methodology to apply the horizontal gaze nystagmus (HGN) examination to trace cannabis influence. Cannabis edibles pose a higher danger due to delayed psychoactive effects, introducing the concept of micro-dosing and possession limits in legalization discussions. Libation, a common method combining THC with alcohol, produces amnestic and sedative properties alongside potential interference with the HGN examination.

Figure 2. Cannabis withdrawal symptoms on human body

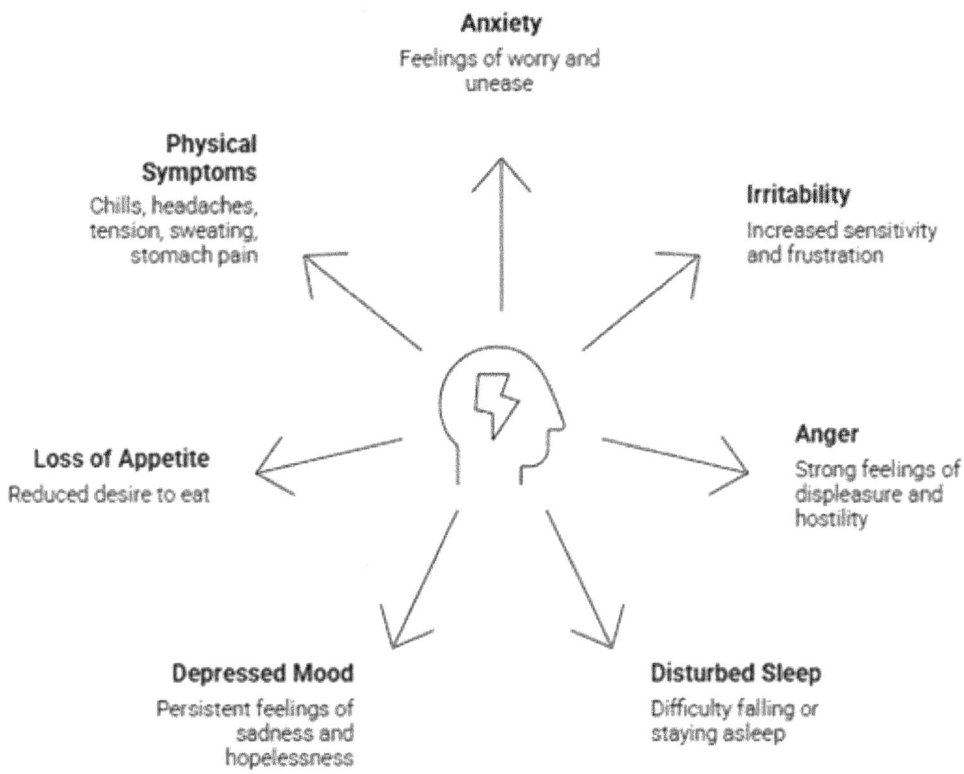

3.2. Cannabinoid Hyperemesis Syndrome

Cannabis is commonly placed in the category of non-addictive drugs, yet users with high frequency and high dosage can develop psychological dependence, physical dependence, and smoking dependence. The chronic use of cannabis can result in cannabis withdrawal syndrome, providing the need for supportive treatment on a clinical and forensic level. Cannabinoid Hyperemesis Syndrome (CHS), a derangement of the normal control of nausea and vomiting, can arise. Patients who develop serious neurological side effects complicate acute cannabis intoxication assessments; forensic cannabis-related examinations are therefore not limited to the physical, somatic, and psychological side effects of cannabis. The use of cannabis and marijuana among adolescents ranges from 10% to 40%, and the escalation these drugs without comprehensible information regarding the health risks contributes to various health and legal problems (Perisetti et al., 2020).

Cannabinoid Hyperemesis Syndrome (CHS) is characterized by cyclical vomiting associated with chronic cannabis use. Science has yet to determine a specific physiological mechanism that explains CHS; however, it is a legally and clinically significant phenomenon. Patients with CHS frequently seek medical advice for prolonged or recurrent vomiting. Administered anti-emetic treatments (e.g. Odansetron) do not alleviate the symptom but patients report some relief of the extreme reflex when they receive medical attention. Abdominal pain is present in some cases. Compulsive bathing even at boiling hot temperatures represents an unusual feature strongly associated with cannabis (Marie Figueroa-Rivera et al., 2015).

Although cannabis hyperemesis syndrome is clinically significant, forensic nurses should evaluate such presentations within broader patient histories and medicolegal circumstances. Excessive focus on isolated adverse effects may not fully reflect contemporary cannabis-related forensic practice.

Cyclic vomiting syndrome, established as an official clinical diagnosis, is defined as recurrent o episodes of nausea and vomiting. Various types of vomiting may have the same underlying cause. Typical cannabis intoxication produces a contrary kind of nausea that is not compatible with CHS diagnostics (Schmid et al., 2018).

3.3. Impact On Comorbid Conditions And Vulnerable Populations

Cannabis has been reported to exacerbate existing mental health conditions such as depression and anxiety and may contribute to the development of new mental health disorders (E. Crocker et al., 2021), including psychosis. Cannabis use is associated with high rates of poly-substance use (Skalisky et al., 2017), negatively impacting patient well-being. The Canadian Association of Emergency Physicians cautions that legalization could cause increased recreational use, especially among vulnerable groups.

Cannabis is the world's most widely used illicit drug. In Canada, cannabis became legal and regulated when Bill C-45 received royal assent on June 21, 2018. Cannabis use prevalence remains elevated among patients presenting with serious mental illness (SMI) and alcohol use disorders, with over 60% of outpatients consuming the substance. The co-occurrence of cannabis and alcohol is concerning because the pathways to intoxication are similar, and alcohol is associated with increased risks of HIV, homelessness, incarceration, and self-harm. Reports show that cannabis can prompt persistent and new-onset psychotic symptoms in this population. The link among cannabis use, worsening of the mental disorder, and increased inpatient care utilization requires further investigation; high consumption in this population may go undisclosed during clinical assessments.

Cannabis use may influence mental health disorders, substance interactions, and chronic medical conditions that can complicate forensic evaluations. Individualized and non-stigmatizing assessment approaches are therefore essential.

4. FORENSIC NURSING ROLES AND RESPONSIBILITIES

Nurses are responsible for collecting and preserving evidence related to potentially criminal activity. Protocol must adhere to standards of care as defined within the profession. Forensic nurses collaborate within interdisciplinary teams to prevent the loss of evidence and continue advocacy for individual rights.

Collection and documentation procedures depend on policy and vary across jurisdictions. Forensic Nursing Association published detailed protocols for guideline development. Evidence is defined as information possessing value for interpretation. Evidence may consist of physical objects, specimens such as blood or hair, statements including patient history and observations, and documentation including photographs. The concept of chain of custody applies to physical and trace evidence. Evidence collected at the time of service and preserved according to protocol preserves integrity through the investigative process. Documentation serves as the basis for complete and accurate record generation (T. Kurtzman et al., 2022). Reports without established supporting documentation raise questions of credibility. Guidance at jurisdictional or organizational level assists compliance with local policy.

Documentation may not adequately address cannabis in the clinical record and preservation of specific types of evidence. Individual-patient cannabis use may arise during patient history, prescribing clinician inquiry on polypharmacy, or associated substance co-morbidity. Forensic Examination report form or equivalent outlines and documents services provided. Cannabis in individual-patient history, clinical records, and documentation must therefore remain consistent with legislation. Falsification, omission, or equivocation regarding cannabis remains ethically acceptable in numerous jurisdictions (Huerne et al., 2022).

Advisors assisting with these challenges across clinical, legal, and ethical lines strengthen policy development input and enhance cannabis-related patient safety.

4.1. Evidence Collection And Chain Of Custody

The forensic nursing standards of practice encompass evidence collection and the chain of custody that accompanies it. The chain of custody, defined as "a record of a person who collected, handled, or transferred a specimen or its container at a specified time" (D'Anna et al., 2023), should follow any collection of evidence from a patient. Documentation containing this information should accompany any evidence transferred to outside agencies. Maintaining a proper chain of custody is critical to the admissibility and credibility of evidence examined in court. Laboratory analysis is an example where a proper chain of custody is required, such as toxicological analyses performed on urine or blood specimens. A record of the chain of custody should therefore be created, capturing information about the specimen and any individuals who handled it (Bartlow, 2009). Forensic nurses must maintain accurate evidence collection procedures and chain-of-custody standards when cannabis-related materials or toxicological samples are involved in legal investigations. Proper documentation supports both patient care and judicial processes.

A contemporary issue with cannabis evidence is the apparent disparity between the existence of cannabis, toxicology tests, and patient denial of use. This situation arises because both the presence of the drug and its metabolites can be determined, though the metabolite specific to such a question is Delta-9-carboxy-THC. Law enforcement officials need to be made aware of this situation during evidence handling to avoid allegations that a sample has been altered and to establish that a screening was conducted for cannabis. A process is required to document such situations in a professional and consistent manner, and an example is offered to meet this need.

4.2. Documentation Standards And Documentation Gaps

Cannabis use impairs cognitive, motor, and sensory functions, presenting public-health challenges. Forensic nurses play a central role in the cannabis-legalization context through a credible, patient centred approach to care that respects individual autonomy and promotes well-being. They contribute competently by documenting clinical manifestations of intoxication, abuse, and dependence while handling evidence and adhering to protocol. Professional standards exist to guide documentation however, gaps in cannabis-specific policy impede nursing practice in legislation where such materials are unavailable (G. Balneaves et al., 2024). Documentation should remain factual, objective, and free from assumptions regarding impairment or criminal behavior. Trauma-informed forensic charting is essential to preserve patient dignity and evidentiary reliability.

Cannabis legalization raises concerns about personal rights. Cannabis use alters perception, concentration, and decision-making, enhancing the risk of abuse. Changing legal and policy contexts warrant consideration of ethical issues concerning patient rights to access medically appropriate care, even when related to intoxication, dependency, or illicit substances. Forensic nurses have an ethical responsibility to acquire and retain pertinent information that enhances patient safety, enabling them to advocate for services directly addressing risk-related issues while remaining within the care-support framework.

4.3. Interdisciplinary Collaboration And Advocacy

Forensic teams must assess and document evidence of cannabis use and other substances in cases involving intoxicated or impaired minors. In legal contexts, forensic nurses frequently assist in collecting and preserving evidence in these situations. The forensic nursing perspective incorporates holistic evidence-centered advocacy, recognizing that individuals of varying ages and backgrounds may consume cannabis and other substances. Ethical considerations and protection of individuals' rights are paramount during evidence acquisition. Forensic nurses should formally advocate for strengthening chain-of-custody documentation, guidance on evidence storage and transfer, and adherence to clinicians' discretion regarding suspected substance categorization. Effective cannabis-related forensic care requires collaboration among forensic nurses, toxicologists, law enforcement personnel, mental health professionals, and legal teams. Interdisciplinary communication enhances patient safety and medicolegal accuracy.

5. LEGAL AND POLICY CONTEXTS

Evidence of cannabis related clinical, legal, and policy concerns motivates exploration of forensic nursing perspectives. Legislative contexts influence, or fail to specify, care obligations; patient safety principles and ethical frameworks provide guidance. As cannabis may contribute to injuries or fatalities, both care and reporting remain relevant. In some jurisdictions nurses may be legally mandated to report cannabis use when prescribed, raising patient rights concerns. Respecting autonomy, privacy, and confidentiality remains paramount; documentation may influence decisions to report or investigate by emphasizing medical cannabis as a therapeutic, not recreational, agent. Involuntary disclosure directly contravenes nurse patient advocacy obligations. Reportable conditions involving cannabis use occur frequently and apply to other prescribed medications. In the absence of legislated obligations, weighing the public interest served against duty to protect privacy is recommended.

Cannabis accessibility and use among older adults requires consideration of complex medical histories and prescription regimens. Adverse cardiovascular effects associated with baseline conditions and drug-drug interactions between polypharmacy treatments and cannabis on patients already using multiple substances may invoke the duty to report. Cannabis also possesses an established therapeutic role in addressing chronic pain and various mental health conditions, where cannabis contributes to the clinical picture yet remains beneficial the reporting equation favours non-disclosure. In cases of prenatal or paediatric cannabis use bordering on neglect or abuse, outreach mechanisms exist to facilitate advocacy without breaching confidentiality.

5.1. Cannabis Legislation By Jurisdiction

Cannabis legislation varies widely across jurisdictions and often includes guidelines for medical access. In Canada, provinces, territories, and municipalities have enacted supplementary laws and restrictions, with institutional regulations further shaping access to safe and effective use. (Kavousi et al., (2022) Research indicates that healthcare professionals require additional education and support to help meet the needs of patients seeking medical assistance, and guidelines for safe prescribing, where permitted have been prepared in several provinces. Prior to the 2023 legalization of recreational cannabis in Canada, the national Cannabis Regulations 5 outlined a framework for the controlled production, distribution, sale, and possession of cannabis for medical purposes, along with physician and nurse practitioner authorization where cannabis still illegal, health professionals would be subject to mandatory disclosure under the Health Information Act if aware of a patient's plan to engage in the unlawful use of the substance. (Shover and Humphreys 2019). Cannabis legislation varies considerably across jurisdictions, influencing forensic investigations, reporting obligations, and healthcare responsibilities. Forensic nurses must remain aware of applicable regional legal frameworks and professional standards.

Cannabis remains illegal in most countries, although some jurisdictions such as ten eastern states of the U.S.A are implementing cannabis legislation. Nevertheless, optional policies, educational requirements, and practice standards for nurses have been constructed in several jurisdictions worldwide. (Smart and Pacula 2019; Hammond et al. 2020). For instance, Canada, where nurse practitioners can prescribe cannabis has issued regulatory policy guidance with associated practice and educational materials. In Manitoba, a practice direction for the use of cannabis, an associated framework for regulation and education, and a supplementary framework specifying nurse standards all exist. While Cannabis-related practices are legally mandated to be documented, inspections to maintain the integrity of the formal proof of documentation must not be overlooked during professional concern inspections and active cannabis education inspection.

Evans (2013), on the other hand, concentrated on the economic aspect and advised policymakers to adopt thorough cost-benefit analyses rather than revenue-centric narratives, pointing out that although legalization may result in fiscal revenue, it also carries social costs related to healthcare, productivity loss, and potential increases in substance misuse. The significance of incorporating hospital surveillance into policy evaluation and preparing health systems for potential increases in cannabis-related acute presentations is highlighted by Fink et al. (2025) most recent clinical evidence from urine toxicology testing in emergency room patients, which showed rising cannabis positivity rates in legalized contexts. Cannabis-related findings may influence reporting requirements, workplace investigations, child welfare assessments, and legal decision-making. Objective clinical evaluation is necessary to avoid bias and ensure appropriate case management.

5.2. Implications For Reporting And Mandatory Disclosure

Cannabis legislation varies across regions and at multiple levels, producing practices and policies for which nurses need to remain informed. Consideration of the legal landscape promulgated by amendments to the Cannabis Act offers further insight into an evolving system that also affects cannabis use, its compelling implications for care and reporting, obligations pertaining to medical use of controlled substances, and ethical concerns surrounding observation, disclosure, and practice regulation based on patient rights and participation. These cannabis-focused aspects of forensic nursing thus frame core interventions interdependent with education, documentation, chain of custody, and other forms of guidance throughout the profession's regulatory and scientific evolution.

In jurisdictions that have legalized cannabis, law enforcement is not a mandatory reporting agency for children, and cannabis, unlike alcohol and many other medications, is not a controlled substance. Mandated reporting is a hospital policy enacted to protect the child until a formal determination can be made about the validity of the report. Mandatory disclosure depends on whether a reported concern of parental cannabis use meets the threshold of a "reasonable belief" that a child may be in need of protection from the parent. As part of safeguarding, Cannabis and clear overhead lighting are required to facilitate optimal clinical observation to determine safety of the treatment vehicle.

In jurisdictions where cannabis is legal, it is not a controlled substance, and law enforcement is not required to report children exposed to cannabis or parental use of cannabis. Except under these circumstances, reporting remains a mandated and supported police function. Emergency departments (EDs) must provide appropriate clinical interventions for substance use issues whether or not the situation is lawful. Mandatory reporting is a facility directed activity that carries significant legal, criminal, and financial consequences if not adhered to Optional disclosure to a next-of-kin is an ethical right of the nurse.

5.3. Ethical Considerations And Patient Rights

Cannabis remains legal to varying degrees in some jurisdictions of Canada but not within Manitoba; notwithstanding, cannabis use remains prevalent across the general population, including certain health care workers. Despite increasing legalization and accessibility, cannabis remains a neglected yet highly relevant substance within nursing and forensic dimensions. It is crucial to ensure that persons using cannabis are treated fairly by the health care system within the forensic context (J III Mootz, 2018). Legislation governing cannabis use be it legal, illegal, decriminalized, or otherwise regulated impacts the degree of mandatory reporting required and the discretion involved in assessing and acting upon suspected impairment, the scope of patient confidentiality, and the ability to refuse consent for breath or blood tests. Furthermore, the notion of cannabis access and associated patient rights must transcend the mere act of medicating to encompass the absence of discrimination in forensic evaluation and the protection of individuals from unnecessary, unfounded, or excessive intervention. Likewise, protection against the disclosure of information that is unrelated to the alleged offence, such as the use of cannabis for extra-medical purposes, is crucial in safeguarding the integrity of professional relationships by preventing systematic bias or targeting by forensic practitioners. Ethical forensic nursing practice requires respect for patient autonomy, confidentiality, informed consent, and culturally sensitive care. Rights-based approaches help reduce stigma associated with cannabis use in medicolegal settings.

6. CANNABIS USE IN SPECIAL POPULATIONS

Cannabis poses unique challenges within the care of special populations, affecting prenatal and pediatric health, older adults with comorbidities and polypharmacy, and those with mental health and substance use disorders. During pregnancy, cannabis use increases the risk of preterm birth, low birth weight, and impaired neurodevelopment; moreover, children with in-utero exposure may exhibit greater difficulty with attention and impulse control. In Canada, 15% of women report access cannabis during and after pregnancy, often to manage nausea, mood, and stress relief. Accurately assessing frequency, amount, and developmental staging cultivates understanding of risk, normalizes discussion, and helps coordinate care children's right of access ought to be protected where children are identified as relevant within the family unit.

Older adults are the most rapidly growing segment of cannabis users, increasing from 2% of the population in 2000 to 22% in 2019. Although, similar to youth, older adults are at high risk of polysubstance use and more frequent misuse of prescribed medications, being more likely than younger age groups to consume cannabis as a substitute for prescribed medications to relieve chronic pain, stress, anxiety, insomnia, or mood. Over 50% of seniors take five or more medications, and polypharmacy substantially increases the risks of serious adverse drug events (ADEs), toxicity, delirium, hospitalisation, and death. Choices regarding the addition of any more agents necessitate careful risk assessment.

Sixteen percent of cannabis users report concurrent mental health or alcohol and other drug (AOD) problems; harm from these comorbidities remains a significant impediment to treatment success. Addressing these interdependencies remains essential for guiding care.

6.1. Prenatal And Pediatric Considerations

Most jurisdictions allow medical cannabis (MC) for cancer, HIV, Crohn's disease, PTSD, seizures, and severe pain. Pregnant persons commonly use cannabis to address nausea and vomiting. Cannabis exposure may adversely affect development. The risk is compounded for foster care applications the decision-maker may not adequately assess cannabis risk. Prenatal cannabis exposure is one of the leading causes of referrals to child protection services (Navarrete et al., 2020). Many women are unaware of the long-term neurodevelopmental effects of prenatal cannabis exposure (Kiel et al., 2022). Children aged 6 and 10 exposed during gestation displayed difficulties in visuospatial working memory. Cannabinoid Hyperemesis Syndrome often remains unrecognized. Literature lacks guidance on evaluating cannabis exposure and documenting potential adverse effects on clinical care, legal context, and research. Cannabis exposure during pregnancy and childhood requires careful forensic and clinical evaluation due to potential developmental and safeguarding concerns. Assessment should remain evidence-based and avoid punitive assumptions.

Older adults may use various cannabis formulations for polypharmacy, especially with psychotropic drugs. The potential complicity of substance use with serious mental illness further elevates risk. Cannabis may potentiate or ameliorate the influence of other substances. Yet hydrocarbon inhalation and vapourizer attributed lung disease remain a concern with illicit products. Although literature concerning early-onset withdrawal is limited, interest among the mentally ill remains substantial. With early-onset theorems gaining attention, early-onset interviews remain necessary. Explaining cannabis, careful consumption, and contextual links to other substances constitute essential elements. The objective is to mitigate widespread miscalculations regarding cannabis safety and seek early assistance as required.

6.2. Older Adults And Polypharmacy

Older adults are a growing population of cannabis users with unique patterns of use and concerns. Although estimates vary, people aged over 65 years represent the fastest-growing segment among medical cannabis patients in the United States and have significant prevalence rates among adult users in formative studies in Canada. Older adults are at greater risk of experiencing adverse effects from cannabis, given polypharmacy and increased physiological susceptibility, yet patterns of cannabis use among older adults are not well understood, and clinical studies on cannabis use among older patients are sparse.

Older patients often consider cannabis for therapeutic use to reduce chronic pain, an increasingly prevalent condition within this demographic. Without appropriate monitoring, older patients considering cannabis to reduce chronic pain could face adverse repercussions; therefore, careful assessment regarding the appropriateness of recommending a medical cannabis consultation is crucial. Cannabis may benefit individuals who also consume alcohol by reducing overall alcohol intake; however, older adults generally exhibit more concerns about substance use than younger adults, demonstrating the need to better understand older patients seeking cannabis to replace their alcohol consumption (Kaskie, 2023). Older adults may experience altered cannabis metabolism and increased interactions with prescribed medications, complicating forensic interpretation. Comprehensive medication review and clinical assessment are therefore important.

6.3. Mental Health And Substance Use Comorbidity

Cannabis use during pregnancy and lactation is a significant public health concern. Observational studies and a meta-analysis suggest potential associations between prenatal cannabis exposure and alterations in child neurodevelopment, cognition, behaviour, and risk of later substance abuse. Cannabis use among older adults is increasing, often in conjunction with prescription medications for chronic conditions. The effects of cannabinoids on the elderly with significant comorbidity and polypharmacy remain poorly understood. Cannabis represents the single most commonly used substance among individuals with serious mental illness (SMI) and is associated with greater risk of developing a substance use disorder. The prevalence of lifetime and past year cannabis use is more than double among adults with serious mental illness than among the general population. Cannabis use among those with SMI is associated with diminished access to treatment and poorer treatment outcomes for co-occurring substance use and mental disorders. It is also linked to more persistent psychotic symptoms among patients with comorbid cannabis use but may facilitate greater engagement with treatment. Clients presenting with current substance use, or having used within the past thirty days, should be asked about substance use history and mental health status, ideally using a standardized assessment tool. Further insights into the epidemiology of cannabis use among outpatients with co-occurring SMI and substance use disorders, and its clinical implications, remain warranted as legalization continues to spread across North America (Hasin & Walsh, 2020). Cannabis use may coexist with mental health disorders and polysubstance exposure, influencing patient presentation and forensic evaluation. Trauma-informed and non-judgmental approaches support more accurate assessment outcomes.

Cannabis-related forensic and neuroclinical research highlighted about the critical issues spanning analyte stability, addiction mechanisms, impairment testing, and perinatal care. Nisbet et al. (2023) highlighted that analyte stability in solvents and biological matrices is essential for precise quantitation in forensic toxicology, with degradation and metabolite formation leading to under or overestimation. Zehra et al. (2018) summarized research on cannabis addiction from a neurobiological perspective using the Koob–Volkow paradigm. They describe dysregulation of reward, stress, and executive-control systems and connect rising prevalence of cannabis use disorders to changing risk perceptions and potent product profiles. In addition to this, Curran et al. (2016) reviewed cognition and addiction discussing the controversial causality and persistence of cognitive changes, the importance of individual vulnerability factors in addition to product potency and routes of administration, and the centrality of addiction over psychosis in public health burden.

The neurochemical underpinnings of cannabis addiction are outlined by Maldonado et al., (2011), who described CB1 receptor-mediated modulation of dopaminergic reward circuitry and plasticity in glutamatergic/GABAergic systems, matching the addictive effects of THC with common substrates of alcohol, nicotine, opioids, and stimulants. Johnson et al., (2022) list current challenges and developments in impairment testing, emphasizing the discrepancy between biological measures and real-time functional impairment, jurisdictional variations in per se limits, and new methods (such as performance-based and brain-derived metrics) intended to enhance forensic and roadside evaluations. Lastly, Sarathy et al., (2023) recommend more focused, evidence-based perinatal screening strategies due to the limited clinical utility of routine toxicology testing at delivery for perinatal cannabis use. They note the low yield of unexpected positives and potential unintended consequences for care.

7. CLINICAL AND FORENSIC ASSESSMENT TOOLS

Federal and state cannabis-related legislation across many countries and jurisdictions frequently challenges traditional legal obligations and responsibilities, particularly in regard to mandatory reporting of suspected impairment while attendance care (A. MacCallum et al., 2022). Such revisions substantiate the identification and assessment of cannabis use, particularly within special clinical populations at increased risk. Examination of multiple cannabis-oriented clinical assessment tools within the subsequent sections fulfills an essential knowledge gap hindering practice-compliant evaluation of cannabis-related risks, thereby facilitating the selection of appropriate documentation and evidence-collection protocols in accordance with guidelines previously delineated.

Accessing, documenting, and safeguarding evidence while preserving the patient-nurse therapeutic relationship remains challenging. The potential for accidental exposure to contaminated products capable of eliciting psychoactive effects, such as cannabis and other new psychoactive substances, poses additional legal, ethical, clinical, and legislative queries. Development of a practice framework permitting comprehensive integration of previously noted cannabis-related governance across nursing domains may inform policy formulations at local, regional, and international levels. Efforts to advocate cannabis inclusive policy enhancing practice further elaborate the multifactorial influences upon cannabis related health risks, identification and assessment requirements, and safeguard provisions needing consideration by nursing personnel.

Numerous critical studies have highlighted the significant clinical significance of cannabis toxicology, which has been well investigated in both acute and chronic dimensions. The intricacy of cannabis chemistry and metabolism was highlighted by Sharma, et al., (2012), who pointed out that while chronic exposure is associated with dependency and psychiatric illnesses, acute toxicity frequently presents as poor cognition, anxiety, tachycardia, and psychomotor dysfunction. To further emphasizes on the need for increased clinical awareness, Schep, et al., (2020) offered a thorough overview of clinical toxicology, identifying both acute presentations like panic attacks, psychosis, and cardiovascular effects as well as chronic complications like respiratory disease and cognitive impairment. Noble, et al., (2019) documented acute cannabis toxicity with symptoms ranging from severe anxiety and psychosis to cannabinoid hyperemesis syndrome and pediatric exposures from edibles, with a specific focus on emergency presentations. This highlighted the significance of preparedness in emergency medicine. Lastly, Reece (2009) looked at chronic toxicity and found that long-term cannabis use is associated with immunological suppression, respiratory disease, cardiovascular hazards, and mental consequences like sadness and psychosis. This suggests that the overall public health burden may be underestimated.

7.1. Screening Instruments And Risk Assessment

Cannabis use and cannabis use disorder (CUD) have serious consequences, including mental and physical health issues, injuries, and poor neonatal outcomes thus, early identification of those at risk is critical. Brief, valid screening instruments to guide diagnosis and treatment recommendations are invaluable as approximately 50 million Americans use cannabis, and CUD remains underreported and untreated despite evidence-based solutions yet screening instruments have yet to be validated in routine care. CUD prevalence is highest among young adults (5% to 14%) and those with co-occurring mental health and substance use conditions (8% to 23%) (E. Matson et al., 2022). The Cannabis Abuse Screening Test (CAST) comprises six items that assess problematic use against DSM-IV criteria, and a cutoff score of ≥ 2 indicates dependence (Thanki et al., 2013). Conversely, short scales measuring dependence and problems related to cannabis use facilitate population-level estimation of the consequences associated with cannabis use and identification of individuals requiring more comprehensive assessment (Piontek et al., 2008). Structured screening tools and risk assessment frameworks may assist forensic nurses in evaluating impairment, vulnerability, and safety concerns related to cannabis exposure. These tools should complement, rather than replace, clinical judgment.

7.2. Forensic Documentation Templates

Despite an increasing demand for forensic nursing practice focused on cannabis, no template for forensic documentation tailored to such cases currently exists. The absence of a clear template hinders evidence collection, documentation, and legal policy development (Tavabi et al., 2023).

Forensic documentation templates for cannabis-related incidents should accordingly incorporate elements related to a detailed understanding of both the clinical and legal aspects of cannabis use. Since advocating for public policy surrounding cannabis remains a central aspect of forensic nursing, documentation templates should reflect these supporting activities. Standardized forensic documentation templates can improve consistency, objectivity, and legal defensibility in cannabis-related cases. Clear recording of observations and patient statements remains essential.

Figure 3. Forensic nursing documentation cycle

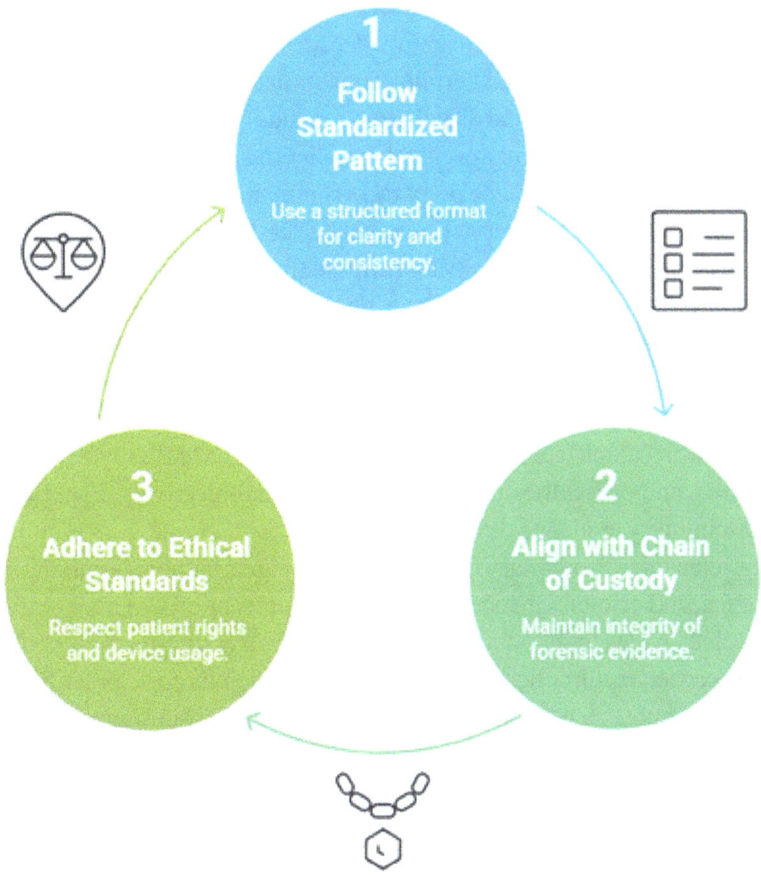
1
Follow Standardized Pattern
Use a structured format for clarity and consistency.
2
Align with Chain of Custody
Maintain integrity of forensic evidence.
3
Adhere to Ethical Standards
Respect patient rights and device usage.

8. RESEARCH GAPS AND FUTURE DIRECTIONS

Methodological challenges surrounding forensic cannabis research complicate the emergence of evidence based policies that might guide nurses practices. Nevertheless, specific policy-informed cannabis innovations could optimize both practice and research. These include establishing cannabis as a policy priority and developing standard questions and evidence-based guidance on cannabis use and employing cannabis focused quality and safety frameworks which broadly disseminating cannabis use resources and information and creating links among nurses interested in cannabis. These types of measures would strengthen the integration of broader ethical considerations in the forensic cannabis domain and reinforce the momentum behind cannabis focused clinical, documentation, and legal innovations already under consideration.

8.1. Methodological Challenges In Forensic Cannabis Research

Advancements in cannabis science and rising cannabis legalization, both medical and recreational, have progressed exponentially during the past several decades. Cannabis remains a Schedule I drug under the federal Controlled Substances Act, and certain cannabis and hemp derivatives remain federally controlled. Hence, cannabis usage, supply, and distribution remains criminalized in many legal jurisdictions. Notably, cannabis remains illegal in numerous legal jurisdictions, whether statewide, county, municipal, or otherwise, or specific compounds and/or preparations remain prohibited.

Cannabis consumption has been observed to engender certain physical and psychological effects. Physicochemical profiles elucidate the toxicity and elimination pathways of these compounds. standards and the policy principles underpinning them; later develops practice innovations that might alleviate some of the ethical and equity challenges stipulated in the previous sections. Legal and policy contexts overlap considerably with the clinical forensic boundaries already addressed, since documentation informs care and constitutes evidence while therapeutic considerations shape forensic narratives and standards. Cannabis-related forensic research faces methodological limitations due to regulatory differences, inconsistent testing standards, and difficulties measuring impairment objectively. These challenges highlight the need for multidisciplinary evidence development.

Forensic nursing, as an interdisciplinary field and specialty area, combines nursing science with public health, forensic science, and criminal justice to facilitate the prevention and intervention of violence and criminality within society. A clear methodological difficulty involves the interpretation of cannabis-related phenomena and their consequent implications, the extent to which forensic practitioners wish to remain inclusive of psychoactive substances, and the extent to which illegal substance usage relates directly to forensic nursing. Reflecting contemporary licensure, policy, and legislative trends, considerable gaps exist within the forensic cannabis literature.

8.2. Policy-Informed Practice Innovations

Research suggests that applying a forensic nursing perspective to cannabis use along with the healthcare continuum reveals substantial knowledge and practice gaps from pharmacology to documentation and highlights distinct clinical considerations when working with specific populations. These knowledge gaps also extend to legal and policy dimensions. At the research policy nexus, the cannabis field presents systematic challenges related to regulatory and methodological frameworks; addressing these requires clearly articulated, policy-informed, and systematic practice innovations. Emerging forensic nursing practices increasingly emphasize evidence-based policy development, digital documentation systems, and trauma-informed cannabis care models. Continued professional education is necessary to support evolving medicolegal practice.

Methodological challenges associated with cannabis are compounded by the complexities of forensic research. As policy develops and forensic nursing patients increasingly request care in cannabis-related contexts without sufficient knowledge or understanding of complex interconnections between cannabis, health, care, documentation, and legal contexts research in these areas becomes ever more critical. Policy-informed practice innovations that address the gaps identified across the cannabis-health-care continuum can respond to these urgent needs.

Suggestions for policy-informed innovations include two focal areas relating to the healthcare continuum are first is establishing documentation mechanisms and clarification of clinical roles consistent with both existing legislation and emergent legal developments and second, enhancing understanding of cannabis-related toxicity among front-line healthcare providers and community-based organizations. By working within available regulatory frameworks to improve cannabis knowledge and advance safe, effective healthcare practices, cannabis-relevant research can contribute to practice innovations that inform future activities concerning both policy and documentation. Guidance obtained from public health agencies and organizations such as the Canadian Federation of Nurses Unions, the Nurses' Union, and local health authorities offers further refinements and recommendations.

9. CONCLUSION

Cannabis focused forensic nursing integrates clinical care, documentation integrity, and interprofessional collaboration to influence practice and policy. Perspectives on cannabis inform acute intoxication, Cannabinoid Hyperemesis Syndrome, withdrawal, and comorbidity management in vulnerable populations or with polypharmacy. These factors guide indications for health-care encounters and shape documentation content. Procedural evidence collection including patient history, photographs, and specimen acquisition requires adherence to chain-of-custody guidelines, as does the legal-sounding nature of the related documentation. Following these procedures enables rigorous documentation that respects patient rights and fosters trust, even when patients express reluctance to provide information. Such considerations clarify legal risks for practitioners and patients, particularly when a forensic examination is sought. Consequently, interprofessional collaboration emerges as a crucial aspect of both forensic nursing and cannabis policy. The growing intersection between cannabis use and medicolegal care highlights the expanding role of forensic nurses in assessment, documentation, patient advocacy, and interdisciplinary collaboration. Contemporary forensic practice requires balanced, evidence-informed, and non-stigmatizing approaches to cannabis-related clinical and legal contexts.

REFERENCES

Adams, I. B., & Martin, B. R. (1996). Cannabis: Pharmacology and toxicology in animals and humans. *Addiction (Abingdon, England), 91*(11), 1585–1614. DOI: 10.1046/j.1360-0443.1996.911115852.x PMID: 8972919

Amin, M. R., & Ali, D. W. (2019). Pharmacology of medical cannabis. *Recent advances in cannabinoid physiology and pathology. Advances in Experimental Medicine and Biology, 1162*, 151–165. DOI: 10.1007/978-3-030-21737-2_8 PMID: 31332738

Arkell, R., Kevin, R. C., Stuart, J., Lintzeris, N., Haber, P. S., Ramaekers, J. G., & McGregor, I. S. (2019). Detection of Δ(9) THC in oral fluid following vaporized cannabis with varied cannabidiol (CBD) content: An evaluation of two point-of-collection testing devices. *Drug Testing and Analysis, 11*(10), 1486–1497. DOI: 10.1002/dta.2687 PMID: 31442003

Ashton, C. H. (2001). Pharmacology and effects of cannabis: A brief review. *The British Journal of Psychiatry, 178*(2), 101–106. DOI: 10.1192/bjp.178.2.101 PMID: 11157422

Balneaves, G., Alraja, A. A., Thompson, G., Penner, J. L., John, P. S., Scerbo, D., & van Dyck, J. (2024). Cannabis use in a Canadian long-term care facility: A case study. *BMC Geriatrics, 24*(1), 467. DOI: 10.1186/s12877-024-05074-2 PMID: 38811895

. Bartlow, N. (2009). Establishing the digital chain of evidence in biometric systems.

Carla Monti, M. (2022). Analysis of Synthetic and Natural Cannabinoids in the Forensic Field Applying High-Resolution. *Mass Spectrometry (Tokyo, Japan).*

. Charitos, I. A., Gagliano-Candela, R., Santacroce, L., & Bottalico, L. (2021). The Cannabis spread throughout the continents and its therapeutic use in history. *Endocrine, Metabolic & Immune Disorders-Drug Targets (Formerly Current Drug Targets-Immune, Endocrine & Metabolic Disorders), 21*(3), 407-417.

Connor, P., Stjepanović, D., Budney, A. J., Le Foll, B., & Hall, W. D. (2022). Clinical management of cannabis withdrawal. *Addiction (Abingdon, England), 117*(7), 2075–2095. DOI: 10.1111/add.15743 PMID: 34791767

Crocker, E., Carter, A. J. E., Emsley, J. G., Magee, K., Atkinson, P., & Tibbo, P. G. (2021). When Cannabis Use Goes Wrong: Mental Health Side Effects of Cannabis Use That Present to Emergency Services. *Frontiers in Psychiatry, 12*, 640222. DOI: 10.3389/fpsyt.2021.640222 PMID: 33658953

Curran, H. V., Freeman, T. P., Mokrysz, C., Lewis, D. A., Morgan, C. J., & Parsons, L. H. (2016). Keep off the grass? Cannabis, cognition and addiction. *Nature Reviews. Neuroscience, 17*(5), 293–306. DOI: 10.1038/nrn.2016.28 PMID: 27052382

D'Anna, T., Puntarello, M., Cannella, G., Scalzo, G., Buscemi, R., Zerbo, S., & Argo, A. (2023). The Chain of Custody in the Era of Modern Forensics: From the Classic Procedures for Gathering Evidence to the New Challenges Related to Digital Data. *Health Care, 11*(5), 634. PMID: 36900637

Djilali, E., Pappalardo, L., Posadino, A. M., Giordo, R., & Pintus, G. (2022). Effects of the storage conditions on the stability of natural and synthetic cannabis in biological matrices for forensic toxicology analysis: An update from the literature. *Metabolites*, *12*(9), 801. DOI: 10.3390/metabo12090801 PMID: 36144208

Evans, D. G. (2013). The economic impacts of marijuana legalization. *The Journal of Global Drug Policy and Practice*, *7*(4), 2–40.

Fink, D. S., Samples, H., Malte, C. A., Olfson, M., Wall, M. M., Alschuler, D. M., Simpson, T., Mannes, Z., Saxon, A. J., & Hasin, D. S. (2025). Cannabis legalization and increasing cannabis use in the United States: Data from urine toxicology testing in emergency room patients. *The International Journal on Drug Policy*, *138*, 104765. DOI: 10.1016/j.drugpo.2025.104765 PMID: 40058102

Giordano, G., Mattia, M., Boracchi, M., Biehler-Gomez, L., Cummaudo, M., Porro, A., Caccianiga, M., Sardanelli, F., Slavazzi, F., Galimberti, P. M., Di Candia, D., & Cattaneo, C. (2023). Forensic toxicological analyses reveal the use of cannabis in Milano (Italy) in the 1600s. *Journal of Archaeological Science*, *160*, 105873. DOI: 10.1016/j.jas.2023.105873

Hammond, D., Goodman, S., Wadsworth, E., Rynard, V., Boudreau, C., & Hall, W. (2020). Evaluating the impacts of cannabis legalization: The International Cannabis Policy Study. *The International Journal on Drug Policy*, *77*, 102698. DOI: 10.1016/j.drugpo.2020.102698 PMID: 32113149

Hasin, D. (2023). Legalization of cannabis for medical and recreational use. *European Psychiatry : the Journal of the Association of European Psychiatrists*, *66*(S1, Suppl 1), S20–S21. DOI: 10.1192/j.eurpsy.2023.83

Hasin, D., & Walsh, C. (2020). Cannabis Use, Cannabis Use Disorder, and Comorbid Psychiatric Illness: A Narrative Review. *Journal of Clinical Medicine*, *10*(1), 15. DOI: 10.3390/jcm10010015 PMID: 33374666

Huerne, K., Ells, C., Grad, R., Filion, B., & Eisenberg, M. J. (2022). Cannabis-Impaired driving: Ethical considerations for the primary care practitioner. *Annals of Medicine*, *55*(1), 24–33. DOI: 10.1080/07853890.2022.2151716 PMID: 36444881

. J III Mootz, F. (2018). Ethical Cannabis Lawyering in California. 9 St. Mary's Journal on Legal Malpractice & Ethics, 2-63.

Johnson, O. E., Miskelly, G. M., & Rindelaub, J. D. (2022). Testing for cannabis intoxication: Current issues and latest advancements. *WIREs Forensic Science*, *4*(4), e1450. DOI: 10.1002/wfs2.1450

Kalant, H. (2001). Medicinal use of cannabis: History and current status. *Pain Research & Management*, *6*(2), 80–91. DOI: 10.1155/2001/469629 PMID: 11854770

Karki, P., & Rangaswamy, M. (2023). A review of historical context and current research on cannabis use in India. *Indian Journal of Psychological Medicine*, *45*(2), 105–116. DOI: 10.1177/02537176221109272 PMID: 36925496

Kaskie, B. (2023). The cannabis and older persons study: What we have learned. *Innovation in Aging*, *7*(Suppl 1), 173. DOI: 10.1093/geroni/igad104.0567

Kavousi, P., Giamo, T., Arnold, G., Alliende, M., Huynh, E., Lea, J., Lucine, R., Tillett Miller, A., Webre, A., Yee, A., Champagne-Zamora, A., & Taylor, K. (2022). What do we know about opportunities and challenges for localities from Cannabis legalization? *The Review of Policy Research, 39*(2), 143–169. DOI: 10.1111/ropr.12460

Kiel, L., Hsu, C., Wartko, D., Albertson-Junkans, L., Ewing, J., & Lapham, G. T. (2022). Perspectives from women who engaged in prenatal and postpartum cannabis use in a U.S. State with legal non-medical use. *Preventive Medicine Reports, 31*, 102075. DOI: 10.1016/j.pmedr.2022.102075 PMID: 36820379

Klein, A., & Clark, C. S. (2022). Therapeutic use of cannabis in the US. *The Nurse Practitioner, 47*(12), 16–25. DOI: 10.1097/01.NPR.0000884880.81603.c5 PMID: 36399143

Kurtzman, T., Greene, J., Begley, R., & Drenkard, K. N. (2022). "We want what's best for patients." nurse leaders' attitudes about medical cannabis: A qualitative study. *International Journal of Nursing Studies Advances, 4*, 100065. DOI: 10.1016/j.ijnsa.2022.100065 PMID: 38745605

MacCallum, C. A., Lo, L. A., Pistawka, C., Christiansen, A., Boivin, M., & Snider-Adler, M. (2022). A Clinical Framework for Assessing Cannabis-Related Impairment Risk. *Frontiers in Psychiatry, 13*, 883517. DOI: 10.3389/fpsyt.2022.883517 PMID: 35832600

Maldonado, R., Berrendero, F., Ozaita, A., & Robledo, P. (2011). Neurochemical basis of cannabis addiction. *Neuroscience, 181*, 1–17. DOI: 10.1016/j.neuroscience.2011.02.035 PMID: 21334423

Marie Figueroa-Rivera, I., Estremera-Marcial, R., Sierra-Mercado, M., Gutiérrez-Núñez, J., & Toro, H. (2015). D. (2015). Cannabinoid Hyperemesis Syndrome: A Paradoxical Cannabis Effect. *Case Reports in Gastrointestinal Medicine*, 405238.

Matson, E., Lapham, G. T., Bobb, J. F., Oliver, M., Hallgren, K. A., Williams, E. C., & Bradley, K. A. (2022). Validity of the Single-Item Screen–Cannabis (SIS-C) for Cannabis Use Disorder Screening in Routine Care. *JAMA Network Open, 5*(11), e2239772. DOI: 10.1001/jamanetworkopen.2022.39772 PMID: 36318205

Nasrin, S. J. W., Watson, C. X., Perez-Paramo, Y., & Lazarus, P. (2021). Cannabinoid Metabolites as Inhibitors of Major Hepatic CYP450 Enzymes, with Implications for Cannabis-Drug Interactions. *Drug Metabolism and Disposition: the Biological Fate of Chemicals, 49*(12), 1070–1080. DOI: 10.1124/dmd.121.000442 PMID: 34493602

Navarrete, F., Salud García-Gutiérrez, M., Gasparyan, A., Austrich-Olivares, A., Femenía, T., & Manzanares, J. (2020). Cannabis Use in Pregnant and Breastfeeding Women: Behavioral and Neurobiological Consequences. *Frontiers in Psychiatry, 11*, 586447. DOI: 10.3389/fpsyt.2020.586447 PMID: 33240134

Nisbet, L. A., DiEmma, G. E., & Scott, K. S. (2023). Drug stability in forensic toxicology. *Wiley Interdisciplinary Reviews: Forensic Science, 5*(4), e1481.

Noble, M. J., Hedberg, K., & Hendrickson, R. G. (2019). Acute cannabis toxicity. *Clinical Toxicology, 57*(8), 735–742. DOI: 10.1080/15563650.2018.1548708 PMID: 30676820

Perisetti, A., Gajendran, M., Shekhar Dasari, C., Bansal, P., Aziz, M., Inamdar, S., Tharian, B., & Goyal, H. (2020). Cannabis hyperemesis syndrome: An update on the pathophysiology and management. *Annals of Gastroenterology*, *33*(6), 571–578. DOI: 10.20524/aog.2020.0528 PMID: 33162734

Piontek, D., Kraus, L., & Klempova, D. (2008). Short scales to assess cannabis-related problems: A review of psychometric properties. *Substance Abuse Treatment, Prevention, and Policy*, *3*(1), 25. DOI: 10.1186/1747-597X-3-25 PMID: 19055741

Reece, A. S. (2009). Chronic toxicology of cannabis. *Clinical Toxicology*, *47*(6), 517–524. DOI: 10.1080/15563650903074507 PMID: 19586351

Roberts, B. (2019). Legalized Cannabis in Colorado Emergency Departments: A Cautionary Review of Negative Health and Safety Effects. *The Western Journal of Emergency Medicine*, *20*(4), 557–572. DOI: 10.5811/westjem.2019.4.39935 PMID: 31316694

Sarathy, L., Chou, J. H., Lerou, P. H., Terplan, M., Mark, K., Dorfman, S., Wilens, T. E., Bernstein, S. N., & Schiff, D. M. (2023). Limited utility of toxicology testing at delivery for perinatal cannabis use. *Hospital Pediatrics*, *13*(4), 317–325. DOI: 10.1542/hpeds.2022-006897 PMID: 36855896

Schep, L. J., Slaughter, R. J., Glue, P., & Gee, P. (2020). The clinical toxicology of cannabis. *The New Zealand Medical Journal (Online)*, *133*(1523), 96–103. PMID: 33032307

Schmid, S., Lapaire, O., Huang, D., Jürgens, F., & Güth, U. (2018). Cannabinoid hyperemesis syndrome: An underreported entity causing nausea and vomiting of pregnancy. *Archives of Gynecology and Obstetrics*, *284*(5), 1095–1097. DOI: 10.1007/s00404-010-1811-8 PMID: 21170540

Sharma, P., Murthy, P., & Bharath, M. M. (2012, Fall). Chemistry, metabolism, and toxicology of cannabis: Clinical implications. *Iranian Journal of Psychiatry*, *7*(4), 149–156. PMID: 23408483

Sharma, P., Rao, V., Kumar Chand, P., & Murthy, P. (2023). Quantification of Δ9-tetrahydrocannabinol in urine as a marker of cannabis abuse. *The Indian Journal of Medical Research*, *158*(5-6), 535–541. DOI: 10.4103/ijmr.IJMR_3899_20 PMID: 37929356

Shover, C. L., & Humphreys, K. (2019). Six policy lessons relevant to cannabis legalization. *The American Journal of Drug and Alcohol Abuse*, *45*(6), 698–706. DOI: 10.1080/00952990.2019.1569669 PMID: 30870053

Skalisky, J., Leickly, E., Oluwoye, O., & McPherson, M. (2017). *S., Srebnik, D., M. Roll, J., K. Ries, R., & G. McDonell, M.* Prevalence and Correlates of Cannabis Use in Outpatients with Serious Mental Illness Receiving Treatment for Alcohol Use Disorders.

Smart, R., & Pacula, R. L. (2019). Early evidence of the impact of cannabis legalization on cannabis use, cannabis use disorder, and the use of other substances: Findings from state policy evaluations. *The American Journal of Drug and Alcohol Abuse*, *45*(6), 644–663. DOI: 10.1080/00952990.2019.1669626 PMID: 31603710

Tavabi, N., Raza, M., Singh, M., Golchin, S., Singh, H., Hogue, D., & Kiapour, A. M. (2023). Disparities in cannabis use and documentation in electronic health records among children and young adults. *NPJ Digital Medicine*, *6*(1), 138. DOI: 10.1038/s41746-023-00885-w PMID: 37553423

Thanki, D., Domingo-Salvany, A., Barrio Anta, G., Sánchez Mañez, A., Llorens Aleixandre, N., Maria Suelves, J., Brime Beteta, B., & Vicente, J. (2013). The Choice of Screening Instrument Matters: The Case of Problematic Cannabis Use Screening in Spanish Population of Adolescents. International Scholarly Research Notices, 723131, 13 pages

Trif, C., Harpaz, D., Eltzov, E., Parcharoen, Y., Pechyen, C., & Marks, S. (2024). Detection of Cannabinoids in Oral Fluid Specimens as the Preferred Biological Matrix for a Point-of-Care Biosensor Diagnostic Device. *Biosensors (Basel)*, *14*(3), 126. DOI: 10.3390/bios14030126 PMID: 38534233

Warf, B. (2014). High points: An historical geography of cannabis. *Geographical Review*, *104*(4), 414–438. DOI: 10.1111/j.1931-0846.2014.12038.x

Wills, S. (1998). Cannabis use and abuse by man: an historical perspective. In *Cannabis* (pp. 16–46). CRC Press. DOI: 10.4324/9780203304228_chapter_1

Zehra, A., Burns, J., Liu, C. K., Manza, P., Wiers, C. E., Volkow, N. D., & Wang, G. J. (2018). Cannabis addiction and the brain: A review. *Journal of Neuroimmune Pharmacology*, *13*(4), 438–452. DOI: 10.1007/s11481-018-9782-9 PMID: 29556883

Chapter 9
From Spirit to Symptom:
A Caring Science Model for Cannabis Nursing

Sherri Mack
http://orcid.org/0009-0007-8503-3125
Holistic Caring, USA & The Green Nurse, USA

ABSTRACT

This chapter examines cannabis nursing as an emerging specialty grounded in caring science, holistic nursing philosophy, and contemporary cannabinoid research, advancing a spirituality-first approach to clinical practice. Drawing upon Jean Watson's Theory of Human Caring, professional nursing standards, and the endocannabinoid system, the chapter asserts that spirituality is not ancillary to cannabis care but foundational to ethical, person-centered nursing practice. A Spirituality-First Clinical Model and the H.I.G.H. Framework (Hope, Inspiration, Growth, and Healing) are introduced to illustrate how cannabis-supported care may influence physical, mental, emotional, social, and spiritual domains of health. Through clinical narratives, the chapter demonstrates how presence, nonjudgment, intention, and relationship-centered care shape therapeutic outcomes. By integrating science and meaning, this work positions cannabis nursing as a relational, ethically grounded specialty that honors human dignity, supports whole-person healing, and advances holistic nursing practice.

INTRODUCTION

Cannabis nursing is an emerging specialty grounded in holistic philosophy, caring science, and the lived experiences of patients who seek relief and healing through plant-based therapeutics. While cannabis is often discussed in terms of pharmacology, policy, or symptom management, its clinical use frequently opens conversations related to identity, trauma, spirituality, and meaning. For some patients, cannabis use is associated not only with symptom relief but also with introspection and emotional regulation.

Nursing, as both a science and a practice of care, has long recognized that healing extends beyond the physical body. From Florence Nightingale's emphasis on environment and presence to Jean Watson's Theory of Human Caring (Watson, 2008), nursing theory has consistently affirmed the interconnectedness of physical, psychological, emotional, relational, and spiritual dimensions of health. Holistic nursing traditions further emphasize the nurse's role in cultivating presence, compassion, and attentiveness to

DOI: 10.4018/979-8-3373-7287-7.ch009

the patient's experience. Cannabis nursing aligns with these traditions by extending assessment beyond symptoms to include the patient's internal and relational context.

Within contemporary healthcare systems, spirituality is often under addressed or treated as optional. Time constraints, biomedical priorities, regulatory complexity, and stigma surrounding cannabis use may limit engagement with spiritual dimensions of care. At the same time, professional nursing standards increasingly identify spirituality, cultural humility, and nonjudgment as components of ethical practice. In cannabis nursing, where patients may present with fear, stigma, trauma, or existential distress, the absence of this dimension may narrow the scope of care.

This chapter advances the position that spirituality functions as a central component of cannabis nursing practice rather than a secondary consideration. Through a spirituality-first lens, cannabis nursing is conceptualized as a relational and ethically grounded practice informed by presence, intention, and clinical judgment. Integrating caring science, holistic nursing philosophy, and contemporary cannabinoid research, this chapter introduces a Spirituality-First Clinical Model alongside the H.I.G.H. Framework (Hope, Inspiration, Growth, and Healing) (Mack, 2026). These frameworks are used to examine how cannabis supported care may influence physical, psychological, emotional, social, and spiritual domains of health while maintaining attention to patient autonomy, cultural context, and clinical boundaries, as well as underlying biological mechanisms such as the endocannabinoid system (Lu & Mackie, 2016).

The objectives of this chapter are to:

- Situate cannabis nursing within a spirituality-first theoretical framework.
- Examine the role of the nurse–patient relationship in shaping therapeutic outcomes.
- Explore how cannabis intersects with emotional, social, and spiritual dimensions of health.
- Illustrate how spirituality, intention, and relationship centered care inform ethical cannabis nursing practice through clinical narratives.

BACKGROUND

Spirituality forms the foundational context for understanding cannabis nursing. Across cultures and throughout history, healing has been understood as a multidimensional process involving the body, mind, emotions, relationships, and spirit. Modern nursing reflects this orientation. The American Holistic Nurses Association defines holistic nursing as "all nursing practice that has healing the whole person as its goal" (American Holistic Nurses Association [AHNA], n.d.). A systematic review and concept analysis further identifies spirituality in healthcare as encompassing meaning, purpose, connection, and transcendence, independent of religious affiliation (de Brito Sena et al., 2021). This perspective supports the position that spirituality is integral to health and healing. Cannabis nursing, grounded in holistic philosophy, extends this foundation.

Spirituality is also embedded within nursing theory. Florence Nightingale described healing as an engagement with environment, presence, and the natural world. Jean Watson later articulated caring as a moral, relational, and transpersonal process that affirms human dignity and wholeness (Watson, 2008). Cannabis nursing reflects this trajectory by recognizing that cannabis use may be associated not only with symptom relief but also with emotional processing, introspection, and meaning making. Patients may describe experiences of reconnection with self, which aligns with Watson's conceptualization of healing as movement toward harmony within the body, mind, and spirit.

One framework for describing the spiritual dimensions of cannabis care is the H.I.G.H. Framework, defined as Hope, Inspiration, Growth, and Healing (Mack, 2026). This model describes shifts that may occur as distress is reduced and patients reconnect with a sense of possibility. Hope may emerge as pain or anxiety diminishes. Inspiration may arise when reduced physiological arousal allows for clarity or creativity. Growth may unfold through emotional insight and changes in self-perception. Healing is characterized by a movement toward coherence, reflected in balance, meaning, and self-compassion. While the endocannabinoid system regulates biological homeostasis, the H.I.G.H. Framework provides a conceptual structure for understanding associated psychological and spiritual experiences.

Professional guidelines further support this integration. The Cannabis Nursing: Scope and Standards of Practice (American Cannabis Nurses Association and American Nurses Association, 2024) incorporates spirituality, cultural humility, and nonjudgment within RN and APRN competencies. Nurses are expected to assess and respond to patients' beliefs, values, and meaning making processes in care planning. Similarly, the National Council of State Boards of Nursing (2018) identifies nonjudgment as an ethical requirement when caring for individuals who use cannabis, particularly those experiencing stigma, trauma, chronic illness, or end of life concerns. These standards reinforce that cannabis nursing involves relational and ethical dimensions in addition to clinical care.

The spiritual foundations of cannabis nursing are also reflected in the plant's historical use as a medicine and consciousness modulating substance across cultures. Shamanic traditions have used botanical medicines to support emotional processing, insight, and healing within relational and ritual contexts (Winkelman, 2010). Although contemporary cannabis nursing is grounded in clinical science, these historical patterns provide context for understanding the human tendency to use plant-based therapies in the context of meaning making and healing.

Viewed within this framework, cannabis nursing can be understood as a relational practice that integrates clinical care with attention to meaning, connection, and patient experience. The nurse–patient relationship, characterized by presence, compassion, cultural humility, and attentiveness, functions as a central component of care. Cannabis may contribute to symptom relief, including reductions in pain, anxiety, or distress, while the nurse's presence supports the patient's interpretive and adaptive processes. This background establishes the conceptual foundation for the Caring Science framework, clinical model, and narratives that follow, and prepares for examination of the ethical, systemic, and clinical considerations that shape contemporary cannabis nursing practice.

Issues, Controversies and Problems

Cannabis nursing exists at the intersection of evolving science, shifting policy, and deeply rooted cultural beliefs. At the same time, it reflects a broader tension between biomedical models of care and the lived human experiences of meaning, suffering, and healing. While evidence supporting the therapeutic use of cannabis continues to grow, nurses often practice within healthcare systems that remain ambivalent, inconsistent, or resistant to its integration. Regulatory ambiguity, institutional risk aversion, and persistent stigma create ethical and professional tensions that shape how cannabis care is delivered, limited, or avoided in clinical practice.

One persistent controversy involves the tension between federal prohibition and state level legalization. Nurses may care for patients who legally use medical cannabis while working in institutions governed by federal regulations or policies that restrict education, documentation, or discussion of cannabis use. This disconnect places nurses in ethically complex positions, requiring them to balance patient advocacy, legal compliance, and professional accountability. Fear of disciplinary action or job loss may discourage nurses from engaging openly with patients about cannabis, even when such conversations are clinically relevant. This tension extends beyond policy into the relational space, where avoidance may limit opportunities for patients to discuss experiences that include emotional or spiritual dimensions of their care.

Importantly, the regulatory landscape surrounding cannabis is beginning to shift. Recent federal actions have initiated a formal review of cannabis classification under the Controlled Substances Act, with the possibility of rescheduling cannabis from Schedule I to Schedule III. While rescheduling would not constitute full legalization, it signals increasing institutional recognition of cannabis's accepted medical use and may reduce barriers related to research, clinical discourse, and professional education (U.S. Department of Health and Human Services, 2023). During this transitional period, nurses must remain informed, ethically grounded, and responsive to evolving regulatory guidance while continuing to prioritize patient centered care.

Stigma surrounding cannabis use represents another significant barrier. Patients who use cannabis, particularly those with chronic pain, mental health conditions, or serious illness, often report feeling judged, dismissed, or misunderstood by healthcare providers. Nurses may carry implicit or explicit biases that influence assessment, communication, and care planning. Without intentional reflection and education, stigma can erode trust and compromise the therapeutic relationship, limiting not only clinical disclosure but also deeper conversations related to meaning, coping, and lived experience.

Educational gaps further compound these challenges. Many nurses report limited formal education related to the endocannabinoid system, cannabis pharmacology, dosing considerations, and potential risks and benefits. As a result, nurses may feel unprepared to answer patient questions or integrate cannabis discussions into holistic assessments. This lack of preparation can perpetuate avoidance, reliance on personal belief systems, or inconsistent clinical guidance, particularly in situations where patients are seeking support for complex physical, emotional, or spiritual concerns.

Ethical considerations also arise in relation to vulnerability and power dynamics. Patients seeking cannabis care may be experiencing significant suffering, fear, or existential distress. In these contexts, nurses must remain attentive to the risks of coercion, overstatement of benefits, or the imposition of personal beliefs. Respect for autonomy, cultural humility, and clear professional boundaries remain essential, particularly when conversations extend into areas of meaning, identity, and spirituality.

Cannabis nursing also unfolds within healthcare systems that prioritize efficiency, productivity, and measurable biomedical outcomes. Time constraints, documentation demands, and task-oriented workflows often limit opportunities for presence, dialogue, and spiritual assessment. When these elements are minimized, care may become fragmented, reducing opportunities for relational engagement and whole person understanding. These systemic pressures continue to challenge the integration of cannabis within holistic nursing practice (American Cannabis Nurses Association & American Nurses Association, 2024; National Council of State Boards of Nursing, 2018).

Taken together, these issues highlight a central tension within cannabis nursing: the integration of therapies that often evoke psychological and spiritual experiences into systems that are not structured to recognize or support them. This tension underscores the need for a clearly defined, spirituality informed framework to guide clinical practice. These challenges point toward the importance of intentional approaches that support nurses in integrating cannabis care with confidence, competence, and compassion.

Solutions and Recommendations

Addressing the issues, controversies, and problems within cannabis nursing requires intentional, systems informed, and ethically grounded solutions. Nurses must be supported in developing both the knowledge and reflective capacity necessary to engage cannabis care with confidence, humility, and compassion. Effective solutions must operate across individual, organizational, educational, and regulatory levels to support the evolution of cannabis nursing as an evidence informed and human centered specialty.

At the individual level, nurses benefit from education that extends beyond pharmacology to include the endocannabinoid system, trauma informed care, cultural humility, and spiritual assessment. Developing self-awareness related to personal beliefs, biases, and comfort with altered states of consciousness supports ethical and relational practice. Reflective practices such as mindfulness, journaling, supervision, and peer dialogue can further cultivate presence, nonjudgment, and clinical discernment in cannabis related encounters.

At the organizational level, healthcare institutions play a critical role in shaping how cannabis care is understood and delivered. Clear policies, scope of practice guidance, and documentation standards can reduce ambiguity and fear among nurses. Institutions that support open, evidence informed dialogue about cannabis create safer environments for both patients and clinicians. Integrating cannabis education into continuing education offerings and interdisciplinary forums can further normalize its role within clinical care.

Educational institutions and professional organizations are well positioned to address persistent knowledge gaps. Incorporating endocannabinoid science, cannabis therapeutics, and ethical considerations into nursing curricula prepares future nurses for informed practice. Continuing education programs, specialty certificates, and mentorship opportunities can support practicing nurses in developing competency while remaining aligned with regulatory requirements. These efforts should emphasize critical thinking, patient centered communication, and respect for diverse cultural and spiritual perspectives.

At the regulatory and policy level, ongoing clarification of nursing roles related to cannabis education, assessment, and documentation is essential. As federal and state policies continue to evolve, nursing leadership must remain engaged in dialogue and advocacy efforts that protect patient access while supporting nurse safety and professional integrity. Nurses are encouraged to practice within current regulations while remaining informed about policy developments that may expand or refine their scope.

The ethical integration of cannabis within nursing practice requires sustained attention to relationship centered care. Presence, trust, and nonjudgment are core clinical competencies. By approaching cannabis as one component of a broader healing process rather than a singular intervention, nurses can support patients in navigating physical symptoms, emotional distress, relational challenges, and spiritual meaning with integrity and compassion.

Clark (2021) emphasizes the need for nurses to understand the function of the endocannabinoid system, cannabinoid interactions, dosing strategies, pharmacokinetics, and harm reduction principles to practice safely and effectively. Blesching (2022) further highlights the holistic and psychospiritual dimensions of cannabis, noting that the plant influences the interconnected mind, body, and spirit in ways that require nuanced understanding. Without this knowledge, nurses may feel unprepared to support patients through emotional, psychological, or spiritual experiences that arise during cannabis related care.

Mack (2020) underscores that many patients are left to navigate cannabis use through trial and error due to limited clinician education. In *Cannabis for Health: Become a Coach,* she identifies the need for competency in the endocannabinoid system, dosing principles, intention setting, and patient centered goal clarification. This coaching framework aligns with a spirituality-first clinical approach, emphasizing that effective cannabis care begins with understanding the whole person, including their fears, values, worldview, beliefs, and readiness for change. In this context, spiritual assessment, presence, and nonjudgment emerge as essential clinical competencies rather than optional enhancements.

While systems level solutions, education, and policy guidance are necessary, they are insufficient without a coherent clinical framework that supports nurses in translating these principles into practice. Emerging global nursing research suggests that spirituality is already integrated into advanced nursing practice, even when it is not formally named or explicitly taught (Rogers et al., 2025).

These recommendations support the ethical and relational integration of cannabis within nursing practice while also highlighting the need for continued inquiry. Ongoing research is needed to evaluate clinical outcomes, refine competencies, and further establish evidence informed frameworks that integrate spirituality, caring science, and cannabinoid therapeutics.

The following section presents spirituality not as an abstract concept, but as the organizing foundation of cannabis nursing care. Through a spirituality-first lens, nurses are invited to integrate presence, intention, and ethical awareness into clinical encounters, setting the stage for a holistic assessment of health across physical, mental, emotional, social, and spiritual domains.

SPIRITUALITY AS THE ROOT OF CANNABIS CARE

Spirituality is not an accessory to cannabis nursing. It is the foundation upon which this specialty is built. While cannabis is often framed through pharmacology, symptom management, or regulatory discourse, its clinical use frequently invites patients into deeper experiences of meaning, identity, emotional integration, and spiritual inquiry. For nurses, this reality requires a shift from task-oriented care toward relational presence that honors the whole person.

Within holistic nursing and caring science traditions, spirituality is understood as the dimension through which individuals seek meaning, purpose, connection, and transcendence, particularly in the context of illness, suffering, or life transitions. Cannabis nursing aligns with this understanding by recognizing that healing unfolds not only through biochemical mechanisms, but also through the patient's lived experience, inner narrative, and relational environment.

Jean Watson's Theory of Human Caring provides a critical theoretical foundation for this orientation. Caring science emphasizes transpersonal relationships, intentional presence, and the moral commitment to honor human dignity (Watson Caring Science Institute, n.d.). In cannabis nursing, these principles become especially relevant, as patients may be navigating stigma, vulnerability, trauma, or existential distress alongside symptom burden. The nurse's role extends beyond information delivery to include the creation of a safe, nonjudgmental space in which patients can explore their experiences with integrity and support.

A spirituality-first approach reframes cannabis not as a stand-alone intervention, but as one component within a broader healing process. When supported by presence, intention, and ethical awareness, cannabis may facilitate emotional regulation, self-reflection, and reconnection. Patients often describe these experiences as meaningful aspects of healing, even when symptoms persist. This perspective invites nurses to attend to what emerges during cannabis related encounters rather than focusing solely on measurable outcomes.

By centering spirituality, cannabis nursing positions healing as relational and contextual. The nurse–patient relationship becomes the primary environment through which trust, meaning making, and integration occur. This orientation prepares the ground for a clinical model that honors the interconnectedness of physical, mental, emotional, social, and spiritual dimensions of health.

A spirituality-first orientation also requires nurses to cultivate reflective and ethical awareness. Because cannabis may influence perception, emotion, or consciousness, nurses must remain attentive to power dynamics, boundaries, and intention. Engaging this work responsibly involves self-reflection, cultural humility, and a willingness to examine personal beliefs about suffering, healing, and altered states. This inner work supports ethical discernment and helps prevent projection, coercion, or overinterpretation of patient experiences.

Within this framework, nonjudgment is understood as an active clinical skill. Patients who use cannabis often carry histories of stigma, marginalization, or dismissal within healthcare settings. A spirituality-first approach calls nurses to meet these patients with curiosity, respect, and openness, recognizing that trust is foundational to therapeutic engagement. When assumptions are suspended and listening is deepened, patients are more likely to share meaningful aspects of their experience that inform holistic assessment and care.

Understanding spirituality as the root of cannabis care also shapes how outcomes are interpreted. Rather than measuring success solely by symptom reduction, this perspective recognizes shifts in meaning, emotional regulation, relational connection, and self-awareness as valid indicators of healing. For some patients, cannabis supported care may not eliminate pain or distress, but it may reduce suffering, restore dignity, or support reconciliation with illness, identity, or life circumstances.

Importantly, centering spirituality does not diminish the role of science or clinical rigor. Instead, it integrates biological understanding, including endocannabinoid system function, within a broader human context. Cannabis nursing therefore bridges physiology and meaning, evidence and experience, and science and lived experience. This integrative stance allows nurses to remain grounded in evidence informed practice while attending to the subjective dimensions of health that are essential to patient care.

The therapeutic use of cannabis is defined as the use of cannabis products for medicinal, wellness, and healing purposes (American Cannabis Nurses Association & American Nurses Association, 2024). While individual experiences of cannabis are subjective, therapeutic use requires clinical discernment and ethical grounding. Within this model, cannabis may be considered therapeutic when its use contributes to improvement in one or more domains of health, including physical, mental, emotional, social, or spiritual, without causing harm or deterioration in others. This multidimensional approach supports holistic evaluation while maintaining professional accountability.

Together, these principles form the foundation of a Spirituality-First Clinical Model. By grounding cannabis nursing in presence, intention, ethical awareness, and relationship centered care, this model provides a coherent framework for practice that reflects the complexity of human healing. The following sections build on this foundation by exploring the interconnected pathways of physical, mental, emotional, social, and spiritual health, translating these domains into clinical applications for holistic, cannabis supported care.

Five Domains of Health

Contemporary models of health recognize that human well-being is multidimensional, interconnected, and relational. Whether described as biopsychosocial-spiritual, whole person, or holistic frameworks, these models converge on five essential domains: physical, mental, emotional, social, and spiritual health. Each domain influences the others in dynamic and bidirectional ways and is shaped by endocannabinoid system tone, lived experience, environment, and meaning making. For cannabis nurses, understanding these domains is a clinical necessity. They provide a structured approach to comprehensive assessment, trauma informed communication, and endocannabinoid system–informed care planning.

Holistic nursing has long recognized that health exists on a continuum shaped by values, beliefs, and meaning rather than symptoms or diagnoses alone (Dossey & Keegan, 2022). The World Health Organization (2022) affirms that well-being includes social, emotional, and spiritual dimensions, while the McKinsey Health Institute highlights that mental, social, and spiritual health are as important as physical health and deeply interconnected (Hartenstein & Latkovic, 2022). Cannabis nursing extends this perspective by acknowledging that phytocannabinoids interact with the endocannabinoid system in ways that influence multiple domains simultaneously.

The Five Domains of Health, physical, mental, emotional, social, and spiritual, provide a foundational assessment framework within cannabis nursing practice. These domains reflect global nursing perspectives, including the World Health Organization's recognition of spirituality as a dimension of well-being (World Health Organization, 2022) and the American Holistic Nurses Association's emphasis on the interconnectedness of body, mind, and spirit (American Holistic Nurses Association, n.d.). Within cannabis care, the Five Domains offer a practical structure for understanding the multidimensional effects of endocannabinoid system dysregulation and cannabinoid therapeutics.

Within the physical domain, cannabis may support the management of pain, inflammation, nausea, muscle tension, and sleep disturbances. Within the mental domain, it may support focus, cognitive flexibility, and a reduction in intrusive thought patterns. Within the emotional domain, cannabis may help reduce hypervigilance and support the expression and processing of emotions that were previously difficult to access. Within the social domain, symptom relief may allow patients to reconnect with relationships, daily activities, and community engagement. Within the spiritual domain, patients may report experiences of restored meaning, inner peace, or a renewed sense of self.

Within the Spirituality-First Clinical Model, these domains are not treated as separate categories but as interconnected pathways through which healing occurs. Nurses assess each domain, identify areas of imbalance or suffering, and support patients in cultivating greater coherence across all dimensions of their lives. This multidimensional approach allows cannabis nursing to move beyond symptom management toward integrated, person-centered care.

Physical Health

Physical health encompasses biological functioning, homeostasis, mobility, sleep, pain modulation, inflammatory balance, and overall physiological resilience. The endocannabinoid system plays a central regulatory role across these processes, influencing nociception, immune response, appetite, and sleep–wake cycles (De Petrocellis & Di Marzo, 2009; Di Marzo et al., 1998). Patients commonly seek cannabis to address pain, inflammation, neuropathy, insomnia, anxiety, and complex symptom clusters associated with chronic or serious illness.

Endocannabinoid scientist Vincenzo Di Marzo described the endocannabinoid system as governing core survival functions, including eating, sleeping, relaxing, forgetting, and protecting, highlighting its role in stress recovery and the restoration of physiological balance following internal or external disruption (Di Marzo et al., 1998). This perspective positions the endocannabinoid system as a biological bridge between stress, physiological regulation, and resilience.

In clinical practice, cannabis may support physical health through modulation of pain perception, reduction of inflammation, improvement in sleep quality, stimulation of appetite, and reduction of somatic tension. Therapeutic response is variable and requires individualized assessment. Nurses evaluate for dose related adverse effects such as dizziness, sedation, orthostatic hypotension, gastrointestinal disturbance, or paradoxical anxiety, while also considering individual differences in metabolism, tolerance, and comorbid conditions.

A holistic nursing approach recognizes that improvement in physical symptoms should not come at the expense of mental, emotional, or social well-being. For example, while cannabis may reduce pain, excessive sedation or cognitive impairment may interfere with daily functioning or relational engagement. Nurses support safe and effective integration through careful titration, ongoing monitoring, and alignment of cannabis use within broader treatment plans.

Within a Spirituality-First Clinical Model, physical health is understood as one expression of the body's capacity to regulate, adapt, and restore balance. Symptom relief may create space for rest, emotional processing, and shifts in perception or meaning. Nurses remain attentive to whether physical interventions support coherence across all domains of health, ensuring that care remains balanced, individualized, and aligned with the patient's overall well-being.

Mental Health

Mental health encompasses cognitive functioning, mood regulation, psychological resilience, and the capacity to process stress and trauma. It includes attention, perception, thought patterns, and executive functioning that influence how individuals interpret and respond to their experiences. Individuals often seek cannabis to support anxiety, depression, posttraumatic stress symptoms, rumination, and sleep related cognitive distress. The endocannabinoid system contributes to the modulation of stress responses, emotional memory, and neural signaling pathways involved in fear, mood, and affect regulation.

In clinical contexts, cannabis may support mental health by reducing anxiety, promoting relaxation, improving sleep continuity, and quieting intrusive thought patterns. Responses are highly individualized and dose dependent. In some individuals, cannabis, particularly products high in tetrahydrocannabinol, may exacerbate anxiety, paranoia, or cognitive disorganization. Nurses remain attentive to mental health history, current diagnoses, and prior responses to cannabis when supporting clinical decision making.

Trauma informed care is essential within cannabis nursing. Patients with trauma histories may demonstrate increased sensitivity to changes in perception or consciousness. While cannabis may reduce hyperarousal or intrusive memories, it may also contribute to dissociation or emotional flooding if not used with intention and support. Nurses assess readiness, provide education, and offer grounding strategies to promote safety and integration.

Mental health assessment within a holistic framework extends beyond symptom reduction to include cognitive clarity, insight, emotional regulation, and functional capacity. Nurses evaluate whether cannabis use enhances or interferes with attention, decision making, and participation in daily life. Therapeutic use supports mental health when it promotes regulation, integration, and adaptive coping rather than avoidance, dependency, or impairment.

Within a Spirituality-First Clinical Model, mental health is understood as interconnected with meaning, identity, and self-awareness. Nurses attend not only to symptom expression but also to how cannabis influences a patient's inner narrative, sense of safety, and capacity for reflection. Presence, nonjudgment, and ethical discernment remain central to supporting mental health within cannabis nursing practice.

Emotional Health

Emotional health involves the capacity to recognize, experience, regulate, and integrate feelings such as fear, grief, anger, joy, and vulnerability. It reflects how individuals process and express affective states in response to internal and external experiences. In healthcare settings, emotional experience is often minimized, yet unprocessed emotion can significantly influence physical symptoms, mental health, and overall well-being. Patients may seek cannabis to soften emotional intensity, facilitate emotional expression, or create space for reflection and self-compassion.

Cannabis supported emotional responses vary widely. For some individuals, cannabis may reduce emotional reactivity, support relaxation, or enhance emotional awareness and insight. For others, it may intensify emotions or bring forward unresolved experiences. Nurses remain attentive to emotional responses that emerge during cannabis use, recognizing when expression supports integration and when it may indicate overwhelm, dysregulation, or distress.

Supporting emotional health requires a balance between allowing authentic expression and maintaining safety. Nurses create environments in which patients can explore emotions without fear of judgment while also providing grounding strategies when emotional experiences become destabilizing. This includes recognizing signs of emotional flooding, dissociation, or avoidance and responding with appropriate clinical support.

A holistic nursing perspective recognizes that emotional health is interconnected with mental clarity, physical comfort, social connection, and spiritual meaning. Therapeutic cannabis use supports emotional health when it fosters integration, resilience, and self-awareness rather than numbing, suppression, or avoidance. Nurses support patients in reflecting on emotional shifts and integrating these experiences into daily life in ways that promote stability and growth.

Within a Spirituality-First Clinical Model, emotional health is understood as a meaningful pathway within the healing process. Emotions are not viewed as problems to eliminate, but as signals that invite attention, compassion, and understanding. Through presence and nonjudgment, nurses support patients in engaging emotional experience as part of a broader process of healing, integration, and self-awareness.

Social Health

Social health reflects the capacity for connection, belonging, communication, and participation within relationships and community. Illness, chronic pain, trauma, and stigma can disrupt social functioning, contributing to isolation, withdrawal, or strained relationships. Patients may seek cannabis to support social engagement, reduce social anxiety, or enhance their sense of connection with others.

Cannabis related social effects vary widely. For some individuals, cannabis may support feelings of connection, empathy, or openness, facilitating communication and relational presence. For others, it may contribute to withdrawal, emotional blunting, or decreased social engagement. Nurses assess how cannabis use influences social roles, relationships, and participation in daily life rather than assuming consistent benefit.

Stigma plays a significant role in shaping social health for individuals who use cannabis. Fear of judgment, concerns about disclosure, and potential legal or workplace consequences may limit access to social support and increase isolation. Nurses help mitigate these effects by fostering nonjudgmental dialogue, validating lived experience, and supporting patients in making thoughtful decisions about disclosure that prioritize safety and personal values.

A holistic nursing approach recognizes that social health is interconnected with physical comfort, mental clarity, emotional regulation, and spiritual meaning. Therapeutic cannabis use supports social health when it enhances connection, communication, and participation without compromising safety, responsibility, or relational trust. Nurses support patients in reflecting on changes in social functioning and integrating cannabis use in ways that align with their values, roles, and relationships.

Within a Spirituality-First Clinical Model, social health is understood as inherently relational and contextual. Healing occurs not only within the individual but also through relationships, community, and shared meaning. Nurses attend to the social dimensions of cannabis use by recognizing cultural context, relational dynamics, and the fundamental human need for belonging and connection.

Spiritual Health

Spiritual health encompasses meaning, purpose, connection, transcendence, and the ways individuals make sense of illness, suffering, and healing. In nursing practice, spirituality is recognized as a core dimension of holistic care, influencing how patients experience symptoms, cope with uncertainty, and navigate life transitions. Patients may engage cannabis as part of reflection, meaning making, or spiritual inquiry, particularly during periods of existential distress, serious illness, or end-of-life care.

Cannabis related spiritual experiences are highly individualized and shaped by cultural, personal, and contextual factors. For some patients, cannabis may support introspection, connection with self or others, or a sense of peace and acceptance. For others, it may evoke discomfort, fear, or confusion. Nurses approach spiritual experience with humility, cultural sensitivity, and respect for diverse belief systems while maintaining clear professional boundaries and avoiding interpretation or validation of spiritual content.

Spiritual assessment within cannabis nursing centers on understanding what provides a patient with meaning, hope, and strength. Rather than directing or shaping spiritual experience, nurses create space for patients to articulate their beliefs, values, and questions. This includes recognizing spiritual distress, loss of meaning, or existential fear, as well as experiences of peace, reconciliation, or acceptance.

A spirituality-first approach emphasizes presence rather than intervention. Nurses offer attentive listening, nonjudgment, and authenticity, recognizing that spiritual processes cannot be prescribed or controlled. Cannabis may support spiritual health when its use is associated with greater coherence, acceptance, or connection, while nurses remain attentive to whether these experiences support integration or contribute to distress.

Within a Spirituality-First Clinical Model, spiritual health is understood as foundational to all other domains. Meaning, purpose, and connection influence physical resilience, mental clarity, emotional integration, and social engagement. By recognizing spiritual health as foundational, cannabis nursing supports whole person care and affirms the importance of meaning and connection within the healing process.

SPIRITUALITY-FIRST CLINICAL MODEL

The Spirituality-First Clinical Model positions spirituality as the central organizing element of cannabis nursing practice rather than an adjunct or optional consideration. Within this model, spirituality informs assessment, presence, ethical discernment, and clinical decision making across all domains of health. Rather than beginning with symptoms or protocols, nurses begin by understanding the patient's meaning making process, values, beliefs, and sources of hope or distress.

This approach reflects principles of holistic nursing and caring science, which recognize the nurse–patient relationship as the primary context for healing. The model emphasizes presence, intentionality, and relational engagement as core clinical competencies. Cannabis is understood not as a stand-alone intervention, but as one component within a broader healing process shaped by relationship, context, and individual experience.

Assessment within the Spirituality-First Clinical Model is dynamic and iterative. Nurses attend to physical symptoms while also exploring emotional patterns, mental clarity, social context, and spiritual meaning. This multidimensional assessment supports identification of imbalance or vulnerability and guides ethical discernment. Nurses evaluate when cannabis use aligns with a patient's values and goals and when it may contribute to harm, avoidance, or dysregulation.

Clinical application of the model requires nurses to cultivate self-awareness and reflective practice. Because cannabis may influence perception, emotion, or consciousness, nurses remain attentive to boundaries, power dynamics, and intention. Engaging a spirituality-first approach involves examining one's own beliefs about healing and suffering while maintaining nonjudgment, humility, and ethical presence in patient interactions.

The Spirituality-First Clinical Model is adaptable across care settings, populations, and stages of illness. Whether supporting symptom management, chronic illness, trauma recovery, or end-of-life care, the model supports nurses in engaging the full complexity of human experience. By centering spirituality, the model affirms that healing extends beyond symptom reduction and includes meaning, dignity, connection, and wholeness.

The H.I.G.H. Framework

The H.I.G.H. Framework, defined as Hope, Inspiration, Growth, and Healing, offers a patient centered lens for understanding the inner experience of healing within cannabis nursing care. While the Spirituality-First Clinical Model guides nursing practice, the H.I.G.H. Framework describes how patients may experience meaning, transformation, and integration throughout the healing process.

Hope reflects the restoration of possibility and forward orientation. Illness, trauma, or chronic suffering may erode hope over time. Therapeutic cannabis use may support moments of relief or ease that reopen a sense of possibility. Nurses support hope by helping patients articulate goals, recognize subtle shifts, and reconnect with meaning without creating unrealistic expectations.

Inspiration involves moments of insight, clarity, or renewed perspective. Cannabis may facilitate reflective states that allow patients to access creativity, reframe experience, or reconnect with personal values. Nurses support inspiration through presence rather than interpretation, allowing insights to emerge while maintaining clinical grounding and safety.

Growth refers to psychological, emotional, or spiritual development that may occur through illness and healing. Cannabis supported experiences may bring forward patterns or emotions that invite reflection and change. Nurses support integration by helping patients process experiences without imposing meaning, direction, or interpretation.

Healing is understood as wholeness rather than cure. It may involve symptom relief, acceptance, reconciliation, or peace, even when disease persists. Nurses assess whether cannabis use supports coherence across domains of health and contributes to dignity and quality of life.

The H.I.G.H. Framework emphasizes that healing is non-linear and deeply individual. Not all patients will experience each element, and no single outcome defines success. By recognizing hope, inspiration, growth, and healing as possible but not prescriptive, cannabis nursing affirms the uniqueness of each patient's experience.

The H.I.G.H. Framework also serves as a reframing tool, using accessible and human centered language to address stigma and fear-based narratives associated with cannabis use. By grounding care in hope, meaning, growth, and healing rather than pathology or judgment, the framework supports more open and compassionate clinical dialogue.

One of the most persistent barriers in cannabis nursing is the fear associated with the term *high*. Many patients, families, and clinicians equate this term with intoxication, impairment, or loss of control. These concerns may be amplified among individuals navigating chronic illness, trauma histories, religious conflict, or the vulnerabilities associated with aging. Misinterpretation of this term may create hesitation or anxiety that limits therapeutic engagement with cannabis.

The H.I.G.H. Framework reframes the term high as an acronym for Hope, Inspiration, Growth, and Healing, restoring a human centered and meaning centered interpretation. Neurobiological research supports this perspective, demonstrating that cannabinoids can influence emotional processing and reduce fear responses (Fusar-Poli et al., 2009; Rabinak & Phan, 2014). These findings suggest that some concerns related to cannabis may be shaped by cultural perception in addition to physiological response.

Nurses play a critical role in helping patients distinguish between therapeutic modulation of consciousness and non-therapeutic use. When approached with education, intention, and individualized dosing, cannabis may support clarity, calm, emotional regulation, and connection while maintaining safety and autonomy.

The Role of Nursing Theory in Cannabis Nursing

Nursing theory provides the conceptual foundation that distinguishes professional nursing practice from task-based care. It offers a shared language for understanding human experience, guiding ethical decision making, and grounding clinical practice in values, relationships, and professional identity. In established specialties, theory shapes education, practice standards, and research agendas. In emerging specialties, it is essential for legitimacy, coherence, and professional integrity.

Cannabis nursing has been recognized as a nursing specialty, yet it continues to evolve within complex clinical, regulatory, and cultural environments. Without a strong theoretical foundation, cannabis related nursing care risks becoming fragmented, protocol driven, or reduced to product knowledge alone. Nursing theory anchors cannabis care within the discipline of nursing, ensuring that practice remains relational, ethical, holistic, and person centered rather than intervention focused.

For emerging specialties, theory serves several critical functions. It clarifies scope and purpose, guides professional standards, supports ethical discernment, and provides a foundation for education and research. Theory also protects nursing practice from being shaped solely by biomedical, commercial, or policy driven influences. In cannabis nursing, where stigma, uncertainty, and rapidly evolving evidence are common, theory offers stability and moral grounding.

Clark (2021) situates cannabis nursing within Watson's Theory of Human Caring in *Cannabis: A Handbook for Nurses*, emphasizing that cannabis therapeutics cannot be separated from presence, intention, relationship, or whole person connection. This work reinforces Caring Science as a foundational framework for cannabis nursing and highlights the importance of grounding practice in relational and ethical principles.

This theoretical grounding aligns with the clinical realities of cannabis nursing, where healing is often reflective, relational, and integrative. Cannabis may support shifts in awareness, emotional processing, and meaning making. When nurses guide patients through cannabis supported care, they are also supporting processes of self-reflection, connection, and personal insight.

According to Watson, healing occurs within a transpersonal caring relationship characterized by authentic presence, empathy, and compassion (Watson, 2008). Within this relational space, patients may feel safe to explore fear, grief, trauma, hope, and meaning. This context is particularly relevant in cannabis nursing, where patients often present with complex symptom burden alongside emotional and existential distress. As physiological regulation improves, some patients may experience increased openness to reflection and communication.

Watson describes meaningful clinical interactions as carative encounters that reflect the essence of nursing as a healing practice (Watson, 2008). In cannabis nursing, these encounters may arise when patients experience relief, insight, or emotional expression within a supportive relational context. While cannabis may influence symptoms, the nurse's presence remains central to facilitating safety, trust, and integration.

Caring science aligns closely with cannabis nursing by emphasizing presence, intentionality, human dignity, and the nurse–patient relationship. By situating cannabis nursing within this framework, the specialty affirms that care extends beyond symptom management to include meaning, wholeness, and ethical engagement.

The following section explores Jean Watson's Caritas Processes as a guiding theoretical framework for cannabis nursing practice, illustrating how caring science informs assessment, presence, and clinical decision making within a Spirituality-First Model of care.

Jean Watson's Caritas Processes Applied to Cannabis Nursing

Jean Watson's Theory of Human Caring provides a foundational nursing framework that centers the moral, ethical, and relational dimensions of care. Central to this theory are the Caritas Processes, which define caring as an intentional, transpersonal practice grounded in compassion, presence, and respect for human dignity. Within cannabis nursing, this framework offers guidance for navigating complex clinical, ethical, and emotional dimensions of care.

The Caritas Processes invite nurses to cultivate loving-kindness, maintain authentic presence, and honor the subjective experiences of patients (Watson, 2008). In cannabis nursing, this includes recognizing patient vulnerabilities related to stigma, fear of judgment, and prior negative healthcare experiences. Nurses practicing within a caring science framework engage cannabis related conversations with openness, humility, and ethical awareness.

Watson's emphasis on the transpersonal caring relationship aligns closely with a spirituality-first orientation. Transpersonal caring extends beyond task-based interactions to engage nurse and patient in a shared human experience that honors meaning, belief, and connection. Within this context, cannabis nursing shifts from a focus on product or intervention toward relational presence, ethical discernment, and patient centered understanding.

The Caritas Processes also support trauma informed care by prioritizing safety, trust, and emotional attunement. Many patients seeking cannabis care have histories of trauma, chronic illness, or marginalization. Watson's framework guides nurses to respond with compassion rather than control, creating environments that support regulation, integration, and healing.

Integrating the Caritas Processes into cannabis nursing practice reinforces that healing is not solely a physiological outcome but a relational and ethical process. Caring science provides a stable theoretical foundation that supports practice grounded in presence, person centered care, and respect for human dignity. Within a Spirituality-First Clinical Model, the Caritas Processes offer a practical pathway for translating theory into everyday clinical encounters.

Caritas Process 1: Practicing Loving-Kindness and Equanimity Within a Caring Consciousness

Jean Watson's first Caritas Process calls nurses to practice loving-kindness and equanimity toward self and others as the ethical foundation of caring (Watson, 2008). Loving-kindness is not sentimentality; it is a disciplined moral stance that recognizes the inherent dignity of every person, regardless of diagnosis, behavior, belief, or circumstance. Equanimity reflects the nurse's capacity to remain emotionally steady, nonreactive, and grounded in the presence of uncertainty, suffering, or difference. Together, these qualities shape the consciousness from which all caring actions emerge.

In cannabis nursing, this Caritas Process is especially relevant. Patients seeking cannabis related care often present with fear, shame, frustration, or mistrust shaped by stigma, legal ambiguity, and prior negative healthcare experiences. Practicing loving kindness requires nurses to suspend judgment, avoid assumptions, and engage each patient with openness and respect. Equanimity supports the nurse's ability to approach cannabis related conversations with steadiness and ethical clarity, even when patient perspectives or goals differ from conventional medical norms.

Loving-kindness in cannabis nursing also extends inward. Nurses practicing in this emerging specialty may encounter moral distress, professional scrutiny, or internal conflict related to policy constraints, institutional culture, or personal beliefs about cannabis. Cultivating self-compassion supports reflective practice, ethical clarity, and professional resilience, reducing the risk of burnout or reactive care. Equanimity allows nurses to hold complexity without urgency to control or correct, fostering thoughtful clinical discernment.

Applied within a Spirituality-First Clinical Model, Caritas Process 1 anchors cannabis nursing practice in presence rather than persuasion. The nurse's grounded and compassionate awareness becomes the therapeutic context within which assessment, education, and shared decision making occur. By embodying loving-kindness and equanimity, cannabis nursing supports an environment of dignity, trust, and psychological safety, creating conditions that support healing across all domains of health.

Caritas Process 2: Being Authentically Present and Enabling Faith–Hope

Jean Watson's second Caritas Process emphasizes the nurse's capacity to be authentically present while enabling faith–hope as a sustaining force in healing (Watson, 2008). Authentic presence extends beyond physical availability and reflects the nurse's willingness to engage fully with the patient's lived experience, uncertainty, and vulnerability. Within caring science, faith–hope is not bound to specific beliefs or outcomes. It reflects an enduring sense of possibility, purpose, and inner orientation toward healing, even in the presence of illness or distress.

In cannabis nursing, authentic presence is especially important, as many patients present with diminished trust in healthcare systems. Prior experiences of dismissal, moral judgment, or symptom minimization may leave patients guarded or hesitant to share openly. By engaging with presence and without agenda, nurses create an environment of safety and respect, allowing patients to express their goals, concerns, and expectations related to cannabis use. This relational presence supports trust and encourages open, meaningful dialogue.

Supporting faith–hope within cannabis care requires careful ethical balance. Nurses do not promise relief, cure, or transformation. Instead, they help patients identify realistic goals and recognize meaningful shifts such as improved sleep, moments of comfort, emotional regulation, or increased engagement in daily life. In this context, faith–hope emerges through acknowledgment of progress, validation of effort, and affirmation of the patient's capacity for self-awareness and informed choice.

Authentic presence also requires nurses to remain engaged when cannabis experiences are uncertain or challenging. Some patients may experience anxiety, disappointment, or unexpected emotional responses. By maintaining presence rather than withdrawing or redirecting prematurely, nurses support patients in processing and integrating these experiences safely. This approach reinforces faith–hope as a form of trust in one's ability to navigate complexity with appropriate support.

Within a Spirituality-First Clinical Model, Caritas Process 2 positions presence as an active therapeutic element of care. The nurse's steady and attentive engagement provides grounding and containment, allowing faith–hope to emerge organically. In cannabis nursing, this Caritas Process supports care that is relational, ethically grounded, and responsive to the patient's evolving experience, while reinforcing resilience, dignity, and the potential for healing.

Caritas Process 3: Cultivating One's Own Spiritual Practices and Transpersonal Self (Going Beyond Ego)

Jean Watson's third Caritas Process calls nurses to cultivate their own spiritual practices and transpersonal self, moving beyond ego-based reactions to engage patients with humility, awareness, and ethical presence (Watson, 2008). This process recognizes that the nurse's inner life, including values, beliefs, assumptions, and emotional regulation, directly influences the quality of care delivered. Cultivating the transpersonal self supports nurses in remaining grounded, open, and responsive rather than reactive.

In cannabis nursing, Caritas Process 3 is particularly important, as conversations about cannabis may evoke strong personal, cultural, and moral beliefs. Nurses may hold implicit assumptions about substance use, altered states of consciousness, or what constitutes appropriate healing. Without reflective awareness, these beliefs may influence communication and clinical judgment, contributing to bias, defensiveness, or premature conclusions. Engaging the transpersonal self allows nurses to recognize internal responses without acting on them, preserving relational safety and ethical integrity.

Cultivating spiritual practices such as reflection, mindfulness, or contemplative inquiry supports nurses in holding space for complex patient experiences. Cannabis related care may surface grief, trauma, existential questioning, or shifts in meaning. Nurses grounded in self-awareness are better prepared to witness these experiences without imposing interpretation, redirecting prematurely, or centering their own comfort or worldview.

Moving beyond ego in cannabis nursing also involves recognizing professional limits and shared humanity. Nurses do not position themselves as authorities over meaning making, spiritual insight, or transformation. Instead, they accompany patients as compassionate witnesses, supporting integration while honoring autonomy and individual belief systems. This approach supports balance within the therapeutic relationship and helps prevent power imbalances.

Within a Spirituality-First Clinical Model, Caritas Process 3 reinforces that ethical cannabis nursing practice begins with self-awareness and humility. By cultivating their own spiritual grounding, nurses strengthen their capacity for discernment, compassion, and presence, supporting care that honors both the patient's lived experience and the nurse's professional responsibility.

Caritas Process 4: Developing and Sustaining a Helping–Trusting Caring Relationship

Jean Watson's fourth Caritas Process emphasizes the development and sustainment of a helping trusting caring relationship as central to healing (Watson, 2008). Trust is not assumed; it is cultivated over time through consistency, transparency, respect, and ethical presence. Within caring science, the helping trusting relationship serves as the relational context in which vulnerability, meaning making, and healing can occur safely.

In cannabis nursing, establishing trust is especially important. Many patients seeking cannabis related care have experienced dismissal, disbelief, or moral judgment within healthcare settings. Others may have concerns related to legal, professional, or social consequences associated with disclosure of cannabis use. A helping trusting relationship begins when nurses communicate reliability and respect, clearly explaining scope of practice, confidentiality, documentation considerations, and clinical boundaries while maintaining a collaborative and patient centered approach.

Sustaining trust requires ongoing relational integrity. Nurses demonstrate trustworthiness by listening attentively, validating lived experience, and honoring patient autonomy, even when clinical recommendations differ from patient preferences. In cannabis nursing, this may involve navigating uncertainty together, adjusting goals, monitoring outcomes across the Five Domains of Health, and responding thoughtfully to both benefit and challenge. Trust deepens when patients experience care as supportive and collaborative rather than directive or controlling.

The helping trusting relationship also supports ethical discernment. When trust is established, patients are more likely to share concerns such as adverse effects, inconsistent use, emotional distress, or changes in motivation. This openness allows nurses to respond proactively, adapting education, safety planning, or referrals as appropriate. In this way, trust functions not only as a relational foundation but also as a component of clinical safety.

Within a Spirituality-First Clinical Model, Caritas Process 4 affirms the nurse patient relationship as the primary medium of care. In cannabis nursing, the helping trusting relationship helps reduce stigma, supports open communication, and anchors care in mutual respect. Through sustained trust, nurses foster therapeutic partnerships that support dignity, safety, and integration within complex and evolving care contexts.

Caritas Process 5: Being Present to, and Supportive of, the Expression of Positive and Negative Feelings

Jean Watson's fifth Caritas Process calls nurses to be present to, and supportive of, the expression of both positive and negative feelings as an essential dimension of caring (Watson, 2008). This process recognizes emotional expression as integral to healing rather than something to be managed, redirected, or minimized. Caring presence invites authenticity, allowing patients to express joy, relief, fear, anger, grief, or disappointment without judgment or urgency to resolve emotion.

In cannabis nursing, Caritas Process 5 is especially relevant because cannabis may influence emotional awareness and reduce emotional defenses. Patients may experience relief, gratitude, or renewed hope, while others may encounter anxiety, sadness, frustration, or unexpected emotional intensity. Nurses remain emotionally attuned, validating a full range of affective experience while maintaining grounding and clinical awareness. Emotional expression is neither pathologized nor idealized but is recognized as meaningful information within holistic assessment.

Supporting emotional expression also requires clinical discernment. Nurses listen for signs that emotions may be becoming overwhelming, dysregulating, or associated with trauma activation. In these moments, presence includes gentle containment through pacing, grounding strategies, and, when appropriate, collaboration on additional support or referral. This balance supports safety while honoring the patient's need for authentic expression.

Caritas Process 5 also invites nurses to reflect on their own relationship with emotion. Cannabis related conversations may evoke strong emotional responses in both patients and nurses, particularly when intersecting with stigma, moral beliefs, or existential concerns. Nurses grounded in self-awareness are better prepared to remain present without defensiveness, avoidance, or premature reassurance, supporting relational safety and trust.

Within a Spirituality-First Clinical Model, Caritas Process 5 affirms emotional expression as a pathway to integration rather than a barrier to care. By remaining present to both ease and distress, cannabis nurses support emotional honesty, resilience, and meaning making. This approach allows emotional experience to inform healing across domains while reinforcing dignity, authenticity, and wholeness.

Caritas Process 6: Creative Use of Self and All Ways of Knowing as Part of the Caring Process

Jean Watson's sixth Caritas Process emphasizes the creative use of self and all ways of knowing, including scientific, experiential, ethical, intuitive, and aesthetic, as integral to the caring process (Watson, 2008). This process affirms that nursing practice is not solely technical or evidence informed, but relational, contextual, and responsive to the uniqueness of each patient encounter. Creative use of self reflects the nurse's ability to integrate multiple forms of knowing while remaining grounded in clinical judgment and ethical responsibility.

In cannabis nursing, Caritas Process 6 is particularly relevant because care unfolds at the intersection of evolving science, lived experience, cultural meaning, and regulatory complexity. Nurses draw upon pharmacological knowledge, endocannabinoid science, symptom assessment, and safety monitoring while also attending to patient narrative, values, intuition, and spiritual context. No single source of knowledge is sufficient; effective cannabis care emerges through thoughtful integration rather than rigid adherence to protocol.

Creative use of self also requires flexibility in communication and patient education. Individuals vary in health literacy, belief systems, and prior experiences with cannabis. Nurses adapt language, metaphors, and teaching approaches to meet patients where they are, translating complex information into meaningful and accessible guidance. This approach supports shared understanding and encourages active patient participation in care.

All ways of knowing are further engaged through reflective practice. Cannabis nursing may involve ambiguity, uncertainty, or multiple interpretations of patient experience. Nurses grounded in Caritas Process 6 reflect on these situations rather than seeking premature resolution, using curiosity and clinical discernment to guide next steps. This reflective stance supports nuanced care and honors the complexity inherent in holistic healing.

Within a Spirituality-First Clinical Model, Caritas Process 6 affirms that integration and creativity are essential components of ethical cannabis nursing practice. By engaging multiple ways of knowing, nurses support individualized care that is informed by science, grounded in experience, and responsive to meaning and context, creating space for healing that is both clinically sound and deeply human.

Caritas Process 7: Engaging in Genuine Teaching Learning Experiences That Attend to Meaning

Jean Watson's seventh Caritas Process centers on engaging in genuine teaching learning experiences that attend to meaning rather than simple information transfer (Watson, 2008). This process reframes education as a relational and reciprocal exchange grounded in respect for the learner's values, readiness, and lived experience. Within caring science, teaching learning is co-created, responsive, and oriented toward understanding rather than compliance.

In cannabis nursing, Caritas Process 7 is especially important because education often determines whether cannabis use is experienced as therapeutic, confusing, or potentially harmful. Patients frequently encounter conflicting information, misinformation, or stigma influenced narratives. Nurses practicing this Caritas prioritize dialogue over directive instruction, inviting patients to share what they understand, what concerns them, and what they hope to achieve. This approach allows education to be tailored to the patient's goals, cultural context, and level of health literacy.

Effective cannabis education includes clarifying intentions and expectations. Nurses support patients in understanding how to use cannabis safely while also exploring the purpose behind its use and evaluating its impact across the Five Domains of Health. Education includes harm reduction principles, dosing considerations, monitoring for adverse effects, and recognizing when adjustments or referrals may be appropriate. Learning becomes meaningful when patients are able to connect information to their lived experience and personal values.

Genuine teaching and learning also requires humility and flexibility. Nurses remain open to patient insight and experience, recognizing that patients are knowledgeable about their own bodies and responses. When outcomes differ from expectations, nurses revisit education collaboratively, framing learning as an ongoing and adaptive process. This approach supports patient empowerment and reduces reliance on directive or prescriptive guidance.

Within a Spirituality-First Clinical Model, Caritas Process 7 affirms education as a relational exchange that honors autonomy, dignity, and meaning. By engaging patients as active participants in learning, cannabis nurses support informed choice, self-awareness, and ethical integration of cannabis into care. This approach strengthens trust and supports healing that is both informed and intentional.

Caritas Process 8: Creating a Healing Environment at All Levels

Jean Watson's eighth Caritas Process emphasizes the creation of a healing environment at physical, emotional, energetic, and relational levels (Watson, 2008). Within caring science, the environment extends beyond the physical setting to include the interpersonal, emotional, and ethical climate in which care occurs. Healing environments support safety, regulation, dignity, and coherence, allowing patients to engage more fully in their healing processes.

In cannabis nursing, Caritas Process 8 is especially relevant because patients may be sensitive to both internal and external stimuli. Cannabis may influence sensory awareness, emotional responsiveness, and sensitivity to environmental stressors. Nurses attend to factors such as privacy, tone of communication, pacing of interaction, and the emotional atmosphere of clinical encounters. Creating a calm and respectful environment supports regulation and grounded engagement, particularly for patients with trauma histories or heightened nervous system sensitivity.

The healing environment in cannabis nursing also extends beyond the clinical setting. Nurses support patients in evaluating home and social environments, including routines, sleep–wake patterns, nutrition, hydration, and sources of emotional support. Guidance may include reducing overstimulation, creating safe and comfortable spaces for use, and incorporating grounding practices that promote stability and regulation. These environmental considerations support assessment of therapeutic impact across the Five Domains of Health.

Relational and ethical environments are equally important. Nurses contribute to healing environments by reducing stigma, maintaining confidentiality, and practicing nonjudgment. When patients experience respect and psychological safety, they are more likely to communicate openly about their experiences, concerns, and challenges. This openness supports clinical monitoring and ethical integration of cannabis into care.

Within a Spirituality-First Clinical Model, Caritas Process 8 affirms that healing environments are co-created through presence, intention, and relationship. By attending to physical, emotional, and relational conditions, cannabis nurses support spaces that foster regulation, meaning making, and dignity, allowing healing to unfold across all domains of health.

Caritas Process 9: Assisting with Basic Needs, with an Intentional Caring Consciousness

Jean Watson's ninth Caritas Process emphasizes assisting with basic human needs while maintaining an intentional caring consciousness (Watson, 2008). This process recognizes that meeting fundamental physiological and functional needs, including comfort, nutrition, rest, mobility, and safety, is inseparable from honoring dignity and wholeness. Caring consciousness transforms routine care into a relational act, ensuring that support for basic needs is delivered with presence, respect, and ethical attentiveness.

In cannabis nursing, Caritas Process 9 is particularly relevant because patients often seek cannabis to address persistent or unmet basic needs such as pain, sleep disturbance, appetite changes, nausea, muscle tension, or autonomic dysregulation. Nurses assess these needs comprehensively and monitor responses carefully, recognizing that cannabis may support function for some patients while presenting risks for others. Intentional caring consciousness guides dosing education, timing, formulation considerations, and safety planning while maintaining a whole person approach to care.

Assisting with basic needs in cannabis nursing also requires attention to adverse effects and functional impact. Nurses monitor for sedation, dizziness, orthostatic changes, cognitive impairment, anxiety, and potential interactions with other therapies. When challenges arise, caring consciousness supports adjustment rather than judgment, encouraging collaborative problem solving, modification of treatment approaches, and incorporation of additional supports that preserve safety and quality of life.

Caritas Process 9 also highlights the interconnected nature of basic needs with emotional, social, and spiritual well-being. Pain, fatigue, and sleep disruption can significantly influence meaning making, relational engagement, and overall resilience. By addressing foundational needs with intention and compassion, nurses support stability across domains and create conditions that allow deeper healing processes to emerge.

Within a Spirituality-First Clinical Model, Caritas Process 9 affirms that attending to basic needs is a relational and ethical responsibility rather than a purely technical task. In cannabis nursing, intentional support of the body reflects respect for the whole person, supporting comfort, function, and dignity while acknowledging the connection between physical experience and inner life.

Caritas Process 10: Opening and Attending to Existential–Spiritual Dimensions of Life and Death

Jean Watson's tenth Caritas Process invites nurses to open and attend to the existential, spiritual, and unknown dimensions of life and death as an integral aspect of caring (Watson, 2008). This process acknowledges that healing extends beyond physical outcomes and includes meaning, mystery, suffering, reconciliation, and transcendence. Caring presence in this domain requires humility, courage, and a willingness to remain with questions that do not have clear or immediate answers.

In cannabis nursing, Caritas Process 10 is especially relevant because patients may seek cannabis during periods of profound existential distress, including serious illness, chronic suffering, trauma recovery, or end-of-life care. Cannabis use may prompt reflection on identity, purpose, mortality, or spiritual beliefs. Nurses do not interpret or validate specific spiritual experiences; rather, they create space for patients to explore and articulate their own meanings, questions, fears, and sources of comfort.

Attending to existential and spiritual dimensions also includes recognizing spiritual distress. Feelings of hopelessness, loss of meaning, fear of death, or disconnection from self or others may arise alongside physical symptoms. Nurses grounded in Caritas Process 10 respond with openness and respect, supporting patients in exploring these concerns while maintaining attention to safety, integration, and appropriate referral when indicated.

Caritas Process 10 also calls nurses to honor the depth and significance of the nurse patient relationship during moments of vulnerability and transition. Presence may take the form of silence, witnessing, gentle inquiry, or compassionate accompaniment. In cannabis nursing, this may include supporting patients as they move through spiritual reflection, emotional reconciliation, or acceptance without imposing belief, direction, or outcome.

Within a Spirituality-First Clinical Model, Caritas Process 10 affirms that existential and spiritual care is foundational to wholeness. By attending to uncertainty and honoring the unknown, cannabis nurses support dignity, meaning, and peace across the continuum of care, particularly when cure is not possible and healing takes quieter and more internal forms.

While the Caritas Processes provide a comprehensive theoretical and ethical framework for cannabis nursing, theory alone does not capture the complexity of lived clinical practice. Nursing knowledge is embodied, relational, and shaped within real encounters influenced by vulnerability, context, and meaning. The following clinical narratives illustrate how a Spirituality-First Clinical Model, the H.I.G.H. Framework, the Five Domains of Health, and Watson's Caritas Processes converge in practice. These examples demonstrate how nurses translate caring science into presence, discernment, and ethical action, revealing cannabis supported care as a relational process grounded in dignity, nonjudgment, and whole person healing.

CLINICAL APPLICATION AND PRACTICE IMPLICATIONS OF THE SPIRITUALITY-FIRST MODEL

Before presenting these narratives, it is important to clarify that they are not formal medical case studies, but clinical vignettes derived from real patient encounters within a national cannabis nursing practice at Holistic Caring & The Green Nurse. These narratives are offered not as prescriptive examples, but as teaching tools that illustrate how spirituality functions as the foundation of cannabis care. All patient names and identifying details have been modified to protect privacy. Each vignette was selected to demonstrate how presence, nonjudgment, cultural humility, the H.I.G.H. Framework, and the Caritas Processes inform healing within cannabis nursing practice.

Viewed through Watson's framework, each narrative reflects a transpersonal caring interaction in which nurse and patient engage beyond traditional clinical roles. The Caritas Processes are evident as nurses establish trust, support emotional expression, facilitate meaning making, and cultivate healing environments that affirm patient dignity and wholeness. Across these vignettes, a consistent pattern emerges in which cannabis care deepens the nurse's capacity for presence, humility, and recognition of patient resilience.

These narratives demonstrate that cannabis nursing extends beyond cannabinoid therapeutics to include relational, ethical, and meaning centered care. Within these encounters, the emergence of Hope, Inspiration, Growth, and Healing, as described in the H.I.G.H. Framework, becomes evident as patients move from distress and fragmentation toward increased coherence, connection, and possibility.

Clinical Exemplar 1: Mabel – From Hospice to Wholeness

When Mabel first entered our care, she was a 70-year-old woman with Stage IV pancreatic cancer who had exhausted conventional treatment options. Her tumor was deemed unresectable, and prior chemotherapy and radiation had not achieved the desired outcomes. She was discharged to hospice care with the understanding that she was nearing the end of life. At the time of her cannabis consultation, she was unable to walk and relied on a wheelchair. Persistent nausea and significant pain limited her ability to eat, and sleep was severely disrupted. Medications intended to reduce symptoms contributed to sedation and disengagement, and she expressed emotional and spiritual distress as she prepared for the possibility of death.

Her stated goal was simple and deeply meaningful: "I just want to sleep and complete my legacy work with my family."

From the initial interaction, care was guided by a Spirituality-First Clinical Model. The encounter began with presence rather than intervention. Time was spent listening to her concerns, fears, and priorities, including unfinished conversations and the meaning she hoped to create in the time remaining.

This approach reflected Caritas Processes in action, including loving kindness, authentic presence, and respect for her lived experience (Watson, 2008).

A comprehensive assessment was conducted that included physical symptoms, emotional and mental state, social context, and spiritual needs. Education was provided regarding the endocannabinoid system and the potential role of cannabinoid-based approaches in symptom support. An individualized, ECS informed care plan was discussed, including general dosing considerations, product types, and safety monitoring. Although her family had previously obtained dispensary products, Mabel chose to wait until she had a clearer understanding and felt prepared to proceed in a structured and informed manner.

Her primary goals included pain management, improved sleep, and the ability to participate meaningfully with her family. She initiated a cannabinoid regimen aligned with these goals, which included CBD dominant formulations, THC containing products for nighttime use, and topical applications for localized discomfort. Education focused on gradual titration, monitoring response, and adjusting use based on tolerance and effect.

This approach supported improved comfort while preserving a sense of agency and participation in her care. Her family was engaged through education on communication, safety considerations, and supportive presence as her symptoms and experiences evolved.

We were never notified of Mabel's passing. Months later, she called from her oncologist's office, her voice trembling with disbelief: "They can't find the cancer. What do I do now?" Mabel reported that imaging obtained through her oncology team showed no evidence of detectable disease. She described improvements in appetite, sleep, and pain, as well as a renewed sense of engagement and purpose. While this outcome was unexpected and cannot be attributed to any single intervention, it represented a significant shift in her clinical course.

From a nursing perspective, this case illustrates the Caritas Processes in practice, including development of trust, support of emotional expression, creation of a supportive environment, and attention to meaning making and spiritual well-being. It also aligns with the Cannabis Nursing Scope and Standards of Practice (American Cannabis Nurses Association & American Nurses Association, 2024), which emphasize relational presence, cultural humility, spiritual assessment, and evidence informed cannabinoid education.

Over time, and in coordination with her medical providers, Mabel reported gradual changes in her use of medications and cannabinoid products. She described learning to adjust her use based on symptom patterns and personal response. As her condition stabilized, she transitioned primarily to hemp derived CBD products, including softgels, tinctures, and topicals, while using small amounts of balanced cannabinoid products as needed for symptom support.

Years into her recovery, Mabel revealed another notable outcome: her husband, who had quietly adopted a similar cannabinoid routine, had also achieved remission from his prostate cancer. They later returned to her native Italy, where Mabel was able to complete the legacy work she had once feared she would never live to finish. These observations reflect individual experiences and are not intended to imply causation or generalizable outcomes.

Mabel's story is not presented as a promise or a prescriptive model of care. It is offered as a teaching narrative, a meaningful example of what may emerge when cannabis nursing embraces spirituality as assessment, presence as intervention, nonjudgment as ethical foundation, intention setting as part of care, and meaning making as medicine. Her journey reflects that cannabis care is not solely about cannabinoids; it is about connection, dignity, and the unfolding of human resilience within a supportive and intentional care context. Through the guidance of the Caritas Processes and the Spirituality-First

Clinical Model, Mabel's story illustrates how presence, intention, and relational care may support a renewed sense of engagement and possibility.

Clinical Exemplar 2: Sister Sally – From Suffering to Sacred Renewal

Sister Sally was a 70-year-old retired nun whose life had long been defined by devotion, service, and spiritual discipline. Her journey, however, was marked by prolonged and misunderstood suffering. Following an incorrect diagnosis of multiple sclerosis years earlier, she endured decades of polypharmacy and invasive interventions, including lidocaine infusions and implantation of a spinal neurotransmitter stimulator. The cumulative trauma from these treatments, combined with unrelenting pain, profoundly altered her life. After experiencing adverse effects from medications prescribed for a condition she did not have, she suffered a fall that resulted in a stroke. She awoke in the hospital with Complex Regional Pain Syndrome, leaving her in chronic, severe pain that no conventional therapy had adequately relieved.

When Sister Sally was referred to Holistic Caring & The Green Nurse, she was using 400 mcg fentanyl patches every 36 hours and continued to experience significant pain. Her suffering affected every domain of her health, limiting her ability to engage in daily life and reducing her time out of bed. Although she remained connected to her faith community, she described a growing sense of disconnection from her church, her purpose, and her identity. Her goals were both simple and profound: relief from pain, a return to prayer within her church, and restoration of her life.

From the beginning, care was guided by a Spirituality-First Clinical Model. The encounter began with presence rather than intervention. Sister Sally shared her experience of suffering, her theological concerns about cannabis, and her desire to heal in a way that aligned with her values. This dialogue reflected multiple Caritas Processes in practice, including loving kindness, authentic presence, and respect for belief systems without judgment (Watson, 2008).

Following this initial engagement, education was provided on a gentle, stepwise titration approach. Sister Sally was introduced to foundational principles of cannabinoid use, including CBD dominant formulations for baseline support, THC containing formulations for breakthrough symptoms, and balanced cannabinoid options for microdosing. She chose not to use inhaled forms of cannabis, instead utilizing tinctures, capsules, and oils as part of her self-directed routine following education and ongoing support.

Approximately three months into her regimen, Sister Sally reported a gradual reduction in pain intensity. As her comfort improved, she expressed readiness to begin tapering her opioid medication. In collaboration with her prescribing physician, her fentanyl patch dosage was reduced over the course of a year. During this time, nursing support focused on education, presence, and guidance in micro titration to help her adjust cannabinoid use based on symptom response. Each stage of this process required careful attention to safety, reassurance, and alignment with her goals.

One moment remains especially meaningful. On the day she removed her final fentanyl patch, she called and said, "It's my last day wearing the fentanyl patch. Do you think I can really do this?" With support and preparation, she successfully completed the taper.

She reported that she did not require escalation of THC or emergency dosing. Her use of cannabinoid formulations supported her comfort and stability during opioid tapering. Over time, she transitioned away from higher THC formulations and primarily used hemp derived cannabinoid products, including full spectrum softgels and broad-spectrum formulations, with occasional use of a balanced cannabinoid full spectrum product for sleep support as needed.

As her physical symptoms improved, other aspects of her life began to shift. She returned to prayer, deepened her meditation practice, resumed gardening, and reengaged with her church community. She described a renewed sense of connection, identity, and purpose. Importantly, she did not experience cannabis as conflicting with her faith, but rather as something that supported her ability to live it.

In a later reflection, Sister Sally shared, "Cannabis is not the devil's lettuce. It's the Lord's kale. God created it, and He would expect us to use His gifts wisely."

This case reflects key elements of the Cannabis Nursing Scope and Standards of Practice (American Cannabis Nurses Association & American Nurses Association, 2024), including cultural humility, respect for worldview, and the integration of spirituality into patient education and care. It also aligns with guidance from the National Council of State Boards of Nursing (2018), emphasizing nonjudgment, patient education, and safety.

At its core, Sister Sally's experience extended beyond pain management and opioid reduction. It reflected a return to wholeness, identity, faith, and self-compassion. Through the integration of presence, trust, intention, and the Caritas Processes within a Spirituality-First Clinical Model, this case illustrates how cannabis nursing may function as a supportive bridge from suffering toward greater stability, meaning, and connection.

Clinical Exemplar 3: My Mother Madeline – From Fear to Freedom

Madeline was 75 years old when she began her cannabis journey, long after she believed such a thing could ever be possible for her. She carried decades of cultural, familial, and religious stigma surrounding the plant and made it clear that she disapproved not only of cannabis, but of me using it as medicine, and even more so of me becoming a cannabis nurse. "What would they think?" she would say, invoking an unnamed audience of neighbors, relatives, and imagined critics whose judgment held more weight than the suffering she endured. No amount of research I shared made a difference. Her answer was always the same: "No. You are sinning."

Ironically, it was Sister Sally's story that softened something in her. Listening to a former nun speak of cannabis as "the Lord's kale," a gift rather than a temptation, opened a door my mother had kept closed for years. She began to wonder whether it was her suffering, rather than the plant, that truly conflicted with her beliefs. "If it could help me," she said hesitantly, "wouldn't it be a sin not to try it?"

Her suffering was longstanding. She lived with chronic pain related to orthopedic injuries, osteoarthritis, multiple procedures, and years of interventions that had not provided sustained relief. She had trialed various opioid medications, which contributed to gastrointestinal distress and cognitive fog without adequately addressing her pain. Her goals were modest and deeply personal: to experience less pain, improve sleep, and feel more present in her life. Despite this, fear remained a significant barrier.

She was afraid of feeling high.

Afraid of losing control.

Afraid of judgment.

Afraid of violating the moral framework she had lived by for decades.

The Caritas Processes were applied with patience and intention. Fear was met with loving-kindness, and trust was built through authentic presence and nonjudgment. Education was offered gradually, and care unfolded in alignment with her readiness. This was not only a clinical interaction, but a relational encounter shaped by generational beliefs, cultural narratives, and spiritual reflection.

The process began with a very small and non-threatening step: a CBD isolate topical. This initial approach avoided psychoactive effects and respected her concerns about safety and control.

When she experienced relief, she quietly asked, "This helps… could it be better?"

That question marked a turning point. Progression occurred gradually and in alignment with her comfort level:

- CBD isolate topical
- CBD isolate topical with CBD isolate tincture used sublingually
- CBD isolate topical with broad spectrum CBD tincture
- Full spectrum CBD topical with full spectrum CBD tincture containing trace THC
- Introduction of a low dose THC product when she expressed readiness

When she became curious about experiencing a mild psychoactive effect, education was provided regarding THC dosing and strategies to reduce potential discomfort. She expressed interest in a THC infused chocolate product and was encouraged to begin with a low dose, monitor her response, and adjust gradually. She was also informed that CBD could be used if the effects felt too intense and was reassured that support was available if needed.

She did not call that evening, so I reached out the next day.

Her voice carried a hint of humor. "Sherri… I didn't take one square. I ate three. Now I know what it feels like to be high. It wasn't awful, but it was too much for me. I didn't like it, but at the same time it was kind of fun. Now I know my dose, and I won't do that much again."

What followed was not simply symptom relief, but meaningful change. Her pain became more manageable. Sleep improved. Irritability decreased. She described feeling more like herself and more engaged in her life.

Her experience was so impactful that she chose to share it publicly. When asked what it meant to feel well without feeling high, she said:

> "I finally feel good. My pain has become background noise. I sleep. I laugh. I'm not as grumpy or mean. I'm not so depressed about my problems. I'm not high, I'm better."

Her journey reflects the principles of the Spirituality-First Clinical Model. She moved through stigma, fear, and moral conflict with support grounded in presence, education, and respect for her beliefs. The process supported not only physical comfort, but also emotional and relational well-being.

This case also aligns with the Cannabis Nursing Scope and Standards of Practice (American Cannabis Nurses Association & American Nurses Association, 2024), including respect for worldview, reduction of stigma, and integration of spirituality into care. It reflects the nonjudgmental approach emphasized by the National Council of State Boards of Nursing (2018), particularly when supporting individuals navigating deeply held belief systems.

For me, this journey became a lesson in humility, patience, timing, and love. It showed me how healing can unfold when patients, especially those we hold close, are given the space to come to it in their own way. Her story reinforced something I have learned again and again in cannabis nursing: that presence matters deeply, and that connection often carries a kind of healing we cannot fully quantify.

Synthesis of Clinical Narratives: Cannabis Nursing as Transpersonal Caring

The stories of Mabel, Sister Sally, and my mother Madeline illustrate what may emerge when cannabis nursing is guided by the Caritas Processes and grounded in the spiritual dimensions of care. Across each narrative, change begins not with cannabinoids, but with presence, a willingness to sit with suffering, listen without judgment, honor fear, and create space for meaning. Within these encounters, the nurse does not solely address symptoms; the nurse contributes to the healing environment through authentic presence, compassion, and relational engagement that extend beyond conventional clinical interactions (Watson, 2008).

Across these narratives, the importance of nonjudgment, as emphasized in the National Council of State Boards of Nursing guidelines (2018), and the integration of spirituality and worldview described in the Cannabis Nursing: Scope and Standards of Practice (American Cannabis Nurses Association & American Nurses Association, 2024), are evident in practice. Whether supporting end-of-life care, opioid tapering, spiritual conflict, or stigma-related barriers, the nurse helps create conditions that support clarity, autonomy, and resilience. By honoring the patient's lived experience and inner world, trust is established, forming the foundation for therapeutic engagement.

The Caritas Processes are reflected throughout these cases, not as isolated steps, but as an integrated approach to care. Loving-kindness helps soften fear, authentic presence reduces isolation, and support for emotional expression restores dignity. Intentionality guides care decisions, and co-created healing environments support patients in reconnecting with themselves, their relationships, and their sense of meaning. Within this context, cannabis may serve as one component of care, supporting comfort, insight, and engagement in ways that align with individual goals and experiences.

Historically and cross-culturally, cannabis has been used in contexts that extend beyond symptom management, including ritual, reflection, and healing practices. Within cannabis nursing, the plant may be understood not only as a pharmacologic agent, but as part of a broader relational and experiential process. When used intentionally and safely, patients may report increased self-awareness, emotional processing, and a greater capacity for reflection, which can support the relational and holistic aims of nursing care.

In many ways, these observations align with Watson's conceptualization of caring as a moral and relational practice rooted in compassion, presence, and authentic engagement (Watson, 2008). Some patients report that cannabis use may reduce fear, enhance interoceptive awareness, and create space for reflection, allowing for greater emotional clarity and meaning making. While these experiences are subjective and not universal, they may support processes that are consistent with transpersonal caring.

These narratives illustrate this variability. Across different clinical contexts, patients described not only changes in physical symptoms, but also shifts in emotional, relational, and existential domains. Many described a return to a sense of self, coherence, or connection, reflecting the interconnected nature of healing across the mind, body, and spirit.

From a holistic nursing perspective, cannabis may function as both a biological and experiential support. Physiologically, cannabinoids may influence pain, sleep, appetite, inflammation, and emotional regulation. Experientially, some patients describe increased awareness of internal states, including emotional needs, unresolved experiences, or areas requiring attention. These responses vary widely and require careful education, monitoring, and individualized support.

These cases also highlight the impact of cannabis nursing on the nurse. The work calls for humility, presence, and deep listening, inviting attunement not only to symptoms, but to meaning, belief, and lived experience. It reinforces the importance of nonjudgmental care and the ethical responsibility to support patients without imposing interpretation or expectation.

To describe cannabis as a meaningful component of care is not to elevate it beyond scientific understanding or assign it inherent transformative properties. Rather, it acknowledges that, within appropriate clinical and relational contexts, cannabis may support experiences that contribute to comfort, reflection, and engagement. The role of the nurse is not to ascribe meaning, but to create a safe, informed, and supportive environment in which patients can explore their own experiences.

Across these narratives, the emergence of Hope, Inspiration, Growth, and Healing, as described in the H.I.G.H. Framework, becomes visible as patients move from distress and fragmentation toward greater coherence, connection, and possibility.

FUTURE RESEARCH DIRECTIONS

Future research is needed to further examine the role of spirituality-centered cannabis nursing and its impact on patient outcomes, provider well-being, and healthcare systems. While emerging evidence supports the therapeutic potential of cannabinoids for symptom management, less is known about how relational, spiritual, and meaning centered approaches influence clinical outcomes, patient satisfaction, and quality of life. Investigating these dimensions may help clarify how cannabis nursing contributes to whole-person care across diverse populations and settings.

Specific areas for future inquiry include evaluation of the H.I.G.H. Framework as a clinical model, including its influence on patient-reported outcomes such as hope, resilience, emotional regulation, and perceived quality of life. Research is also needed to examine how the integration of spiritual assessment and caring science principles into cannabinoid education and care planning affects patient engagement, adherence, and safety. Mixed-methods and qualitative studies may be particularly valuable in capturing the lived experience of patients, as well as the relational and existential aspects of healing that are not easily measured through traditional biomedical approaches.

Further investigation into nursing practice is warranted, including the impact of cannabis nursing on provider well-being, moral distress, and professional fulfillment. As nurses navigate evolving regulatory landscapes and ethically complex care environments, understanding how spirituality-informed practice influences burnout, resilience, and job satisfaction will be important for workforce sustainability. Additionally, research exploring competency development, educational standards, and scope-of-practice clarity will support the continued professionalization of cannabis nursing as an emerging specialty.

There is also a need for research that addresses health equity and access. Cannabis-based care remains shaped by regulatory variability, socioeconomic barriers, and persistent stigma. Future studies should examine disparities in access to cannabinoid therapies, culturally responsive care models, and the role of nurses in advocating for safe, equitable, and informed use across communities. Inclusion of diverse populations in research, including older adults, patients with complex chronic conditions, and those from historically marginalized groups, is essential.

Advances in cannabinoid science, including minor cannabinoids, terpene profiles, and personalized dosing strategies, present additional opportunities for research. Integrating this evolving science with nursing frameworks such as the Caritas Processes and the Five Domains of Health may support more individualized and effective care models. Interdisciplinary collaboration among nurses, clinicians, researchers, and patient advocates will be critical in translating emerging evidence into practice.

As the field continues to evolve, future research should aim not only to evaluate outcomes, but also to define best practices that honor both scientific evidence and the relational, ethical, and spiritual dimensions of care. Through continued inquiry and collaboration, cannabis nursing has the potential to contribute to a more integrative, patient-centered approach to health and healing. This emerging body of research will be essential in shaping the ethical, clinical, and educational foundations of cannabis nursing as a recognized specialty within professional nursing practice.

CONCLUSION: SPIRITUALITY IS THE ROOT OF CANNABIS CARE

"From spirit to symptom, healing begins the moment we remember that spirit leads the way. Cannabis may open the door, but it is our presence, our love, and our willingness to truly see the human before us that makes the journey meaningful." Nurse Sherri Mack

Spirituality is not an accessory or enhancement to cannabis nursing; it is a foundational dimension upon which this specialty is grounded. Across cultures, histories, and clinical encounters, a consistent theme emerges: healing is not solely the reduction of pain, distress, or disease. Healing also involves the restoration of meaning, identity, connection, agency, dignity, and a sense of wholeness.

Cannabis nursing, when practiced with intention and integrity, may be understood as both a clinical and relational discipline. It invites nurses to meet patients at deeper levels of experience, where suffering is contextualized, fear may soften in the presence of compassion, and individuals reconnect with aspects of self that illness or stigma may have obscured. This work requires humility, curiosity, cultural sensitivity, and a willingness to engage with the complexity of human experience.

Throughout this chapter, spirituality is woven through each dimension of cannabis nursing. The Five Domains of Health highlight the interconnectedness of physical, emotional, mental, social, and spiritual well-being. The H.I.G.H. Framework, Hope, Inspiration, Growth, and Healing, offers a structure for understanding the internal shifts that may occur as patients reconnect with themselves through ECS informed care. These frameworks align with professional nursing standards, including the Cannabis Nursing: Scope and Standards of Practice (American Cannabis Nurses Association & American Nurses Association, 2024) and NCSBN guidelines (2018), which emphasize the importance of meaning making, worldview, and nonjudgment in ethical nursing care.

Jean Watson's Theory of Human Caring and the Ten Caritas Processes provide the ethical and philosophical grounding for this work. Watson describes caring as a relational and moral practice rooted in authentic presence, loving kindness, and respect for the whole person (Watson, 2008). When integrated with cannabinoid-based care, these principles may support a shift from task-oriented interventions toward more holistic, person-centered engagement. Within a caring relationship, cannabis may serve not only as a therapeutic agent, but also as part of a broader process that supports insight, emotional integration, and self-awareness.

The clinical narratives of Mabel, Sister Sally, and my mother Madeline illustrate these principles in practice. In each case, change began with presence, listening, humility, and nonjudgment. These stories demonstrate that cannabis nursing is inherently relational and that meaningful outcomes are often shaped by the quality of the nurse patient interaction as much as by the interventions themselves.

Whether supporting end-of-life care, opioid tapering, or the resolution of long held stigma, these narratives reflect the importance of addressing both physiological and existential dimensions of care. They demonstrate how the Caritas Processes may be expressed through practice, including the cultivation of trust, support of emotional expression, creation of healing environments, and openness to meaning making.

In some patient experiences, cannabis is described as facilitating reflection, emotional awareness, or a renewed sense of connection. While these responses are subjective and vary across individuals, they may contribute to processes of coping, adaptation, and integration. From a nursing perspective, the role is not to assign meaning to these experiences, but to support patients in exploring them safely and within an appropriate clinical and relational context.

Ultimately, spirituality may be understood as a foundational element of cannabis nursing because it reflects a core principle of nursing itself: the recognition of the person as more than a diagnosis. Historical and contemporary nursing frameworks, from Nightingale to Watson to modern professional standards, emphasize the importance of presence, connection, and respect for the individual's inner experience.

Cannabis nursing exists at the intersection of science and lived experience, integrating neurobiological understanding with relational and ethical care. When nurses lead with presence, uphold nonjudgment, and respect the patient's worldview, cannabis-based care may support not only symptom management, but also broader dimensions of well-being.

This is the essence of the specialty.

This reflects the core of caring science.

This represents an evolving direction for holistic nursing practice.

REFERENCES

American Cannabis Nurses Association & American Nurses Association. (2024). *Cannabis nursing: Scope and standards of practice* (2nd ed.). American Nurses Association. https://www.nursingworld.org/nurses-books/cannabis-nursing-scope-and-standards-of-practice

American Holistic Nurses Association. (n.d.). *What is holistic nursing?* https://www.ahna.org/About-Us/What-is-Holistic-Nursing

Blesching, U. (2022). *The cannabis health index: Mind, body, spirit guide to a healthy endocannabinoid system* (3rd ed.). North Atlantic Books.

Clark, C. S. (2021). *Cannabis: A handbook for nurses* (1st ed.). Wolters Kluwer Health.

de Brito Sena, M. A., Moreira-Almeida, A., Koenig, H. G., Vallada, H., & Lucchetti, G. (2021). Defining spirituality in healthcare: A systematic review and concept analysis. *Frontiers in Psychology*, *12*, 756080. DOI: 10.3389/fpsyg.2021.756080 PMID: 34867654

De Petrocellis, L., & Di Marzo, V. (2009). An introduction to the endocannabinoid system: From the early to the latest concepts. *Best Practice & Research. Clinical Endocrinology & Metabolism*, *23*(1), 1–15. DOI: 10.1016/j.beem.2008.10.013 PMID: 19285257

Di Marzo, V., Melck, D., Bisogno, T., & De Petrocellis, L. (1998). Endocannabinoids: Endogenous cannabinoid receptor ligands with neuromodulatory action. *Trends in Neurosciences*, *21*(12), 521–528. DOI: 10.1016/S0166-2236(98)01283-1 PMID: 9881850

Dossey, B. M., & Keegan, L. (2022). *Holistic nursing: A handbook for practice* (9th ed.). Jones & Bartlett Learning., https://www.jblearning.com/catalog/productdetails/9781284196528

Fusar-Poli, P., Crippa, J. A., Bhattacharyya, S., Borgwardt, S., Allen, P., Martin-Santos, R., Seal, M., Surguladze, S. A., O'Carroll, C., Atakan, Z., Zuardi, A. W., McGuire, P. K., & Stone, J. M. (2009). Distinct effects of Δ9-tetrahydrocannabinol and cannabidiol on neural activation during emotional processing. *Archives of General Psychiatry*, *66*(1), 95–105. DOI: 10.1001/archgenpsychiatry.2008.519 PMID: 19124693

Hartenstein, L., & Latkovic, T. (2022). *The secret to great health? Escaping the healthcare matrix.* McKinsey Health Institute. https://www.mckinsey.com/mhi/our-insights/the-secret-to-great-health-escaping-the-healthcare-matrix

Lu, H. C., & Mackie, K. (2016). An introduction to the endogenous cannabinoid system. *Biological Psychiatry*, *79*(7), 516–525. DOI: 10.1016/j.biopsych.2015.07.028 PMID: 26698193

Mack, E. (2020). *Cannabis for health: Become a coach.* AuthorHouse. https://www.authorhouse.com/en/bookstore/bookdetails/805950-cannabis-for-health

Mack, S. (2026). Medical, recreational, and wellness: Understanding cannabis use across contexts. Ask The Green Nurse Substack https://thegreennurse.substack.com/p/medical-recreational-and-wellness

National Council of State Boards of Nursing. (2018). The NCSBN national nursing guidelines for medical marijuana. *Journal of Nursing Regulation*, *9*(2, Suppl.), S5–S46. DOI: 10.1016/S2155-8256(18)30082-6

Rabinak, C. A., & Phan, K. L. (2014). Cannabinoid modulation of fear extinction brain circuits: A novel target to advance anxiety treatment. *Current Pharmaceutical Design*, *20*(13), 2212–2217. DOI: 10.2174/13816128113199990437 PMID: 23829364

Rogers, M., Stephenson, J., Ali, G., Andrews, C., Curran, S., Gulliksen, E., Kra-Friedman, A., Ali, N., Lamarche, K., Niu, Y., Slater, H., & Pike, J. (2025). Advanced practice nurse perceptions of spirituality: A global quantitative perspective in everyday life and practice settings. *Journal of Holistic Nursing*, 08980101251377815. Advance online publication. DOI: 10.1177/08980101251377815 PMID: 41148204

U.S. Department of Health and Human Services. (2023). *Basis for the recommendation to reschedule marijuana under the Controlled Substances Act.* https://www.hhs.gov/about/news/2023/08/30/hhs-recommends-marijuana-rescheduling.html

Watson, J. (2008). *Nursing: The philosophy and science of caring* (Rev. ed.). University Press of Colorado., https://upcolorado.com/university-press-of-colorado/item/1849-nursing-revised-edit

Watson Caring Science Institute. (n.d.). *The 10 Caritas Processes®*. In *Caring science theory*. Retrieved December 1, 2025, from https://www.watsoncaringscience.org/caring-science-theory/10-caritas-processes/

Winkelman, M. (2010). *Shamanism: A biopsychosocial paradigm of consciousness and healing* (2nd ed.). Praeger., https://api.pageplace.de/preview/DT0400.9780313381829_A24399361/preview-9780313381829_A24399361.pdf DOI: 10.5040/9798216014133

World Health Organization. (2022). *Achieving well-being: A draft global framework for integrating well-being into public health utilizing a health promotion approach*. World Health Organization. https://www.who.int/publications/m/item/achieving-well-being

KEY TERMS AND DEFINITIONS

Cannabinoid Therapeutics: The clinical application of cannabinoids and related compounds to support physiological regulation, symptom management, and overall well-being within an evidence informed and patient centered framework.

Cannabis Nursing: A nursing specialty focused on the ethical, evidence informed, and holistic integration of cannabis and cannabinoid therapeutics into patient centered care across diverse populations and clinical settings.

Caring Science: A nursing philosophy grounded in Jean Watson's Theory of Human Caring that emphasizes transpersonal relationships, intentional presence, compassion, and a moral commitment to honoring human dignity and wholeness.

Caritas Processes: Ten guiding principles within Jean Watson's Theory of Human Caring that describe caring as a moral, relational, and transpersonal practice that supports healing, dignity, and meaning making.

Endocannabinoid System (ECS): A complex biological regulatory system composed of endogenous cannabinoids, receptors, and enzymes that supports homeostasis across physiological, emotional, cognitive, and immune functions.

Five Domains of Health: An integrated framework encompassing physical, mental, emotional, social, and spiritual dimensions of well-being, used in cannabis nursing to guide holistic assessment and evaluation of therapeutic outcomes.

H.I.G.H. Framework: A spirituality centered framework describing the inner dimensions of healing, Hope, Inspiration, Growth, and Healing, that may emerge during ethically guided therapeutic cannabis care.

Spirituality First Clinical Model: A holistic nursing model that places spirituality, meaning making, and relational presence at the foundation of cannabis nursing assessment, clinical decision making, and care planning.

Therapeutic Use of Cannabis: The use of cannabis products for medicinal, wellness, or healing purposes, supported by professional nursing guidance and evaluated through changes in one or more domains of health while prioritizing safety.

Transpersonal Caring: A caring relationship that extends beyond physical interaction, engaging nurse and patient in authentic presence, shared humanity, and connection beyond roles, diagnoses, or tasks.

Trauma Informed Cannabis Care: An approach to cannabis nursing that recognizes the prevalence and impact of trauma, prioritizes safety and autonomy, and integrates presence, nonjudgment, and ethical discernment into care delivery.

Chapter 10
Cannabis Nursing Administration:
U.S. Workplace Regulations and Cannabis Case Management

Janice Putnam
http://orcid.org/0009-0003-6211-2411
American Cannabis Nurses Association, USA

Michelle Zang
http://orcid.org/0009-0006-4527-981X
American Cannabis Nurses Association, USA

ABSTRACT

This chapter will focus on nursing leadership, particularly nursing administration, as a critical component of fostering safety, quality, collaboration, and policy in the evolving specialties of cannabis nursing care and case management. Significant nursing administrative actions for cannabis care are from within the framework of the core values of the 2024 Cannabis Nursing Scope and Standards of Practice: Evidence-Based Practice Application Of Caring And Social Justice Ethics Cannabis Health Care Consumer-Centered Care Interprofessional Health Care Teamwork The chapter will provide cannabis nurse leaders with distinct legal, ethical, and practice considerations for navigating cannabis nursing care. Specifically, this chapter will address the conflict between federal and state laws and how these regulations continue to impact the policy landscape of cannabis healthcare operations, including regulation, administrative leadership, ethics, and advocacy, as well as the management of cannabis nursing education, competence, and stigmas.

DOI: 10.4018/979-8-3373-7287-7.ch010

INTRODUCTION

To support patients using cannabis legally, nurse leaders are addressing evidence-based knowledge gaps, creating safe hospital policies, advocating for clarity in legal regulations between federal and state laws, and enhancing nursing education through the development of standards for curricula.

Cannabis administration is crucial for promoting safety, quality, collaboration, and effective policy. The role of nursing administration leadership in cannabis care is to address the challenges created by the conflict between federal and state laws by developing clear, evidence-based policies within the framework of the values outlined in the Cannabis Nursing Scope and Standards of Practice (American Nurses Association and American Nurses Association, 2024).

This chapter provides cannabis nurse administrators with distinct legal, ethical, and practice considerations for cannabis care nursing administration. Various issues surrounding the current state of nursing administration for cannabis care, including the conflict between federal and state laws and their impact on workplaces, are presented.

This chapter then explores the future of hybrid case management, which combines case management with cannabis care nursing, as a bridge for nursing administration through legal, ethical, and advocacy issues. This is particularly true as the landscape of medicinal cannabis use evolves. Specialty cannabis case managers provide evidence-based, client-centered care. Cannabis case managers navigate legal intricacies by educating patients, health teams, and advocating for cannabis harm reduction (Clark, 2022).

After reading this chapter, one should be able to discuss the impact cannabis care has on nursing administration for:

1. Creating policy to address the legal challenges of the federal vs. state laws conflict,
2. Demanding new protocols for medical cannabis safety and use documentation,
3. Increasing the need for patient access to medication advocacy
4. Highlighting significant and ongoing staff education gaps for medicinal cannabis

5. Supporting cannabis care case management

BACKGROUND

In 2017, *The Health Effects of Cannabis and Cannabinoids* reported strong evidence for cannabis in treating chronic pain, nausea and vomiting from chemotherapy, and spasticity in multiple sclerosis. Today, in many places across the United States, nurse administrators are managing facility policies for cannabis use by patients and employees. Nurse administrators play a critical role in monitoring federal regulations, balancing patient rights, promoting workplace safety, enforcing dispensing standards, strategizing case management, and ensuring insurance coverage (American Nurses Association [ANA], 2016; Ryan, 2021).

Nurse administrators are encountering barriers caused by federal illegality conflicting with state-level legalization. These barriers exist for inpatients using cannabis and may be a risk for opioid use (Kurtzman, 2022). Medical cannabis use varies significantly by state-level legalization status, while legal concerns and education deficits deter patients from disclosing cannabis use or concerns with healthcare providers (Perlman et al., 2021; Ryan & Sharts-Hopko, 2017).

Federal Cannabis Law Landscape

In 1970, President Nixon signed Title II of the Comprehensive Drug Abuse Prevention and Control Act (CSA) into law, unifying drug laws into a single, unified framework for regulating controlled substances (U.S.C. § 824) (Comprehensive Drug Abuse Prevention Control Act of 1970, 1970). The CSA established a federal control system over the manufacture, importation, possession, and distribution of controlled substances with a five-tiered scheduling system that classifies drugs based on risk for abuse and medical use. Cannabis is a Schedule I drug under federal law because the U.S. government has determined cannabis has a high potential for abuse, no accepted medical use, and no safe administration guidelines (Department of Justice/Drug Enforcement Agency Drug Fact Sheet: Marijuana/Cannabis, 2020). Soon after, all states also adopted either the model Uniform Controlled Substances Act or a similar piece of legislation that aligned state and federal drug laws (Braun, 1991; King, n.d.). Having aligned state and federal drug laws prevented the types of policy gaps and conflicts seen today.

Why do the federal authorities not actively supersede state law? It is a matter of policy, constitutional principle, and the 2013 "Cole" memo. In the 2013 memo, the Department of Justice narrowed law enforcement to marijuana and gangs, distribution to minors, and transport across state lines (*Guidance Regarding Marijuana Enforcement*, 2013). This ongoing federal classification prohibition creates a "conflict of law" with state legislated cannabis use laws (Lampe et al., 2024). The federal status of cannabis creates barriers to its integration into the mainstream healthcare system. This conflict causes a disconnect between state-level legal access and federal-level legal access, as well as financial and operational compliance. Schedule I classification of cannabis has also hindered cannabis-related research (Mead, 2019; Ryan, 2021).

State Cannabis Law Landscape

The state of state cannabis laws encompasses a diverse set of differing regulations (Bryan, 2024). Historically, Colorado legalized medical use in 2000 and recreational use in late 2012. In 1996 and 2026, California legalized medical and then recreational cannabis.

Each state has laws legalizing cannabis for medical and recreational use, medical use only, or complete prohibition. Decriminalized cannabis means it is still illegal, but penalties are reduced, typically from criminal charges to civil fines (2019 State of States Report, 2019). One of the most restrictive states is North Carolina, where both medical and recreational use are illegal (Bryan, 2024).

In medicinal marijuana states, doctors and nurse practitioners make a *recommendation* for cannabis if the patient presents with a qualifying condition according to the state's law. The US Court of Appeals for the Ninth Circuit in *Conant v. Walters* ruled that a physician discussing medicinal marijuana and making recommendations is protected speech under the First Amendment (*Conant v Walters*, 309 F. 3d 629, 636 (9th Cir 2002)). Nurse practitioners should always consult their state board for practice considerations in states with full scope of practice as a well as in states with restrictive advanced practice registered nurse authority. Since every U.S. state has laws defined in the Nursing Practice Act (NPA), state nursing boards enforce different NPA laws in their respective state (Boehning & Haddad, 2023; Ryan et al., 2021).

Main FOCUS OF the CHAPTER

Issues, Controversies, Problems

There are many issues, controversies, and problems with cannabis use under the Federal Controlled Substances Act (CSA). The CSA prevents federal healthcare reimbursement for cannabis from Medicare and Medicaid. The CSA poses risks for facility operations funding, licensing, and accreditation. In addition, the CSA creates operational challenges by prohibiting the use of federal funds for cannabis-related treatments (Lawler, 2025).

Reimbursement for Cannabis Use is Against Federal Law: Because cannabis lacks U.S. Food and Drug Administration (FDA) drug approval, federal programs such as Medicare and Medicaid do not cover or reimburse costs for medical marijuana (Lawler, 2025). Private insurers generally follow federal guidelines and do not reimburse for cannabis products due to the federal prohibition and lack of FDA approval, which could expose them to legal liability. A federal judge has dismissed a proposed class-action lawsuit that aimed to require insurers in New Mexico to cover medical cannabis as a behavioral health treatment (Emerson, 2025). Therefore, patients must cover all related expenses (evaluations, application fees, products) out-of-pocket. The only exceptions for coverage are FDA-approved synthetic or cannabis-derived medications (e.g., Epidiolex, Marinol, Ceramet), which may be a benefit under Medicare Part D. (*Medicare to test coverage of medical marijuana*, n.d.)

Facility Risks: Facility premises that permit the use or possession of marijuana could violate federal law, risking loss of federal funding, licensing, and accreditation (*The Evolution of Marijuana as a Controlled Substance and the Federal-State Policy Gap*, 2022; Kellogg, Anderson, & Michiels, 2022). Under 21 U.S.C. § 824(a): Denial, revocation, or suspension of registration: The DEA may take disciplinary action against providers, including revoking their DEA registration, which can result in fines or criminal charges (Diversion Control Division, n.d.).

Some state laws protect healthcare providers from state-level discipline for certifying patients for medical cannabis use. For example, Minnesota: The state's medical cannabis law specifies that the Commissioner of Health, staff, agents, and any healthcare practitioner are not subject to any civil or disciplinary penalties by their respective licensing boards (including the Board of Medical Practice and Board of Nursing) solely for participating in the state's registry program. According to the Marijuana Policy Project, several states (including Arizona, Arkansas, Connecticut, Delaware, Maine, Massachusetts, etc.) have anti-discrimination provisions in their medical cannabis laws or have had court rulings that generally prohibit professional or occupational licensing boards from penalizing registered patients and, in many cases, the associated healthcare providers for permissible conduct under the state's medical cannabis program (*Federal Policies*, n.d.; Marijuana Policy Project, 2022; *State Policies*, n.d.).

Operational Challenges: Maintaining a drug-free workplace as required for federal contractors under the Drug-Free Workplace Act of 1988 (Pub. L. 100-690, Title V, Subtitle D; 41 U.S.C.) while navigating state-level employment protections for medical cannabis patients is a considerable operational challenge. An MMP is a jurisdictional resource for medical cannabis. Medical Marijuana Programs (MMPs) include for-fee state-issued cannabis identification cards (medical marijuana identification or medical marijuana card) enabling patients to obtain, possess, or cultivate cannabis (*Medical Cannabis Glossary*, n.d.).

Healthcare facilities providing cannabis care need to implement risk-reducing policies and procedures. These procedures include maintaining a qualified workforce for state Medical Marijuana Programs (MMP) certification, medication management, including drug interactions, and post-surgical complications.

Cannabis related operational challenges for nurse administrators may include:

- Managing MMP certification by Nurse Practitioners (NPs) who may certify patients and provide required guidance on legal responsibilities and best practices. An official cannabis policy that clearly states the roles and responsibilities of healthcare providers within the institution can help alleviate concerns of licensed professionals working in the institution (Ryan, 2021).
- Managing Medications, including how to safely store, manage, and administer substances that are illegal under federal law (Temple et al., 2019).
- Managing potential drug interactions, monitoring adverse effects (such as sedation and dizziness), and ensuring safe administration protocols fall under the nursing purview (Temple et al., 2019).

SOLUTIONS AND RECOMMENDATIONS

NCSBN National Nursing Guidelines for Marijuana

National organizations, including the American Nurses Association (ANA), the National Council of State Boards of Nursing (NCSBN), and the American Cannabis Nursing Association (ACNA), have published practice guidelines that collectively support nurse administrators in cannabis care.

- *Nursing Administration: Scope and Standards of Practice* (2016) is an ANA guideline that assists nursing administrators in decision-making and fulfilling their responsibilities to the system and organization.
- *NCSBN National Nursing Guidelines for Medical Marijuana* (2018) guides nurses caring for patients using medical cannabis, addresses the evidence gaps, emphasizes non-judgmental care, and standards of non-impaired job performance. See Table 1. NCSBN National Nursing Guidelines for Marijuana (2018).
- *Cannabis Nursing: Scope and Standards of Practice* (2024) aids in decision-making regarding the quality and validity of competencies relevant to cannabis nursing.

Table 1. NCSBN National Nursing Guidelines for Marijuana (2018)

NCSBN National Nursing Guidelines for Marijuana (2018)
● Legal and policy awareness: Nurses should be aware of cannabis legalization in their jurisdiction and their facility's specific policies on medical marijuana administration. ● Knowledge of cannabis and patient care: ○ Understand the basics of the endocannabinoid system and the pharmacology of cannabis. ○ Have a general understanding of medical marijuana programs. ○ Be aware of the limited and often conflicting research on cannabis for medical use, which can pose challenges for evidence-based practice. ● Clinical approach: ○ Assess and gather data about the patient's specific health situation to guide their care. ○ Avoid judgment regarding the patient's choice of treatment, providing care without personal bias or prejudice. ○ Be mindful that many patients with medical cannabis use may conceal their use due to fear of stigma or legal consequences, which can increase stress and impact their healthcare access. ● Professional conduct: ○ Cannabis use by a nurse that interferes with job performance may result in disciplinary action, regardless of employee protections. ○ Nurses should understand their state and federal laws, as marijuana remains illegal at the federal level. ● Education and curriculum: ○ The National Council of State Board of Nursing created NCSBN guidelines to address an educational gap and provide direction for educators and licensees. ○ The guidelines provide a foundation for curriculum development in prelicensure and advanced practice registered nurse (APRN) education programs. (NCSBN National Nursing Guidelines for Medical Marijuana, 2018).

Clinical Policies for Nursing Care: Ryan's Law

Ryan Bartell was diagnosed with stage four pancreatic cancer and was using cannabis medicines for pain relief when the hospital prohibited their use (Ryan's Law Foundation, n.d.). California's 2021 Ryan's Law, named for Ryan, now requires medical facilities to allow patients with a prognosis of life of one year or less to use their own medical cannabis.

Facilities have developed formal procedures allowing terminally ill patients to use medical cannabis on-site. These procedures focus on safety, documentation, and patient responsibility, ensuring respect for the patient's treatment plan without disrupting the facility (*Physicians Guide to Ryan's Law*, 2021), as outlined in Table 2. Standard operating procedure (SOP) considerations for medical cannabis compassionate care laws. Real-world implementation of Ryan's Law has been reported as successful (McKaig et al., 2025). ACNA supports California's model as safe and compassionate and recommends that it be adopted nationally (2025).

Table 2. Standard operating procedure (SOPs) considerations for medical cannabis compassionate care laws

Standard operating procedure (SOPs) considerations for medical cannabis compassionate care laws
● Adopt a policy banning smoking or vaporizing cannabis on premises ● Train staff on verifying the status of a Medical Marijuana Identification Card (MMIC) or a doctor's recommendation ● Include medicinal cannabis use within the patient's medical records ● Create a plan for cannabis storage ● Create a waiver of liability of a health care facility for lost or stolen medical cannabis goods ● Develop educational materials around the pharmacodynamics and pharmacokinetics of cannabinoid therapeutics, safety training, and written guidelines for the healthcare team and staff (ACNA, 2025; ASA, 2025; Sobel, 2025)

Ryan's law applies to terminally ill patients, typically with a prognosis of one year or less. It allows for medical cannabis use in hospitals, skilled nursing facilities, and hospices, but not emergency departments. Patients must have a physician's recommendation or a medical cannabis identification card for medical cannabis use. Smoking and vaping products are prohibited on the premises. Patients are responsible for their own cannabis supply, storage, and administration. The law protects healthcare facilities with a "safe harbor clause" if federal agencies attempt to interfere with their operations (*Physicians Guide to Ryan's Law, 2021*).

The University of California, Los Angeles (UCLA), Santa Monica Medical Center shares this clinical workflow, as described in the inpatient oncology unit (McKaig et al., 2025). "A medical provider assesses the patient and determines eligibility under Ryan's Law. The provider places an order to approve the patient's self-administration of the medication. The patient signs a consent and liability form. Nursing staff contact the pharmacy, which delivers a lockbox for storage. The patient self-administers the medical cannabis product and notifies the nurse of each dose. The nurse documents the administration in the patient's electronic medical record." See Table 3. Nursing procedures for patient cannabis use present guidance for nursing procedures for patient cannabis use.

Table 3. Nursing procedures for patient cannabis use

Nursing Procedures for Patient Cannabis Use:	
Patient admission and intake procedures	**A copy of a physician's medical cannabis recommendation or a valid MMIC, eligibility screening upon admission, and a signed agreement acknowledging the patient's responsibility for the procurement, storage, and self-administration of medicinal cannabis. The agreement also prohibits hospital staff from assisting with administration.**
Storage and handling procedures	Storing the patient's cannabis in a locked container provided by the hospital pharmacy, which is kept at the patient's bedside, a non-smoking/vaping facility policy, and self-administration, notifying nursing staff before each use.
Electronic medical records and monitoring procedures	Medical record entry of cannabis use and the reason for use, and its effects on the patient, nursing assessments, patient-administered cannabis documented on the Medication Administration Record (MAR), and outcome evaluation for improvements in symptoms such as anxiety and insomnia.
Facility guidelines and professional development	Written guidelines for medical cannabis use available to patients and staff, education to train nurses and other staff on the procedures and policies for Ryan's Law, and a "safe harbor" clause if facing federal enforcement action. (ACNA, 2025)

Nurses reported being comfortable implementing the cannabis policy, noting improvements in patient symptom management and a positive effect on the patient stay. UCLA's oncology unit reported zero safety incidents, intense nurse satisfaction, and improved symptom management (McKaig et al., 2025).

The California Hospital Association initially had liability concerns, including documentation, drug interactions, oversedation, and liability for lost belongings. There were also conflicts with federal law (Schedule I, risk to federal funding, jeopardizing professional licenses) (Armentano, 2021). Provisions to mitigate these concerns included a "safe harbor" provision that allows facilities to suspend compliance if directly threatened by federal enforcement action, providing reassurance against loss of funding or licensure (*Ryan's Law Foundation,* n.d.).

The advocacy group Compassionate Oregon reintroduced Ryan's Law legislation as Oregon Bill 3214 in 2025. Areas of concern for passage include problems cannabis nurses are familiar with - insufficient research data on cannabis, inconsistent regulatory oversight, dosing, administration, informed consent procedures, as well as potential for harm, and ongoing stigmas (*Cannabis Use in Hospice and Palliative Care*, 2025).

Nursing administrators and cannabis care nurses are being called upon to lead medical facilities in integrating state cannabis laws into clinical practice. When a nurse helps the facility to develop a policy for cannabis use and evidence-based staff education, the plan should include a legal consultation to ensure compliance with federal, state, and case law (Borgelt & Franson, 2017). With proper guidelines, hospital staff and patients will feel comfortable with the process of extending compassionate use of cannabis to more patients (McKaig et al., 2025).

Academic Workplace Policies on Cannabis Use

Academic nurse administrators manage nursing programs, overseeing faculty and students, with responsibilities that include budget and financial management, policy strategy, development and implementation, quality assurance, collaboration, communication, and the professional development of themselves and their staff (*CareRev,* 2024). Their roles involve a blend of clinical, educational, and administrative skills, fostering collaboration both within and outside their institutions (Greenway & Acai, 2024). Academic nurse administrators have opportunities to influence the medicinal cannabis curriculum by assessing the challenges, implementing strategies that enable success, scanning key external educational and healthcare environments, monitoring trends and forecasting their direction, and evaluating how to respond to the opportunities (Birkhead et al., 2022). Challenges for academic nurse managers include heavy workloads, navigating internal conflicts, and inadequate organizational support (Javeed, 2024).

Academic workplace cannabis policies remain restrictive due to the federal Drug-Free Workplace Act of 1988 (Drug-Free Workplace Act of 1988, 41 U.S.C. § 8101 et seq. (2018)). This Act mandates that any organization receiving a federal grant of any size must have a drug-free workplace policy prohibiting the use of controlled substances, which includes cannabis (Drug-Free Workplace Act of 1988, 41 U.S.C. § 8101 et seq. (2018)). Failing to adhere to these federal guidelines can result in a loss of funding, making compliance a necessity for most higher education institutions (Drug-Free Workplace Act of 1988, 41 U.S.C. § 8101 et seq. (2018)). Therefore, on-campus possession, use, or distribution of cannabis is generally prohibited, even in states where it is legal for recreational or medicinal use. Executive Order 12564 (1986) directly banned federal employees from using drugs, on or off duty. The Drug Free Workplace Act reinforced that federally funded institutions are prohibited from using cannabis, even when off-duty (Drug-Free Workplace Act of 1988, 41 U.S.C. § 8101 et seq. (2018)).

Higher education has concerns for impaired mental health, dependence, and blunted academic engagement and achievement in students who use cannabis regularly. Cannabis can seriously impact student development, especially when started at an early age. Institutional leadership must clearly articulate the risks associated with regular use and the optimal conditions for student success (Porter, 2016). Klimer (2018) makes the following recommendations for campuses regarding student cannabis use:

1. Stay compliant with the Drug Free Schools and Communities Act.
2. Consider that marijuana potency has changed in the last several decades.
3. Construct messages regarding marijuana in campus coverage mindfully.
4. Consider survey-based screening for cannabis use disorder.
5. Campus professionals can help identify struggling students using the Cannabis Use Disorders Identification Test – Revised.

6. Correct misperceived norms on campus.
7. Provide services for those contemplating a change in their substance use.
8. Investment in staff education on campus (Kilmer, 2018).

If the Drug Enforcement Administration (DEA) reschedules cannabis to Schedule III, the change in level would not legalize cannabis outright. Academic institutions would still be required to maintain drug-free policies for federally funded activities. However, California's Department of Cannabis Control offers research grants to expand scientific knowledge and inform future policy. This funding activity indicates a shift toward a more evidence-based approach to policy, although the underlying academic restrictions remain (Department of Cannabis Control, n.d.).

The ban on cannabis leads to various outcomes, both positive and negative. On the one hand, it upholds a drug-free environment as required by federal law and potentially reduces incidents related to drug use. On the other hand, it may drive cannabis use underground, leading to unsafe consumption practices and reluctance to seek help for fear of disciplinary action (Delatte, 2024).

Employee Workplace Policies on Cannabis Use

Cannabis regulatory framework complexities may extend to workers who are medical cannabis users (Perlman et al., 2021). Nurses who use any cannabis must not work if they are unable to meet the requirements of safe nursing practice (Clark, 2021). Nurses who use cannabis should be cautious of conflicts in state and federal law, individual employer policies, and state nursing board regulations (Do Nurses Get Drug Tested for Marijuana in Today's Healthcare Settings, 2025). Cannabis nurses who provide care or use cannabis have historically faced penalties (American Nurses Association and American Cannabis Nurses Association, 2024; Clark, 2021). Cannabis use causing impairment may result in professional disciplinary action as outlined on the NCSBN Discipline webpage https://www.ncsbn.org/nursing-regulation/discipline.page.

The National Council of Boards of Nursing (2018) acknowledges that current lab tests cannot indicate when the individual has consumed cannabis, nor can they establish a level of THC or its metabolites to determine impairment. Further research for valid testing tools is widely supported (Fitzgerald et al., 2023; Marcotte et al., 2023; McNichol, 2025; Ramaekers et al., 2023). The American Nurses Association (2025) opposes cannabis drug testing for healthcare workers (1994) and holds nurses ethically responsible for reporting impairment in others (*2025 Code of Ethics for Nurses*, 2025, Provision 3.5).

According to Right-Touch Regulation for nurses testing positive for THC, regulatory discipline should be proportionate, consistent, targeted, transparent, accountable, and agile (Gowen et al., 2018). This ensures that a regulatory body's decisions affecting public safety strike a balance between mitigating the risk of harm and applying discipline fairly and consistently.

Nursing administrators must have policies covering employee cannabis use for on-the-job possession, use, and impairment. These policies should outline the types of drug testing as pre-employment, random, post-accident, and "reasonable suspicion" testing. Policy development should include training requirements for identifying cannabis impairment, concerns for patient safety, and justifying reasonable suspicion drug tests (*Employer drug-testing policies must evolve with state law—Troutman Pepper Locke*, July 19, 2023). There should be a reasonable accommodation process for employees with medical conditions who use cannabis, guided and in compliance with disability laws (Marijuana Policy Project, n.d.).

Nurse administrators also need to modernize drug testing policies, replacing outdated THC-based testing methods with validated ones, protecting nurses who lawfully use cannabis off-duty, updating institutional policies to eliminate discrimination, and advocating for national standards (American Cannabis Nurses Association, 2025).

It is an ongoing concern that there is a lack of consistency from state to state, and there is a lack of transparency within states about nurses' ability to use medical cannabis and maintain a nursing license (American Cannabis Nurses Association, 2024). California and Washington have passed legislation protecting employees from off-duty cannabis use. New York bans cannabis testing for many professions. However, these laws may exclude nurses because of the "potential to significantly impact the health or safety of employees or members of the public" (*New Marijuana Laws have companies questioning current drug testing policies*, n.d., *New York City Council Passes Trailblazing Bill to Ban all Preemployment Marijuana Testing,* 2019). Nursing professionals must consult their State Board of Nursing for specific cannabis-use policies and regulations.

ADMINISTRATIVE LEADERSHIP, ETHICS, AND ADVOCACY

Ethical Challenges in nursing, cannabis nursing, and administrative nursing

The ANA's Scope and Standards of Cannabis Nursing Practice emphasizes four ethical challenges cannabis nurses face in practice:

- The legal ambiguity caused by federal and state-level cannabis laws
- Cannabis stigma causes patient and provider fear of prosecution, negatively impacting care
- Lack of cannabis nursing education leaves patients with unreliable information
- Lack of objective impairment detection (2024)

The ethical obligations of nursing administrators to their patients, employees, and the broader healthcare system in leading cannabis health policy change will be discussed. Resolving conflicts between federal and state cannabis laws will improve patient access and consistency of care (Comprehensive Pain Management, n.d.; Perlman et al., 2021; *Physicians, Medical Marijuana, and the Law,* 2014; Ryan, 2021; *Utah Canna*, 2025). A call to action by nursing administrators through advocacy activities is needed to ensure patients can continue legally using cannabis while inpatients and at home.

Nursing ethics: Nursing practice, cannabis nursing, and administrative nursing all have values grounded in the community, tradition, and practices of nursing (2025 Code of Ethics for Nurses, 2025). These values are justice, equity, inclusiveness, integrity, dignity, cultural humility, care, comfort, compassion, trust, commitment, and health. The values are in ten provisions describing nursing relationships as nurse-to-patient, nurse-to-nurse, nurse-to-self, nurse-to-profession, nurse-to-others, nurse/nursing-to-society, and nursing-to-the global community (2025 Code of Ethics for Nurses, 2025).

Cannabis is not mentioned in the ANA Code of Ethics; however, the American Nurses Association (ANA) has a position statement on the therapeutic use of marijuana. The American Nurses Association (ANA) (ANA Position Statement: Therapeutic Use of Marijuana and Related Cannabinoids, 2022) approaches cannabis ethics from a perspective of patient advocacy and evidence-based practice, supporting the safe, legal, and therapeutic use of cannabis:

1. Patient advocacy to choose cannabis for symptom management and approaching patients without judgment regarding their treatment choices.
2. There is a need for further research into the therapeutic use.
3. Protection for patients and nurses from criminal or civil penalties for using, discussing, or administering cannabis according to professional standards and state laws.
4. Professional competence on the endocannabinoid system, cannabis pharmacology, and safe usage guidelines.
5. Social justice recognizes that specific communities have been disproportionately affected by cannabis prohibition and its related healthcare inequities (American Nurses Association, 2016).

Cannabis nursing ethics, as outlined by the American Cannabis Nursing Association, are approached from a patient-centered, nursing-focused standpoint (American Cannabis Nursing Association, 2024). Their ethical framework is rooted in principles of care, social justice, and advocacy.

1. Patient advocacy: ACNA nurses act as advocates and educators for patients, helping them navigate the complex and often stigmatized world of medicinal cannabis. Advocating includes ensuring patients have access to safe, regulated, and tested products.
2. Ethical principles: Cannabis nurses apply the foundational ethical principles of nursing, balancing these principles while considering legal restrictions and navigating ethical dilemmas related to cannabis care.
3. Social justice: The ACNA emphasizes social justice by acknowledging that marginalized communities have been disproportionately affected by health disparities and the criminalization of cannabis.
4. Evidence-based practice: The ACNA encourages cannabis nurses to stay informed about the latest scientific evidence regarding therapeutic cannabis use and real-world patient data to counter misinformation. (American Nurses Association, 2021; American Cannabis Nurses Association, 2024)

However, ***administrative ethics*** involve a broader focus on the organization, populations, and systems, rather than the individual patient. Organizational leaders are responsible for promoting organizational well-being, effective resource allocation, and fostering a supportive work environment (ANA Position Statement: Nurses' Professional Responsibility to Promote Ethical Practice Environments, 2023). Nursing administrative ethics focuses on system-level issues, including the health of entire populations, the organization, and the nursing workforce (Aroskar, 1998). Therefore, cannabis nursing administrators extend nursing ethics to an even broader context, requiring administrators to consider how their decisions impact the entire system, including both patients and employees.

The 2009 ANA Nurse Administration: Scope and Standards of Practice, in its latest version titled "Nursing Leadership: Scope and Standards of Practice, 3rd Edition" (2024), reflects changes in the role and terminology. This third edition, a collaboration between the ANA and the American Organization for Nursing Leadership (AONL), includes 19 national standards. "The committee organized these standards in a way that emphasizes Leadership as the first standard. The standard of Just and Equitable Practice requires the nurse leader to promote an inclusive, shared governance structure aimed at reducing barriers to care, enhancing the delivery of care, and addressing inequities. DEI is threaded throughout the accountabilities and standards of practice and is a key cornerstone" (American Organization for Nursing Leadership, 2024).

The Nursing Leadership Ethics Performance Competencies include maintaining and improving the ethical environments of the work setting for safe and quality healthcare. They do this by promoting staff and patient health and safety; recognizing that a nurse's commitment is to the patient can be to the individual, family, group, community, or population; disparities in healthcare are essential to acknowledge; advancing the profession through research, professional standards development, and the generation of nursing and health policies; using an ethical, DEI- and values-driven, evidence-based framework to improve the health index of the ecosystem (Cadmus et al., 2024).

The administrative nurse's role in cannabis care advocacy

Advocacy is the process by which stakeholders speak to policymakers on issues that affect their lives at the local, state, and national levels. It also means helping policymakers find specific solutions to persistent problems. Most nonprofits can and do engage in significant advocacy to achieve their goals (ACNA Lobbying/Advocacy with 501c3 status, n.d.).

Nursing administrators can advocate for cannabis care by educating policymakers about cannabis health policy needs related to cannabis. There are several ways to do this, including emailing or calling elected officials, organizing meetings with legislators and their staff, and sharing views with policymakers and the community through media campaigns. Keep in mind that these activities cross the line into lobbying if they call for action on introduced legislation or a pending regulation (ACNA Lobbying/Advocacy with 501 (c) (3) status, n.d.).

CSA Rescheduling and Hemp Prohibition: U.S. Nursing Advocacy Strategies

What does rescheduling cannabis mean for the nurse and patient? If cannabis becomes a level III drug, cannabis as a medicine would still be a controlled substance (MPP, n.d.). States would still have a conflict with their own medical and recreational cannabis programs. Reduced research restrictions would allow access to conducting more evidence-based medical studies (*Federal Marijuana Rescheduling*, n.d.). Financially, rescheduling could expand cannabis business access to banking/financial services. Moreover, eliminate the Internal Revenue Code Section 280E requirement, allowing regular business expenses to be deducted (Sacco, 2024).

There has been activity towards rescheduling. In 2023, the U.S. Department of Health and Human Services (HHS) recommended moving cannabis from Schedule I to Schedule III. In 2024, the DEA issued a proposed rule to transfer cannabis to Schedule III. In 2025, a hearing on the proposal was indefinitely postponed, and the DEA had a new administrator, Terrance Cole. Political factors and legal challenges could cause further delays in 2026 (*Federal Marijuana Rescheduling*, n.d.).

Powerful legislative events have occurred in 2025 that will impact the future of these types of clinical policy-making activities. In November 2025, Congress passed the Agriculture, Rural Development, Food and Drug Administration, and Related Agencies Appropriations Act of 2026 (P.L. 119-37, Division B). This law effectively bans most intoxicating hemp products by amending the definition of hemp in the Agricultural Marketing Act of 1946 (*Continuing Appropriations, Agriculture, Legislative Branch, Military Construction and Veterans Affairs, and Extensions Act, 2026*, Pub. L. No. 119-37, 139 Stat. 495, 2025). Then, on December 18, 2025, President Donald Trump signed an executive order *Increasing Medical Marijuana and Cannabidiol Research* (Trump, 2025). The executive order orders the acceleration of the rescheduling of cannabis and expands cannabis-related research.

When it comes to hemp, Section 781 of the Continuing Appropriations, Legislative Branch, Military Construction and Veterans Affairs, and Extensions Act, 2026, establishes a new limit for tetrahydrocannabinol (THC) content in products of 0.4 milligrams combined total per container of total THC. This change has significant implications for the hemp industry, outlawing mainstream drinks, creams, gummies, oils, and vapes. The provision closes a loophole in the 2018 Farm Bill that allowed the sale of hemp-derived products containing tetrahydrocannabinol. US Senator Mitch McConnell, a Republican from Kentucky, said the bill prohibits intoxicating products and protects children from products marketed to them. The ban takes effect on Nov. 13, 2026 (Schermele, 2025).

The U.S. Hemp Roundtable, a coalition for safe hemp and CBD products, is working with bipartisan legislators on regulating high or irregular THC content, synthetic ingredients, copycat products, and marketing or packaging meant to appeal to minors. U.S. Hemp Roundtable says the new rules would ban more than 95% of all hemp-extract products – including many CBD products that have no intoxicating effect (Meckes, 2025).

In response, Republican South Carolina U.S. House Rep. Nancy Mace has filed draft legislation, the "American Hemp Protection Act of 2025," which would repeal Section 781. U.S. House Reps. Thomas Massie, R-Ky., Zoe Lofgren, D-Calif., and James Baird, R-Ind., signed on as original co-sponsors for this bill (*Cannabis Business Times*, 2025). In December 2025, Senators Ron Wyden (D-OR) and Jeff Merkley (D-OR) introduced the Cannabinoid Safety and Regulation Act. Key provisions of this act include cannabinoid testing, age restriction for individuals under 21 years of age, THC caps for products, prohibition on flavored e-vaping, amending the FFDCA to make cannabinoids permitted for human consumption, and regulating cannabinoid beverages (Samuel et al., 2025).

American Nurses Association Position

The American Nurses Association (ANA) supports moving cannabis from a Schedule I drug to Schedule III of the Controlled Substances Act (ANA, 2024). It cites evidence of cannabis's therapeutic qualities and believes it meets the criteria for "currently accepted medical use," justifying reclassification. The ANA contends that rescheduling would lead to expanded research opportunities, allowing healthcare providers, particularly nurses, to better care for patients. The association has also expressed a desire to see cannabis eventually removed from the CSA entirely. By supporting reclassification, acknowledging cannabis nursing as a specialty, and providing ethical guidelines, the ANA is helping to shape a more ethical and safer environment for therapeutic cannabis use.

American Cannabis Nurses Association Position

The American Cannabis Nurses Association (ACNA) is a strong proponent of rescheduling cannabis (ACNA, 2025). While Schedule III reclassification marks progress, it remains insufficient because of persistent legal contradictions between federal and state laws, barriers to equitable patient access, lack of protection for patients in employment, housing, and parental rights contexts, and continued DEA oversight, which may impede research expansion (Americans for Safe Access [ASA], 2025; NASEM, 2017).

The ACNA is exploring alternative regulatory models, such as the Schedule VI framework proposed by Americans for Safe Access (ASA) (ASA, 2025). The ASA Schedule VI Proposal outlines a regulatory structure designed explicitly for cannabis-based medicine to support safe and legitimate medical use while addressing gaps unresolved by Schedule III reclassification. ACNA, in alignment with Americans for Safe Access, recommends: Adoption of a dedicated Schedule VI classification tailored to cannabis medicine and the creation of the Office of Medical Cannabis & Cannabinoid Control to oversee national standards, patient protections, and research facilitation.

Rescheduling of cannabis represents a significant milestone in U.S. drug policy reform. Proposed rescheduling frameworks offer viable paths to address access, equity, research, and patient safety. See Table 4. Resources for related website resources.

Table 4. Resources

Marijuana in the Workplace: Guidance for Occupational Health Professionals and Employers	**https://www.scribd.com/document/392195043/jurnal-hoammmmmmmmmmmmmmmmmm**
ANA Code of Ethics, 2025	https://codeofethics.ana.org/home
American Organization for Nursing Leadership Guiding Principles	https://www.aonl.org/resources/guiding-principles
NCSBN National Nursing Guidelines for Medical Marijuana	https://www.ncsbn.org/nursing-regulation/practice/marijuana-guidelines.page
ANA Official Position Statements	https://www.nursingworld.org/practice-policy/nursing-excellence/official-position-statements/
Society of Cannabis Clinicians (SCC)	https://www.cannabisclinicians.org/
Americans for Safe Access (ASA)	https://www.safeaccessnow.org/#gsc.tab=0
Drug Policy Alliance	https://drugpolicy.org/
Healer / Leaf411	https://leaf411.org/
International Association for Cannabis as Medicine (IACM)	https://www.cannabis-med.org/
Marijuana Policy Project (MPP)	https://www.mpp.org/
NORML (National Organization for the Reform of Marijuana Laws)	https://norml.org/
Veterans for Medical Cannabis Access (VMCA)	http://www.veteransformedicalmarijuana.org/content/about-vmma

MANAGING CANNABIS NURSING EDUCATION, COMPETENCE, AND STIGMAS

Nurse Managers' competencies include being responsible for employing and appraising employees (ANA, 2016). The competencies include overseeing nurses who should have a solid foundation in essential cannabis knowledge and use non-judgmental approaches to ensure they can provide safe and effective care (ACNA, 2024; National Council of State Boards of Nursing, 2018). Two major cannabis education issues are impacting US health systems for which nursing administrators are responsible. One issue affecting the workforce is the nursing school curriculum deficits that impact practice competence in cannabis nursing (Clark, 2021; Parmalee & Clark, 2022; Zolotov et al., 2021). The second issue is an ongoing, pervasive stigma that impacts both providers and patients (King et al., 2024).

Curriculum Deficit: Training Requirements for Medical Cannabis Knowledge

Cannabis education is largely absent from nursing school curricula, requiring administrators to seek and implement continuing education for nurses on cannabis properties, dosing, side effects, and interactions (Theisen & Konieczny, 2019). The NCSBN National Nursing Guidelines for Medical Marijuana (2018) recommendations for curriculum content provide principles of safe and knowledgeable practice for patient safety when certifying or caring for patients using marijuana. Table 5. contains the NCSBN Six Principles of Essential Knowledge for medical marijuana, which create a solid foundation for safe and knowledgeable nursing care for patients using medical and recreational cannabis (National Council of State Boards of Nursing, 2018).

Table 5. Six principles of essential knowledge

1. The nurse shall have a working knowledge of the current state of legalization of medical and recreational cannabis use
2. The nurse shall have a general knowledge of the principles of an MMP.
3. The nurse should have a general understanding of the endocannabinoid system, including cannabinoid receptors, cannabinoids, and their interactions.
4. The nurse shall have an understanding of cannabis pharmacology and the research associated with the medical use of cannabis.
5. The nurse shall be able to identify the safety considerations for patients' use of cannabis.
6. The nurse shall approach the patient without judgment regarding the patient's choice of treatment or preferences in managing pain and other distressing symptoms.

(National Council of State Boards of Nursing, 2018)

NCSBN's pre-licensure recommendations incorporate awareness of medical marijuana administration considerations into the Six Principles of Essential Knowledge.

NCSBN's Advanced Practice Registered Nurse recommendations build upon the pre-licensure,

- Able to recognize signs and symptoms of cannabis use disorder and cannabis withdrawal syndrome,
- Aware of the medical marijuana administration considerations,
- Aware of the ethical considerations related to the care of patients using medical marijuana, and
- Follow specific employer policies and procedures, terms of the collaborative agreement, standard care arrangement, and facility policy and procedures regarding certifying a qualifying condition (National Council of State Boards of Nursing, 2018, pp 40-42).

The ACNA's Cannabis Nursing Scope of Practice supports the NCSBN's 2018 Six Principles of Essential Knowledge (2024). Cannabis nursing courses have not always been available. Nursing education programs are now available in various forms, including undergraduate and graduate degrees, certifications, and continuing education (ACNA, 2024). The ACNA recommends the development of specialized cannabis nursing curricula, nationally standardized certification, and ongoing education programs (ACNA, 2024). ACNA is developing a new credentialing process to provide a national certification for cannabis nursing.

The NCSB's Six Principles of Essential Knowledge are not universally recognized or implemented in US Nursing education programs (Parmalee & Clark, 2022). Recently, core competencies for undergraduate medical education addressing medical cannabis were developed by Zolotov et al. (2025). Using a modified Delphi process (N = 23), six core competencies were identified, including cannabis pharmacology, legal frameworks, clinical evidence, risks, and clinical management. The curricular framework has a spiral approach to cannabis therapeutics reappearing at increasing levels of complexity in the academic curriculum across multiple contexts rather than existing as a stand-alone add-on (Kogan, et al., 2025).

The Cannabis Nursing Workforce has a Critical Knowledge Gap

Zolotov et al. report that these competencies are needed to enhance clinical preparedness, to support counseling, and to help promote informed discussions with patients about cannabis use (Zolotov et al., 2025). Simulated patients may also have a role in resolving the cannabis care education gap.

Papanagnou et al. (2021) reported on a process to develop standardized patient-based cases for communication training for medical residents. The simulation program aimed to improve the quality of graduate medical communication with ER patients. The process included facilitator and standardized patient training, technology, debriefing, and engagement of all involved stakeholders. Papananou outlined an 11 step proces for developing such a standardized patient. This approach has potential for combating cannabis stigma and unconscious bias through deliberate cannabis case generation.

Education for a Non-Judgmental Nursing Approach (NCSBN Guidelines, 2018)

Providers will look towards nursing administrators for cannabis care support and education to accompany clinical guidelines and guidance from regulatory authorities, decreasing the stigma surrounding cannabis use, which may encourage patients to engage in conversations about use and promote safe care (Wiese et al., 2024). The 2018 NCSBN guidelines emphasize the development of non-judgmental decision-making as a core competency of safe practice (National Council of State Boards of Nursing, 2018).

A non-judgmental approach in cannabis care training may incorporate the principles of the NCSBN Clinical Judgment Measurement Model (CJMM) into a program that emphasizes empathy, self-awareness, and the objective appraisal of patient data (National Council of State Boards of Nursing, 2018). Supervisors can use the following methods to foster non-judgmental care:

- Values Training/Self-Awareness: Initiate training with "values training" to help nurses recognize their own personal values, biases, and stereotypical beliefs that may lead to judgmental attitudes.
- Active Listening and Empathy: Encourage active listening and the expression of empathy. The supervisor should model this by actively listening to the nurse's concerns and providing support.
- Cultural Competence: Provide opportunities to enhance cultural knowledge and skills, thereby improving the ability to interact with diverse patients without judgment.
- Patient-Centered Care: Emphasize patient-centered care, focusing on the patient's emotional, spiritual, mental, and cultural needs as primary, while maintaining professional boundaries.
- Role-Playing/Simulation: Utilize clinical scenarios and simulation with structured debriefing to practice handling sensitive situations and ethical dilemmas in a safe environment.

Appraisal of a Cannabis Nurse's Training

A nursing administrator should use a systematic process when appraising a nurse's understanding of cannabis pharmacology, the endocannabinoid system, and their knowledge of state and federal laws regarding cannabis against established standards, competencies, and institutional goals (Chen, 2025).

A nurse's training appraisal should be objective, competency-based, focused on clinical judgment, and aligned with the organization's goals and best practices (Chen, 2025). The nurse should be able to provide patient education, assess safety risks, and approach the topic without judgment (National Council of State Boards of Nursing, 2019). Table 6 outlines the six cognitive steps of the NCSBN CJMM (NCLEX, n.d.). Supervisors may use these to evaluate the nurse's reasoning process during training scenarios or actual patient care.

Table 6. Six cognitive steps of the NCSBN Clinical Judgment Measurement Model (CJMM)

1. Recognize Cues: Evaluate if the nurse is gathering all relevant data, including non-verbal cues and patient requests, without being sidetracked by personal feelings or biases. 2. Analyze Cues: Evaluate how the nurse organizes and interprets the collected data, ensuring their reasoning is grounded in evidence and knowledge, rather than personal opinions. 3. Prioritize Hypotheses: Evaluate the nurse's ability to identify and rank client concerns objectively, with a focus on patient safety and needs. 4. Generate Solutions: Evaluate the nurse's ability to develop evidence-based solutions for the prioritized concerns. 5. Take Action: Observe the implementation of the chosen interventions. The supervisor should ensure the nurse's actions are professional and respectful. 6. Evaluate Outcomes: Utilize reflection and feedback to enable nurses to assess the effectiveness of their actions and learn from their experiences, promoting continuous self-improvement in providing non-judgmental care.

Nursing administrators promote professional and non-judgmental nursing in a supportive environment using direct observation, guided reflection, performance improvement, and feedback (Lewis, 2025). The gap in cannabis care education can be filled in as competencies and educational tools are being designed. These tools need the attributes of reliability and validity to make accurate decisions about cannabis learning and competency (Gupta, 2023). Nurse administrators who demonstrate support for the implementation of an innovation, such as cannabis care education, can positively influence staff involvement and encourage prioritization of innovation implementation (Birken, Lee & Weiner, 2012; Chuang et al., 2011).

FUTURE RESEARCH DIRECTIONS

Cannabis Case Management Nurses

Case management nursing is a specialty focused on coordinating patient care and services within the healthcare setting and connecting patients with community resources. Cannabis patients have unique health care needs that go beyond what mainstream healthcare provides, which includes social and emotional treatment that are also barriers preventing these patients from getting the proper care they need. Cannabis patients have care needs with distinct streams for cannabinoid therapy and adult cannabis use (Costiniuk et al., 2023). Cannabis nursing is a new specialty (ANA, 2023), and cannabis case management for patients who use cannabis is an upcoming subspecialty. Cannabis case management nurses help patients understand the legal framework and access the appropriate care, especially for complex conditions (Commission for Case Manager Certification, n.d.).

Case Management Nursing

Case management nurses assist patients and their families in navigating services available within their benefit plan, organization, and community, and in optimizing healthcare and psychosocial goals and outcomes cost-effectively (Giardino & De Jesus, 2023). Case managers' seminal references include the CMSA's Standards of Practice (n.d.), the NASW Standards for Social Work Case Management (n.d.), and publications from the Commission for Case Manager Certification (CCMC, n.d.) and NIH/NCBI (Giardino & De Jesus, 2023).

Case management responsibilities center on assessment, care coordination/planning, advocacy, and communication (CCMC, n.d.). Health education is another significant case management activity. Case managers work with an interdisciplinary healthcare team, monitoring, evaluating, and transitioning between care settings (Giardino & De Jesus, 2023). Case management goals include patient-centered care that enhances the experience, supporting healthier populations through education and resources, and reducing healthcare costs (Belitung, 2021).

Health systems have not adequately addressed patients who self-reported marijuana use or provided sufficient resources for assistance. For example, healthcare provider and client discussions may be negatively impacted by appointment time constraints. Other barriers include a lack of standardized clinical practice guidelines or the inability to refer patients to specialized treatment for substance use disorders or specialists (Bosley et al., 2023). For example, one study reports patient-reported medical cannabis use as 35.1% compared to 4.8% in the electronic health record, which has significant clinical implications (Lapham, Matson & Carrell, 2022).

How Does it Work?

Case management already includes many specialty areas. According to the Commission for Case Manager Certification, 95% of certified case managers have specialty experience in one or more areas (Commission for Case Manager Certification, n.d.). It is a natural progression to see case managers now specializing in therapeutic and adult-use cannabis nursing.

Cannabis nurses apply evidence-based research to educate, care, reduce harm, and coach cannabis consumers, caregivers, family members, and other health care providers on cannabis and cannabis therapeutics (Clark, 2021). When integrating the principles of case management with the practice of cannabis nursing care, a variety of services also become available for supporting the cannabis patient. These services include an interdisciplinary team addressing disease management, behavioral health, and addiction issues (Giardino & De Jesus, 2023). Cannabis case management uses a referral system for multi-provider care available within health plans. The patient receives a comprehensive network of services, providers, and treatments at a much more reasonable cost (Giardino & De Jesus, 2023). These case management identified resources remove barriers such as searching for providers, draining financial resources, and losing hope (CMSA, n.d.)

Integrating case management and cannabis care nursing creates a subspecialty grounded in ethical roots in the Nursing Code of Ethics, specifically the Autonomy Provisions 1, 3, and 4 (American Nurses Association, 2025). This ensures the patient's right to self-determination and decision-making, as well as nonmaleficence, thereby securing the patient's safety. The importance of utilizing an interdisciplinary team, providing evidence-based information, and educating the patient to support harm reduction leads to positive patient outcomes (American Nurses Association, 2025). These shared commonalities with the ACNA *Scope and Standards of Practice* (2024) may reduce health care costs for consumers, health plans, and other stakeholders across the health care continuum.

Table 7. Integrated Hybrid Model of Case Management and Cannabis Care Nursing presents a visual synthesis of Case Management Nursing with Cannabis Care Nursing as a subspecialty. This framework illustrates how foundational case management integrates assessment, coordination, advocacy, and evaluation with advanced cannabinoid science, patient education, and harm reduction principles. This cannabis nursing practice model offers a contemporary approach to measurable competencies, ensuring safety in cannabis nursing care, fostering interdisciplinary communication, and providing guidance for enhancing health system outcomes in nursing practice.

Table 7. Integrated hybrid model of case management and cannabis care nursing

Case Management Nursing	Cannabis Care Nursing	Hybrid Subspecialty Outcomes	Research Support
Comprehensive assessment • Holistic biopsychosocial assessment • Identification of risk factors, SDOH, and care gaps • Evaluation of readiness for change	ECS physiology • Understanding endocannabinoid signaling • Awareness of ECS dysregulation and clinical implications	Improved patient experience • Increased trust and engagement • Reduced stigma and improved communication	Giardino & De Jesus (2023): Case management improves navigation, outcomes, and patient-centered care.
Care coordination • Linking patients to medical, behavioral health, and community services • Facilitating interdisciplinary communication	Cannabinoids, terpenes, flavonoids • Knowledge of therapeutic profiles • Understanding entourage effects and product variability	Reduced readmissions • Prevention of unnecessary ED visits • Alignment with CMS, HEDIS, and NCQA transition-of-care standards	CCMC (2019): Case managers must understand cannabis to guide clients effectively.
Resource optimization • Maximizing health plan benefits • Reducing unnecessary utilization • Identifying cost-effective care pathways	COA interpretation • Evaluating potency, contaminants, and product safety • Teaching patients how to select safe, evidence-informed products	Enhanced safety and early risk identification • Early detection of CHS, misuse, or adverse effects • Prevention of drug–drug interactions	Clark (2021c): ACNA Scope & Standards require evidence-based cannabis education and safety competencies.
Advocacy • Supporting patient autonomy and informed decision-making • Addressing stigma and systemic barriers	Drug–drug interaction awareness • Understanding CYP450 interactions • Monitoring polypharmacy risks	Increased access to BH + SDOH services • Improved linkage to therapy, grief support, nutrition, and community resources	Campo (2025): Providers lack cannabis training; education improves safety and access.
Transition planning • Ensuring safe movement between care settings • Preventing gaps in follow-up care	Harm reduction • Teaching safer use practices • Supporting dose titration, product selection, and risk mitigation	Cost savings and ROI • Reduced ED utilization • Lower inpatient costs • Prevention of avoidable complications	Temple et al. (2019): Identifies barriers; structured cannabis education reduces harm and improves outcomes.
Monitoring & evaluation • Ongoing assessment of progress and barriers • Adjusting care plans based on outcomes	Motivational interviewing • Supporting behavior change • Enhancing adherence and self-efficacy	Strengthened interdisciplinary communication • Improved collaboration between medical, behavioral health, and community teams	Bates (2023): Stigma reduction improves communication, engagement, and patient outcomes.

Cannabis case management is a valuable intervention to overcome barriers to treatment and support services (Doucette et al., 2025). Cannabis case management and educational programming lead to positive social, health, and legal outcomes (Vederhus et al., 2022). Proposed measures and outcomes of cannabis case management include preliminary data that builds a robust database, return on investment by offering care management and attracting more patients, and a patient transition system with dosing guidelines and patient monitoring for new users to promote safe and effective use of medical cannabis (Langley, 2019). Although data is limited due to legal conflicts and other barriers, cannabis care case management may be used in different health care settings, potentially decreasing cost and utilization of benefits lowering premiums (Cook et al., 2023), decreasing readmissions per Centers for Medicare and Medicaid Services (CMS, 2025) Guidelines, and improving Healthcare Effectiveness Data and Information Set (HEDIS) measures (*Follow-Up After Emergency Department Visit for Substance Use (FUA) - NCQA,* 2025) by the National Committee for Quality Assurance (*Diagnosed Substance Use Disorders (DSU) - NCQA,* 2025). Since medicinal cannabis is obtained through dispensaries, it has been suggested that specific outcome-related data be collected on measures through state-level dispensary registries (Langley, 2019).

Barriers and Limitations

Cannabis case management is experiencing the same types of barriers and limitations as other nurse management areas. These include

- evidence-based knowledge gaps,
- the need for new or updated facility policies,
- the lack of legal clarity between the federal and state laws,
- and gaps in nursing education on cannabis, with standards for curricula.

Evidence-based knowledge gaps exist for cannabis effectiveness, dosage, delivery, indications, and drug interactions. Additionally, there is a lack of education and medical staff training, inadequate communication and coordination regarding patient care, dosing options complexity and lack of information, and access barriers for patients seeking treatment and therapy (Temple et al., 2019; Kocis et al., 2024). A recent study from the College of Osteopathic Medicine found that most health care providers lack education and training to discuss medical cannabis with their patients. At the same time, multiple specialties also had differentiating views (Campo, 2025).

There is a need for safe facility policies for cannabis safe management (Borgelt & Franson, 2017). Lack of these may be an obstacle to developing cannabis education programs and care (National Academies of Sciences, Engineering, and Medicine, 2017). As discussed earlier in this chapter, policy conflicts and healthcare operations have known issues, including reimbursement, the risks of maintaining a drug-free workplace, facility risks, and operational challenges. Risk-reducing policies and procedures, maintaining a qualified workforce for MMP certification, medication management, and addressing drug interactions and post-surgical complications, are necessary (Borgelt & Franson, 2017).

Gaps exist between federal and state law. Federally funded organizations may lose federal funding due to federal regulations. Managed Care Organizations with Medicare recipients in their membership have previously not been receptive to cannabis education and care for members because of the risk and are not required to do so (*Federal law preempts state coverage rules for medical cannabis*, 2025). Future federal funding may be addressed through changes in cannabis rescheduling (Federal Marijuana Rescheduling: Process and Impact, 2025). Further regulations or directives may be created to address this new change.

Scope of practice discrepancies may exist between cannabis case management nurses and state professional licensing bodies because of the difference in state and federal cannabis laws (Fleider, 2025). State Nursing Boards are currently evaluating cannabis-related complaints on a case-by-case basis. This process results in varied and sometimes stringent policies, which can result in disciplinary action for nurses, even in states where cannabis use is legal (Writer, 2024). As a result, access to nursing education for cannabis specialization integrated with case management, especially in rural communities, across different states, may be difficult. For now, many Americans are relying on untrained dispensary staff to explain medical product options and healthcare choices (Maynard, 2025).

The conflict in laws has promoted cannabis stigmas. Cannabis use has been deeply stigmatized as an illegal gateway drug since the 1930s prohibition, and this stigma continues. However, an executive order by the President ordered cannabis rescheduled to a Schedule III drug in 2025 (Whitehouse, 2025). Patients report they are apprehensive about notifying their providers about their cannabis use, as providers are not well educated and do not provide much guidance or treatment (King et al., 2024). Cannabis users have been negatively categorized, and misconceptions have resulted in cultural biases, racial prejudice, and baseless fears with media depictions that continually perpetuate this damaging belief (Bates, 2023).

Gaps between federal and state law have impacted community collaborations. Health plan companies and managed care organizations have difficulty with cannabis community and dispensary relationships due to legal restrictions and federal funding mechanisms (*Medical Cannabis Insurance Coverage: Are We Getting Closer?*, 2025). Changes in these areas may be occurring soon as cannabis patients increase access to their health care, and services may be necessary to achieve a better understanding of the cannabis patient needs and better health outcomes (*Federal Marijuana Rescheduling: Process and Impact*, 2025).

Gaps in nursing education on cannabis, with standards for curricula, are impacting the current cannabis case management workforce (Moore, 2024). Cannabis case management education needs include cannabis education, nursing assessments, available resources and treatments, referral systems, either health plan-based or available community resources, IDT approach including medical teams, health and wellness, behavioral health, social work, urgent care teams and auxiliary medical teams, including infusion centers (*Ethics- Cannabis and Case Management: Medical Marijuana Updates*, n.d.). Cannabis case managers must understand the logistical, medical, and ethical implications of medical cannabis to guide clients. "One of the most important things for case managers to do is keep learning," says Vivian Campagna, MSN, RN-BC, CCM, chief industry relations officer, Commission for Case Manager Certification. "The lifelong learning so valued by professional case managers is particularly vital when it comes to cannabis." (Commission on Certified Case Managers, 2019).

Cannabis case management is an upcoming subspecialty. Cannabis case management nurses help patients understand the legal framework and access the appropriate care (Commission for Case Manager Certification, n.d). However, significant limitations and barriers are affecting growth in the cannabis case management workforce development.

Case Study

J.M., a 22-year-old female, presented to the Emergency Room (ER) with complaints of intractable nausea, vomiting, and abdominal pain. She has been unable to tolerate any food or fluid intake and has stopped any intake by mouth for over 24 hours. She reports feeling weak and exhausted from consistent vomiting episodes. The patient has no known previous medical history but reports consistent use of cannabis via joint multiple times daily for anxiety, sleep, and to increase her appetite. The hospital's gastrointestinal workup showed bloodwork and negative imaging results within normal limits. Urine toxicology results showed positive for cannabinoids. J.M. was stabilized, given intravenous hydration therapy, and prescribed antiemetics and antianxiety medications.

J.M. was referred to the Case Manager/Cannabis Nurse Educator for education and coordination of a multidisciplinary team. The patient reports that she lost both parents at the age of 16 and started using cannabis to decrease her anxiety. She uses a joint with an indica flower to help her calm down whenever she feels anxious, which she states can be at least 20 inhalations daily. Patient reports she purchases her product at a local dispensary. Still, she is unable to determine the THC dose, presence of other cannabinoids, terpene profile, flavonoids, and states she has not heard about a Certificate of Analysis (COA). The patient also said she takes a couple of inhalations before sleeping, and cannabis is effective in increasing her appetite until recently. She also reports she has been growing her frequency of use throughout the years, has attempted to stop using cannabis after losing her previous employment due to use, but has not been successful, and resumes use after 8 weeks, stating she "gets shaky, and I start craving it."

J.M. verbally agreed to cannabis related services for 60 days. During this time, the cannabis case manager provided education on the cannabis plant, including cannabinoids, terpenes, flavonoids, and the importance of understanding the Certificate of Analysis (COA). Patient was educated on the effects of cannabis use on the developing brain, which is considered not fully developed until the age of 25 years, along with cardiac and pulmonary effects with increased use. The patient was educated on the complications of use, including possible cannabinoid hyperemesis syndrome (CHS), adverse effects like scromiting, dehydration, risks, and medication interactions. The patient was educated on the Endocannabinoid System (ECS), effects of cannabis use on the ECS, and identified ways to upregulate the ECS that include food intake, stress reduction, exercise, meditation, yoga, and lifestyle changes.

Social Work evaluated the Social Determinants of Health (SDOH) needs, community resources for added support, behavioral health evaluation to address her anxiety, loss of parents at a young age, lack of emotional support, and positive results from the Adverse Childhood Experience Screening (ACES).

A registered dietitian was included for weight loss of three pounds since the onset of nausea and vomiting before her ER presentation, stating she was afraid to eat or drink water, as food irritates her stomach and increases her nausea and vomiting episodes.

The primary care provider was notified regarding the patient's use of cannabis and the available outpatient infusion treatment for intravenous hydration. Intravenous hydration can help decrease readmission rates for patients who present to the hospital within 30 days and are discharged with needs that can be addressed in the outpatient setting. An order is needed for the infusion center, and the cannabis care manager coordinated the process, which was covered in the patient's health plan benefits.

By the end of the program, the patient reports continued cessation of cannabis use, reports seeing her therapist consistently, and has also been participating in a grief support group. She is stable in her new job and has new responsibilities. She also denies any further episodes of nausea and vomiting, and she is looking forward to spending time with her younger sister, who has been neglected as she was more focused on using cannabis and recovering from the effects of use than spending quality time with her. J.M. is planning to return to the local community college. She hopes to be employed in the healthcare setting someday.

J.M. was grateful for the extensive education she received about cannabis, her use, and how it affected her. She decided to discontinue her use but was optimistic that she is more informed and able to choose her cannabis medication correctly, along with dosing, frequency, and type of components, after she turns 25 years old. She is focusing on addressing her medical needs, including her anxiety and insomnia, through therapy, support groups, and providers. She is excited and looks forward to a closer, supportive relationship with her sister and plans to visit other family members. She was grateful for the full support she received without stigma and thankful that services were available to her through her health plan benefits; otherwise, she would not have been able to afford them on her own.

Since this interaction, this patient has not been readmitted to the hospital, fulfilling requirements to reduce future readmissions (*Follow-Up After Emergency Department Visit for Substance Use (FUA) - NCQA,* 2025) and decreasing healthcare costs (*Diagnosed Substance Use Disorders (DSU) - NCQA,* 2025).

CONCLUSION

This chapter examined the roles of nursing leaders and administrators involved in cannabis nursing care and integrated hybrid case management and cannabis care in the United States. Nursing administrators and leaders are at the forefront of the conflict between state and federal cannabis laws. These laws are impacting cannabis healthcare operations, regulation, and administrative leadership. Nursing administrators have an obligation to develop clear, evidence-based cannabis management policies and to contribute to cannabis nursing education, competence, and stigma reduction. Significant administrative actions are necessary to promote safe and high-quality cannabis care policies in collaborative environments, such as healthcare facilities, college campuses, and workplace settings, for case management.

ACKNOWLEDGMENT

We thank the American Cannabis Nurses Association (ACNA) for their support and mentorship.

On a personal note, we would like to dedicate this chapter to our inspirational forces, our mothers, Marie and Lydia. We also thank our supportive families, Christina, Joe, Scott, and Z.

REFERENCES

2019. State of States Report. (2019). Americans for Safe Access. Retrieved January 6, 2026, from https://www.safeaccessnow.org/sos

2025. Code of Ethics for Nurses. (2025). American Nurses Association. Retrieved January 7, 2026, from https://codeofethics.ana.org/

Agriculture Improvement Act of 2018, S.3042, 115th Cong. (2018). Congress.gov. June 18, 2018. https://www.congress.gov/bill/115th-congress/senate-bill/3042?q=%7B%22search%22%3A%22farm+bill%22%7D&s=3&r=1

American Cannabis Nurse Association. (2025). Clinical Cannabis Policies in Compassionate Care Position Paper. https://cannabisnurses.org/statements

American Cannabis Nurses Association. (2025). American Cannabis Nurses Association Position on Cannabis Rescheduling: Advocating for Schedule VI Position & Policy Statement of the American Cannabis Nurses Association. ACNA.https://cannabisnurses.org/statements

American Cannabis Nurses Association. (n.d.). Lobbying/Advocacy with 501 (c) (3) status. https://docs.google.com/document/d/132J3taSi4QnXMR_JFW3hnemQcusZaEdF/edit?usp=sharing&ouid=107587315507364884473&rtpof=true&sd=true

American Nurses Association. (2025). Code of ethics for nurses. American Nurses Association.https://codeofethics.ana.org/home

American Nurses Association. (2016). Nursing Administration: Scope and Standards of Practice, 2nd Edition eBook. Nursesbooks. https://api.pageplace.de/preview/DT0400.9781558106444_A30487125/preview-9781558106444_A30487125.pdf

American Nurses Association. (1994, December 8). Drug Testing for Health Care Workers. https://www.nursingworld.org/practice-policy/nursingexcellence/official-position-statements/id/drug-testing-forhealth-care-workers

American Nurses Association. (2024). *Nursing Leadership: Scope and Standards of Practice* (3rd ed.). American Nurses Association.

American Nurses Association. (2024). Re: Schedules of Controlled Substances: Rescheduling of Marijuana [DEA–1362; A.G. Order No. 5931– 2024]. Letter to Attorney General Garland: Submitted electronically at www.regulations.gov https://www.nursingworld.org/globalassets/docs/ana/comment-letters/ana-cannbbis-eschedule-comments-final-2024-07-17.pdf

American Nurses Association and American Cannabis Nurses Association. (2024). *Cannabis Nursing Scope and Standards of Practice* (1st ed.).

American Nurses Association Center for Ethics and Human Rights. (2016). Therapeutic Use of Marijuana and Related Cannabinoids. ANA Silver Spring.https://www.nursingworld.org/globalassets/docs/ana/therapeutic-use-of-marijuna-and-related-cannabinoids.pdf

American Nurses Association Center for Ethics and Human Rights. (2021). Therapeutic Use of Marijuana and Related Cannabinoids Position Statement. ANA.https://www.nursingworld.org/globalassets/practiceandpolicy/nursing-excellence/ana-position-statements/therapeutic-use-of-marijuana-and-related-cannabinoids-position-statement-final-2021.pdf#:~:text=Position%20Statement%3A%20Providing%20patients%20safe,marijuana%2Fcannabis.&text=Code%20of%20ethics%20for%20nurses,interpretive%20statements.%20Silver%20Spring%2C%20MD%3A

American Nurses Association Position Statement: Therapeutic use of marijuana and related cannabinoids. (2022). *OJIN: The Online Journal of Issues in Nursing, 27*(1). https://doi.org/10.3912/OJIN.Vol27No01PoSCol01

American Nurses Association Position Statement: Nurses' professional responsibility to promote ethical practice environments. (January 23, 2023) . OJIN: The *Online Journal of Issues in Nursing 28(1).* https://ojin.nursingworld.org/table-of-contents/volume-28-2023/number-1-january-2023/responsibility-to-promote-ethical-practice-environments/

Organization of Nurse Executives and American Organization for Nursing Leadership. (2022). AONL Nurse Leader Core Competencies, Chicago, IL; AONE, AONL.

Americans for Safe Access. (2025). California healthcare facility implementation guide for the compassionate access to Medical Cannabis Act Ryan's Law SB 311(2021), SB 988 (2022), SB 302 (2023). https://www.safeaccessnow.org/ryanslaw_facilityresources#gsc.tab=0

Armentano, P.A. (2021, September 13). *California: Lawmakers advance legislation providing for medical cannabis use in hospitals,* NORML. https://norml.org/blog/2021/09/13/california-lawmakers-advance-legislation-permitting-medical-cannabis-use-in-hospitals/

Aroskar, M. (1998, December 31). Administrative Ethics: Perspectives on Patients and Community-Based Care. *Online Journal of Issues in Nursing*, *3*(3). Advance online publication. https://doi.org/10.3912/OJIN.Vol3No03Man04DOI: 10.3912/OJIN.Vol3No03Man04

Birken, S.A., Lee, S.D., & Weiner, B.J. (2012). Uncovering middle managers' role in healthcare innovation implementation. *Implementation Science, 7*(1), 28. doi.org/10.1186/1748-5908-7-28

Birkhead, S., Edwards, P., Nettleton, M., Oppenlander, J., & Stapleton, M. (2022). Roles and Skills for Effective Academic Nurse Leaders. *Journal of the American Nurses Association.*, *3*(1), 22–32.https://doi.org/10.47988/janany.28237684.3.1

Board-certified case manager | Commission for Case Manager Certification (CCMC). (2024). Ccmcertification.org. https://ccmcertification.org/about-commissiontm/differences-between-certified-case-managers-and-case-managers/board-certified

Boehning, A. P., & Haddad, L. M. (2023). Nursing Practice Act. [Updated 2023 Jul 17]. In: StatPearls [Internet]. Treasure Island (FL): StatPearls Publishing; 2026 Jan-. Available from: https://www.ncbi.nlm.nih.gov/books/NBK559012/

L.M., & BorgeltFranson, K.L. (2017). Considerations for Hospital Policies Regarding Medical Cannabis Use. *Hospital Pharmacy. 52*(2), 89–90. https://doi:10.1310/hpj5202-89

Bosley, H. G., Peña, J. M., Penn, A. D., Sorensen, J. L., Tierney, M., & Flentje, A. (2023). A Pragmatic, Person-Centered View of Cannabis in the United States: Pursuing Care That Transcends Beliefs. *Substance Abuse*, *44*(4), 337–347.https://doi.org/10.1177/08897077231202836

Braun, R.L. (1991). Uniform Controlled Substances Act of 1990. Campbell Law Review Volume 13 Issue 3 Summer Article 5 Uniform Controlled Substances Act of 1990. Retrieved January 6, 2026, from https://scholarship.law.campbell.edu/cgi/viewcontent.cgi?article=1222&context=clr#:~:text=The%201990%20Uniform%20Controlled%20Substances%20Act%20also%20provides%20for%20emergency,analogs%20or%20other%20dangerous%20substances.&text=prohibiting%20a%20substance%20becomes%20necessary,be%20scheduled%20without%20any%20delay

Bryan, K. (2024). Cannabis Overview 2025 by the National Conference of State Legislatures. https://www.ncsl.org/civil-and-criminal-justice/cannabis-overview

Cadmus, E., Dempsey, C., Boston-Leary, K., & Bates, M. (2024).. . *Nursing Leadership Scope and Standards and Pathway to Excellence Nursing Management*, *55*(6), 7–12.https://doi.org/10.1097/nmg.0000000000000139

Cannabis academic research grants—Department of Cannabis Control. (n.d.). Retrieved January 6, 2026, from https://www.cannabis.ca.gov/about-us/grant-funding/cannabis-academic-research-grants/

Cannabis use in hospice and palliative care – Compassionate Oregon. (n.d.). Retrieved January 6, 2026, from https://compassionateoregon.org/cannabis-use-in-hospice-and-palliative-care/

Management Society of America. (2024, May 31). *The Impact of Case Management on the Healthcare System: A CMSA Perspective.* Cmsa.org. https://cmsa.org/the-impact-of-case-management-on-the-healthcare-system-3/

Certification principles | Commission for Case Manager Certification (CCMC). (n.d.). Ccmcertification.org. https://ccmcertification.org/about-ccmc/about-case-management/certification-principles

Chen, R. (2025, April 15). Evaluation of Nurses' Performance: Key Metrics to Track Bucketlist Blog https://bucketlistrewards.com/blog/evaluation-nurses-performance/#:~:text=By%20assessing%2vvarious%20aspects%20of%20a%20nurse's,to%20transform%20your%20healthcare%20organization%20%C2%B7%20Performance

Chuang, E., Jason, K., & Morgan, J. C. (2011). Factors influencing middle manager support. *Health Care Management Review*, *36*(4), 369–379.https://doi.org/10.1097/HMR.0b013e3182100cc2

Clark, C. S. (2021). *Cannabis: A handbook for nurses* (1st ed.). Wolters Kluwer.

Clark, C. S. (2021). *Legal, ethical, and advocacy concerns: Cannabis from the federal to the state level. Cannabis: A handbook for nurses* (1st ed.). Wolters Kluwer.

Clark, C. S. (2021). Cannabis Science Education: Meeting the Need for Cannabis Care Competencies. American Association of Colleges of Nursing.https://www.aacnnursing.org/portals/0/pdfs/conferences-webinars/presentations/2021/Clark_Carey.pdf

Clark, C. S. (2022). Three questions about the nurse's role and medical cannabis. Blogpost.Nursing-center.comhttps://www.nursingcenter.com/blogs-plus/blogs/blogs-post?identifier=the-Nurses-Role-and-Medical-Cannabis#/post/the-Nurses-Role-and-Medical-Cannabis

for Medicare and Medicaid Services. (2024). *Hospital readmissions reduction program (HRRP).* Www.cms.gov https://www.cms.gov/medicare/payment/prospective-payment-systems/acute-inpatient-pps/hospital-readmissions-reduction-program-hrrp

Code of professional conduct | Commission for Case Manager Certification (CCMC). (2024). Ccmcertification.org. https://ccmcertification.org/about-commissiontm/code-professional-conduct

Comprehensive Drug Abuse Prevention and Control Act of 1970, Pub. L. 91–513, 84 Stat. 1236 (1970)

Comprehensive Pain Management. (n.d.). Understanding Ethical and Regulatory Issues in Prescribing Medical Cannabis: A Comprehensive Overview. Comprehensive Pain Management Associates.https://www.cpmany.org/understanding-ethical-and-regulatory-issues-in-prescribing-medical-cannabis-a-comprehensive-overview/

Conant v Walters, 309 F. 3d 629, 636 (9th Cir 2002).

, A. C., Sirmans, E. T., & Stype, A. (2023). Medical cannabis laws lower individual market health insurance premiums. *International Journal of Drug Policy, 119*, 104143. https://doi.org/10.1016/j.drugpo.2023.104143

Costiniuk, C. T., MacCallum, C. A., Boivin, M., Rueda, S., Lacasse, G., Walsh, Z., Daeninck, P. J., Margolese, S., Mandarino, E., Jagpaul Kaur Deol, Sanchez, T., & Bell, A. D. (2023). *Why a distinct medical stream is necessary to support patients using cannabis for medical purposes. 5*(1), 25–25. https://doi.org/10.1186/s42238-023-00195-8

Cronin, S.P., Cruz, J., Cameron, E., Azemar, S., Dudley, S., Largent-Milnes, T.M., Brady, B.R., Wallace, J.S., Arnett, M.R., Dahmer, S.M., Ibrahim, M.M., Padilla, A.R., Vanderah, T.W., & De La Rosa, J.S. (2025). "It's legal, now what?" development, implementation, and evaluation of interdisciplinary cannabis education for healthcare trainees. *Journal of Cannabis Research;7*(1),68. https://doi.org/10.1186/s42238-025-00321-8

Delatte, G. (2024, May 29). Why is cannabis not allowed on college campuses? Campus rules vs. State freedom. *Eminent.* https://www.eminentconsultingfirm.com/why-cant-you-bring-cannabis-to-college-campuses/

Diagnosed Substance Use Disorders (DSU) - NCQA. (2025, August). NCQA. https://www.ncqa.org/report-cards/health-plans/state-of-health-care-quality-report/diagnosed-substance-use-disorders-dsu

Dickison, P., Haerling, K. A., & Lasater, K. (2019). Integrating the National Council of State Boards of Nursing Clinical Judgment Model into nursing educational frameworks. *The Journal of Nursing Education, 58*(2), 72–78.https://doi.org/10.3928/01484834-20190122-03

Diversion Control Division. (n.d.). United States Department of Justice. Usdoj.gov. Retrieved January 7, 2026, from https://www.deadiversion.usdoj.gov/administrative_actions.html

, M. L., Fisher, E., Chin, J., & Panagiota Kitsantas. (2025). Medical Cannabis Use and Healthcare Utilization Among Patients with Chronic Pain: A Causal Inference Analysis Using TMLE. *Pharmacy, 13*(4), 96–96. https://doi.org/10.3390/pharmacy13040096

Drug-Free Workplace Act of 1988, 41 U.S.C. § 8101 et seq. (2018).

Emerson, J. (2025, April 25). *Insurers not required to cover medical marijuana, federal judge rules.* Becker's Payers Issues, Payer News. https://www.beckerspayer.com/policy-updates/insurers-not-required-to-cover-medical-marijuana-federal-judge-rules/

Employer drug-testing policies must evolve with state law—Troutman Pepper Locke. (2023, July 27). https://www.troutman.com/insights/employer-drug-testing-policies-must-evolve-with-state-law/

Engle, R. L., Lopez, E. R., Gormley, K. E., Chan, J. A., Charns, M. P., & Lukas, C. V. (2017). What roles do middle managers play in implementation of innovative practices? *Health Care Management Review*, *42*(1), 14–27.https://doi.org/10.1097/HMR.0000000000000090

Ethics- cannabis and case management: Medical marijuana updates | Commission for Case Manager Certification (CCMC). (2023, December 29). Ccmcertification.org. https://ccmcertification.org/courses/ethics-cannabis-and-case-management-medical-marijuana-updates#

Federal law preempts state coverage rules for medical cannabis. (2025, May 9). Reedsmith.com. https://www.reedsmith.com/articles/federal-law-preempts-state-coverage-rules-for-medical-cannabis/

Federal marijuana rescheduling | Moritz College of Law. (n.d.). The Ohio State University. Retrieved January 6, 2026, from https://moritzlaw.osu.edu/faculty-and-research/drug-enforcement-and-policy-center/research-and-grants/policy-and-data-analyses/federal-marijuana-rescheduling#:~:text=What%20would%20rescheduling%20marijuana%20from,opportunities%20to%20participate%20in%20research

Federal Policies. (n.d.) Marijuana Policy Project. Retrieved January 6, 2026, from https://www.mpp.org/policy/federal/

Fitzgerald, R. L., Umlauf, A., Hubbard, J. A., Hoffman, M. A., Sobolesky, P. M., Ellis, S. E., Grelotti, D. J., Suhandynata, R. T., Huestis, M. A., Grant, I., & Marcotte, T. D. (2023). Driving under the influence of cannabis: Impact of combining toxicology testing with field sobriety tests. *Clinical Chemistry*, *69*(7), 724–733.https://doi.org/10.1093/clinchem/hvad054

Fleider, E. (2025, October 6). *Medical Marijuana: Implications for nurses in Ohio.* UC News. https://www.uc.edu/news/articles/2025/10/medical-marijuana--implications-for-nurses-in-ohio.html

Follow-Up After Emergency Department Visit for Substance Use (FUA) - NCQA. (2025, August). NCQA. https://www.ncqa.org/report-cards/health-plans/state-of-health-care-quality-report/follow-up-after-emergency-department-visit-for-substance-use-fua/

, A. P., & De Jesus, O. (2023, August 14). *Case management.* PubMed; StatPearls Publishing. https://www.ncbi.nlm.nih.gov/books/NBK562214/

Greenway, M., & Acai, A. (2024). Academic leadership in nursing: A concept analysis. *Nurse Education Today*, *141*, 106338.https://doi.org/10.1016/j.nedt.2024.106338

González-García, A., Pinto-Carral, A., Pérez-González, S., & Marqués-Sánchez, P. (2021). Nurse managers' competencies: A scoping review. *Journal of Nursing Management*, *29*(6), 1410–1419.https://doi.org/10.1111/jonm.13380

Gowen, K., Cahill, M., Russell, K., & Cronquist, R. (2018). Medical Marijuana and Nursing Practice: Legislation, Scientific Literature review, and nursing implications. National Council of State Board of Nursing.https://www.ncsbn.org/public-files/presentations/2018DCM_Medical-Marijuana.pdf

Guidance Regarding Marijuana Enforcement. (2013, August 23). U.S. Department of Justice Office of the Deputy Attorney General. https://www.justice.gov/iso/opa/resources/3052013829132756857467.pdf

Gupta, K. (2023). Validity and Reliability of Students' Assessment: Case for Recognition as a Unified Concept of Valid Reliability. *International Journal of Applied & Basic Medical Research*, *13*(3), 129–132. https://doi.org/10.4103/ijabmr.ijabmr_382_23

Javeed, M. (2024, February 28). Confronting the Crisis: Exploring the Challenges of Nurse Educator Shortages Today. Top content on LinkedIn. https://www.linkedin.com/pulse/confronting-crisis-exploring-challenges-nurse-edccator-javeed-0eh4f#:~:text=1

Kellogg, A., Anderson, C., & Michiels, M. (2022, April). A Cannabis Conflict of Law: Federal vs. State Law Business Law Today American Bar Association, https://www.americanbar.org/groups/business_law/resources/business-law-today/2022-april/a-cannabis-conflict-of-law-federal-vs-state-law/#:~:text=As%20we%20examined%20in%20the,substance%20is%20a%20federal%20offense

Kilmer, J. (2018, November 13). Cannabis and the college campus: Considering the impact on students in a changing legal climate. *Higher Education Today*. https://www.higheredtoday.org/2018/11/13/cannabis-college-campus-considering-impact-students-changing-legal-climate/

King, R. (1972). The drug hang-up: America's fifty-year folly. W.W. Norton.https://www.google.com/url?q=https://www.druglibrary.net/special/king/dhu/dhu28.htm&sa=D&source=docs&ust=1765298703276722&usg=AOvVaw3-RFfIpiJtPV-UD2Ax05Uz

King, D. D., Gill, C. J., Cadieux, C. S., & Singh, N. (2024). The role of stigma in cannabis use disclosure: An exploratory study. *Harm Reduction Journal*, *21*(1), 21.https://doi.org/10.1186/s12954-024-00929-8

Kocis, P. T., Mallinson, D. J., & Servinsky Jr., T. J. (2024). Cannabinoid Awareness, Reporting Use to Health Care Providers, and Perceptions Regarding Safety – Pennsylvania, March 2023–April 2023. *Medical Cannabis and Cannabinoids,* *7*(1), 119–124. https://doi.org/10.1159/000539956

Kurtzman, E. T., Greene, J., Begley, R., & Drenkard, K. N. (2022). "We want what's best for patients." Nurse leaders' attitudes about medical cannabis: A qualitative study. *International Journal of Nursing Studies Advances*, *4*, 100065.https://doi.org/10.1016/j.ijnsa.2022.100065

Kogan, M., Temple, L. M., Zolotov, Y., & Isralowitz, R. (2025). 2025 International Congress Abstract Supplement. *Global Advances in Integrative Medicine and Health*, *14*, 27536130251324543.https://doi.org/10.1177/27536130251324543

Lampe, J. R., Sacco, L. N., & Sheikh, H. Z. (2024, May 2). The Federal Status of Marijuana and the Policy Gap with States. LIBRARY OF CONGRESS https://www.congress.gov/crs-product/IF12270

Lange, T. (2025, November 19). US Congresswoman Unveils Bill to Repeal Federal Hemp Product Ban. Cannabis Business Times. https://www.cannabisbusinesstimes.com/hemp/news/15772220/us-congresswoaan-unveils-bill-to-repeal-federal-hemp-product-ban

Langley, P. C. (2019). Tracking and Reporting Outcomes in Medical Marijuana: Establishing Condition-Specific State-Level Registries. *Innovations in Pharmacy*, *10*(2), 4. https://doi.org/10.24926/iip.v10i2.1800

Lapham, G. T., Matson, T. E., Carrell, D. S., Bobb, J. F., Luce, C., Oliver, M. M., Ghitza, U. E., Hsu, C., Browne, K. C., Binswanger, I. A., Campbell, C. I., Saxon, A. J., Vandrey, R., Schauer, G. L., Pacula, R. L., Horberg, M. A., Bailey, S. R., McClure, E. A., & Bradley, K. A. (2022). Comparison of Medical Cannabis Use Reported on a Confidential Survey vs Documented in the Electronic Health Record Among Primary Care Patients. *JAMA Network Open*, *5*(5), e2211677–e2211677. https://doi.org/10.1001/jamanetworkopen.2022.11677

Lawler, Z. (2025). Medical Cannabis & Cannabinoid Regulation 2025. Last Updated May 29, 2025. USA https://practiceguides.chambers.com/practice-guides/comparison/1003/17057/25531-25538-25540#:~:text=Under%20federal%20law%2C%20cannabis%20is,Enforcement%20Policies:%20The%20Cole%20Memorandum

Lewis, K. (2025, May 29). The Vital Role of Performance Reviews and Appraisals in Nursing. ACI Training and Consultancy LTD. https://www.acitrainingandconsultancy.co.uk/post/the-vital-role-of-performance-reviews-and-appraisals-in-nursing#:~:text=Foster%20a%20supportive%20environment:%20Focus,support%20nurses%20with%20NMC%20revalidation.

Marcotte, T. D., Umlauf, A., Grelotti, D. J., Sones, E. G., Mastropietro, K. F., Suhandynata, R. T., Huestis, M. A., Grant, I., & Fitzgerald, R. L. (2023). Evaluation of field sobriety tests for identifying drivers under the influence of cannabis: A randomized clinical trial. *JAMA Psychiatry*, *80*(9), 914–923. https://doi.org/10.1001/jamapsychiatry.2023.2345

Marijuana Policy Project. (n.d.) *Medical Cannabis Laws and Employment Protections. MPP.* Retrieved January 6, 2026, from https://www.mpp.org/issues/medical-marijuana/medical-cannabis-laws-and-employment-protections/

Marijuana Policy Project. (n.d.). *DEA moves to reschedule marijuana to Schedule III: questions and answers*. MPP. Retrieved January 6, 2026, from https://www.mpp.org/policy/federal/dea-moves-to-reschedule-marijuana-to-schedule-iii-questions-and-answers/

Marijuana Policy Project. (2022, February 7). *Medical Cannabis Laws and Anti-Discrimination Provisions.* MMP. Retrieved January 6, 2026, from https://www.mpp.org/issues/medical-marijuana/medical-marijuana-laws-anti-discrimination-provisions/

M, F. (2025, March 31). *Cannabis and healthcare: Complicated policies and laws.* American Nurse. https://www.myamericannurse.com/cannabis-and-healthcare-complicated-policies-and-laws/

McKaig, A., Ridad, A., Bell, A., McParlane, R., & Quirch, M. (2025). Implementing Ryan's Law on an Inpatient Medical Oncology Unit, *Clinical Journal of Oncology Nursing 20;29*(1), 86–90. https://doi.org/10.1188/25.CJON.86-90

McNichol, W. J. (2025). Pseudoscience and the Detection of Marijuana-Based Impairment: We Can and Must Do Better, 86. *Journal of Studies on Alcohol and Drugs*, *86*(4), 503–509.https://doi.org/10.15288/jsad.24-00307

Mead, A. (2019). Legal and Regulatory Issues Governing Cannabis and Cannabis-Derived Products in the United States. *Frontiers in Plant Science*, (10), 679.https://doi.org/10.3389/fpls.2019.00697

Meckes, K. (2025, November 24). *This is an inflection point for hemp. U.S. Hemp Roundtable.* https://hempsupporter.com/news/this-is-an-inflection-point-for-hemp/

Medical Cannabis Glossary. (n.d.) MM411. https://medicalmarijuana411.com/glossary/medical-marijuana-program-mmp/#:~:text=Definition:%20An%20official%20jurisdictional%20resource,medical%20marijuana%20(MMJ)%20card

*Medical Cannabis Insurance Coverage: Are We Getting Closer? (*2025, August 27). MedCard.com https://getmedcard.co/medical-cannabis-insurance-coverage-are-we-getting-closer/#:~:text=Key%20Takeaways,hindered%20by%20its%20federal%20status

Medicare to test coverage of medical marijuana. (n.d.). AARP. Retrieved January 6, 2026, from https://www.aarp.org/medicare/faq/does-medicare-cover-medical-marijuana/

Moore, E. (2024, July 2). *Connecting the dots with cannabis care.* American Nurse. https://www.myamericannurse.com/connecting-the-dots-with-cannabis-care/

NASW Practice Standards & Guidelines. (2025). Socialworkers.org. https://www.socialworkers.org/Practice/NASW-Practice-Standards-Guidelines/SASW-Standards%20for%20Social-Work-Case-Management

National Academies of Sciences, Engineering, and Medicine. (2017). *The health effects of cannabis and cannabinoids: The current state of evidence and recommendations for research.* The National Academies Press. DOI: https://doi.org/10.17226/24625

National Academies of Sciences, Engineering, and Medicine, Health and Medicine Division, & Board on Population Health and Public Health Practice. (2017, January 12). *Challenges and Barriers in Conducting Cannabis Research.* Nih.gov; National Academies Press (US). https://www.ncbi.nlm.nih.gov/books/NBK425757/

National Council of State Boards of Nursing. (2018). *The NCSBN national nursing guidelines for medical marijuana.* Journal of Nursing Regulation, *9(2).* DOI.https://www.ncsbn.org/marijuana-guidelines.htm10.1016/S2155-8256(18)30094-2

National Council of State Boards of Nursing. (2019, Winter). *Clinical judgment measurement model. Next Generation NCLEX News.* https://www.ncsbn.org/NGN_Winter19.pdf

NCLEX. (n.d.). Clinical Judgment Measurement Model: A framework to measure clinical judgment & decision making. https://www.nclex.com/clinical-judgment-measurement-model.page

New marijuana laws have companies questioning current drug testing policies. (n.d.). Reference Services. Retrieved January 6, 2026, from https://www.referenceservices.com/new-marijuana-laws-have-companies-questioning-current-drug-testing-policies/

New York City Council passes trailblazing bill to ban all preemployment marijuana testing. (2019). Genova Burns LLC. https://www.genovaburns.com/news/labor-law/2019-04-16-new-york-city-council-passes-trailblazing-bill-to-ban-all-preemployment-marijuana-testing

Parmalee, R. A., & Clark, C. S. (2022). Nursing students' knowledge, skills, and attitudes regarding medical cannabis care: A national study. *Journal of Nursing Regulation, 13*(3), 13–23.https://doi.org/10.1016/S2155-8256(22)00082-5

Perlman, A. I., McLeod, H. M., Ventresca, E. C., Salinas, M. G., Post, P. J., Schuh, M. J., & Dabrah, A. M. A. (2021). Medical Cannabis State and Federal Regulations: Implications for United States Health Care Entities. *Mayo Clinic Proceedings, 96*(10), 2671–2681.https://doi.org/10.1016/j.mayocp.2021.05.005

Physicians' Guide to Ryan's Law. (2021). *Americans for Safe Access.* https://d3n8a8pro7vhmx.cloudfront.net/americansforsafeaccess/pages/17096/attachments/original/1640099846/Physician's_Guide_to_Ryan's_Law.pdf?1640099846

Physicians, medical marijuana, and the law. (2014). *AMA Journal of Ethics, 16*(9), 732–738. https://doi.org/10.1001/virtualmentor.2014.16.9.hlaw1-1409

Papanagnou, D., Klein, M. R., Zhang, X. C., Cameron, K. A., Doty, A., McCarthy, D. M., Rising, K. L., & Salzman, D. H. (2021). Developing standardized patient-based cases for communication training: Lessons learned from training residents to communicate diagnostic uncertainty. *Advances in Simulation (London, England), 6*(1), 26.https://doi.org/10.1186/s41077-021-00176-y

Porter, J. (2016, November 16). Cannabis and the mission of higher education. *Inside Higher Ed.* https://www.insidehighered.com/views/2016/11/17/dangers-students-regular-marijuana-use-essay

Putra, A. D. M., & Sandhi, A. (2021). Implementation of nursing case management to improve community access to care: A scoping review. *Belitung Nursing Journal, 7*(3), 141–150. https://doi.org/10.33546/bnj.1449

Ramaekers, J. G., Vinckenbosch, F., & Gilman, J. M. (2023). High traffic—The quest for a reliable test of cannabis impairment. *JAMA Psychiatry, 80*(9), 871–872.https://doi.org/10.1001/jamapsychiatry.2023.2309

Ryan, J., & Sharts-Hopko, N. (2017). The experiences of medical marijuana patients: A scoping review of the qualitative literature. *The Journal of Neuroscience Nursing : Journal of the American Association of Neuroscience Nurses, 49*(3), 185–190.https://doi.org/10.1097/JNN.0000000000000283

Ryan, J. E., McCabe, S. E., & Boyd, C. J. (2021). Medicinal Cannabis: Policy, patients, and providers. *Policy, Politics & Nursing Practice, 22*(2), 126.https://doi.org/10.1177/1527154421989609

Ryan's Law Foundation. (n.d.). Retrieved January 6, 2026, from https://ryanslawfoundation.org/

Samuel, A., O'Brien, J., & Pontious, A. (2025). Lawmakers Introduce Bill to Regulate Hemp Products Ahead of an Impending Ban. Husch Blackwell Cannabis Law Now.https://www.cannabislawnow.com/2025/12/lawmakers-introduce-bill-to-regulate-hemp-products-ahead-of-an-impending-ban/?utm_source=Husch+Blackwell+-+Cannabis+Law+Now&utm_campaign=99e716313a-RSS_EMAIL_CAMPAIGN&utm_medium=email&utm_term=0_6a9bb772e1-99e716313a-73179189

Sacco, L. N. (2024, July 23). Rescheduling Marijuana: Implications for Criminal and Collateral Consequences. *In Focus.* https://www.congress.gov/crs-product/IF12715#:~:text=If%20marijuana%20is%20rescheduled%20to,costs%20of%20selling%20their%20product.&text=As%20with%20other%20controlled%20substances,alcohol%20by%20students%20and%20employees

Schermele, Z. (2025, November 11). *Inside the details of the shutdown deal, from new cannabis rules to a Jack Smith jab.* USA TODAY. Retrieved January 6, 2026, from https://www.usatoday.com/story/news/politics/2025/11/11/inside-shutdown-deal-cannabis-charlie-kirk-jack-smith/87214014007/

State Policies. (n.d.). Marijuana Policy Project. Retrieved January 6, 2026, from https://www.mpp.org/states/

Temple, L.M., Lampert, S.L., & Ewigman, B. (2019). Barriers to Achieving Optimal Success with Medical Cannabis: Opportunities for Quality Improvement. *The Journal of Alternative and Complementary Medicine, 25*(1), 5–7. https://doi.org/10.1089/acm.2018.0250

The Evolution of Marijuana as a Controlled Substance and the Federal-State Policy Gap (Updated April 7, 2022) (R44782). https://www.congress.gov/crs_external_products/R/HTML/R44782.html#:~:text=91%2D513).,for%20purposes%20of%20sanctioned%20research.&text=(A)%20The%20drug%20or%20other,other%20substance%20under%20medical%20supervision.&text=The%20CSA%20was%20enacted%20as,and%20Control%20Act%20of%201970.&text=It%20regulates%20the%20manufacture%2C%20possession,unauthorized%20activities%20involving%20controlled%20substances.&text=whether%20the%20substance%20is%20an%20immediate%20precursor%20of%20an%20already%20scheduled%20substance

Theisen, E. & Konieczny, E. (2019, November 4). Medical cannabis: What nurses need to know. *American Nurse.* American Nurses Association. https://www.myamericannurse.com/medical-cannabis-what-nurses-need-to-know/#:~:text=of%20cannabis%20impossible.-,Cannabis:%206%20essential%20principles,pain%20and%20other%20distressing%20symptoms.

Trump, D. (2025, December 18). *Increasing medical marijuana and cannabidiol research* (Executive Order 14370). The White House. https://www.whitehouse.gov/presidential-actions/2025/12/increasing-medical-marijuana-and-cannabidiol-research/

United States Congress. (2025). Agriculture, Rural Development, Food and Drug Administration, and Related Agencies Appropriations Act, 2026, Pub. L. No. 119-37, div. B (2025). https://www.congress.gov/119/plaws/publ37/PLAW-119publ37.pdf

Utah Canna (2025, September 10). The Federal-State Divide: Why Medical Cannabis Remains Complex. https://utahcanna.org/the-federal-state-divide-why-medical-cannabis-remains-complex/

Vederhus, J.-K., Rørendal, M., Skårdal, M., Næss, M. O., Clausen, T., & Kristensen, Ø. (2022). Successful outcomes with low–threshold intervention for cannabis use disorders in Norway - an observational study. *PLOS ONE, 17*(6), e0269988. https://doi.org/10.1371/journal.pone.0269988

What is a nurse administrator? Responsibilities & qualifications. (2024, September 11). Retrieved January 6, 2026, from https://www.carerev.com/blog/the-role-of-nurse-administrators

Wiese, J.L., Watson, T.M., Bozinoff, N., Rush, B., Stergiopoulos, V., Le Foll, B., & Rueda, S. (2024, December). "Like the Wild West": Health care provider perspectives on impacts of recreational cannabis legalization on patients and providers at a tertiary psychiatric hospital in Ontario, Canada. *Journal of Substance Use and Addiction Treatment 167*, 209487. https://doi.org/10.1016/j.josat.2024.209487

Writer, C. (2024, July 16). *Can Nurses Legally Use Cannabis Across Different States?* Marijuana Packaging. https://marijuanapackaging.com/blogs/questions/can-nurses-legally-use-cannabis-across-different-states

Zolotov, Y., Temple, L. M., Isralowitz, R., Gorelick, D. A., Abraham, R., Abrams, D. I., Barich, K., Boehnke, K. F., Dahmer, S., Friedman, B. R., Wilson-King, G. S., Arnsten, J. H., & Kogan, M. (2025). Developing Medical Cannabis Competencies: A Consensus Statement. *JAMA Network Open*, *8*(10), e2535049.https://doi.org/10.1001/jamanetworkopen.2025.35049

Zolotov, Y., Metri, S., Calabria, E., & Kogan, M. (2021). Medical cannabis education among healthcare trainees: A scoping review. *Complementary Therapies in Medicine*, *58*, 102675.https://doi.org/10.1016/j.ctim.2021.102675

KEY TERMS AND DEFINITIONS

Rescheduling: A federal administrative process to move cannabis from a Schedule I controlled substance to another level under the Controlled Substances Act (CSA).

Medical Cannabis Compassionate Care: State-regulated programs providing patients with severe, debilitating, or terminal medical conditions an in or outpatient cannabis treatment option.

Safe Harbor: Legal provision offering protection from facing severe consequences when following established cannabis guidelines.

Right Touch Regulation: A framework for decision making focusing on risk assessment and positive outcomes, intervening with proportionate action only when necessary.

Cannabis Care Advocacy: Promoting access to cannabis for therapeutic and general wellness using education, policy, and patient support to reduce stigma and barriers.

Non-judgmental Care: A nursing approach creating a safe space for patients to feel valued and respected.

Cannabis Case Management: Client-based collaboration involving assessment, planning, facilitation, and advocating on choices and services for the clients' comprehensive health, social, and occasional legal needs.

Integrated Hybrid Model of Case Management and Cannabis Care Nursing: a combination of case management nursing and cannabis care nurse education providing harm reduction information, coordination of health care benefits to address complications of cannabis use, and reduction of health care costs.

Coordination of Care: an intended, organized, and collaborative approach to manage a patient's health care, incorporating different providers and facility settings, certifying systematic, safe, and high-quality care.

Chapter 11
Equity, Access, and Social Determinants in Medical Cannabis Use:
A Public Health Lens

Thomas A. Clobes
http://orcid.org/0000-0003-1287-5421
California State University Channel Islands, USA

Carey S. Cadieux
http://orcid.org/0000-0001-8812-2667
Binghamton University, USA

ABSTRACT

This chapter examines medical cannabis equity through a public health lens, emphasizing how access to cannabinoid therapeutics in the United States is shaped by structural, historical, and policy-driven determinants rather than individual choice alone. Drawing on social determinants of health frameworks, the chapter analyzes how federal prohibition, state-level policy variation, financial barriers, stigma, and limited clinical guidance contribute to inequitable access and patient experiences. Particular attention is given to the role of stigma and implicit bias within healthcare settings and their effects on disclosure, clinical guidance, and trust. The chapter highlights nurses as critical actors positioned at the intersection of policy, practice, and patient experience, with unique responsibilities in advocacy, education, and harm reduction. Policy and system-level strategies, including health system integration, data surveillance, and equity-oriented reform, are presented as essential for advancing equitable medical cannabis care.

INTRODUCTION

Framing Cannabis Equity as a Public Health Issue

The expansion of legal access to medical cannabis in the United States has created meaningful opportunities for symptom management and patient autonomy; however, these benefits are unevenly distributed

DOI: 10.4018/979-8-3373-7287-7.ch011

given the varying legal status throughout the country (National Conference of State Legislatures, 2025; South et al., 2025). Structural inequities, social determinants of health, and pervasive stigma influence who gains access to medical cannabis and who encounters barriers within both the healthcare and regulatory systems (Hulaihel et al, 2023). These inequities mirror larger patterns of disparate access to healthcare services in the United States, with uneven regulatory environments further shaping eligibility, affordability, and the informational support available to patients (Grbic et al., 2017).

Medical cannabis policy has increasingly been framed as a mechanism to expand therapeutic options for patients with chronic and complex conditions, including cancer-related symptoms, chronic pain, neurological disorders, and palliative care needs (National Academies of Sciences, Engineering, and Medicine [NASEM], 2017; Hossain & Chae, 2024; Perlman et al., 2021). However, from a public health perspective, access to a therapeutic intervention is not determined solely by its legal status, but by the conditions under which it is implemented, regulated, and integrated into healthcare systems. As with other health interventions, uneven implementation of medical cannabis policy risks reproducing existing inequities if social context, economic barriers, and structural determinants are not explicitly addressed (National Academies of Sciences, Engineering, and Medicine, 2017; Orenstein & Glantz, 2020).

Public health scholarship consistently demonstrates that policy changes can yield differential benefits across populations depending on how they intersect with preexisting disparities in healthcare access, education, income, and neighborhood context (Mennis et al., 2016; National Academies of Sciences, Engineering, and Medicine, 2017; Orenstein & Glantz, 2020). In the case of medical cannabis, these disparities are further shaped by stigma, regulatory complexity, and the legacy of cannabis criminalization, which has disproportionately affected racially economically marginalized communities (Martin-Willett et al., 2023). Without intentional equity-oriented design, medical cannabis programs may inadvertently advantage individuals who already possess greater healthcare access, health literacy, and financial resources.

Compounding these systemic challenges is the limited scientific and clinical guidance available to frontline providers. Federal Schedule I classification has historically impeded comprehensive research, producing gaps in dosing protocols, treatment indications, and patient education frameworks (Cooper et al., 2021; Gardiner et al., 2019). In practice, nurses often encounter patients using cannabis for chronic illness, cancer-related symptoms, or psychological distress without adequate institutional resources to guide evidence-informed conversations (Kurtzman et al., 2022; Rice et al., 2022). As a result, patients from marginalized groups, those already more likely to experience mistrust, fragmented care, and financial barriers, may be at heightened risk of receiving incomplete or stigmatizing guidance (Ho et al., 2022; Jaiswal, 2019; Rami et al., 2023).

These challenges position medical cannabis squarely within broader debates about health equity and the social responsibilities of healthcare systems. Similar to earlier policy transitions involving opioids, tobacco, and emerging pharmacotherapies, the absence of standardized clinical guidance and uneven provider education has placed a disproportionate burden on patients to self-navigate risk, benefit, and legality (Barry & Glantz, 2016; Pacula & Smart, 2017). For patients with limited access to consistent primary care or specialty services, this burden is often compounded by mistrust of healthcare institutions and concern about judgment or surveillance (Ho et al., 2022; Jaiswal, 2019; Nayak et al., 2022).

Nurses, who frequently serve as the most accessible point of contact within healthcare systems, encounter the downstream effects of these systemic gaps in routine clinical practice (Kurtzman et al., 2022; Nadzam, 2009; Newell & Jordan, 2015). While registered nurses in the United States are not typically responsible for authorizing medical cannabis use, they are often tasked with symptom assessment, medication reconciliation, patient education, and care coordination. In the absence of clear institutional frameworks, nurses must navigate competing ethical obligations related to patient autonomy, safety, and professional accountability, often without sufficient training or policy support (Gardiner et al., 2019; Kurtzman et al., 2022).

Framing cannabis equity as a public health issue situates these barriers within a broader context of structural determinants (Mennis et al., 2016; National Academies of Sciences, Engineering, and Medicine, 2017; Orenstein & Glantz, 2020). This underscores the essential role of nurses in shaping equitable, patient-centered care (Kurtzman et al., 2022; Nadzam, 2009; Newell & Jordan, 2015). Through culturally responsive communication, advocacy, and systems-level engagement, nurses can help ensure that the evolving landscape of cannabis therapeutics advances rather than undermines health equity.

A public health approach to cannabis equity emphasizes population-level outcomes, prevention of harm, and the reduction of avoidable disparities rather than a narrow focus on individual choice or market access. This approach draws on established frameworks used in tobacco and alcohol control, which highlight the importance of regulation, surveillance, education, and community engagement in shaping health outcomes over time (Barry & Glantz, 2016; Schauer, 2021). Applying these principles to medical cannabis requires attention to who benefits from policy change, who remains excluded, and how healthcare systems mediate these effects.

Within this framework, equity is not an ancillary consideration but a core criterion for evaluating the success of medical cannabis programs. Equity-oriented policy analysis asks whether medical cannabis access is distributed according to need, whether patients receive consistent and evidence-informed guidance, and whether healthcare institutions are equipped to support safe and informed use across diverse populations. Framing cannabis equity as a public health issue thus establishes the conceptual foundation for examining historical policy decisions, social determinants of access, stigma within healthcare settings, and the role of system-level reform explored in the sections that follow.

HISTORICAL & POLICY CONTEXT OF MEDICAL CANNABIS IN THE U.S.

Evolution of Cannabis Policy: From Prohibition to Medical Legalization

The contemporary medical cannabis landscape reflects decades of political, scientific, and regulatory tensions (Zarhin et al., 2020). Although cannabis was widely used as a medicinal product through the early 20th century, prohibitionist policies culminated in its classification as a Schedule I substance under the Controlled Substances Act of 1970, asserting no accepted medical use and severely restricting research (Eddy, 2010; Grbic et al., 2017). This federal stance has persisted despite emerging evidence of therapeutic benefit and increasing public acceptance (Hossain & Chae, 2024).

Early federal cannabis policy was not only shaped by scientific uncertainty, but also by moral, political, and racialized narratives that framed cannabis as a social threat rather than a therapeutic substance (Eddy, 2010; Martin-Willett et al., 2023). Historical analyses of drug policy have documented how cannabis prohibition emerged alongside broader efforts to regulate marginalized populations, particularly immigrants and communities of color, during the early to mid-twentieth century (Martin-Willett et al., 2023). These narratives persisted into the modern era, influencing the placement of cannabis in Schedule I and reinforcing assumptions that it lacked legitimate medical value despite its prior inclusion in the U.S. Pharmacopeia.

For healthcare professionals, including nurses, the consequences of this history extend beyond legality into professional socialization and education. Cannabis has long been excluded from formal health sciences curricula, leaving generations of clinicians without foundational training in cannabinoid pharmacology or therapeutic application (Gardiner et al., 2019; Parmelee & Clark, 2022). This omission has contributed to clinical silence around cannabis use, particularly in institutional settings where legal ambiguity and professional risk aversion discourage proactive engagement with patients. As a result, historical policy decisions continue to shape contemporary clinical practice in subtle but consequential ways (Gardiner et al., 2019; Martin-Willett et al., 2023; Perlman et al., 2021).

State-Level Frameworks and Federal–State Conflict

Research shows that scientific evidence has played a limited role in shaping medical cannabis policy (Zarhin et al., 2020). Policymakers, health professionals, and researchers interviewed across several U.S. states emphasized that political ideology, advocacy pressure, and public sentiment frequently outweighed scientific considerations during legislative development (Grbic et al., 2017). As a result, state-level medical cannabis programs differ markedly in qualifying conditions, clinical oversight, dispensary regulation, and patient certification processes (Hong et al., 2024; Perlman et al., 2021).

Variation in state medical cannabis programs reflects differing policy priorities rather than consistent interpretations of clinical evidence. Some states have adopted highly "medicalized" models characterized by narrow qualifying condition lists, stringent physician oversight requirements, and limited dispensary access, while others have implemented more permissive frameworks that emphasize patient autonomy and broader clinical discretion (Pacula & Smart, 2017). These differences have direct implications for accessibility, particularly for patients with chronic conditions that are more prevalent among older adults, low-income populations, and communities of color.

Comparative policy analyses suggest that restrictive programs may inadvertently suppress legitimate medical use by increasing administrative burden on clinicians and patients alike (Perlman et al., 2021). In contrast, more flexible programs can increase access but may do so without adequate public health safeguards, such as standardized product testing, consistent patient education, or integration with healthcare systems (Orenstein & Glantz, 2020). For nurses working across state lines or within multi-jurisdictional health systems, this variability complicates care coordination and contributes to uneven patient experiences.

Federal research barriers continue to impede clinical guidance and therapeutic standardization (Cooper et al., 2021). Even as states build their own regulatory infrastructures, researchers must navigate a restrictive federal registration process and rely on limited, federally authorized cannabis sources that do not reflect real-world potency or product variation (Donahue et al., 2023). This misalignment between state practice and federal oversight contributes to uncertainty among clinicians and reinforces inconsistency in patient experiences.

Federal restrictions on cannabis research have compounded these challenges by limiting the development of robust clinical evidence to guide practice. Researchers must navigate a complex approval process involving multiple federal agencies and rely on cannabis products that do not reflect the diversity or potency of those available in state-regulated markets (Cooper et al., 2021). This disconnect has slowed progress toward evidence-based dosing guidelines, standardized formulations, and comparative effectiveness research, leaving clinicians to rely on observational data and patient-reported outcomes.

From a nursing perspective, the absence of clear clinical standards places additional responsibility on frontline providers to manage uncertainty while maintaining patient safety. Nurses are frequently tasked with monitoring symptom response, identifying adverse effects, and reconciling cannabis use with other medications, often without formal institutional guidance. These realities highlight how federal research policy functions as an upstream determinant of clinical ambiguity, with downstream effects on patient education and continuity of care.

Policy Design as a Structural Determinant of Access

Taken together, these historical and policy dynamics have produced a fragmented medical cannabis system in which access, clinical guidance, and product safety are shaped less by standardized medical need than by jurisdictional design, political priorities, and regulatory capacity (Pacula & Smart, 2017; Perlman et al., 2021). Federal prohibition has constrained research, delayed the development of clinical standards, and shifted regulatory authority to states, resulting in wide variation in qualifying conditions, provider participation requirements, product formulations, and dispensary oversight. These variations are not merely administrative; they function as structural determinants of access that intersect with existing social and economic inequities. Conceptualizing cannabis policy as a structural determinant of health aligns with broader public health frameworks that recognize laws, regulations, and institutional practices as foundational drivers of health outcomes. Policy design determines who can legally access medical cannabis, which providers are willing or able to participate, and whether patients encounter supportive or punitive clinical environments (National Academies of Sciences, Engineering, and Medicine, 2017). In this sense, cannabis policy operates upstream of individual behavior, shaping risk and opportunity before patients ever enter the healthcare system.

Such policy-driven inequities tend to mirror existing patterns of disadvantage (Mennis et al., 2016; National Academies of Sciences, Engineering, and Medicine, 2017). Individuals with stable insurance coverage, consistent primary care relationships, and higher health literacy are better positioned to navigate complex certification systems, while those facing economic insecurity or fragmented care encounter greater barriers (Ashare et al., 2023; Pacula & Smart, 2017). Recognizing policy as a determinant of access underscores the need to evaluate medical cannabis programs not only on legal compliance or market performance, but on their capacity to reduce or exacerbate health inequities.

Consequently, patients' experiences with medical cannabis are mediated by where they live, their ability to navigate complex certification systems, their access to knowledgeable clinicians, and their financial resources. States with more restrictive programs tend to limit provider participation, impose higher out-of-pocket costs, and offer fewer patient protections, while more permissive programs may increase availability without adequate public health safeguards (Orenstein & Glantz, 2020; Schauer, 2021). This uneven policy landscape creates predictable patterns of inequity, reinforcing disparities along lines of race, income, geography, and health literacy. Understanding medical cannabis through this policy history is therefore essential for situating access disparities within a broader framework of social determinants of health. Importantly, these policy dynamics do not operate in isolation. They interact with social, economic, and geographic factors to produce cumulative disadvantage for certain patient populations (Mennis et al., 2016; National Academies of Sciences, Engineering, and Medicine, 2017). Patients residing in states with restrictive programs may simultaneously face limited provider participation, higher out-of-pocket costs, and reduced access to reliable information, creating layered barriers to care. Conversely, patients in more permissive states may experience increased availability without corresponding clinical integration, placing greater responsibility on individuals to self-manage risk (Barry & Glantz, 2016; Orenstein & Glantz, 2020; Schauer, 2021).

Situating these dynamics within a public health lens emphasizes that inequitable outcomes are not accidental but structurally produced. Understanding how historical prohibition, federal research constraints, and state-level variation converge provides critical context for examining the role of social determinants of health in shaping medical cannabis access. This perspective is essential for nurses and other healthcare professionals seeking to address inequities through both clinical practice and system-level advocacy. The following section builds on this foundation to examine how social determinants of health (SDOH), such as economic stability, neighborhood context, healthcare access, and social marginalization, shape who benefits from medical cannabis policy and who remains excluded.

SDOH & CANNABIS ACCESS

Economic Stability and Financial Barriers to Medical Cannabis

Economic stability is a foundational determinant of medical cannabis access, as nearly all aspects of participation in state programs require out-of-pocket expenditures. Patients typically must pay for physician certification visits, annual registration fees, and cannabis products themselves, none of which are covered by federal insurance programs due to cannabis's Schedule I status (Alexander, 2020). These costs disproportionately affect low-income patients, older adults on fixed incomes, and individuals with disabilities, for whom medical cannabis may be clinically indicated but financially inaccessible Alexander, 2020; Ashare et al., 2023).

Research indicates that when legal medical cannabis is unaffordable, patients are more likely to seek cannabis from unregulated sources, increasing exposure to products with inconsistent potency or contamination risk (Ashare et al., 2023). This pattern mirrors disparities observed with other non-covered therapies and underscores how financial barriers can undermine the safety goals of medical cannabis regulation. For nurses, understanding economic constraints is essential when assessing patients' cannabis use, as financial limitations may shape both access pathways and adherence to safer use recommendations.

SDOH profoundly shape how individuals access and utilize medical cannabis (Martins et al., 2021; Mennis et al., 2016; National Academies of Sciences, Engineering, and Medicine [NASEM], 2017; Pacula & Smart, 2017). A large cross-sectional study of cancer patients found significant racial and socioeconomic disparities in medical cannabis certification, modes of use, and patterns of product acquisition (Ashare et al., 2023). Black/African American patients were less likely to be medically certified and more likely to obtain cannabis from unlicensed sellers, while lower-income groups prioritized affordability and accessibility when making decisions about use. These disparities reflect broader patterns of unequal access to healthcare resources and underscore the intersection of cannabis policy with long-standing inequities related to race, income, and healthcare discrimination.

From a public health standpoint, SDOH provide a critical framework for understanding why legalization alone does not ensure equitable access to medical cannabis (Orenstein & Glantz, 2020). The World Health Organization (WHO) and U.S. public health agencies have long emphasized that health outcomes are shaped by the conditions in which individuals are born, live, work, and receive care, rather than by clinical interventions alone (National Academies of Sciences, Engineering, and Medicine, 2017; World Health Organization, 2008). In the context of medical cannabis, these conditions influence not only whether patients are legally eligible, but also whether they can successfully navigate certification processes, afford products, and receive reliable guidance from healthcare professionals (National Academies of Sciences, Engineering, and Medicine, 2017). As a result, cannabis access reflects broader structural inequities embedded within healthcare systems and social policy.

SDOH operate cumulatively, meaning that patients facing multiple forms of disadvantage often experience layered barriers to access (Mennis et al., 2016; National Academies of Sciences, Engineering, and Medicine, 2017). For example, economic instability may coincide with limited transportation options, fragmented healthcare access, and lower health literacy, compounding the difficulty of obtaining regulated medical cannabis. Recognizing this cumulative effect is essential for understanding why disparities persist even in states with relatively permissive cannabis policies.

Neighborhood Context, Geography, and Dispensary Access

Neighborhood and geographic context further shape medical cannabis access by influencing the physical availability of regulated and, thus, safe products. Studies of dispensary distribution consistently demonstrate that cannabis retailers are unevenly distributed, often clustering in socioeconomically disadvantaged areas while remaining sparse or absent in rural communities (Unger, 2022). While proximity to dispensaries can increase access for some patients, it may also expose certain neighborhoods to heightened public health risks if regulatory oversight and community resources are insufficient.

Conversely, patients living in rural or restrictive jurisdictions may face long travel distances, limited transportation options, and fewer participating providers, effectively excluding them from legal access (Pacula & Smart, 2017; Perlman et al., 2021). Geographic barriers are particularly salient for patients with mobility limitations, chronic illness, or limited caregiving support. Nurses working in rural or underserved settings frequently encounter patients who express interest in medical cannabis but lack feasible pathways to obtain regulated products, highlighting how geography operates as a structural access barrier rather than an individual choice.

Furthermore, proximity of one's residence to cannabis dispensaries is correlated with more positive attitudes toward medical cannabis, meaning those who live closer are more likely to hold negative attitudes toward it (Clobes et al., 2025). Attitudinal differences tied to geographic proximity also have implications for patient engagement and disclosure. Patients who perceive medical cannabis as socially stigmatized or controversial within their community may be less likely to discuss its use with healthcare providers, even when legally permitted. These dynamics underscore the importance of contextualizing cannabis attitudes within place-based social norms rather than treating beliefs as purely individual preferences. For nurses, sensitivity to local community attitudes can inform more effective patient education and trust-building strategies. While increased retail presence may enhance access for some patients, these clustering patterns may expose disadvantaged communities to disproportionate risks such as youth exposure, impaired driving concerns, and inconsistent enforcement of safety regulations. Conversely, patients in rural areas or jurisdictions with restrictive cannabis policies may lack reasonable access to regulated products, driving them toward informal supply chains with greater safety variability.

Healthcare Access, Provider Participation, and System Navigation

Healthcare access represents a critical intermediary between cannabis policy and patient utilization. Even in states with legal medical cannabis programs, access depends on provider willingness to participate, institutional policies, and availability of certifying clinicians (Perlman et al., 2021). Patients without stable primary care relationships or those relying on safety-net systems may encounter limited opportunities to receive evidence-informed guidance or certification, reinforcing disparities rooted in broader healthcare access inequities.

Navigating medical cannabis programs often requires multiple steps, including identifying eligible providers, completing documentation, and understanding state-specific regulations (Pacula & Smart, 2017; Perlman et al., 2021). Patients with fragmented care histories or limited experience navigating healthcare bureaucracies may struggle with these requirements, increasing reliance on informal sources of information. Nurses frequently serve as navigators within complex healthcare systems, making their awareness of cannabis policy and access pathways particularly important for mitigating these barriers (Kurtzman et al., 2022).

Health Literacy, Information Access, and Misinformation

Health literacy and information access further shape the patient experience. In the absence of standardized clinical education, patients with limited educational or digital resources may struggle to navigate the certification process or evaluate product potency and safety (Gardiner et al., 2019). These dynamics highlight the essential role of nurses and other clinicians in helping patients interpret complex policy environments and make informed decisions within structurally constrained contexts.

Health literacy plays a central role in shaping how patients interpret information about medical cannabis, assess risk, and make decisions about use. In the absence of standardized clinical education materials, patients often rely on dispensary staff, online forums, or peer networks for guidance, sources that vary widely in accuracy and consistency (Gardiner et al., 2019). Lower health literacy and limited digital access can exacerbate misinformation, particularly among older adults and individuals with limited formal education.

For nurses, addressing health literacy gaps involves translating complex regulatory and clinical information into accessible, patient-centered guidance. This may include clarifying differences between medical and recreational cannabis, discussing dosing and administration in understandable terms, and correcting misconceptions rooted in stigma or marketing claims. Integrating health literacy considerations into cannabis-related conversations is essential for promoting safer and more equitable use.

Cumulative Disadvantage and Equity Implications

Cumulatively, economic, geographic, healthcare, and informational barriers interact to produce cumulative disadvantage in medical cannabis access (Martin-Willett et al., 2023). Patients who experience multiple forms of marginalization are more likely to encounter fragmented access pathways, inconsistent guidance, and heightened exposure to risk (Ashare et al., 2023; Perlman et al., 2021). These patterns reflect broader inequities within the healthcare system and underscore the limitations of policy reforms that do not explicitly address social context.

Viewing cannabis access through an SDOH lens highlights the need for equity-oriented interventions that extend beyond legalization (Mennis et al., 2016; National Academies of Sciences, Engineering, and Medicine, 2017). For nurses and other healthcare professionals, this perspective emphasizes the importance of situating cannabis-related care within a broader understanding of patients' lived environments

(Kurtzman et al., 2022). The following section builds on this analysis by examining how stigma and implicit bias within healthcare settings further shape patient experiences and access to medical cannabis.

STIGMA, IMPLICIT BIAS, & HEALTHCARE PROVIDER GUIDANCE

Stigma as a Barrier to Disclosure and Care

Stigma remains a central determinant of inequitable cannabis use and access. In a qualitative study of cancer survivors, participants described medical cannabis–related stigma as more pervasive in clinical settings than in personal or professional contexts, often leading to secrecy, hesitancy to disclose use, or avoidance of conversations about symptom management (Nayak et al., 2022). Stigmatizing responses from clinicians, including dismissal, moral judgment, or discomfort, can hinder open communication and compromise care quality.

Stigma surrounding medical cannabis operates at multiple levels, including individual attitudes, professional norms, and institutional policies (Dahlke et al., 2024; Nayak et al., 2022). Unlike stigma associated with some other therapies, cannabis-related stigma is shaped by its dual identity as both a therapeutic agent and a historically criminalized substance. This duality creates ambiguity in clinical settings, where cannabis may be perceived as less legitimate than other symptom-management options despite comparable or emerging evidence bases (Zarhin et al., 2020). For patients, this ambiguity can translate into uncertainty about whether cannabis use will be viewed as a reasonable health choice or as a marker of deviance (King et al., 2024).

Institutional stigma may further manifest through silence or omission, such as the absence of cannabis from patient education materials, clinical guidelines, or documentation practices (Perlman et al., 2021). When healthcare systems fail to normalize cannabis discussions, patients may infer that disclosure is risky or unwelcome (Nayak et al., 2022). Nurses, who often establish the tone for patient communication, are therefore positioned at the intersection of individual and institutional stigma, navigating how and when cannabis is acknowledged in care conversations.

Provider Knowledge Gaps and Clinical Uncertainty

Healthcare provider knowledge gaps represent a critical mechanism through which stigma is reproduced in clinical practice. Systematic reviews indicate that while many clinicians express openness toward medical cannabis, they simultaneously report limited formal education, uncertainty about dosing and safety, and discomfort initiating conversations with patients (Gardiner et al., 2019; Parmelee & Clark, 2022). These gaps are not evenly distributed across disciplines, contributing to inconsistent messaging and fragmented guidance within healthcare teams.

For nurses, limited access to evidence-based education can result in reliance on informal knowledge sources or deference to institutional silence (Gardiner et al., 2019; Kurtzman et al., 2022). In such contexts, avoidance of cannabis-related discussions may be interpreted as a safer professional stance, even when patients would benefit from guidance. Over time, this pattern reinforces stigma by positioning cannabis as outside the bounds of legitimate clinical care, rather than as a topic warranting informed discussion and monitoring (Zarhin et al., 2020).

Provider-level factors further intensify these inequities. A comprehensive systematic review found that while many healthcare professionals express support for medicinal cannabis, they consistently report low levels of knowledge regarding cannabinoid pharmacology, therapeutic applications, and safety considerations (Gardiner et al., 2019). Such gaps can inadvertently reinforce stigma or lead clinicians to rely on personal beliefs rather than scientific evidence when responding to patient inquiries.

Clinical uncertainty is further amplified by the absence of standardized practice guidelines and institutional policies. Unlike other pharmacologic therapies, cannabis lacks universally accepted dosing frameworks, contraindication lists, and monitoring protocols, leaving clinicians to navigate risk without clear benchmarks (Perlman et al., 2021). This uncertainty can lead providers to adopt overly cautious or dismissive approaches, particularly in settings where legal liability or professional scrutiny is perceived as high.

Nurses frequently encounter the downstream effects of this uncertainty during routine care activities, such as symptom assessment, medication reconciliation, and patient education (Kurtzman et al., 2022; Nadzam, 2009). When cannabis use is excluded from formal care plans, nurses may struggle to integrate it into holistic assessments, increasing the risk of unrecognized interactions or unmet patient concerns (Gardiner et al., 2019; Perlman et al., 2021). Addressing knowledge gaps and uncertainty is therefore essential for reducing stigma and improving care quality.

Implicit Bias and Racialized Assumptions in Clinical Decision-Making

Implicit bias represents a distinct but interrelated barrier to equitable medical cannabis access. Research across healthcare settings demonstrates that racially marginalized patients are more likely to have their symptoms undertreated, their credibility questioned, and their health behaviors scrutinized through a lens of suspicion (Jaiswal, 2019). When applied to cannabis, these biases may shape assumptions about misuse, nonadherence, or criminality, even in states where medical use is legal.

These dynamics are particularly salient in pain management and substance use contexts, where racial disparities in prescribing, monitoring, and trust are well documented (Martins et al., 2021). Patients who anticipate biased treatment may choose not to disclose cannabis use or may disengage from care altogether, undermining opportunities for safe, guided use. For nurses, recognizing how implicit bias influences both provider behavior and patient disclosure is critical for fostering equitable clinical environments.

Implicit bias, particularly toward racially marginalized patients, may also influence provider attitudes and decisions (Dahlke et al., 2024; Jaiswal, 2019; Nayak et al., 2022). These biases intersect with known disparities in pain management, substance use treatment, and patient trust, potentially shaping assumptions about misuse, adherence, or criminality (King et al., 2024; Lucas, 2012; Martins et al., 2021; Perlman et al., 2021). When combined with structural inequities in access and affordability, stigma and bias can meaningfully restrict the ability of marginalized patients to obtain safe, guided, and effective cannabis care (Ashare et al., 2023; Martin-Willett et al., 2023; Mennis et al, 2016; National Academies of Sciences, Engineering, and Medicine, 2017).

Bias and stigma rarely operate independently of structural conditions. When combined with financial barriers, limited provider participation, and inconsistent policy implementation, implicit bias can intensify inequities in medical cannabis access. Patients from marginalized backgrounds may encounter multiple reinforcing obstacles, including skepticism from clinicians, lack of insurance coverage, and reliance on unregulated products (Ashare et al., 2023; Martin-Willett et al., 2023). These intersecting factors contribute to patterns of inequitable access that persist even in ostensibly permissive policy environments.

Understanding stigma and bias as structurally embedded phenomena rather than isolated attitudes shifts responsibility from individual patients to healthcare systems. This perspective underscores the importance of institutional interventions, including training, policy reform, and accountability mechanisms, to address inequities. Nurses play a central role in operationalizing these interventions through daily practice and advocacy.

Nursing Ethics, Patient Autonomy, and Professional Responsibility

Ethical nursing practice requires attention to how stigma and bias constrain patient autonomy and informed decision-making. Principles of beneficence, nonmaleficence, and justice demand that patients receive accurate information and respectful engagement, regardless of the legal or social status of a therapy. When cannabis-related stigma limits open communication, patients may be deprived of opportunities to make fully informed choices about symptom management (Nadzam, 2009; Newell & Jordan, 2015).

Nurses often serve as advocates for patient-centered care, particularly for individuals navigating complex or stigmatized health decisions (Kurtzman et al., 2022). By fostering nonjudgmental dialogue, acknowledging structural barriers, and supporting informed disclosure, nurses can mitigate the effects of stigma within clinical encounters (Nayak et al., 2022). These ethical commitments provide a foundation for broader system-level reforms aimed at promoting equity in medical cannabis care.

For nurses who often serve as primary communicators, symptom-management specialists, and patient advocates, addressing these barriers is both an ethical imperative and a professional responsibility (Nadzam, 2009; Newell & Jordan, 2015). Equitable guidance requires awareness of one's own assumptions, engagement with emerging evidence, and commitment to fostering clinical environments where patients feel safe discussing cannabis use.

Some nurses report experiencing moral distress when institutional policies or professional norms conflict with perceived patient needs (Prompahakul et al., 2021). In the context of medical cannabis, this may arise when nurses believe a patient could benefit from guided use but feel constrained by policy ambiguity or lack of institutional support. Moral distress can contribute to disengagement, burnout, and reduced advocacy over time. Addressing stigma at the organizational level may therefore have implications not only for patient outcomes but also for workforce well-being. Supporting nurses through education, clear policy guidance, and ethical dialogue can help align professional identity with equitable care practices.

THE NURSE'S ROLE IN PROMOTING EQUITY AND ACCESS

The following section will review how the cannabis care nurse can support patient equity and cannabis access, including clinical practice approaches, education in nursing curricula, involvement in policy development, community partnerships, and research dissemination.

Cannabis equity refers to three primary issues in the medical cannabis space, including: Medical cannabis patient access disparities, treatment outcomes, and participation in the legal cannabis space for populations who have been harmed by cannabis prohibition. An ad hoc committee from the National Academies of Science, Engineering, and Medicine (NASEM) (2024) is currently studying the impact of state-level cannabis policies on cannabis access and assessing regulatory access through a social equity lens. Some of their assigned tasks are to determine the:

- Economic impact on state tax revenue, employment, and other economic indicators.
- Environmental impact of cannabis and hemp production within the states.
- Number of encounters with the justice system related to cannabis regulation
- Impact of policy on the unregulated market,
- Availability of cannabis use disorder community treatment options
- Key public health outcomes and the adequacy of state surveillance methods, and
- The equity and social impacts of decriminalization and incarceration rates for cannabis possession.
- Use of a harm-reduction approach to the regulatory process and the impact within the social, employment, and educational spheres.

Lastly, the committee will make recommendations for policy research for the next 5 years (National Academies of Sciences, Engineering, and Medicine, 2024).

Cannabis care nurses are committed to improving health outcomes in communities and implementing health education, promotion, and prevention efforts for vulnerable populations. To better understand the nurse's role in this area, the Cannabis Nursing: Scope and Standards of Practice (American Nurses Association & American Cannabis Nurses Association, 2024) guides the competencies cannabis care nurses should focus on related to equity. For instance, Standard 9: Respectful and Equitable Practice, focuses on developing the skills to provide culturally competent care and advocate for policies that promote health and prevent harm for underserved/ vulnerable populations. Under Standard 18, Environmental Health, the nurse must analyze the impact of social, political, and economic influences on consumers and the environment (ANA & ACNA). There is an expectation that the nurse will be involved in local, state, and federal advocacy efforts to ensure that medical cannabis patients have access to safe, tested medicines and that vulnerable populations who use cannabis are cared for (Clark, 2021a). Examples of this include the efforts nurses have made to support the legal process of allowing medical cannabis patients to be used in inpatient settings, such as occurred with Ryan's Law in California and other states' processes of enacting similar laws. Nurses in many states have supported the emergence of medical cannabis and adult use laws by connecting with legislators and partnering with organizations, while also educating communities about the benefits and challenges of regulating cannabis for these purposes (Clark, 2021a). These efforts help to support equity in medical cannabis spaces and in healthcare as well, with increased patient access to medical cannabis.

Other examples of nurses working toward equity include the Cannabis Nurses of Color hosted *A Day at the Capitol: Health Policy Summit* in 2023 in Washington, D.C. The focus of this day was to explore how nurses can help shape cannabis policy (Cannabis Nurses of Color, n.d.). ACNA also partnered with ANA to ensure that policy and advocacy are incorporated into the development of the scope and standards of practice, and that compassion and equity are embedded in the organization's mission. ACNA developed an organizational equity rider to help foster the inclusion and voice of LGBTQIA+, BIPOC, and people with disabilities.

Many cannabis nurses form partnerships within communities to ultimately support population well-being and access to medical cannabis, whether this is consulting with dispensaries and cannabis growers, working with cannabis companies to white-label products, consulting with patients by coaching and educating them toward safe and effective cannabis use, running small farms that focus on hemp production, or consulting with local, state, or federal regulators and legislators. All of these efforts play a role in helping to ensure that cannabis stigma is addressed, populations are cared for, disparities are reduced, and advocacy for better medical and adult use policy and regulations are emerging (Clark, 2021a).

Nursing education has been slow to include medical cannabis care content in curricula. A study by Parmelee & Clark (2022) found that nursing students across the United States are desirous of receiving medical cannabis care content. Still, the vast majority of the students surveyed were not getting much, if any, medical cannabis knowledge, attitude, or skill support. The over 1300 surveyed nursing students relied on learning about cannabis from patients, the media, and by attempting to analyze the available research. Despite the National Council of State Boards of Nursing (2018) call to include at least six essential areas of medical cannabis knowledge into all nursing curricula, the barriers to implementing medical cannabis care into curricula remain and include lack of time to learn about cannabis and the endocannabinoid systems, lack of administrative support, lack of discussion amongst faculty regarding the importance of cannabis care content, and crowded curricula (Parmelee, 2025). Additionally, a lack of alignment of required related content by accrediting organizations and organizations like the American Association of Colleges of Nursing (AACN) and the Quality, Safety, and Education for Nurses (QSEN) Institute may impact nursing faculty's desire to take the steps to include not only content about the endocannabinoid system and cannabinoid therapeutics, but also about the importance of social justice issues and equity and access related to cannabis and underserved, vulnerable populations.

There is a dearth of evidence regarding the nurse's preparation to address equity and access in medical cannabis spaces, public health seetings, and with policy development, but education and reduction of stigma may help play a role in development of the nurse's voice in the medical cannabis space. Medical cannabis care proficency and being prepared to advocate for medical cannabis patients' needsare steps toward ensuring nurses' voices are heard and help to address the issues of equity, access, and social justice concerns (King et al., 2024).

Research dissemination and analysis of medical cannabis plays an enormous role in the nurse's ability to support patients' safe and effective use of cannabis. Unfortunately, many nurses, healthcare providers, and patients rely heavily on the media for their information about cannabis research, and often the research is reduced to short summaries that are unlikely to capture the complexity of the research, including the limitations of the study, the level of quality of the study, and calls for future research. For more information about supporting nursing students and nursing with applying the research analysis process to the medical cannabis body of evidence, review Clark (2021a), where an example of this length process is provided. Clark (2019a; 2019b) provides the full example of the detail required to fully analyze an article in the *Lancet Psychiatry* that linked cannabis use to first time psychosis in large scale multi county population, where the author examines the details of the issues with the research process including relying on participant recall, no testing of cannabis products uses, and no follow-up to see if the cannabis users went on to have a formal mental health diagnosis related to the psychotic episode. An aspect of working toward equity in cannabis care is identifying poor quality research, which is rampant in the medical cannabis field (Clark, 2021a).

Until cannabinoid therapeutics and the ECS are included on the NCLEX and AANP/AACN board certification exams, there will be little incentive to include medical cannabis content. However, the ethical implications should be motivating: How can we ensure the 25% of the population who use cannabis do so safely and effectively if faculty are not committed to including the information in curricula? How can nurses have a voice in policy development at the local, state, and federal levels that ensures equity for vulnerable populations?

POLICY & SYSTEM-LEVEL STRATEGIES

While clinical education and individual provider attitudes are critical to improving equitable cannabis care, durable change requires policy and system-level strategies that address upstream structural barriers (Alexander, 2020; Ruheel et al., 2021). A public health–oriented approach to medical cannabis emphasizes regulation, data infrastructure, and institutional accountability, rather than reliance on individual clinicians or patients to navigate a fragmented system. Drawing on lessons from tobacco, alcohol, and pharmaceutical regulation, scholars and public health organizations have identified several policy domains that are particularly salient for advancing equity in medical cannabis access (Barry & Glantz, 2016; National Academies of Sciences, Engineering, and Medicine, 2017; Orenstein & Glantz, 2020).

From a systems perspective, policy and regulatory frameworks shape not only who can access medical cannabis, but also how responsibility for risk management is distributed across patients, clinicians, and institutions. When policies emphasize individual authorization without corresponding system supports, patients are often left to navigate complex markets and clinical uncertainty independently. Public health–oriented strategies instead seek to embed safeguards within regulatory and healthcare infrastructures, reducing reliance on individual knowledge or resources (Orenstein & Glantz, 2020). For nurses, this distinction is critical, as system-level design determines whether equitable care is feasible in everyday practice. Nurses receive little education about how these systems work, and it can be a challenge for them to build their policy and advocacy skills.

Equity-Grounded Policy Reform

One of the most significant barriers to equitable access is the limited participation of healthcare providers in medical cannabis programs (Alexander, 2020). State policies which require burdensome registration processes, expose clinicians to legal ambiguity, or prohibit meaningful clinical guidance have been shown to suppress provider engagement, particularly in safety-net and community-based settings (Perlman et al., 2021). Reform efforts should prioritize clarifying scope of practice protections, standardizing clinician participation requirements, and explicitly recognizing medical cannabis counseling as a legitimate component of patient care.

Provider participation barriers have implications beyond workforce engagement; they directly influence the equity of patient access. When clinicians are discouraged from participating in medical cannabis programs, patients with limited provider choice, including those in safety-net or rural settings, face compounded obstacles. In these contexts, patients may rely on nonclinical sources for guidance or forego regulated access altogether, undermining the intent of medical cannabis policy (Perlman et al., 2021). Addressing provider participation through policy reform is therefore an equity intervention as much as professional accommodation.

Insurance coverage represents a second critical equity lever. Because medical cannabis is excluded from federal insurance programs and most private plans, patients must pay out of pocket for certification visits and products (Alexander, 2020). This cost burden disproportionately affects low-income patients and contributes to reliance on unregulated markets, which carry greater safety risks (Ashare et al., 2023; National Academies of Sciences, Engineering, and Medicine, 2024). While federal rescheduling would be required for full insurance integration, states can mitigate inequities through fee waivers, subsidized certification programs, and targeted patient assistance initiatives. The exclusion of medical cannabis from insurance coverage also limits the ability of healthcare systems to integrate cannabis use into standard care pathways (Alexander, 2020). Without coverage, cannabis remains peripheral to formal treatment plans, reducing opportunities for coordinated monitoring and follow-up. This separation reinforces a two-tiered system in which patients who can afford cannabis receive informal or parallel care, while those who cannot are excluded entirely. From a public health standpoint, integrating coverage considerations into policy reform is essential for aligning medical cannabis with principles of equity and continuity of care.

Research funding policy is also central to equity. The National Academies and other bodies have emphasized that current research restrictions have produced evidence gaps that disproportionately affect marginalized populations, whose experiences are underrepresented in clinical studies (National Academies of Sciences, Engineering, and Medicine, 2017; Martin-Willett et al., 2023). Equity-focused policy reform should expand access to research materials, incentivize community-engaged studies, and support investigators from historically excluded backgrounds to ensure that scientific gains are broadly distributed. A call may be made to provide funding emphasis on exploring how nurses can influence policy and address equity and SDOH related to medical cannabis.

Health System Integration and Clinical Infrastructure

Beyond legislative reform, health systems play a decisive role in shaping patient experiences with medical cannabis (National Academies of Sciences, Engineering, and Medicine, 2017; Perlman et al., 2021). Many institutions lack standardized documentation protocols, leaving cannabis use inconsistently recorded in electronic health records or excluded from medication reconciliation processes (Perlman et al., 2021; Gardiner et al., 2019).

Public health approaches to tobacco and alcohol regulation offer instructive parallels for medical cannabis policy (World Health Organization, 2024). Evidence from these domains demonstrates that taxation, marketing restrictions, and reinvestment in prevention can reduce population-level harms while preserving access for those who benefit (Barry & Glantz, 2016). Applying similar principles to medical cannabis requires careful adaptation to avoid unintended barriers to patients with legitimate therapeutic need. Nonetheless, these frameworks underscore the importance of proactive system design rather than reactive regulation.

Standardized documentation practices are foundational to patient safety and equitable care. When cannabis use is inconsistently recorded in electronic health records, clinicians may lack critical information needed to assess interactions, monitor outcomes, or provide coordinated care (Perlman et al., 2021). This gap is particularly concerning for older adults and patients with multiple chronic conditions, who are more likely to use cannabis alongside other medications.

Health systems that fail to establish clear documentation protocols effectively shift responsibility to individual providers, increasing variability and risk. Developing standardized approaches to recording cannabis use within medication reconciliation processes can support safer care and reduce reliance on informal disclosure. For nurses, consistent documentation frameworks facilitate more accurate assessments and enable continuity across care settings. This omission undermines care coordination and increases the risk of drug–drug interactions, particularly among older adults and patients with complex comorbidities (Perlman et al., 2021).

Interprofessional communication is equally important (National Academies of Sciences, Engineering, and Medicine, 2017; Orenstein & Glantz, 2020). Nurses, pharmacists, physicians, and behavioral health providers often operate with differing levels of cannabis knowledge, resulting in fragmented or contradictory guidance (Gardiner et al., 2019; Moustaqim et al., 2019; Perlman et al, 2021; Philpot et al., 2019). Health systems should develop interprofessional education models and clinical pathways that clarify roles, promote shared decision-making, and integrate cannabis discussions into routine symptom management and chronic disease care (Barry & Glantz, 2016; National Academies of Sciences, Engineering, and Medicine, 2017; Perlman et al., 2021).

Interprofessional education initiatives offer a practical mechanism for addressing fragmented cannabis guidance (Perlman et al., 2021; National Academies of Sciences, Engineering, and Medicine, 2017). Training models that bring together nurses, pharmacists, physicians, and behavioral health providers can promote shared understanding of roles, legal boundaries, and evidence limitations (Philpot et al., 2019; Moustaqim-Barrette et al., 2019). Such models are consistent with broader trends in healthcare education emphasizing team-based care and collaborative decision-making. Embedding cannabis-related content within existing interprofessional frameworks may be more effective than siloed training approaches.

Cultural competency training is essential to these efforts. Given the racialized history of cannabis criminalization and ongoing stigma in clinical settings, providers must be equipped to recognize how bias and mistrust influence patient disclosure and engagement (Nayak et al., 2022; Jaiswal, 2019). Training that explicitly addresses structural racism, stigma, and patient autonomy can help ensure that public health realted medical cannabis conversations support, rather than undermine, equitable care.

Data, Surveillance, and Community-Engaged Research

Robust data systems are foundational to equitable policy design (Wang et al., 2025). Public health surveillance should track not only utilization and adverse outcomes, but also access indicators such as provider availability, dispensary distribution, patient demographics, and affordability. Anderson and Rees (2023) emphasized that without longitudinal, state-level data, policymakers risk drawing incomplete or misleading conclusions about cannabis policy impacts.

Data systems that prioritize equity must also be attentive to how data are collected, interpreted, and used. Surveillance efforts that fail to disaggregate outcomes by race, income, or geography risk obscuring disparities and limiting policy responsiveness. Incorporating equity metrics into cannabis surveillance can help identify unintended consequences and guide targeted interventions. Nurses, as contributors to clinical documentation and quality improvement initiatives, play an important role in ensuring that data reflect patient diversity and lived experience.

Community-based participatory research (CBPR) offers a particularly powerful tool for equity-oriented policy development (Freudenberg & Tsui, 2014). Engaging patients and communities most affected by criminalization and healthcare exclusion can surface barriers that are invisible in administrative data alone (Martin-Willett et al., 2023). Historically, community-controlled health initiatives have demonstrated how local governance and patient leadership can transform access for marginalized populations, offering a relevant model for contemporary cannabis policy design (Brown, 2016; Martin-Willett et al., 2023; Mennis et al., 2016).

State-Level Variation as Policy Laboratories

Finally, state-level variation in medical cannabis utilization provides natural policy laboratories for identifying best practices. Research comparing states with differing regulatory frameworks demonstrates that policy design influences patterns of use, provider participation, and patient outcomes (Martins et al., 2021). States that emphasize public health oversight, limit commercialization pressures, and reinvest revenues into prevention and education tend to align more closely with equity goals than those that prioritize market expansion.

For nurses, understanding these variations is critical. Nurses are uniquely positioned to translate policy into practice, advocate for system-level reforms, and contribute to data-driven evaluation efforts (Nadzam, 2009). By engaging with policy processes at institutional, state, and national levels, nurses can help shape a medical cannabis landscape that is clinically sound, ethically grounded, and responsive to the needs of diverse patient populations.

RECOMMENDATIONS FOR NURSING EDUCATION AND PRACTICE

Nurses must be supported when considering their competency development and cannabis care literacy. This section will briefly review competencies for cannabis care nurses, define cannabis-related continuing education and professional development opportunities for nurses, and discuss the need for interprofessional educational approaches that include collaborations between schools of nursing, pharmacy, health sciences, psychology, and social work.

The ANA and ACNA (2024) *Cannabis nursing: Scope and standards of practice* is the primary tool defining the roles and responsibilities of the cannabis nursing specialty. While cannabis nursing is a newly recognized subspecialty in nursing, it also aligns well with holistic nursing, and the evidence clearly demonstrates that many holistic modalities upregulate the ECS (McPartland et al., 2014). It is clear that holistic nurses care for the ECS, and the cannabis care nurse is also ultimately a holistic nurse, supporting patients towards quality of life and the use of all available medical, integrative, and self-care tools to potentiate that quality of life (Clark, 2021a). Cannabis care nurses strive to create a caring, healing presence and practice on a foundation of social justice and an ethic of care, while also considering ethical and legal concerns (ANA & ACNA, 2024).

ANA and ACNA (2024) aligned the standards and practice for cannabis nurses, including standard I assessment, standard II diagnosis, standard III outcomes identification, standard IV planning, standard V implementation, and standard VI evaluation. These standards align with the ANA (2021) *Nursing: Scope and standards of practice* (fourth edition), which defined the who, what, where, when, and why of general nursing practice. Standards VII-XVII focus on professional performance competencies. Historically, some of the challenges faced by cannabis nurses include the role of being an advocate for populations during the prohibition era, and many nurses have lost their license or have had their license threatened for simply educating people about safe cannabis use. Any nurse working with medical cannabis patients and supporting their safe and effective use of cannabis must follow the standards, develop their competencies, document appropriately, follow hospital and/or organizational policies, and always focus on using the skills of educating and coaching their patients.

Cannabis related learning opportunities abound for nurses. The ACNA offers ongoing educational opportunities, as do organizations such as the Cannabis Clinicians Society and Patients Out of Time. AHNA often offers cannabis-related educational opportunities, including at their annual conferences, and many nursing journals and podcasts have cannabis-related content. *Cannabis: A handbook for nurses* (Clark, 2021b) is a textbook written for and by nurses that covers the role of the cannabis nurse and the advanced practice cannabis nurse, along with chapters on history, the ECS, pharmacology, and evidence related to cannabis's effectiveness. It is a tool that can be used by educators to guide cannabis curriculaum development and by any nurse interested in supporting patients with medical cannabis use.

Many institutions of higher learning have focused on creating cannabis certificate or degree programs, including John Patrick University of Health and Human Services, Thomas Jefferson University, Cal Poly Humboldt, and the University of Maryland/Baltimore. Many community colleges and universities offer cannabis microcredentials or certificates, with some focusing on the cannabis business or cannabis agriculture, and others concentrating on care for populations.

Interprofessional education that focuses on the roles of the healthcare team can be fruitful in supporting patient equity and access, though there is a dearth of research in this area. It is known that medical cannabis education decreases cannabis stigma and it is viewed as professional and moral obligation (Metha, 2025), but there is little data to show how medical cannabis education, ending stigma, and taking a lens to policy development with equity in mind can shift outcomes.

Ideally, in educational settings for healthcare professionals, there would be opportunities to participate in coursework, applied practice simulations, or clinical placements that place cannabis care at the forefront with an emphasis on public health, social determinants of health, equity, access, social justice issues, and policy development (Clark, 2021a). For instance, medical, nursing, pharmacology, nutrition/health studies, social work, and psychology students come together to discuss patient care, current related public health policies, how the team can collaborate, and define their roles. Nursing is at the forefront of defining the cannabis care scope and standards of practice, and other professions are beginning to follow suit (ANA &ACNA, 2024).

Interprofessional Education

While there is a strong need for this type of educational experience, and the reality of medical cannabis care is that it does not occur in a silo within a single discipline, meaningful interprofessional collaboration in academia remains rare. A scoping review of interpreofessional education found that interprofessional collaboration is hindered by scheduling logistics, instructor training, role definition, and program collaboration (Chávez-Valenzuela et al., 2025). These researchers suggested that simulation experiences involving the interprofessional team may be helpful. Another approach is to hold grand rounds presentations and student-faculty research presentations, and to define interdisciplinary teams interested in studying medical cannabis care collaboratively, particularly around public health concerns and equity.

As nurses are the largest group of healthcare professionals, they likely spend the most time with the greatest number of patients, and they were the first to establish a cannabis subspecialty, nursing should lead in developing educational opportunities for both nurses and interprofessional teams. Supporting the other professions in defining their specific scopes and standards of practice is a role that nurses must consider. The following is a scenario of how the nurse leads the interprofessional team with cannabis care of an oncology patient in a community setting. Oncology patients often suffer from adverse effects of thier prescribed treatments, and medical cannabis access may depend greatly on their healthcare team's knowledge, attitudes, and experiences.

Interprofessional Cannabis Care Scenario in Community Oncology

Table 1. Interprofessional cannabis care in community oncology

Patient Profile: Patient: Mr. J., 62-year-old Hispanic male. Diagnosis: Stage III colorectal cancer **Current Treatment:** FOLFOX chemotherapy regimen **Symptoms**: Chemotherapy-induced nausea and vomiting, peripheral neuropathy, decreased appetite, anxiety, and weight loss. **Subjective data**: Mr. J. reports persistent nausea and appetite loss despite antiemetics and discloses unsupervised cannabis use. The oncologist refers the case to the cannabis care nurse to guide interprofessional planning. **Current Cannabis Use**: Occasional edibles without medical guidance **Interprofessional Team Members**: Include the oncologist, cannabis care nurse (CCN), clinical pharmacist, social worker, dietitian, primary oncology nurse, and chaplain. **The goal**: Mr. J. experiences improved nausea and appetite with no adverse effects. Mr. J's trust has been enhanced, and he reports satisfaction with palliative care measures.
Role of the Cannabis Care Nurse: The cannabis care nurse conducts a comprehensive cannabis assessment following the ANA and ACNA (2024) standard of practice, screens for contraindications, and reframes cannabis as a therapeutic adjunct focused on safety and symptom control. The nurse uses motivational interviewing to set palliative goals with the patient guided by an ethic of care. **Interprofessional Collaboration: The team must define their roles and role-play outcomes driven scenarios** **EG:** The oncologist supports cautious adjunctive use and verifies for any contraindications to current oncological care.
The pharmacist reviews drug–drug interactions and dosing safety. The cannabis care nurse (CCN) supports foundational education about the ECS and cannabis therapeutics, the self-titration process, accessing cannabinoids, storing cannabinoids, adverse effects, and upregulation of the ECS through holistic modalities. The CCN provides ongoing coaching, and remains culturally sensitive, respectful, and aware in all of her interactions with Mr. J. The dietitian aligns cannabis timing with culturally preferred nutrition and educates patients about cannabinoids and nutritional products. The social worker addresses legal access and cost and assesses the family situation and structure. The social worker approaches the patient using a cultural competency lens and considers the impact of prohibition on the population she is working with. The chaplain discusses spiritual care needs and the role cannabis can play in spiritual healing, though the nurse has introduced this concept in the initial assessment process. The chaplain may support the creation of rituals around cannabinoid therapeutic use and aligning cannabis use with the patient's spiritual and/or religious preferences. The chaplain works with the patient to understand how cultural concerns and experiences may shape spiritual needs. The oncology nurse monitors outcomes and reinforces education through coaching and motivational interviewing techniques. The oncology nurses provides culturally competent care. **Outcomes: The team must work together to support outcomes and overcoming challenges and barriers, defining any policy related issues at the workplace, local, state, and/or federal level.**

Additionally, the case can be converted to a simulation experience, where the team works to support the patient in the context of community and public health settings. The following is an example of a case study scenario, based on Mr J.'s care from Table 1.

Table 2. Interprofessional Education (IPE) simulation: Cannabis care in oncology

Interprofessional Education Collaborative (IPEC) core competencies alignment:
- Values/Ethics: Respect for patient autonomy, harm reduction, and shared decision-making
- Roles/Responsibilities: Clear delineation of professional roles in cannabis-supported oncology care
- Interprofessional Communication: Structured team dialogue and patient-centered communication
- Teams/Teamwork: Collaborative planning led by the cannabis care nurse

Simulation Overview (Brief)
Setting: Outpatient oncology clinic
Learners: Nursing, medicine, pharmacy, social work, dietetics, chaplain
Duration: 20–30 minutes

Patient Scenario
Mr. J., a 62-year-old patient with stage III colorectal cancer receiving chemotherapy, reports uncontrolled nausea, poor appetite, and anxiety. He discloses unsupervised cannabis edible use.
Simulation Objectives: Upon completion of the simulation, the learners will:
- Demonstrate safe, team-based cannabis care planning
- Apply role-specific expertise to symptom management
- Practice shared decision-making and harm reduction
- Define team member's implicit biases
- Communicate effectively across disciplines

Roles in Simulation
Cannabis Care Nurse (Team Lead):
- Conducts cannabis assessment
- Educates patient and team; coaches patient using motivational interviewing to set goals, provides ongoing coaching and education, supports upregulation of the ECS
- Facilitates interprofessional discussion: helps to define policy related challenges, barriers, ethical concerns.

Oncologist:
- Confirms appropriateness of adjunct cannabis use. Considers the ECS and reinforces information around self-titration/ dosing of cannabinoid therapeutics.

Pharmacist:
- Reviews drug interactions and dosing considerations

Dietician:
- Aligns cannabis use with nutritional goals and discusses

Social Worker:
- Addresses access, legality, cultural, equity, and psychosocial factors

Primary Oncology Nurse:
- Monitors symptoms and reinforces education using culturally competent care approaches.

Chaplain:
- Assesses spiritual healing needs, defines patient's spiritual care preferences, supports development of cannabis-related spiritual care rituals alongside the nurse, considers cultural care needs, and provides ongoing spiritual care.

Simulation Flow
1. Patient disclosure of cannabis use
2. Team huddle led by cannabis care nurse, with consideration of patient's cultural needs, ethical concerns, and policies that may support or hinder equitable access.
3. Patient education and agreement on next steps. How, when, where will the patient access cannabinoid therapeutics? Does the patient need a medical cannabis recommendation and how is that procured in the state? What level of caocahing, education, and support does the patient need?
4. Collaborative care plan developed.
5. Debrief and next steps.

Debriefing Points
- How did each role contribute to patient safety?
- How did interprofessional collaboration improve care?
  - What ethical concepts were employed?
  - How was culturally competent care provided?
  - What policies at the workplace, local, state, or federal level hinder or support the patient's equitable access.
- What challenges arose in discussing cannabis use? Were biases present? What are the policy (specific setting, state, and federal regulations) concerns to be considered, and how could the team address them to ensure more equitable access?

Outcomes
Learners demonstrate collaborative, ethical, and patient-centered cannabis care within oncology practice. Their own biases are checked and they come up with an interprofessional plan to address the barriers they discovered.

Finally, Table 3 depicts an approach to teaching about cannabis policy from an interprofessional perspective.

Table 3. Interprofessional cannabis policy education experience: Cannabis in healthcare: Policy, practice, and interprofessional decision-making

<table>
<tr><td>

Learners: Nursing, Medicine, Pharmacy

- Social Work, Public Health
- Behavioral Health, Health Administration
- Law/Policy or Ethics students (optional but valuable)

Objectives: By the end of this experience, students will be able to:

1. Explain federal, state, and institutional cannabis policies and their implications for healthcare practice.
2. Compare professional scope-of-practice differences related to cannabis across disciplines.
3. Analyze ethical, legal, and equity considerations related to medical and recreational cannabis.
4. Apply interprofessional collaboration to patient scenarios involving cannabis use.
5. Demonstrate policy-informed clinical decision-making and patient education.

</td></tr>
<tr><td>

Duration: 3-4 hours, may be split over multiple weeks

Outline of Content

Lecture: Cannabis Policy Foundations (45 minutes):

- Federal vs. state cannabis law (Schedule I status, DEA, FDA)
- Medical vs. recreational cannabis frameworks
- Institutional policies (hospitals, clinics, schools)
- Employment, licensure, and liability considerations

Activity: Each discipline discusses how cannabis policy affects their role (e.g., prescribing limits, patient counseling, documentation, reporting)

Scope of Practice & Professional Roles (Panel or Breakout – 45 min)

- Nursing: Patient assessment, education, advocacy, harm reduction, coaching, holistic modalities and approaches, spirituality, ECS, cultural care, equity
- Medicine/Advanced Practice Nursing: Certification/recommendation authority, dosing
- Pharmacy: Drug interactions, dosing considerations, product safety
- Social Work: Legal navigation, access barriers, stigma reduction, cultural concerns, equity
- Public Health: Population-level impacts, health equity, surveillance, racism, stigma

</td></tr>
<tr><td>

Activity:

Students map who can do what legally and ethically in cannabis-related care.

Ethics, Equity, and Social Justice (Small Groups – 30 min)

- Racial disparities in cannabis enforcement
- Access to medical cannabis
- Informed consent and patient autonomy
- Vulnerable populations (pregnancy, adolescents, older adults)

Activity: Reflection or written assignment: "How do cannabis policies support or harm patient-centered care?"

Interprofessional Case-Based Simulation (75–90 min)

Case Example:

A 55-year-old patient with chronic pain, PTSD, and hypertension uses state-approved medical cannabis while employed in a federally regulated job.

Student Roles Assigned:

- Nurse
- Physician/APRN
- Pharmacist
- Social Worker
- Health Administrator/Policy Advisor

</td></tr>
<tr><td>

Tasks:

- Identify policy constraints: workplace, local, state, and federal levels
- Assess clinical risks and benefits
- Address medical cannabis patient education, coaching, and safety
- Develop a unified interprofessional care plan

Activity:

Develop one-page policy-informed care plan with recommendations

Policy-to-Practice Reflection & Debrief (30 min)

Guided Reflection Prompts:

- How did policy influence your clinical decisions?
- Where did professional roles overlap or conflict?
- What advocacy opportunities exist for healthcare professionals?

Activity: group submits a one-page summary of the learning experience.

</td></tr>
</table>

While there may be resistance to including cannabis care in nursing and interprofessional education efforts, we are ethically obligated to support patients in our communities toward safe and effective cannabinoid therapeutics use and examining issues of equity and access. Nursing faculty have many resources available to support cannabis science learning and curriculum development efforts, including linking to professional cannabis organizations, attending continuing education events, and supporting the inclusion of cannabis science in nursing education. Whether cannabinoid science is included across the curriculum, in short seminars, or via interprofessional experiences, both the providers and the patients will benefit from an increased level of knowledge and shifts in attitudes and skills (King, et al, 2024). Public health and community efforts can build upon interprofessionals cannabis care knowledge to address the many policy and social determinants of health issues that are impacting patients ability to access both quality cannabis and cannabis care, though more research is needed in this area.

CONCLUSION

This chapter has examined medical cannabis equity through a public health lens, demonstrating that access to cannabinoid therapeutics in the United States is shaped far less by individual choice than by structural, historical, and policy-driven determinants. While the expansion of state-level medical cannabis programs has created new therapeutic opportunities, these benefits remain unevenly distributed across populations. Federal prohibition, fragmented state policies, financial barriers, stigma, and limited clinical guidance collectively function as upstream determinants of access, reproducing long-standing inequities rooted in race, income, geography, and healthcare access.

Situating medical cannabis within established public health and social determinants of health frameworks underscores that legalization alone is insufficient to ensure equitable outcomes. Instead, policy design, healthcare system integration, provider education, and community context mediate whether patients can obtain safe, regulated products and receive evidence-informed guidance. The chapter highlights how economic instability, geographic isolation, fragmented healthcare access, and limited health literacy intersect with stigma and implicit bias in clinical settings, creating cumulative disadvantage for marginalized populations. These dynamics mirror inequities observed across other areas of healthcare and reinforce the necessity of addressing cannabis access as a systems-level issue rather than an individual behavior.

Nurses emerge throughout this analysis as critical actors at the intersection of policy, practice, and patient experience. As frontline clinicians, educators, advocates, and system navigators, nurses are uniquely positioned to mitigate inequities through culturally responsive communication, harm-reduction–oriented education, and ethical advocacy. The development of cannabis nursing as a recognized specialty, alongside the establishment of scope and standards of practice, reflects an important professional response to longstanding gaps in clinical guidance and education. However, realizing the full equity-promoting potential of nursing requires sustained investment in curricula, interprofessional education, research dissemination, and institutional policy reform.

At the policy and system levels, the chapter underscores the importance of equity-grounded reforms that expand provider participation, reduce financial barriers, integrate cannabis into healthcare infrastructure, and strengthen surveillance and data systems. Drawing on lessons from tobacco, alcohol, and pharmaceutical regulation, a public health–oriented approach to medical cannabis emphasizes proactive system design, accountability, and reinvestment in prevention and education. State-level variation offers valuable opportunities to evaluate which regulatory models best align with equity goals, particularly when informed by community-engaged research and disaggregated data.

Taken together, the evidence presented in this chapter reinforces that cannabis equity is neither ancillary nor aspirational, but a core criterion for evaluating the success of medical cannabis policy and practice. Advancing equity in this space requires coordinated action across policy, education, healthcare systems, and professional practice, with nurses playing a central role in translating structural change into meaningful patient outcomes. As medical cannabis continues to evolve within the United States, grounding future efforts in public health principles, ethical nursing practice, and social justice will be essential to ensuring that access to cannabinoid therapeutics advances, rather than undermines, health equity.

REFERENCES

Alexander, S. P. (2020). Barriers to the wider adoption of medicinal Cannabis. *British Journal of Pain, 14*(2), 122–132. DOI: 10.1177/2049463720922884 PMID: 32537151

American Nurses Association. (2021). *Nursing: Scope and standards of practice* (4th ed.). American Nurses Association.

American Nurses Association & American Cannabis Nurses Association. (2021). Cannabis Nursing: Scope and standards of practice. American Nurses Association.

Anderson, D. M., & Rees, D. I. (2023). The public health effects of legalizing marijuana. Journal of Economic Literature, 61(1), 86–143. doi:10.1257/jel.20211635

Ashare, R. L., Turay, E., Worster, B., Wetherill, R. R., Bidwell, L. C., Doucette, A., & Meghani, S. H. (2023). Social determinants of health associated with how cannabis is obtained and used in patients with cancer receiving care at a cancer treatment center in Pennsylvania. *Cannabis (Research Society on Marijuana), 6*(2), 1–12. DOI: 10.26828/cannabis/2023/000151 PMID: 37484056

Barry, R. A., & Glantz, S. (2016). A public health framework for legalized retail marijuana based on the US experience: Avoiding a new tobacco industry. *PLoS Medicine, 13*(9), e1002131. DOI: 10.1371/journal.pmed.1002131 PMID: 27676176

Brown, T. M. (2016). Working with the panthers to transform health care for poor black communities. *American Journal of Public Health, 106*(10), 1756–1757. DOI: 10.2105/AJPH.2016.303402 PMID: 27552281

Cannabis Nurses of Color. (n.d.). *1st 'Day at the Capital': Health policy summit.* https://cannabisnursesofcolor.com/capitalday/

Chávez-Valenzuela, P., Kappes, M., Sambuceti, C. E., & Díaz-Guio, D. A. (2025). Challenges in the implementation of inter-professional education programs with clinical simulation for health care students: A scoping review. *Nurse Education Today, 146*, 106548. DOI: 10.1016/j.nedt.2024.106548 PMID: 39740591

Clark, C. S. (2019 a). *Evaluating the evidence: Cannabis and psychosis, Part I.* https://nursemanifest.com/2019/03/21/evaluating-the-evidence-cannabis-and-psychosis-part-i/

Clark, C. S. (2019b). *Evaluating the evidence: Cannabis and psychodid, Part II.* https://nursemanifest.com/2019/03/26/evaluating-the-evidence-cannabis-and-psychosis-part-ii/

Clark, C. S. (2021a). The nurse's role: Providing cannabis care. In Clark, C. S. (Ed.), *Cannabis: A handbook for nurses* (pp. 268–312). Wolters Kluwer.

Clark, C. S. (2021b). *Cannabis: A handbook for nurses.* Wolters Kluwer.

Clobes, T. A., Himebaugh, S., Gamez, S. A., & Torres, M. (2025). Relationship between cannabis dispensary density, proximity, and attitudes toward medical cannabis: A cross-sectional study. *Health Science Reports, 8*(4), e70685. DOI: 10.1002/hsr2.70685 PMID: 40260030

Cooper, Z. D., Abrams, D. I., Gust, S., Salicrup, A., & Throckmorton, D. C. (2021). Challenges for clinical cannabis and cannabinoid research in the United States. *Journal of the National Cancer Institute. Monographs*, *2021*(58), 114–122. DOI: 10.1093/jncimonographs/lgab009 PMID: 34850896

Dahlke, S., Butler, J. I., Hunter, K. F., Toubiana, M., Kalogirou, M. R., Shrestha, S., Devkota, R., Law, J., & Scheuerman, M. (2024). The effects of stigma: Older persons and medicinal cannabis. *Qualitative Health Research*, *34*(8-9), 717–731. DOI: 10.1177/10497323241227419 PMID: 38305270

Donahue, D. M., Metzger, M., Baker, M., & Rosenof, L. (2023). Let's match: Making cannabis policy guided by research. *Clinical Therapeutics*, *45*(6), 515–520. DOI: 10.1016/j.clinthera.2023.03.011 PMID: 37414501

Eddy, M. (2010). Medical marijuana: Review and analysis of federal and state policies. Congressional Research Service. https://files.iowamedicalmarijuana.org/imm/RL33211_20100402.pdf

Freudenberg, N., & Tsui, E. (2014). Evidence, power, and policy change in community-based participatory research. *American Journal of Public Health*, *104*(1), 11–14. DOI: 10.2105/AJPH.2013.301471 PMID: 24228677

Gardiner, K. M., Singleton, J. A., Sheridan, J., Kyle, G. J., & Nissen, L. M. (2019). Health professional beliefs, knowledge, and concerns surrounding medicinal cannabis: A systematic review. *PLoS One*, *14*(5), e0216556. DOI: 10.1371/journal.pone.0216556 PMID: 31059531

Grbic, J., Goddard, P., & Ryder, D. (2017). Observations of the role of science in the United States medical cannabis state policies: Lessons learnt. *The International Journal on Drug Policy*, *42*, 109–114. DOI: 10.1016/j.drugpo.2016.12.019 PMID: 28190671

Ho, I. K., Sheldon, T. A., & Botelho, E. (2022). Medical mistrust among women with intersecting marginalized identities: A scoping review. *Ethnicity & Health*, *27*(8), 1733–1751. DOI: 10.1080/13557858.2021.1990220 PMID: 34647832

Hong, G., Sideris, A., Waldman, S., Stauffer, J., & Wu, C. L. (2024). Legal and regulatory aspects of medical cannabis in the United States. *Anesthesia and Analgesia*, *138*(1), 31–41. DOI: 10.1213/ANE.0000000000006301 PMID: 38100798

Hossain, M. K., & Chae, H. J. (2024). Medical cannabis: From research breakthroughs to shifting public perceptions and ensuring safe use. *Integrative Medicine Research*, *13*(4), 101094. DOI: 10.1016/j.imr.2024.101094 PMID: 39640076

Hulaihel, A., Gliksberg, O., Feingold, D., Brill, S., Amit, B. H., Lev-ran, S., & Sznitman, S. R. (2023). Medical cannabis and stigma: A qualitative study with patients living with chronic pain. *Journal of Clinical Nursing*, *32*(7-8), 1103–1114. DOI: 10.1111/jocn.16340 PMID: 35488381

Jaiswal, J. (2019). Whose responsibility is it to dismantle medical mistrust? Future directions for researchers and health care providers. *Behavioral Medicine (Washington, D.C.)*, *45*(2), 188–196. DOI: 10.1080/08964289.2019.1630357 PMID: 31343959

King, D. D., Gill, C. J., Cadieux, C. S., & Singh, N. (2024). The role of stigma in cannabis use disclosure: An exploratory study. *Harm Reduction Journal*, *21*(1), 21. DOI: 10.1186/s12954-024-00929-8 PMID: 38273362

Kurtzman, E. T., Greene, J., Begley, R., & Drenkard, K. N. (2022). "We want what's best for patients." Nurse leaders' attitudes about medical cannabis: A qualitative study. *International Journal of Nursing Studies Advances*, *4*, 100065. DOI: 10.1016/j.ijnsa.2022.100065 PMID: 38745605

Lucas, P. (2012). It can't hurt to ask: A patient-centered quality of service assessment of Health Canada's medical cannabis policy and program. *Harm Reduction Journal*, *9*(1), 2. DOI: 10.1186/1477-7517-9-2 PMID: 22214382

Martin-Willett, R., Stanger, M., James, W., Bryan, A. D., & Bidwell, L. C. (2023). Effects of historical inequity and institutional power on cannabis research: Moving toward equity and inclusion. *PNAS Nexus*, *2*(12), pgad383. Advance online publication. DOI: 10.1093/pnasnexus/pgad383 PMID: 38089600

Martins, S. S., Segura, L. E., Levy, N. S., Mauro, P. M., Mauro, C. M., Philbin, M. M., & Hasin, D. S. (2021). Racial and ethnic differences in cannabis use following legalization in US states with medical cannabis laws. *JAMA Network Open*, *4*(9), e2127002–e2127002. DOI: 10.1001/jamanetworkopen.2021.27002 PMID: 34570205

McPartland, J. M., Guy, G. W., & Di Marzo, V. (2014). Care and feeding of the endocannabinoid system: A systematic review of potential clinical interventions that upregulate the endocannabinoid system. *PLoS One*, *9*(3), e89566. DOI: 10.1371/journal.pone.0089566 PMID: 24622769

Mennis, J., Stahler, G. J., & Mason, M. (2016). Risky substance use environments and addiction: A new frontier for environmental justice research. *International Journal of Environmental Research and Public Health*, *13*(6), 607. DOI: 10.3390/ijerph13060607 PMID: 27322303

Metha, D. H. (2025). Cannabis education: A professional and moral obligation for physicians. *JAMA Network Open*, *8*(10), e2536224. DOI: 10.1001/jamanetworkopen.2025.36224 PMID: 41055911

Moustaqim-Barrette, A.. (2019). Healthcare provider knowledge, attitudes, and practices related to cannabis. *Cannabis and Cannabinoid Research*, *4*(3), 204–212. DOI: 10.1089/can.2018.0054 PMID: 31579835

Nadzam, D. M. (2009). Nurses' role in communication and patient safety. *Journal of Nursing Care Quality*, *24*(3), 184–188. DOI: 10.1097/01.NCQ.0000356905.87452.62 PMID: 19525757

National Academies of Sciences, Engineering, and Medicine. (2017). *The health effects of cannabis and cannabinoids.* https://nap.nationalacademies.org/catalog/24625/the-health-effects-of-cannabis-and-cannabinoids-current-state-of-evidence

National Academies of Sciences, Engineering, and Medicine; Health and Medicine Division; Board on Population Health and Public Health Practice; Committee on the Public Health Consequences of Changes in the Cannabis Policy Landscape. (2024). *Cannabis policy impacts public health and health equity.* National Academies Press (US). https://www.ncbi.nlm.nih.gov/sites/books/NBK609489/

National Conference of State Legislatures. (2025). *State medical cannabis laws.* https://www.ncsl.org/health/state-medical-cannabis-laws

Nayak, M. M., Revette, A., Chai, P. R., Lansang, K., Sannes, T., Tung, S., & Braun, I. M. (2022). Medical cannabis-related stigma: Cancer survivors' perspectives. *Journal of Cancer Survivorship: Research and Practice*, *17*(3), 951–956. DOI: 10.1007/s11764-022-01297-7 PMID: 36435953

Newell, S., & Jordan, Z. (2015). The patient experience of patient-centered communication with nurses in the hospital setting: A qualitative systematic review protocol. *JBI Evidence Synthesis*, *13*(1), 76–87. DOI: 10.11124/jbisrir-2015-1072 PMID: 26447009

Orenstein, D. G., & Glantz, S. A. (2020). Cannabis legalization in state legislatures: Public health opportunity and risk. *Marquette Law Review*, *103*(4), 1313–1340. PMID: 34376874

Pacula, R. L., & Smart, R. (2017). Medical marijuana and marijuana legalization. *Annual Review of Clinical Psychology*, *13*(1), 397–419. DOI: 10.1146/annurev-clinpsy-032816-045128 PMID: 28482686

Parmelee, R. A. (2025). *Nurse educators' experiences with medical cannabis education* (Doctoral dissertation, Walden University). Walden University ScholarWorks. https://scholarworks.waldenu.edu/cgi/viewcontent.cgi?article=18960&context=dissertations

Parmelee, R. A., & Clark, C. S. (2022). Nursing students' knowledge, skills, and attitudes regarding medicinal cannabis care. *Journal of Nursing Regulation*, *13*(3), 13–23. DOI: 10.1016/S2155-8256(22)00082-5

Perlman, A. I., McLeod, H. M., Ventresca, E. C., Salinas, M. G., Post, P. J., Schuh, M. J., & Abu Dabrh, A. M. (2021). Medical cannabis state and federal regulations: Implications for United States health care entities. *Mayo Clinic Proceedings*, *96*(10), 2671–2681. DOI: 10.1016/j.mayocp.2021.05.005 PMID: 34607636

Philpot, L. M., Ebbert, J. O., & Hurt, R. T. (2019). A survey of the attitudes, beliefs and knowledge about medical cannabis among primary care providers. *BMC Family Practice*, *20*(1), 17. DOI: 10.1186/s12875-019-0906-y PMID: 30669979

Prompahakul, C., Keim-Malpass, J., LeBaron, V., Yan, G., & Epstein, E. G. (2021). Moral distress among nurses: A mixed-methods study. *Nursing Ethics*, *28*(7-8), 1165–1182. DOI: 10.1177/0969733021996028 PMID: 33888021

Rami, F., Thompson, L., & Solis-Cortes, L. (2023). Healthcare disparities: Vulnerable and marginalized populations. In Searight, H. R. (Ed.), *COVID-19: Health disparities and ethical challenges across the globe*. Springer International Publishing., DOI: 10.1007/978-3-031-26200-5_6

Rice, J., Hildebrand, A., Waslo, C. S., Cameron, M. H., & Jones, K. D. (2022). Cannabis for medical purposes: A cross-sectional analysis of health care professionals' knowledge. *Journal of the American Association of Nurse Practitioners*, *34*(1), 100–106. DOI: 10.1097/JXX.0000000000000590 PMID: 33767121

Ruheel, M. A., Gomes, Z., Usman, S., Homayouni, P., & Ng, J. Y. (2021). Facilitators and barriers to the regulation of medical cannabis: A scoping review of the peer-reviewed literature. *Harm Reduction Journal*, *18*(1), 106. DOI: 10.1186/s12954-021-00547-8 PMID: 34649577

Schauer, G. L. (2021). Cannabis policy in the United States: Implications for public health. *Journal of the National Cancer Institute. Monographs, 2021*(58), 39–52. DOI: 10.1093/jncimonographs/lgab016 PMID: 34850901

South, A. M., Babalonis, S. L., Fanucchi, L. C., & Lofwall, M. R. (2025). "Medical Cannabis": Advising patients while navigating medical ethics and limited evidence. *Journal of General Internal Medicine, 1-5.* Advance online publication. DOI: 10.1007/s11606-025-09680-7 PMID: 40624323

Unger, J. B. (2022). Regulation of cannabis retailers: Facilitating responsible adult use and promoting health equity while preventing access to minors. *American Journal of Public Health, 112*(11), 1532–1534. DOI: 10.2105/AJPH.2022.307102 PMID: 36223589

Wang, Y., Boyd, A. E., Rountree, L., Ren, Y., Nyhan, K., Nagar, R., Higginbottom, J., Ranney, M. L., Parikh, H., & Mukherjee, B. (2025). *Towards enhancing data equity in public health data science.* Cornell University. https://doi.org//arXiv.2508.20301DOI: 10.48550

World Health Organization. (2008). *Closing the gap in a generation: health equity through action on the social determinants of health - Final report of the commission on social determinants of health.* https://www.who.int/publications/i/item/WHO-IER-CSDH-08.1

World Health Organization. (2024). *Global status report on alcohol and health and treatment of substance use disorders.* https://www.who.int/publications/i/item/9789240096745

Zarhin, D., Negev, M., Vulfsons, S., & Sznitman, S. R. (2020). "Medical cannabis" as a contested medicine: Fighting over epistemology and morality. *Science, Technology & Human Values, 45*(3), 488–514. DOI: 10.1177/0162243919862866

KEY TERMS AND DEFINITIONS

Cannabis Equity: The principle that access to cannabis-related healthcare, information, and legal protections should be distributed according to need and without discrimination, particularly for populations historically harmed by prohibition.

Cannabis Nursing: A recognized nursing subspecialty focused on patient education, harm reduction, advocacy, and clinical guidance related to cannabis and cannabinoid therapeutics within ethical and legal frameworks.

Harm Reduction: A public health approach that prioritizes minimizing adverse health, social, and legal consequences of substance use without requiring abstinence as a precondition for care.

Health Equity: The attainment of the highest possible level of health for all individuals through the elimination of avoidable and unjust differences in access, quality, and outcomes of healthcare.

Implicit Bias: Unconscious attitudes or stereotypes held by individuals that influence understanding, decision-making, and behavior, often contributing to inequitable healthcare treatment.

Medical Cannabis: Cannabis used under state-authorized programs for the management of specific health conditions, typically requiring clinician certification and regulatory oversight.

Social Determinants of Health: The social, economic, and environmental conditions in which individuals live and receive care that shape health risks, access to services, and overall outcomes.

Stigma: Social disapproval or devaluation directed toward individuals or practices, which in health-care settings can restrict disclosure, communication, and access to appropriate care.

Structural Determinants of Health: Upstream legal, political, and institutional systems, including laws and policies, that systematically shape patterns of health advantage and disadvantage.

Chapter 12
Medical Cannabis Curricula for Nurses:
Integrating Content

Carey Shannon Cadieux
http://orcid.org/0000-0001-8812-2667
Binghamton University, USA

ABSTRACT

This chapter focuses on the development of curricula on medical cannabis for nursing students. It follows the National Council of State Boards of Nursing (2018) call for six essential areas of medical cannabis knowledge, attitudes, and skills to be addressed in academia. The chapter will expand on the implications of developing medical cannabis curricula for nurses that include the role of the cannabis nurse from the perspectives of the Cannabis nursing scope and standards of practice (American Nurses Association & American Cannabis Nurses Association, 2024), advocacy, ethics, safety issues, spiritual concerns, and common challenges and barriers that nurses providing care for medical cannabis patients may face.

INTRODUCTION

In 2018, the National Council of State Boards of Nursing (NCSBN) called for nurses to gain knowledge in six essential cannabis areas to prepare them to care for patients using medical cannabis. At that time, a rapid movement of states enacted rights to legalize cannabis for both medical and adult/recreational use. At the forefront of the scene, the author had the pleasure in 2019 of leading the development and launching of the first medical cannabis certificate program offered at an accredited 4-year university in the United States (US). We initially developed the program at Pacific College of Health and Science (PCHS) for nurses to address the NCSBN six essentials; they soon found that all healthcare providers were interested in enrolling in the certificate program. In addition to educating nurses at all levels, we provided education for physicians, osteopaths, pharmacists, nutritionists, health coaches, and massage therapists. Many other universities subsequently established their own programs. PCHS has since closed its program, and the author is developing a new graduate-level interprofessional medical cannabis credential at Binghamton University. This chapter will draw on evidence and the author's knowledge and

DOI: 10.4018/979-8-3373-7287-7.ch012

experience in curriculum development, with a focus on helping the reader integrate medical cannabis education for nurses into the mainstream curriculum.

The need for nursing programs to include medical cannabis science in their curricula continues to grow. 25-40% of all oncology patients use cannabis (Worster et al., 2022). While 85% of patients want their medical cannabis education and coaching information from their providers, only 15% receive any medical cannabis support (Pergam et al., 2017).

In 2022, the author co-authored a study demonstrating that, despite the NCSBN's call for nursing students to be educated on the six essentials, more than 1,300 nursing students who completed the survey indicated that they were not receiving the education they needed to care for patients with medical cannabis (Parmelee & Clark, 2022). While more than 90% of the participants agreed that medical cannabis has therapeutic effects, 74% stated that their nursing schools do not include any medical cannabis content. Most of the students had a great desire for medical cannabis inclusion in their educational content and clinical experience; however, they generally received information about medical cannabis from the media/news, research articles, and patients. There has likely been little shift in the number of schools providing adequate medical cannabis education for nursing students across all levels.

Schools of nursing have not been including medical cannabis into their curricula for a variety of reasons, including lack of accreditation standards that specifically include cannabinoid science, lack of NCLEX questions addressing medical cannabis care, stigma, and nursing faculty's own knowledge deficits in these areas (Clark, 2021a). Regardless of the reasons why, nursing faculty are ethically obligated from the perspectives of patient autonomy and the nurse's duty of nonmaleficence and beneficence to include this content, as patients are using cannabis, and they need support, education, and coaching to use the medicine effectively while avoiding adverse effects.

This chapter will guide the reader through the key components for developing and implementing a medical cannabis curriculum. Whether the course is a one-hour lecture or a standalone elective, nurses across the specialty areas must be prepared and confident to guide patients in the safe and effective use of cannabis. The chapter will review the NCSBN (2018) six essentials for medical cannabis education for nurses, explore how the American Nurses Association/ American Cannabis Nurses Association (2023) *Cannabis nursing: Scope and standards of practice* can guide the learner and educator, and review the importance of addressing ethics, advocacy, legal concerns, and cannabis as a spiritual plant entheogen. Consideration for inclusion in undergraduate and graduate nursing programs is provided, with differentiation across several short lectures, semester-long courses, or certificate programs, and the integration of medical cannabis curriculum components across the curriculum.

As the world moves out of the global cannabis prohibition era and into an era of regulation, it is increasingly vital that nurse educators take steps to end stigma and include medical cannabis care across all levels of education so that nurses may effectively act as advocates for patients' access to quality cannabinoid therapeutics and safe use. The objectives for this chapter are that the reader will:

- Explore the National Council of State Boards of Nursing (2018) six essentials of the medical cannabis curriculum for nurses.
- Define the importance of an extended medical cannabis curriculum for nurses that also includes historical implications, advocacy, ethics, a holistic approach, and the entheogenic nature of the plant.
- Consider the benefits of a medical cannabis curriculum delivered through short lectures, semester-long courses, certificate programs, and/or curricular integration.

BACKGROUND

This section provides a review of the literature on issues with including medical cannabis in nursing curricula. This section aims to strengthen the reader's understanding of the importance of including medical cannabis care in all nursing curricula.

As we move out of the global cannabis prohibition era and into an era of regulation, it is increasingly vital that nurse educators take steps to end stigma and include medical cannabis care across all levels of education so that nurses may effectively act as advocates for patients ' access and safe use (Clark, 2021a).

Cannabis is now readily accessible for many people in the US. According to the Pew Research Center (2024), 74% of the US population now resides in states where cannabis is legal for either medical or adult use cannabis, 54% live in states with legal adult use cannabis, 79% live in a county with at least one cannabis dispensary, and there are over 15,000 cannabis dispensaries in the US. 88% of adults in the US believe that cannabis should be legal for medical use (59%) or for adult legal use (30%). Interestingly, US cannabis dispensary locations often cluster on the border with states where cannabis is not legal, likely increasing access across state lines (please note that it is federally illegal to cross state lines with cannabis at the time of this writing). With such a large percentage of the population now being able to access cannabis, it becomes more important than ever that healthcare professionals strive to provide education and coaching around safe and effective cannabis use to lower the incidence of adverse effects, which saves healthcare dollars.

The National Academies of Science, Engineering, and Medicine's (NASEM)(2017) report found that medical cannabis use is evidence-based and demonstrated to be effective for a limited number of health concerns, including chronic pain. Even though evidence generation has been impacted by prohibition and cannabis being a Drug Enforcement Administration (DEA) Schedule I medicine for decades, many patients with a wide variety of illnesses and wellness concerns use cannabis to palliate their symptoms. The NASEM report also found that prohibition has greatly impacted cannabis research and stigmatized medical cannabis patients.

Patients are using and inquiring about medical cannabis, as the data demonstrates that 50-79% of clinicians reported a patient had inquired about medical cannabis (Ziemianski et al., 2015; Balneaves et al., 2018; St. Pierre et al., 2020). The American Society of Regional Anesthesia and Pain Medicine surveyed 334 physicians from October 2019 to March 2020 and found that 76% cared for patients using medical cannabis (Narouze et al., 2020). Two hundred eighty-eight pediatric oncology providers from Illinois, Massachusetts, and Washington, 30% reported at least one patient request in the past month for medical cannabis (Ananth et al., 2018). One study found that the use of medical cannabis among pediatric patients with severe illness and palliative care needs resulted in lower resource utilization rates, reduced polypharmacy, increased quality of life scores, and overall positive outcomes with symptoms (Free et al., 2025).

Stigma and social justice issues related to cannabis use and cannabis patients and cannabis and cannabinoid-related research have been challenging to conduct during this era of prohibition (National Academies of Science, Engineering, and Medicine, 2017). This lack of emphasis on medical cannabis science in healthcare providers' educational experience leads providers not to be well-versed in the action of cannabinoid therapeutic interactions with the endocannabinoid system, the adverse effects of cannabinoids, and approaches to ensuring safe and effective use of cannabinoids (Clark, 2021a). Healthcare providers may avoid discussing medical cannabis use with their patients as they lack both the confidence and knowledge to do so. Melnikov et al. (2021) found that from a sample of 221 healthcare professionals, attitudes towards medical cannabis use, intention to recommend cannabis, and stigma towards medical cannabis users were correlated (2021). Knowledge and skills shape the practitioner's attitudes and beliefs, and most healthcare providers have mostly learned about medical cannabis through media and other clinicians (Carlini et al., 2017).

A survey conducted of 451 U.S. neurologists, nurses, and pharmacists indicated that 80% of the respondents perceive cannabis as providing a potential therapeutic opportunity, and over half of them were unfamiliar with both cannabis clinical applications and cannabinoid pharmacology (Szaflarski et al., 2020). Another study found that with 310 Washington State health care professionals, 58% did not have adequate knowledge and skills to provide medical authorizations for patients to use cannabis (Kaplan et al., 2020). In another study, 91% of 310 hospice professionals supported medical cannabis use for hospice patients, and 84% believed their organization and patients would benefit from clear policies around medical cannabis use. However, less than a third of those surveyed provided medical cannabis education to their patients (Costantino et al., 2019).

Canada federally legalized cannabis nationwide in October 2018, and they still have similar issues with education for healthcare providers. (Government of Canada, 2021). Of 189 Canadian nurse practitioners, 76.3% reported educational needs about cannabis for therapeutic purposes (Balneaves et al., 2019). A survey of 103 Canadian oncology healthcare professionals found that 84% reported a lack of sufficient knowledge in cannabis to support patients' therapeutic purposes (McLennan et al., 2020). Ninety-three Canadian physicians-in-training reported receiving less education than necessary, though their patients often inquire about medical cannabis (St. Pierre et al., 2020). This research demonstrates that legalization does not automatically lead to providers receiving the education they need to support patients' safe and effective use of cannabis.

Without healthcare providers' training, patients have limited reliable guidance in safely using cannabis for their medical needs. Patients may rely on entry-level employees or "budtenders" at dispensaries when purchasing cannabis for a medical condition. They may use the undertrained dispensary staff in an attempt to learn about safe and effective cannabinoid use, which is problematic in that a recent analysis of 434 cannabis dispensary staff interactions found that 74% based their recommendations on medical conditions, whereas only 40% relied on clinician input; the sample included 40% budtenders, 32% managers, and 13% pharmacists (Merlin et al., 2021).

Medical cannabis education can help to increase nursing students' knowledge, attitudes, and skills with medical cannabis. A pilot study by King et al. (2023) found that teaching on cannabis pharmacology and the physiology of the endocannabinoid system (ECS) directly influenced advanced practice nursing (APRN) students' clinical practice, and the students agreed that faculty should include medical cannabis content in APRN curricula.

A 2025 qualitative dissertation focused on eleven nurse educators' experiences with medical cannabis education (Parmelee, 2025). Parmelee (2025) found that the educators who lived in legal medical cannabis states and had two years of experience teaching in accredited nursing programs felt guided by their own understanding of cannabis's therapeutic potential, their journeys with learning more about medical cannabis, a lack of time to learn more about medical cannabis and a lack of time within the curriculum to include medical cannabis, defining where medical cannabis aligns within the nursing curriculum, and implications around updating the overall curriculum to include medical cannabis content. Having limited discussions with colleagues impacted the educator's ability to include medical cannabis content, with federal legality and stigma issues around prohibition being a consideration and changing laws may be difficult to keep up with.

There is very little evidence around the outcomes from medical cannabis curricula endeavors, and I am currently conducting a study around this, as are colleagues in Canada and elsewhere. However, the evidence is clear that there is both a need for medical cannabis curricula in nursing education and that faculty need guidance around creating the educational experience for their learners. Nurses have an ethical obligation to uphold beneficence (doing good) and nonmaleficence (doing no harm) in serving their patients and providing education and support to ensure patients can use cannabis safely and effectively (Clark, 2021a). The following section will review the steps for developing medical cannabis curricula, identify the inclusions of undergraduate and graduate programs, and discuss delivery options.

DEVELOPING MEDICAL CANNABIS CURRICULA

Because there has been a historical dearth of education on the National Council of State Boards of Nursing (2018) essentials, faculty have the conundrum of lacking the requisite knowledge, attitudes, skills, and confidence to integrate this content effectively into their learners' education. Barriers and challenges include limited knowledge, the process of implementing curricular change, the absence of clearly aligned accreditation requirements, and the absence of medical cannabis content on prelicensure and APRN licensing exams (Clark, 2021a). Nursing faculty can undertake this task using the clearly defined process outlined below.

Buy-In

Initial steps include getting buy-in from the faculty and administration. Things to bring to the table during the buy-in process include the National Council of State Boards of Nursing (2018) National Nursing Guidelines for Medical Marijuana, available for download at https://www.ncsbn.org/public-files/The_NCSBN_National_Nursing_Guidelines_for_Medical_Marijuana_JNR_July_2018.pdf. Other items include Parmelee and Clark's (2022) study around the lack of nursing students' medical cannabis educational experience and their desire for such education, and the *Cannabis: A handbook for nurses* (Clark, 2021a) textbook. The Clark textbook can be used in curricula, as can this textbook. Many of the articles mentioned above in the literature review may also be helpful in this process. One selling point that can help convince faculty to proceed with including medical cannabis in the nursing curriculum is framing the discussion from an ethical perspective, including supporting patient autonomy (right to self-determination), and the beneficence of providing patients the education and coaching they need to use cannabis in ways that avoid harm to self and others.

Educating the faculty can also be challenging, but numerous resources are available, including Clark (2021) and materials from the American Cannabis Nurses Association and the Cannabis Clinicians Society. The areas in which faculty require education largely align with the National Council of State Boards of Nursing's (2018) guidelines, which provide a baseline for faculty education. Additionally, reviewing the American Nurses Association (ANA) and American Cannabis Nurses Association (ACNA) (2024) *Cannabis nursing: Scope and standards of practice* ensures that the educator has a sound understanding of what cannabis care nursing entails. One of the concerns for many faculty will be the prohibition-induced issue of stigma that lingers around the use of the plant and the people who use cannabis.

Part of overcoming this stigma is educating nurses and nursing faculty. Having educated thousands of people at professional nursing conferences over the years, I have witnessed many nurses change their minds about cannabis once they learn about two key areas: The human endocannabinoid system (ECS) being the body's master regulator system, and the lack of one's own endocannabinoids leading to health issues and illness, which helps to overcome the stigma related to the "mystery" of how cannabis can support the healing process and palliative needs for so many different issues. It is possible to influence people's viewpoints once they understand the basic science of cannabinoid therapeutics. I also tend to introduce the idea that there has been nothing logical about cannabis prohibition; cannabis was once a first-line over-the-counter medication produced by companies like Eli Lily and available at the corner pharmacy, and the American Medical Association protested the prohibition. Additionally, highlighting cannabis use as an integrative approach can be helpful, as most people will still need other medications, healthcare system support, and to care for their bodies in ways that upregulate the ECS. Drawing attention to the need to examine one's own bias and aligning ethical concepts with the rationale for including the content are also key.

Another area of resistance for faculty may be the packed curriculum (Clark, 2021a). One way to address this is to again refer to the ethical considerations and the desire for an updated curriculum that prepares nursing students to provide truly integrative care. We would not consider leaving out teaching about alcohol and its impact on the body. For a large percentage of the population, cannabis is used recreationally in a similar manner to alcohol.

Once there is some level of buy-in about including medical cannabis in the curriculum, we can begin to discover and discuss how nursing faculty can include medical cannabis.

Topics For All Levels: Addressing Align 6 Essentials and More

The following section reviews the key National Council of State Boards of Nursing (2018) defined essentials and expands on them to include the American Nurses Association (ANA) and the American Cannabis Nurses Association (ACNA) (2024) scope and standards elements that may be relevant to supporting the achievement of competency in medical cannabis. This section will further delineate the expansion of competencies at the graduate level and resources provided with each topic. Additionally, the educator should consider how learners can apply the *Cannabis nursing standards of practice* (American Nurses Association and American Cannabis Nurses Association, 2024) as the nurses consider the tone and health of the patient's ECS, and the standards of cannabis nursing practice, including standard I assessment, standard II diagnosis, standard III outcomes identification, standard IV planning, standard V implementation, and standard VI evaluation.

The Human Endocannabinoid System (ECS)

> *"The nurse shall have an understanding of the endocannabinoid system, cannabinoid receptors, cannabinoids, and the interactions between them"* (National Council of State Boards of Nursing, 2018, p. S20).

The ECS is a master regulatory system in the body that supports homeostasis, prevents disease, and modulates aging. The ECS comprises endocannabinoids, endocannabinoid receptors embedded in cellular membranes throughout the body, and enzymes that synthesize and degrade endocannabinoids (Foster et al., 2021). The two principal endocannabinoids produced by the body are anandamide (*N*-arachidonoylethanolamine) and 2-arachidonoylglycerol (2-AG), which interact with the cellular receptors CB1 and CB2. These chemicals are synthesized and degraded through multiple complex pathways (Foster et al., 2021).

Cannabinoid science remains relatively young, with the identification of the first receptor, CB1, in 1988 by Howlett & Devane, and the discovery of anandamide as the first endocannabinoid in 1992 by Mechoulam, Devane, and Lühr-Hansen (Crocq, 2020). The ECS has two primary receptors: CB1, found primarily in the nervous system, and CB2, involved in inflammation and immunity. The ECS uses retrograde transmission, whereby anandamide and 2AG are released at the postsynaptic membrane and activate presynaptic receptors, thereby reducing neurotransmitter release at the postsynaptic cell (Foster et al., 2021; Crocq, 2020).

Unfortunately, ECS science is not generally included in courses such as anatomy, physiology, and pathophysiology, likely due to crowded curricula, lingering prohibition-era stigma, and its absence from licensing exams. The content for the levels of education includes the following:

Prelicensure

The nurse should have a working knowledge of the components of the ECS and how endocannabinoids and phytocannabinoids found in the cannabis plant (such as THC and CBD) work in the body on a systemic level (National Council of State Boards of Nursing, 2018). In addition to the historical context provided above, the content should include the main components of the ECS, the system's anatomy and physiology, and the implications of endocannabinoid deficiency. Holistic modalities upregulate the ECS, and this should be important information for learners to link how patients can upregulate the ECS through exercise, diet, massage, acupuncture, cold therapy, and mindfulness techniques (Clark, 2021a). Include this content in biology pre-requisite classes, such as anatomy and physiology. The ECS's functions can then be reviewed as appropriate during related content modules across the curriculum when population care is discussed, particularly related to populations who are likely to use medical cannabis (i.e., oncology care, end of life care, and neurological conditions such as seizures, Parkinson's disease, and multiple sclerosis).

APRN

The APRN curriculum may wish to deepen APRN knowledge and consider the broader picture of how endocannabinoids and phytocannabinoids interact with the ECS. APRNs in many states may also be writing recommendations for medical cannabis use, and they may require an expanded knowledge level. Additional content may include non-CB1/CB2 receptors, G protein-coupled receptors, and endocannabinoid-metabolizing compounds.

Evaluate Learning

Faculty can scale content to learners' levels. Tools may include quizzes on the ECS, discussion boards related to functioning, care, and upregulation of the ECS, written assignments or presentations about ECS involvement with a specific disease process or wellness/ health topic, ECS-related case studies using standards I-VI, with consideration of supporting the patient's ECS tone through upregulation of the system.

Resources: American Nurses Association and American Cannabis Nurses Association (2024, pp. 5, 7, 12; Standards I-VI), Clark (2018; 2021a), Crocq (2020), Foster et al. (2021), National Council of State Boards of Nursing (2018), Theisen (2021).

Pharmacokinetics/ Pharmacodynamics

"The nurse shall have an understanding of cannabis pharmacology and the research associated with the medical use of cannabis" (National Council of State Boards of Nursing, 2018, p. S20).

Pharmacokinetics and pharmacodynamics are likely one of the easiest aspects to include in a medical cannabis curriculum, as faculty can integrate this into a cannabinoid therapeutics category within a pharmacology class at both the prelicensure and APRN levels.

Prelicensure

The National Council of State Boards of Nursing (2018) stated that nurses need to be familiar with the body of evidence of medical cannabis effectiveness, which is constantly shifting. Specifics to be covered include: adverse effects of cannabis, populations at risk for adverse effects, cannabis substance use disorder, drug-to-drug interactions, contraindications, dependence versus tolerance and withdrawal, and analysis of medical cannabis Certificates of Analysis (COA). Learners should also be introduced to the benefits of whole plant medicine and the entourage effect, coaching around the self-titration process (starting low, going slow, and staying low with THC dosing), the major cannabinoids, the effect of terpenes and flavonoids, and analyzing COAs which delineate the cannabinoid, terpene, and contaminants like heavy metals, mold, and fungus in cannabinoid products (Parmelee et al., 2021). Routes of administration should include information on variability across type I, II, and III chemovars, as well as the onset of effects by route: vaporization, smoking, oral, sublingual, dermal, ophthalmic, and rectal (Parmelee et al.). Coaching and educating techniques should be used by faculty when working with patients to use the least amount of cannabis to the greatest effectiveness as they learn to self-titrate cannabinoids (Parmelee et al.). Additionally, learners should be aware of workplace drug testing and related state and federal policies (Clark, 2021b; American Nurses Association and American Cannabis Nurses Association, 2024).

APRN

In addition to the material above, the APRN may be interested in cannabinoid therapeutic science, analyzing research on cannabis's effectiveness in specific populations, and how they may become a cannabis medicine recommender in their state for medical cannabis patients (this generally requires some education and a DEA number). The curriculum can address dosing and self-titration processes, with a focus on high-quality research on cannabinoid therapeutics and their effects.

Evaluate Learning

Quiz questions, designing an educational or coaching model about self-titration, presentations on self-titration, analyzing COAs, and/or interviewing patients, providers, and dispensary workers on experiences with either receiving or offering information around self-titration.

Resources: American Nurses Association and American Cannabis Nurses Association (2024, p. 15, 23, 25, 31), Clark (2021a, 2021b), Parmelee et al. (2021), Dr. Dustin Sulak's dosage programs: https://healer.com/dosage-programs/

Evaluating the Evidence

Learners often struggle with evaluating the evidence, and there are thousands and thousands of articles about medical cannabis, in addition to the media often offering short sound bites of information about medical cannabis that may be erroneous. Teaching learners how to evaluate the evidence aligns with both NSBCN (2018) essential 5 ("The nurse shall be able to identify the safety considerations for patient use of cannabis" [p. S20]) and essential 4 ("The nurse shall have an understanding of cannabis pharmacology and the research associated with the medical use of cannabis" [p. S20]).

Prelicensure and Graduate

The NCSBN states that the best research around medical cannabis comes from randomized controlled trials (RCTs). At the time of this writing, cannabis, remaining a Schedule I drug in the US with a potential forthcoming rescheduling to State Schedule III, has made RCTs extremely difficult to complete. Additionally, this fails to recognize other credible sources for cannabis science research and evidence, including qualitative studies related to medical cannabis users' experience, surveys of cannabis users and providers, epidemiological studies, and so on. Regardless, learners need to be able to interpret the evidence, and a structured approach is essential.

Clark (2021a, p. 297-298) stated that a structured approach, such as the following, can be used to guide students in their efforts to analyze research:

- Does the title accurately describe the article?
- Is the abstract representative of the content and findings in the article?
- Does the opening include a clear purpose statement?
- Is there a theoretical framework, and is it used to describe the findings?
- Is the literature review comprehensive and relevant?
- Does the methods section provide an approach that aligns with answering the research question?
- Is the analytical approach aligned with the research design?
- Are the results presented clearly, and do the tables and figures align with them?
- What is the level and quality of the evidence?

Evaluate Learning

Related assignments may include analyzing and presenting one or more articles, and/or synthesizing evidence on a specific disease or health/wellness issue, and on cannabinoid therapeutics.

Resources: Clark (2021a, p. 299-306); Clark (2019); American Nurses Association and American Cannabis Nurses Association (2024, p. 83-84) standards of professional practice # 14.

Legal, Ethical, and Advocacy Concerns

The National Council of State Boards of Nursing (2018) principle 1, "The nurse shall have a working knowledge of the current state of legalization of medical and recreational cannabis use" (p. S19), and principle 2, "The nurse shall have a working knowledge of the jurisdiction's MMP" (p. S19), require that learners understand the legal issues with cannabis, which is particularly important as we leave the prohibition era and make our way into an era of cannabis regulation; laws and regulations will evolve, and the nurse is obligated to ensure that patients understand any legal ramifications related to their cannabis use. Nurses, as well, must be educated regarding any ramifications to their nursing practice or licensure related to education provided to patients and/or their own personal use of cannabis.

Because cannabis laws vary by state, faculty must train nursing students to locate information on state and federal laws, analyze state laws from patients' and providers' perspectives, and consider their role as advocates. While there are global issues related to this topic, the nurse must first understand what is happening in the US before addressing global issues and implications. Providing students with tools to access information and analyze laws and proposed legislation is key. A basic overview of the history of prohibition, how cannabis became a Schedule I drug, and recent efforts to reclassify cannabis as a Schedule III drug should be included, along with discussions about states' rights versus federal government oversight and the implications for patients, providers, and legislators. This content provides an excellent opportunity to discuss social justice issues and institutional racism as related to incarceration rates of people of color (Clark, 2021b).

Ethical considerations include caring and social justice concerns, and the principles of autonomy, beneficence, nonmaleficence, justice, and integrity can be applied in the nurse's work with cannabis patients and in advocacy efforts (American Nurses Association and American Cannabis Nurses Association, 2024; Clark, 2021b). Cannabis nurses strive to create a caring-healing presence with patients, and they recognize that communities of color suffer greater health inequality and ramifications from both prohibition and regulation.

Prelicensure

Provide students with resources to locate their state medical cannabis laws, state representatives, and policy analysis frameworks. Consideration of social justice issues and the ethical implications of prohibition and regulatory efforts is warranted. Statistical considerations of how drug regulation policies and prohibition have adversely impacted communities of color.

APRN

Additional considerations for the APRN include advanced ethical analysis, including application of specific ethical concepts and considerations, state and nationwide expertise and leadership, caring ethics, and social justice considerations (American Nurses Association and American Cannabis Nurses Association, 2024)

Evaluate Learning

Assignments may include interviewing cannabis policy leaders, legislators, and/or nurses who have acted as cannabis advocates. Students may develop educational modules and presentations on cannabis policy to inform the public, healthcare providers, and lawmakers about policy implications. A group discussion on how best to support system-level change and work with lawmakers may be enlightening. Case studies on the ethical obligations of the cannabis care nurse that explore social justice issues, social determinants of health (SDOH), and the impact of cannabis prohibition may help deepen understanding of these larger issues.

Resources: American Nurses Association and American Cannabis Nurses Association (2024, p. 13-14, 71-75, 80-82, 87) standards of professional practice # 7 ethics, # 8 advocacy, #12 leadership. Bryan, (2024); Clark (2021b); Last Prisoner Project: https://www.lastprisonerproject.org/

Safety/ Adverse Effects

When it comes to the consideration of safety and avoiding adverse effects of cannabis, the nurse has multiple considerations. The nurse shall "Be able to identify safety concerns for patient use of cannabis" (National Council of State Boards of Nursing, 2018, p. S20), and standard V Implementation includes the competency that the nurse monitors cannabis consumers for side effects, adverse effects, and cannabis use disorder (American Nurses Association and American Cannabis Nurses Association, 2024, p. 64). The nurse also ensures that the medical cannabis patient explores safety concerns and the self-titration process by providing education and using techniques such as motivational interviewing (Clark, 2021a).

Medical cannabis patients must be coached to use the least amount of THC to palliate symptoms to avoid issues of increasing tolerance and/or adverse effects (Parmelee et al., 2021). Additionally, they should know their state laws, how to read cannabis COAs, how to choose safe, tested cannabinoid products, and how to track their cannabis use in a cannabis diary (Clark, 2021a). Upregulation of the ECS also helps to ensure that folks can use the least amount of cannabis for the greatest benefit. Patients must know how to safely store cannabinoid medicines out of reach or accessibility of pets, children, and/or from those who may divert the medicines (Parmelee et al, 2021).

Prelicensure

Teach the adverse effects of THC, the self-titration process, and the concept of start low, go slow, and stay low with THC dosing. Faculty must address drug-drug interactions and how to look these up on drugs.com should be included. Assessing the patient's knowledge of self-titration and their ability to use and store the medication safely can be practiced. Educational approaches include educating patients about keeping a cannabis diary, how to access cannabis medicine in their state from trusted sources, and avoiding adverse events. Learners should practice using motivational interviewing to assess a patient's goals and set priorities. Follow-up and evaluation should be addressed to ensure patients are not experiencing adverse events and are aware of how to use the medication safely and effectively. Students should be familiar with cannabis as a harm reduction tool, cannabis use disorder, and cannabis hyperemesis syndrome.

APRN

In addition to the information, the APRN learner needs to take a deeper dive into the self-titration process, drug-drug interactions, metabolic pathways, types and quality of products, and full health/medical assessment parameters.

Evaluate Learning

Assignments may include case studies related to adverse events, simulations focused on educating patients, the public, and providers about adverse events and/or drug-drug interactions, and quizzes on drug-drug interactions.

Resources: ANA & ACNA (2024, p. 20, 28-30), Clark (2021a), Parmelee et al. (2021), Theisen (2021).

Holism: Upregulation of the ECS

While the National Council of State Boards of Nursing (2018) recommendations did not focus directly on coaching patients to upregulate the ECS, it is important to note that for patients to use the least amount of THC and avoid adverse effects, they must also focus on the well-being of the ECS (Clark, 2021a). Given that diet, exercise, sleep, and holistic modalities can affect the ECS, we are ethically obligated (autonomy and beneficence) to support patients in optimizing ECS function through holistic modalities (ANA & ACNA, 2024; Clark, 2021a).

We have data to show that exercise is important for supporting the health of the ECS; dietary components such as Omega 3 and 6 fatty acid balance and inclusion of flavonoids support ECS regulation as does losing weight for obese people; sleep and stress reduction help the ECS function; exercise, singing, meditation, yoga, massage, acupuncture, and osteopathy upregulate the ECS (Clark, 2021a).

Prelicensure

At this level, faculty must support nursing students in learning about motivational interviewing and the tenets of coaching. Reviewing with patients the reasons for making lifestyle changes, exploring the benefits and challenges, and encouraging and coaching them toward success are key. Education can focus on why lifestyle changes are key to using cannabis effectively and how the ECS functions optimally given the right lifestyle choices. The focus should be on partnering with the patient and supporting them in progressing toward their health-related goals.

APRN

The APRN can educate and coach medical cannabis patients toward steps to regulate the ECS. In addition, they may consider the medication and drug-drug interactions more closely, where folks may end up using less of all medications from upregulating the ECS. Additionally, there may be times when upregulating the ECS, changing lifestyles, and the use of other herbs or medications may be preferable to cannabis use.

Evaluate Learning

Presentations on educating patients or providers on how to upregulate the ECS. Literature reviews of specific illnesses and research around how holistic interventions may lead to better healthcare outcomes, self-care experiences, and exploring the upregulation of their own ECS.

Resources: ANA & ACNA (2024, p. 4, 12, 39), Clark (2021a), Dr. Dustin Sulak's wellness approaches: https://healer.com/wellness/

Sacred Medicine: Plant Entheogens

Cannabis in our Westernized culture has become a "recreational" drug and is moving toward a regulation-like alcohol approach for adult use, not related to medical care. However, with an intent toward spiritual growth and a mindfulness approach, people can use cannabis to facilitate spiritual healing (Clark, 2021a), which is in direct contrast to the prohibition era demonization of cannabis as a profane Other, with much of this prohibition era racism mindset related to immigration of Others, including those from African, Asian, and South American cultures, from which the prohibition era 'Reefer Madness' idea emerged, and notions that cannabis leads to mental illness, criminal acts, and immorality have created a lasting stigma related to the plant (Partridge, 2024).

Cannabis is an entheogen as it has the potential to create a mind-manifesting experience and to generate the divine within, and, as such, facilitates non-ordinary experiences (Clark, 2021a). Cannabis use can lead to a deep state of relaxation, which can help the cannabis user to enter into a sense of inner stillness, awareness, and peace, and to experience an awakening to the nature of love (Gray, 2016). Partridge (2024, p. 3) described the spiritual experience of cannabis use as, "It is a state of immersive intoxication, trance, and ecstasy, during which the boundary between the self and the observed everyday objects breaks down". Cannabis has a historical role in many religious traditions, including Hinduism, Taoism, Sikhism, Buddhism, Zoroastrianism, and Judaism (Clark, 2021a).

Although nursing has a long history of providing spiritual care, contemporary nursing curricula often overlook this aspect of practice, making it challenging to incorporate the plant's spiritual nature into the curriculum. However, it may also introduce nursing students to the potential for nurses to enhance their patients' healing journeys. Clark (2021a) described the importance of cannabis care nurses guiding patients toward spiritual use of the cannabis plant by considering the set (patients' mindset and past experiences), setting (environment and conditions, setting an intention for healing), and ritual (using potentially sacred objects and processes during the process of ingesting cannabis).

Prelicensure

Assessing the patient's need for spiritual growth and healing, as well as the patient's religious background, can be helpful, as can educating the patient about the plant's entheogenic properties and the importance of spiritual healing (Clark, 2021a).

APRN

The APRN likely has more experience than prelicensure nurses, so creating discussion forums on patients' spiritual needs and the inclusion of plant entheogens could support deeper learning in this area. APRNs may also be interested in other plant entheogens, and cannabis can pave the way for those explorations.

Evaluating Learning

To evaluate learning, faculty may use simulations involving the spiritual needs of medical cannabis patients, case studies requiring spiritual assessments and nursing interventions, quiz questions, and presentations on the historical use of medical cannabis in religious rituals.

Resources: Clark (2021a), Gray (2016), and Patridge (2024).

The Nursing Process, Motivational Interviewing, and Coaching

Students can apply the nursing process to interactions with medical cannabis patients, and cannabis care nurses work primarily to educate and coach patients toward successful use of cannabinoid therapeutics while keeping THC doses low, upregulating the ECS, and avoiding the adverse effects of cannabinoids. The cannabis care nurse can select a guiding nursing theory; for example, Watson's Human Caring Theory aligns with cannabis care nursing (Clark, 2021a).

The following table, based on Clark (2021a) and ANA & ACNA (2024), outlines how the nurse working with a medical cannabis patient uses the nursing process.

Table 1. Using the nursing process and Cannabis nursing: Scope and standards to guide cannabis care practice

Assessment	Objective: medical history, pertinent diagnoses, labs, test results, vital signs, current medications and treatment regimes, lifestyle, religious/spiritual needs and concerns
	Subjective: patient's knowledge about medical cannabis, history of medical or recreational cannabis use, cannabis law knowledge, healing and palliative goals, support system, financial capacity to pay for cannabis, knowledge about: safety, adverse effects, drug-drug interactions, and holistic modalities to upregulate the ECS. Applies Standard I approaches from *Cannabis nursing: Scope and standards of practice.* Motivational interviewing techniques are used to help the patient set goals during the assessment phase.
Diagnoses	Derives diagnoses from assessment data and applies Standard II approaches from *Cannabis nursing: Scope and standards of practice.* Any number of the over 240 NANDA diagnoses may be appropriate including activity intolerance, anxiety, comfort impaired, deficient knowledge, disturbed energy field, dry mouth (risk for), falls (risk for), fatigue/ activity intolerance, fear, health literacy (readiness for enhanced), imbalanced nutrition (more or less than body requirements), impaired resilience, ineffective coping, ineffective role performance, insomnia, moral distress, pain (acute), pain (chronic), nausea, nutrition (readiness for enhanced), risk for injury, self care (readiness for enhanced), sleep deprivation, spiritual distress, spiritual well-being (readiness for enhanced), stress overload.
Planning and Outcomes	Nurses work alongside patients to establish goals using motivational interviewing and coaching techniques. Areas that may be addressed include: medical recommendation processes, use of holistic modalities, ECS/ how cannabis works in the body, accessing evidence around cannabis effectiveness for patients' health concerns, ingestion methods, cannabis chemovars and purchasing products, reading the certificate of analysis, self-titration approaches, adverse effects, cannabis diary, and cannabis as a spiritual tool. Applies Standard III and Standard IV approaches from *Cannabis nursing: Scope and standards of practice*
Interventions and Implementation	The primary role of the cannabis care nurse is to coach the patient toward reaching their goals. The nurse partners with patients; the patient is their own expert; the nurse empowers and motivates. Motivational interviewing techniques are used to empower patients and to review goals, successes, and challenges. The cannabis care nurse partners with the patient's family and significant others to ensure the plan of care is implemented safely and effectively. Provides evidence-based education for patients and families. Considers coordination of care, health teaching, and health promotion efforts to support the patient's ECS health. Supports the self-titration process and use of a cannabis diary. Educates the patients about local cannabis resources and supports them on their journey toward discovering what cannabinoid therapeutics may be used. Applies Standard V approaches from *Cannabis nursing: Scope and standards of practice*
Evaluation	This process is completed alongside the patient. Has the plan of care been effective, and is it being shared with the interdisciplinary team? Is the patient experiencing any adverse effects, and are they able to use cannabinoids safely and effectively? Can the patients afford the cannabinoid therapeutics? Is the patient using modalities to upregulate the ECS? The cannabis diary is reviewed. The nurse reviews goal attainment and determines whether the nursing diagnoses were resolved. Applies Standard VI approaches from *Cannabis nursing: Scope and standards of practice*

Prelicensure

Motivational interviewing (MI) is a skill used in the cannabis coaching process. MI includes expressing empathy through reflective listening, highlighting discrepancies between a patient's goals/ values and current behaviors, avoiding confrontation or arguments, rolling with resistance, supporting self-efficacy, and fostering optimism (Clark, 2021a). The OARS technique includes asking **o**pen-ended questions, using affirmations to enhance positivity, reflecting to the patient what the nurse had heard, and summarizing the patient's thoughts, concerns, and goals.

APRN

The APRN can learn the OARS technique and order specific diagnostic tests as part of their assessment practice. Additionally, the APRN must recognize that a qualifying condition does not guarantee a medical cannabis recommendation. Instead, the APRN must base the recommendation on the patient's goals and individual, specific factors, such as drug-drug interactions and safety concerns.

Evaluate Learning

Students work in triads or participate in simulations to practice MI using the OARS technique to support the nursing process. APRNs may have more in-depth case scenarios and simulations relevant to their role.

Resources: Clark (2021a), ANA & ACNA (2024).

FUTURE RESEARCH

The biggest challenge of taking a full integration approach is that many, if not all, faculty members will need to educate themselves in this area. Given that 25% of people use cannabis regularly, this is a topic that should not be up for discussion. However, rather than solving the problem, the focus is on how this education will be delivered, whether through full or minimal integration. Faculty can evaluate the outcomes from the two approaches to determine which is more effective.

Full Integration

A complete integration of medical cannabis into nursing education is the ideal delivery approach, in which medical cannabis content is addressed early and threaded throughout the curriculum. Biology faculty can incorporate the endocannabinoid system into curricula in anatomy and physiology, pharmacodynamics, and pharmacokinetics. They can also integrate endocannabinoid deficiency syndrome into pathophysiology content and cover the scope and standards of cannabis nursing within courses on pain management, mental health, neurology, oncology, advocacy, ethics, and legal concerns. Clinical courses provide an opportunity for learners to assess for cannabis use in ways that avoid stigma or indications of judgment and provide education around safe and effective use of cannabis. Clinical assignments can focus on the evidence for cannabis's effectiveness given a specific health or illness issue. Educators can include medical cannabis care in simulation exercises. Leadership classes can discuss the issues of legality, ethics, and advocacy. The curriculum can revisit this topic, introducing and reinforcing it while faculty verify student learning multiple times.

Below is a typical 4-year BSN sample curriculum plan with medical cannabis content fully integrated.

Table 2. Typical 4-year BSN curriculum structure, including medical cannabis content

Year	Focus Area	Courses	Medical Cannabis Content
Freshman Year	General Education & Prerequisites	English Composition I & II	
		Anatomy & Physiology I (with lab)	Introduce ECS
		Anatomy & Physiology II (with lab)	Reinforce ECS content
		Chemistry	
		Psychology or Sociology	Cannabis and mental health issues and cannabinoid use Historical and religious or spiritual content related to cannabis use across cultures
Sophomore Year	Foundational Nursing & Health Sciences	Microbiology	
		Nutrition	Define how diet and supplements upregulate the ECS.
		Introduction to Professional Nursing	Begin discussions about ethics and advocacy as part of the role of the nurse
		Health Assessment (Theory & Lab)	How to assess for medical or adult use cannabis in a way that is not stigmatizing
		Pathophysiology	Include information on how ECS deficiency leads to illness and health issues
Junior Year	Core Nursing Specialties & Clinical Rotations	Pharmacology	Cannabinoid therapeutics, adverse effects, self-titration process of cannabis products, drug-drug interactions, populations known to use cannabis (ie, oncology, geriatrics, multiple sclerosis, Parkinson's disease)
		Adult Health / Medical-Surgical Nursing	Opportunities to assess for cannabis use in clinical settings and simulation
		Parent-Child Nursing / Maternal-Newborn	Opportunities to assess for cannabis use in clinical settings and simulation
		Pediatric Nursing	Consider pediatric medical use and adolescent potential harm vs harm reduction.
		Geriatric Nursing	Special precautions for the geriatric population

continued on following page

Table 2. Continued

Year	Focus Area	Courses	Medical Cannabis Content
Senior Year	Advanced Practice & Leadership	Population / Community Health Nursing	Cannabis use in the community and public health considerations, such as education and policy development, and social justice issues.
		Nursing Research	Generation of new knowledge and analysis of the evidence.
		Leadership & Management in Healthcare	Opportunities for advocacy.
		Critical Care Nursing	
		Senior Capstone / Preceptorship	Consider leadership and advocacy issues, including social justice concerns.

Table 3. Typical 3-year DNP/FNP curriculum structure, including medical cannabis content

Year	Focus Area	Courses	Notes
Year 1	Foundations & Core Advanced Nursing	Advanced Pathophysiology	Define how ECS deficiency impacts health and disease potential
		Advanced Pharmacology (Pharmacology in Health Management)	Drug-drug interactions, dosing, and self-titration of cannabinoids, adverse effects, and the medical cannabis recommendation process
		Advanced Health Assessment & Diagnostic Reasoning	Assessing for cannabis use and its impact on tests and patient health outcomes
		Theoretical Foundations of Nursing	How can theory guide the cannabis care nurse?
		Evidence-Based Practice and Research	Analyzing medical cannabis research using a structured approach
		Biostatistics	
Year 2	FNP Specialty & Clinical Management	Primary Care I: Health Promotion & Disease Prevention	Coaching and motivational interviewing concepts
		Primary Care I Practicum (Clinical hours)	Applied coaching and motivational interviewing concepts
		Primary Care II: Management of Chronic Health Problems	
		Primary Care II Practicum (Clinical hours)	Applied coaching and motivational interviewing concepts

continued on following page

Table 3. Continued

Year	Focus Area	Courses	Notes
		Pharmacology for Advanced Practice Nurses	Cannabinoid therapeutics, dosing, and self-titration processes
		Health Policy and Population Health	Current controversies in medical cannabis policy: state vs federal rights, social justice issues, social determinants of health, and cannabis
Year 3	DNP Project & Residency	DNP Project Planning & Implementation	
		Primary Care III: Acute & Complex Care Management	
		Primary Care III Practicum (Clinical hours)	Applied coaching and motivational interviewing concepts
		DNP Residency / Clinical Rotation	
		Leadership in Advanced Nursing Roles	Advocacy around medical cannabis policy, SDOH, and social justice issues.
		Evaluation of Outcomes & Quality Improvement	Supporting patients to use self-titration and tools such as the cannabis diary

Partial Integration

A partial integration approach may prove effective in increasing nursing students' knowledge, attitudes, and skills around medical cannabis. At the time of this writing, some of my colleagues and I are gathering data around devoting one 2-hour class period to discussing the 6 essential areas of knowledge in an anatomy and physiology pre-licensure course and a graduate-level pharmacology course. Using the Clark & Parmelee (2022) *Medical cannabis knowledge, attitudes and skills* (KAS) survey, the initial data have demonstrated that in a prelicensure nursing anatomy and physiology class, students enhanced their KAS related to medical cannabis after the 2-hour session that covered the National Council of State Boards of Nursing (2018) six essential areas of medical cannabis care (Cadieux et al., 2025).

Suggestions for partial or minimal integration include providing the above content in anatomy and physiology (the endocannabinoid system), pharmacology (including cannabinoid therapeutics as a drug class, ethics of supporting patient choice, review of legal issues), the nursing process as applied to working with medical cannabis patients, and providing clinical opportunities to assess patients for cannabis use and educate them on safe and effective use. Faculty can use this approach in nearly every clinical class in which patients with life-threatening illnesses or high palliative needs will be present. Faculty can convey this information in a short period of time, over several hours, and then students can apply it in the clinical setting. There is a need for more evidence on the effectiveness of this approach.

In a pilot study with 17 DNP/CRNA students, King et al. (2023) sought to determine whether addressing the National Council of State Boards of Nursing (2018) essentials for educating APRN students about medical cannabis resulted in significantly higher post-cannabis survey scores than pre-survey scores after a single synchronous class. It is possible to impart medical cannabis care knowledge in a singular, focused, and effective manner.

In Healthcare Settings

There is little research about supporting practicing nurses' knowledge, attitudes, and skills regarding medical cannabis in workplace settings. However, focusing on changing how medical cannabis use is assessed and charted could be one practical approach to helping to end the stigma around cannabis use. Additionally, specific nursing specialty populations, such as those working in oncology, chronic pain, and neurological settings, may be receptive to continuing education offerings on the topic. I have worked with several small hospitals on individual medical cannabis educational offerings, which they received well. The challenge is finding local experts who can provide such offerings and follow up with nurses as needed.

Issues, Controversies, Problems

Due to the lingering stigma associated with the prohibition era of cannabis, cannabis remains a misunderstood and often taboo topic. Historically, some schools will refuse to include cannabis as a legitimate topic or offer meaningful content as they erroneously believe that discussing cannabis care could impact their federal funding streams. Though National Council of State Boards of Nursing (2018) made the call to include medical cannabis essentials in all levels of nursing education, they have failed to include NCELX content on the topic and in test plans, even though the public consumes cannabis. We may also consider how accrediting bodies and groups, such as QSEN and the American Association of Colleges of Nursing, could help steer curricula toward the meaningful inclusion of medical cannabis care.

Cannabis remains a federal Schedule I drug in the US despite a recent 2025 executive order to move cannabis to a State Schedule III, which could pave the way toward more quality research about cannabis's effectiveness. Even with a Schedule III designation, there is little to no defined funding stream for medical cannabis research. This move also creates uncertainty for medical cannabis patients regarding access and future federal regulations. It does not change the federal illegality of cannabis.

Challenges and Barriers

Other barriers and challenges include the lack of faculty education regarding the ECS and cannabinoid therapeutics, overloaded curricula, and the failure of nursing academia to recognize its ethical obligation to ensure patients can make informed autonomous decisions about medical cannabis care and to be then guided on its safe and effective use (Clark, 2021a). Disregarding the prevalence of cannabis use and the role of the nurse puts a large percentage of the population in harm's way. It potentially also denies patients who could benefit from cannabinoid therapeutics the opportunity to use these medicines effectively.

CONCLUSION

This chapter has examined the essentials of medical cannabis knowledge, attitudes, and skill development across nursing education levels. When considering how and when to add this content to an existing nursing curriculum, it is important to secure faculty buy-in and carefully plan its integration. Administration that remains rigidly connected to prohibition-era thinking, along with stigma, challenges nursing faculty and hinders their ability to include cannabis content in schools. It's important that we continue to research the challenges and barriers to including cannabis science in nursing curricula, just as we continue to research outcomes from curricula that integrate cannabis science.

As cannabis enters an era of post-prohibition regulation, and the development of new evidence-based knowledge and cannabinoid therapeutics emerges, the specialty of cannabis care nursing will also continue to evolve. Patients who are interested in palliating symptoms with whole plant cannabis, in using the medicine for spiritual evolution, and learning to upregulate the ECS will remain at the forefront of the cannabis care nurse's concern. All schools of nursing must recognize that nurses can incorporate cannabis care into all areas of specialty care, from birth to the end of life. The ANA & ACNA (2024) officially recognized cannabis nursing as a subspecialty, making the omission of this content from nursing curricula equivalent to omitting oncology, cardiology, or other specialized areas. This requirement is crucial because patients and the public continue to use cannabis for symptom management, regardless of whether healthcare providers recognize it or are adequately educated to ensure they can coach and educate patients to safe and effective use of cannabis.

ACKNOWLEDGMENT

This research received no specific grant from any funding agency in the public, commercial, or not-for-profit sectors.

REFERENCES

American Nurses Association and American Cannabis Nurses Association. (2024). *Cannabis nursing: Scope and standards of practice* (1st ed.). American Nurses Association.

Ananth, P., Ma, C., Al-Sayegh, H., Kroon, L., Klein, V., Wharton, C., Hallez, E., Braun, I., Michelson, K., Rosenberg, A. R., London, W., & Wolfe, J. (2018). Provider perspectives on use of medical marijuana in children with cancer. *Pediatrics, 141*(1), e20170559. DOI: 10.1542/peds.2017-0559 PMID: 29233937

Balneaves, L. B., & Alraja, A. A. (2019). "Guarding their practice": A descriptive study of Canadian nursing policies and education related to medical cannabis. *BMC Nursing, 18*(1), 1–10. DOI: 10.1186/s12912-019-0390-7 PMID: 31827392

Balneaves, L. G., Alraja, A., Ziemianski, D., McCuaig, F., & Ware, M. (2018). A national needs assessment of Canadian nurse practitioners regarding cannabis for therapeutic purposes. *Cannabis and Cannabinoid Research, 3*(1), 66–73. DOI: 10.1089/can.2018.0002 PMID: 29588917

Bryan, K. (2024). *Cannabis overview*. National Conference of State Legislators. https://www.ncsl.org/civil-and-criminal-justice/cannabis-overview

Cadieux, C. S., Garrett, J., & Ewen, H. (2025). Unpublished pilot study data: Nursing students' medical cannabis knowledge, attitudes, and skills (unpublished, raw data). Binghamton University, Decker College of Nursing and Health Sciences.

Carlini, B. H., Garrett, S. B., & Carter, G. T. (2017). Medicinal cannabis: A survey among health care providers in Washington State. *The American Journal of Hospice & Palliative Care, 34*(1), 85–91. DOI: 10.1177/1049909115604669 PMID: 26377551

Clark, C.S. (2018). Medical cannabis: The oncology nurse's role in patient education about the effects of marijuana on cancer palliation. *Clinical Journal of Oncology Nursing*, 22(1), E-1E-6. https://doi.org/. CJON.E1-E6DOI: 10.1188/18

Clark, C. S. (2019). High-potency cannabis and incident psychosis: Correcting the causal assumption. *The Lancet. Psychiatry, 6*(6), e14. DOI: 10.1016/S2215-0366(19)30178-6 PMID: 31122483

Clark, C. S. (2021a). The nurse's role: Providing cannabis care. In Clark, C. S. (Ed.), *Cannabis: A handbook for nurses* (pp. 268–312). Wolters Kluwer.

Clark, C. S. (2021b). Legal, ethical, and advocacy concerns. In Clark, C. S. (Ed.), *Cannabis: A handbook for nurses* (pp. 363–401). Wolters Kluwer.

Costantino, R. C., Felten, N., Todd, M., Maxwell, T., & McPherson, M. L. (2019). A survey of hospice professionals regarding medical cannabis practices. *Journal of Palliative Medicine, 22*(10), 1208–1212. DOI: 10.1089/jpm.2018.0535 PMID: 31094609

Crocq, M. A. (2020). History of cannabis and the endocannabinoid system. *Dialogues in Clinical Neuroscience, 22*(3), 223–228. DOI: 10.31887/DCNS.2020.22.3/mcrocq PMID: 33162765

Foster, K. T., Arterberry, B. J., Zucker, R. A., & Hicks, B. M. (2021). Differences in child and adult biopsychosocial characteristics associated with regular cannabis use in individuals with and without cannabis use disorder. *Drug and Alcohol Dependence, 226*, 108887. DOI: 10.1016/j.drugalcdep.2021.108887 PMID: 34216859

Free, T., Grossoehme, D. H., Richner, G., Brown, M. F., & Friebert, S. (2025). Characterizing the population of a medical cannabis clinic in a pediatric hospital. *Journal of Palliative Medicine, 28*(8), 1020–1028. DOI: 10.1089/jpm.2024.0533 PMID: 40180570

Government of Canada. (2021, December 15). Cannabis Act (S.C. 2018, c. 16). https://laws-lois.justice.gc.ca/PDF/C-24.5.pdf

Gray, S. (2016). *Cannabis spirituality: An explorer's guide to an ancient plant spirit*. Park Street Press.

Kaplan, L., Klein, T., Wilson, M., & Graves, J. (2020). Knowledge, practices, and attitudes of Washington State health care professionals regarding medical cannabis. *Cannabis and Cannabinoid Research, 5*(2), 172–182. DOI: 10.1089/can.2019.0051 PMID: 32656349

King, D. D., DeCarlo, M., Mylott, L., & Yarossi, M. (2023). Cannabis knowledge gaps in nursing education: Pilot testing cannabis curriculum. *Teaching and Learning in Nursing, 18*(4), 474–479. DOI: 10.1016/j.teln.2023.06.012

McLennan, A., Kerba, M., Subnis, U., Campbell, T., & Carlson, L. E. (2020). Health care provider preferences for, and barriers to, cannabis use in cancer care. *Current Oncology (Toronto, Ont.), 27*(2), e199–e205. DOI: 10.3747/co.27.5615 PMID: 32489269

Melnikov, S., Aboav, A., Shalom, E., Phriedman, S., & Khalaila, K. (2021). The effect of attitudes, subjective norms, and stigma on healthcare providers' intention to recommend medicinal cannabis to patients. *International Journal of Nursing Practice, 27*(1), 1–10. DOI: 10.1111/ijn.12836 PMID: 32237017

Merlin, J. S., Althouse, A., Feldman, R., Arnsten, J. H., Bulls, H. W., Liebschutz, J. M., Nugent, S. M., Orris, S. R., Rohac, R., Starrels, J. L., Morasco, B. J., & Kansagara, D. (2021). Analysis of state cannabis laws and dispensary staff recommendations to adults purchasing medical cannabis. *JAMA Network Open, 4*(9), e2124511. DOI: 10.1001/jamanetworkopen.2021.24511 PMID: 34524435

Narouze, S., Hakim, S. M., Kohan, L., Adams, D., & Souza, D. (2020). Medical cannabis attitudes and beliefs among pain physicians. *Regional Anesthesia and Pain Medicine, 45*(11), 917–919. DOI: 10.1136/rapm-2020-101658 PMID: 32759172

National Academies of Science, Engineering, and Medicine. (2017). *The health effects of cannabis and cannabinoids: The current state of evidence and recommendations for research*. National Academies Press.

National Cancer Institute. (2025). *Cannabis and cannabinoids: Health professional version.* https://www.cancer.gov/about-cancer/treatment/cam/hp/cannabis-pdq

National Conference of State Legislators. (2025). *More* https://www.ncsl.org/health/state-medical-cannabis-laws

National Council of State Boards of Nursing. (2018). The NCSBN nursing guidelines for medical marijuana. *Journal of Nursing Regulation*, *9*(2), S2–S60.

Parmelee, R., & Clark, C. S. (2022). Nursing students' knowledge, skills, and attitudes regarding medicinal cannabis care. *Journal of Nursing Regulation*, *13*(3), 13–23. DOI: 10.1016/S2155-8256(22)00082-5

Parmelee, R., Clark, C. S., & Sommers, D. (2021). Cannabis pharmacology: From the whole plant to pharmaceutical applications. In Clark, C. S. (Ed.), *Cannabis: A handbook for nurses.* Wolters Kluwer.

Parmelee, R. A. (2025). *Nurse Educators' Experiences With Medical Cannabis Education* (Doctoral dissertation, Walden University).

Partridge, C. (2024). *Cannabis, sacred and profane.* Bloomsbury Academic. DOI: 10.5040/9781350116238

Pergam, S. A., Woodfield, M. C., Lee, C. M., Cheng, G. S., Baker, K. K., Marquis, S. R., & Fann, J. R. (2017). Cannabis use among patients at a comprehensive cancer center in a state with legalized medicinal and recreational use. *Cancer*, *123*(22), 4488–4497. DOI: 10.1002/cncr.30879 PMID: 28944449

Pew Center for Research. (2024). *Most Americans now live in a legal marijuana state – and most have at least one dispensary in their county.* https://www.pewresearch.org/short-reads/2024/02/29/most-americans-now-live-in-a-legal-marijuana-state-and-most-have-at-least-one-dispensary-in-their-county/

St. Pierre, M., Matthews, L., & Walsh, Z. (2020). Cannabis education needs assessment among Canadian physicians-in-training. *Complementary Therapies in Medicine, 49.* https://doi-org/DOI: 10.1016/j.ctim.2020.102328

Szaflarski, M., McGoldrick, P., Currens, L., Blodgett, D., Land, H., Szaflarski, J. P., & Segal, E. (2020). Attitudes and knowledge about cannabis and cannabis-based therapies among US neurologists, nurses, and pharmacists. *Epilepsy & Behavior*, *109*, 107102. Advance online publication. DOI: 10.1016/j.yebeh.2020.107102 PMID: 32442891

Theisen, E. (2021). Advanced practice nursing considerations. In Clark, C. S. (Ed.), *Cannabis: A handbook for nurses* (pp. 313–362). Wolters Kluwer.

Worster, B., Hajjar, E. R., & Handley, N. (2022). Cannabis use in patients with cancer: A clinical review. *JCO Oncology Practice*, *18*(11), 743–749. DOI: 10.1200/OP.22.00080 PMID: 35749680

Ziemianski, D., Capler, R., Tekanoff, R., Lacasse, A., Luconi, F., & Ware, M. A. (2015). Cannabis in medicine: A national educational needs assessment among Canadian physicians. *BMC Medical Education*, *15*(1), 52. DOI: 10.1186/s12909-015-0335-0 PMID: 25888752

KEY TERMS AND DEFINITIONS

Cannabis Care Nursing: Cannabis care nursing is a specialized nursing practice focused on the safe, ethical, and evidence-informed care of patients who use cannabis for therapeutic purposes. It involves patient assessment, education, coaching, monitoring of effects and interactions, and harm reduction strategies. The practice emphasizes patient-centered care, legal awareness, advocacy, and interdisciplinary collaboration.

Cannabis Nursing Scope and Standards: This 2024 publication from the American Nurses Association and the American Cannabis Nurses Association defines the roles, responsibilities, and professional expectations that guide nurses caring for patients using cannabis therapeutically. The book outlines the boundaries of nursing practice, including assessment, education, monitoring, documentation, and collaboration, while ensuring care is evidence-based, ethical, and compliant with legal and regulatory requirements. These standards promote patient safety, consistency of practice, and accountability within cannabis-related nursing care.

Endocannabinoid System: The endocannabinoid system (ECS) is a complex cell-signaling system in the human body that helps regulate balance and stability, known as homeostasis. It comprises endocannabinoids, cannabinoid receptors (primarily CB1 and CB2), and enzymes that synthesize and degrade these compounds. The ECS plays a role in regulating pain, mood, appetite, sleep, immune function, and stress responses.

Entheogen: An entheogen is a psychoactive substance, typically derived from plants or fungi, used in spiritual, religious, or ceremonial contexts to induce altered states of consciousness. These substances are traditionally employed to facilitate introspection, healing, or a sense of connection with the sacred. Examples include ayahuasca, peyote, psilocybin-containing mushrooms, and specific preparations of cannabis.

Motivational Interviewing: A collaborative, person-centered communication approach designed to strengthen an individual's motivation and commitment to change. It uses open-ended questions, reflective listening, and empathy to explore ambivalence and support self-directed behavior change.

National Council of State Boards of Nursing (NCSBN): A nonprofit organization that provides leadership and regulatory support for nursing licensure and practice in the United States and its territories. It develops and administers the NCLEX examinations that state boards of nursing use to license nurses. NCSBN also promotes public safety through research, policy development, and evidence-based regulatory standards.

Nurse Coaching: A holistic, patient-centered nursing practice that supports individuals in achieving health and wellness goals through partnership, education, and behavior change strategies. It emphasizes motivational interviewing, self-awareness, and empowerment to promote sustainable lifestyle changes. Nurse coaching integrates evidence-based practice with the patient's values, strengths, and readiness for change.

Pharmacodynamics: The study of how a drug affects the body and produces its therapeutic and adverse effects. It examines the mechanisms of action, receptor interactions, dose–response relationships, and drug potency. Pharmacodynamics helps clinicians understand how medications achieve desired outcomes and cause side effects.

Pharmacokinetics: The study of how a drug moves through the body over time. It includes the processes of absorption, distribution, metabolism, and excretion, which determine the onset, intensity, and duration of a drug's effects.

Chapter 13
Medical Cannabis Curriculum for Nursing Students:
An Evidence-Based, Ready-to-Teach Framework

Elisabeth A Mack
http://orcid.org/0009-0008-1418-6201
Holistic Caring, USA & The Green Nurse, USA

ABSTRACT

This chapter presents an evidence-informed, ready-to-implement curriculum for integrating medical cannabis education into undergraduate and graduate nursing programs. Grounded in the NCSBN's 2018 national guidelines and the 2024 ACNA/ANA Cannabis Nursing Scope & Standards of Practice, it translates essential competencies—legal literacy, endocannabinoid system physiology, cannabinoid pharmacology, dosing principles, product literacy, a whole-person assessment, and harm-reduction strategies—into an instructional model that aligns with contemporary nursing education frameworks. Despite widespread patient use, most graduates receive no formal preparation to counsel on cannabis use, assess safety risks, or evaluate drug–drug interactions. This chapter addresses that gap by providing modular content, case-based learning tools, and competency-based evaluation methods. The curriculum equips faculty to teach confidently, supports safe and nonjudgmental patient care, and provides a scalable foundation for all programs seeking to incorporate cannabis therapeutics into modern nursing practice.

INTRODUCTION

Why Cannabis Belongs In Nursing Education

Nurses have long served on the front lines of patient care, functioning as educators, advocates, and coordinators positioned closest to individuals managing chronic and complex conditions. As medical cannabis becomes increasingly integrated into symptom management across the United States, the need for structured cannabis education in nursing programs has become more urgent. Although 40 states permit medical cannabis and 64 million Americans report recent use (Statista, 2025), patients often struggle to navigate product types, dosing strategies, drug interactions, and safety considerations. Many turn to

DOI: 10.4018/979-8-3373-7287-7.ch013

dispensaries staffed by retail personnel who are knowledgeable about products but not trained or authorized to provide medical guidance. In the absence of clinician-led education, patients frequently rely on the internet, peer networks, or trial and error experimentation, resulting in gaps in safety, efficacy, and continuity of care (Mack, 2020; MacCallum & Russo, 2018).

Cannabis-based therapies are increasingly used by patients with cancer, chronic pain, anxiety, insomnia, neurodegenerative disease, and other conditions for which conventional treatments may provide incomplete relief (National Academies of Sciences, Engineering, and Medicine, 2017; National Cancer Institute, n.d.). Many of these individuals also experience polypharmacy, adverse drug effects, and diminishing benefit from standard approaches (Bridgeman & Abazia, 2017). Within a healthcare system often perceived as fragmented, costly, and time constrained, patients are turning toward adjunctive, integrative, and plant-based strategies. Nurses, who are uniquely skilled in holistic assessment, patient education, and care coordination, are well positioned to address these gaps. However, despite increasing patient demand, most nursing students receive little to no formal instruction on the endocannabinoid system (ECS), cannabinoid pharmacology, dosing principles, safety considerations, or legal frameworks (Zolotov, 2021; National Council of State Boards of Nursing, 2018).

Medical education has similarly lagged. Recent consensus work published in JAMA highlights the need for standardized cannabis competencies across health professions. An interdisciplinary panel identified six core domains: (1) understanding ECS physiology; (2) describing cannabis plant components and their biological effects; (3) reviewing legal and regulatory frameworks; (4) evaluating evidence related to clinical indications; (5) recognizing potential risks; and (6) applying principles of clinical management. These domains are further supported by sub competencies addressing patient safety, vulnerable populations, structural inequities, and interprofessional collaboration (Zolotov, 2025).

The absence of cannabis content in nursing curricula is increasingly inconsistent with modern practice. The National Council of State Boards of Nursing (NCSBN) addressed this gap in its 2018 National Nursing Guidelines for Medical Marijuana, identifying six essential knowledge areas for all nurses: legal and regulatory literacy, medical program understanding, ECS function, cannabinoid pharmacology, safety and monitoring, and nonjudgmental patient care (National Council of State Boards of Nursing, 2018). Without competency in these domains, new graduates enter practice unprepared to counsel patients who are already using, or considering, cannabis therapeutically.

This educational gap is compounded by more than a century of stigma and prohibition. Cannabis remains federally classified as a Schedule I substance, limiting research, restricting clinical training, and shaping persistent misconceptions within healthcare (Drug Enforcement Administration, n.d.; Alcohol Policy Information System, n.d.). As a result, many patients hesitate to disclose cannabis use due to fear of judgment or potential consequences related to treatment access. This lack of disclosure contributes to incomplete clinical histories, missed drug interaction screening, and fragmented care (Griffith et al., 2025).

At the same time, the scientific evidence base for cannabis therapeutics continues to evolve. While substantial evidence supports certain indications, such as chronic pain and chemotherapy induced nausea, many clinical applications remain characterized by variability in dosing, formulation, and study design (National Academies of Sciences, Engineering, and Medicine, 2017). Consequently, clinical guidance often requires integration of emerging evidence, consensus recommendations, and patient reported outcomes. For nurses, this underscores the importance of developing not only knowledge, but also critical appraisal skills and clinical judgment when guiding cannabis related care.

A modern, evidence informed nursing curriculum must therefore extend beyond pharmacology to include historical context, legal and ethical considerations, and health equity. Cannabis has been used medicinally for thousands of years and remains embedded in cultural and community-based healing practices (Crocq, 2020). As its role in healthcare expands, nursing education must evolve accordingly.

Cannabis also introduces a framework for whole person care. Its clinical applications often span five domains of health: biological, mental, emotional, social, and spiritual. This multidimensional influence aligns closely with nursing's holistic model of care and reinforces the profession's role in integrating complex, patient centered therapies.

This chapter presents a comprehensive, modular curriculum designed to integrate cannabis science, therapeutics, safety, and ethics into undergraduate and graduate nursing programs. By defining core competencies and providing structured educational strategies, it aims to prepare nurses to deliver safe, evidence informed, and patient centered care within a rapidly changing healthcare landscape.

BACKGROUND

The Endocannabinoid System and Its Clinical Relevance

The endocannabinoid system (ECS) is a sophisticated neuromodulatory network essential for maintaining physiological homeostasis across multiple organ systems. The ECS was first identified by Dr. Raphael Mechoulam and Dr. Lumir Hanus through their research into tetrahydrocannabinol (THC) and cannabidiol (CBD). Their characterization of early phytocannabinoids contributed to the discovery and understanding of this system (Mechoulam & Hanus, 2000).

First characterized in the late twentieth century, the ECS is now recognized as a master regulatory system involved in pain modulation, immune function, mood regulation, appetite, sleep, stress response, and neuroprotection (Alger, 2013; Pertwee, 2015). Unlike many receptor systems traditionally emphasized in nursing curricula, the ECS functions dynamically, responding to internal and external stressors by modulating signaling pathways to restore physiological balance.

The therapeutic relevance of cannabis arises from its ability to interact directly with the ECS through biologically active compounds known as phytocannabinoids. These plant-derived molecules engage endogenous cannabinoid receptors, influence enzymatic activity, and modulate neurotransmitter release. Through these mechanisms, cannabis-based therapies may exert effects across multiple physiological domains simultaneously (Mackie, 2008; Pisanti et al., 2017). This systems-level activity distinguishes cannabinoids from single-target pharmaceutical agents and contributes to their potential utility in complex, multi-symptom conditions frequently encountered in nursing practice.

At the core of the ECS are three interdependent components: cannabinoid receptors, endogenous cannabinoids, and metabolic enzymes. Cannabinoid receptors, primarily CB1 and CB2, are G protein coupled receptors distributed throughout the central nervous system, peripheral organs, connective tissue, immune cells, and the enteric nervous system (Gertsch, Pertwee, & Di Marzo, 2010). CB1 receptors are highly expressed in the brain and spinal cord, where they influence pain perception, mood, memory, appetite, and motor coordination. CB2 receptors are predominantly located in immune tissues and peripheral organs, where they regulate inflammation, immune signaling, and tissue repair. Receptor expression is dynamic, with CB1 and CB2 receptors often upregulated during illness or injury as part of the body's effort to restore equilibrium (Mackie, 2008).

Endogenous cannabinoids, primarily anandamide (AEA) and 2-arachidonoylglycerol (2-AG), function as internal signaling molecules within the ECS. Anandamide, named after the Sanskrit word Ananda meaning "bliss," primarily interacts with CB1 receptors and is associated with mood regulation, emotional processing, and stress modulation. In contrast, 2-AG binds to both CB1 and CB2 receptors and plays a critical role in immune regulation, neuroprotection, and inflammatory control. Unlike classical neurotransmitters, endocannabinoids are synthesized on demand from membrane-derived lipid precursors, reflecting the influence of nutrition, metabolic health, and lifestyle factors on ECS tone (Di Marzo et al., 2014).

Endocannabinoid activity is tightly regulated by metabolic enzymes, primarily fatty acid amide hydrolase (FAAH), which degrades anandamide, and monoacylglycerol lipase (MAGL), which degrades 2-AG. These enzymes ensure that signaling remains transient and responsive to physiological needs. Cannabidiol (CBD), a non-intoxicating phytocannabinoid, has been shown to inhibit FAAH, thereby slowing the breakdown of anandamide and prolonging its anxiolytic and analgesic effects. This mechanism provides a biologically plausible explanation for CBD's observed clinical effects in anxiety, pain, and inflammatory conditions (Aizpurua-Olaizola et al., 2017).

Phytocannabinoids such as THC, CBD, cannabigerol (CBG), cannabinol (CBN), and cannabichromene (CBC) can activate or modulate ECS pathways in context-dependent ways. Depending on dose, receptor distribution, and individual physiology, cannabinoids may function as agonists, partial agonists, antagonists, or allosteric modulators. The ECS has therefore been described as a biological system capable of fine-tuning physiological responses toward homeostasis (Pisanti et al., 2017). This adaptive capacity helps explain variability in patient response, including differences in pain relief, sleep improvement, anxiety reduction, appetite stimulation, and inflammatory control.

Emerging evidence suggests that dysregulation of the ECS may contribute to a range of chronic, treatment-resistant conditions. The concept of clinical endocannabinoid deficiency (CECD), proposed by Russo (2016), links reduced endocannabinoid tone or impaired signaling to disorders such as migraine, fibromyalgia, irritable bowel syndrome, and certain anxiety conditions. Chronic stress, trauma exposure, poor sleep, sedentary behavior, and nutritional deficiencies may further compromise ECS function. While this framework continues to evolve and requires ongoing investigation, it offers a biologically grounded model for understanding symptom clusters that span physical, psychological, and emotional domains.

For nursing education, understanding ECS physiology is foundational rather than optional. ECS literacy enables nurses to conduct accurate assessments of cannabis use, anticipate potential drug interactions, guide safe titration and product selection, and manage patient expectations related to onset, duration, and therapeutic response. It also supports stigma reduction by grounding cannabis discussions in established physiology rather than ideology. Given the ECS's role in pain regulation, immune modulation, neuroprotection, gastrointestinal function, sleep, and stress response, its inclusion in nursing curricula is essential to safe, holistic, and patient centered care.

CANNABINOID PHARMACOLOGY & EVIDENCE OF BENEFITS

Phytocannabinoids and Clinical Pharmacology

Phytocannabinoids are biologically active compounds produced by the Cannabis sativa plant that interact with the human endocannabinoid system (ECS). To date, more than one hundred phytocannabinoids have been identified, each with distinct pharmacological properties, receptor affinities, and potential clinical implications. Among these, delta-9-tetrahydrocannabinol (THC) and cannabidiol (CBD) are the most extensively studied and clinically utilized. A growing body of research has also begun to examine the therapeutic relevance of minor cannabinoids, including cannabigerol (CBG), cannabinol (CBN), cannabichromene (CBC), tetrahydrocannabivarin (THCV), and cannabidivarin (CBDV).

For nursing practice and education, competency in cannabinoid pharmacology is essential to safe patient assessment, clinical decision making, and therapeutic monitoring. Nurses are uniquely positioned and increasingly expected to interpret cannabinoid effects, guide safe use, and integrate these therapies within broader, patient centered care plans.

THC is the primary psychoactive constituent of cannabis and acts predominantly as a partial agonist at CB1 receptors within the central nervous system, as well as CB2 receptors in peripheral and immune tissues. Through these interactions, THC influences pain perception, appetite, mood, sleep, memory, and motor coordination (Pertwee, 2007). Clinically, THC demonstrates biphasic dose response effects, in which lower doses may reduce anxiety, pain, and nausea, while higher doses are more likely to produce anxiety, dizziness, tachycardia, or cognitive impairment. This dose dependent variability underscores the importance of conservative titration, particularly in cannabis naive patients, older adults, and individuals with psychiatric or cardiovascular vulnerabilities. From a nursing perspective, the therapeutic use of THC requires careful balancing of potential benefits with psychoactive effects, emphasizing patient education, individualized dosing, and ongoing risk assessment.

CBD, in contrast, is non intoxicating and exhibits a complex pharmacological profile that extends beyond direct cannabinoid receptor activation. Rather than binding strongly to CB1 or CB2 receptors, CBD modulates ECS activity indirectly by influencing the breakdown of endogenous cannabinoids such as anandamide, as well as interacting with transient receptor potential channels, serotonin receptors, and inflammatory signaling pathways. These mechanisms are associated with anxiolytic, anti-inflammatory, anticonvulsant, and neuroprotective effects observed in preclinical and clinical studies (Pertwee, 2007). Clinically, CBD is often used as a foundational component of cannabinoid based regimens, particularly for patients seeking symptom relief without psychoactive effects or for those sensitive to THC. In nursing practice, CBD is frequently introduced as an initial intervention or used alongside THC to improve tolerability and support safety.

While emerging research continues to expand understanding of both major and minor cannabinoids, the evidence base remains variable across conditions, dosing strategies, and formulations. As a result, clinical application requires integration of available evidence, consensus guidance, and patient response. For nurses, this reinforces the importance of clinical judgment, critical appraisal, and careful titration when incorporating cannabinoid therapies into patient care.

Chemotypes and Phytocannabinoid Classification

Phytocannabinoids are most accurately classified using a chemotype framework that reflects dominant cannabinoid composition rather than traditional strain names. Contemporary cannabis science recognizes three primary chemotypes: Chemotype I (THC dominant), Chemotype II (balanced THC and CBD), and Chemotype III (CBD dominant). This classification system provides a standardized and reproducible method for understanding therapeutic effects and safety profiles, and it aligns with modern laboratory testing practices and clinical decision making (Pertwee, 2007; Reimann-Philipp et al., 2019).

For nursing practice and education, chemotype literacy is essential. Nurses are increasingly expected to move beyond strain-based language and guide patients using objective cannabinoid profiles, supporting safer and more individualized clinical decision making.

Chemotype I products are characterized by high concentrations of delta-9-tetrahydrocannabinol (THC) with minimal CBD. THC is the principal psychoactive cannabinoid and exerts its effects primarily through partial agonism at CB1 receptors in the central nervous system, with additional activity at CB2 receptors in peripheral tissues. Clinically, THC dominant chemotypes are associated with therapeutic effects related to pain, spasticity, sleep disturbance, nausea, appetite stimulation, and post-traumatic stress symptoms. However, psychoactive effects require careful titration and monitoring, particularly in cannabis naive patients, older adults, and individuals with psychiatric or cardiovascular vulnerabilities (CannaKeys, 2020).

Chemotype II products contain relatively balanced proportions of THC and CBD. This chemotype is commonly utilized in clinical practice because CBD moderates THC's psychoactive effects through negative allosteric modulation of the CB1 receptor, while still allowing THC to contribute to analgesic, antispasmodic, and sleep related benefits. For many patients, Chemotype II formulations provide a balance between efficacy and tolerability, making them well suited for chronic pain, anxiety with comorbid insomnia, and conditions requiring longer term symptom management (CannaKeys, 2020).

Chemotype III products are CBD dominant and contain minimal THC. Cannabidiol does not produce intoxication and interacts with the endocannabinoid system through multiple mechanisms, including serotonin (5-HT1A), TRPV1, and inflammatory signaling pathways. CBD is associated with anxiolytic, anti-inflammatory, anticonvulsant, and neuroprotective effects observed across preclinical and clinical studies (Pertwee, 2007). Its therapeutic relevance is further supported by the FDA approval of Epidiolex, a purified CBD formulation indicated for refractory pediatric seizure disorders. Due to its favorable safety profile, Chemotype III products are often considered appropriate initial options, particularly in pediatric and geriatric populations (CannaKeys, 2020).

The chemotype framework represents a significant advancement over traditional strain nomenclature such as "OG Kush" or "Trainwreck," which lacks scientific consistency and does not reliably predict pharmacological effects. Chemovars are defined by their complete biochemical profile, including cannabinoids, terpenes, flavonoids, lipids, and waxes, as quantified through laboratory testing and certificates of analysis. This shift enables nurses to guide patients using measurable data rather than marketing driven labels, strengthening safety, consistency, and clinical reasoning (Reimann-Philipp et al., 2019).

Beyond THC and CBD, minor cannabinoids contribute to the pharmacological complexity of cannabis. CBG, often described as a precursor cannabinoid, has demonstrated potential antimicrobial, anti-inflammatory, and neuroprotective properties. CBC appears to influence pain and inflammation through non CB1 pathways and may support mood regulation. CBN, a degradation product of THC, is commonly associated with sedative effects, although emerging evidence suggests its actions are more nuanced and dose dependent. Varin cannabinoids such as THCV and CBDV exhibit distinct pharmacokinetic profiles and receptor interactions that may be relevant in metabolic disorders, seizure conditions, and neurodevelopmental syndromes (Pertwee, 2007). While clinical evidence for these compounds remains more limited than for THC and CBD, their presence reinforces the importance of individualized response and formulation selection.

Cannabinoids also exist in acidic precursor forms, including tetrahydrocannabinolic acid (THCA) and cannabidiolic acid (CBDA). These compounds are produced in the raw plant and convert to THC and CBD through decarboxylation when exposed to heat or prolonged light. Acidic cannabinoids are not psychoactive in their native form but may demonstrate anti-inflammatory, anti-nausea, and neuroprotective properties (Russo & Marcu, 2017). Their clinical relevance highlights the importance of preparation methods, routes of administration, and patient preference in therapeutic outcomes.

The pharmacological diversity of phytocannabinoids supports the understanding that cannabis functions as a multi target therapeutic agent rather than a single mechanism drug. This complexity aligns with models of chronic disease management in which symptoms often span physical, psychological, and emotional domains. For nurses, phytocannabinoid literacy supports accurate assessment of patient experience, anticipatory guidance regarding expected effects, and informed collaboration with interdisciplinary care teams. As cannabis use continues to expand across medical, wellness, and self-directed contexts, nursing education must equip clinicians with the knowledge required to apply cannabinoid pharmacology safely, ethically, and effectively.

Terpenes and the Entourage Effect

Terpenes are aromatic compounds produced by many plants, including Cannabis sativa, and contribute to both the sensory characteristics and potential therapeutic effects of cannabis-based products. In cannabis, terpenes are synthesized in the same glandular trichomes as cannabinoids and are responsible for the plant's characteristic aromas and flavors. Beyond these properties, terpenes exhibit independent pharmacological activity and may influence cannabinoid effects through synergistic interactions, a phenomenon commonly referred to as the entourage effect (Russo & Marcu, 2017).

The concept of the entourage effect suggests that cannabinoids and terpenes act together to influence pharmacological outcomes in ways that differ from isolated compounds. Rather than functioning as inert flavoring agents, terpenes may affect receptor signaling, influence blood brain barrier permeability, and interact with neurotransmitter systems involved in mood, pain perception, inflammation, and arousal (Russo & Marcu, 2017; Russo, 2019). From a clinical perspective, this interaction helps explain why patients may experience different therapeutic responses from products with similar cannabinoid concentrations but distinct terpene profiles.

Several terpenes commonly found in cannabis have been studied for their potential clinical relevance. Myrcene, one of the most prevalent cannabis terpenes, has been associated with sedative and muscle relaxant effects and may contribute to the calming properties reported with certain formulations. Limonene has been linked to mood elevation and stress modulation, while linalool demonstrates anxiolytic and sedative properties that may support sleep and relaxation. Beta caryophyllene is unique among terpenes in that it selectively binds to CB2 receptors, suggesting a role in immune modulation and anti-inflammatory activity (Russo & Marcu, 2017). Pinene has been associated with alertness and memory support and may counterbalance some of the cognitive effects of THC.

For nursing practice, terpene literacy strengthens patient education and supports more nuanced clinical guidance in product selection and expected effects. Nurses are increasingly expected to interpret terpene profiles in conjunction with cannabinoid content, helping patients understand variability in therapeutic response. While terpene effects should not be interpreted deterministically, awareness of their influence allows for more individualized, patient centered care.

Terpene expression is influenced by cultivation methods, processing, storage conditions, and formulation. This variability reinforces the importance of laboratory testing and certificates of analysis when evaluating product quality, consistency, and safety.

Despite growing interest, the clinical evidence base for terpenes remains less robust than that for major cannabinoids, with much of the available data derived from preclinical or observational studies. As such, terpenes are best understood as modulators within a broader pharmacological framework rather than primary therapeutic agents (Russo, 2019). Nursing education should emphasize critical interpretation, patient centered assessment, and integration of terpene knowledge within comprehensive cannabinoid pharmacology.

Routes of Administration and Clinical Implications

The route of administration plays a critical role in determining the onset, intensity, duration, and overall clinical effect of cannabis-based therapies. Unlike many pharmaceutical agents that follow standardized dosing and delivery pathways, cannabinoids exhibit marked variability depending on how they are introduced into the body. For nursing practice, understanding these differences is essential for patient education, safety monitoring, and individualized care planning, particularly given the wide range of products available across medical and consumer markets (Mack, 2020).

Inhalation, including smoking and vaporization, results in rapid absorption of cannabinoids through the alveoli of the lungs, producing effects within minutes. This route bypasses first-pass hepatic metabolism, leading to higher bioavailability of THC compared to oral ingestion. The rapid onset allows patients to titrate doses more precisely based on immediate symptom relief, which may be beneficial for acute pain, nausea, or breakthrough anxiety. However, inhalation is associated with shorter duration of action and variability in dosing, and smoking introduces respiratory risks that must be considered in patients with pulmonary or cardiovascular conditions (Bridgeman & Abazia, 2017).

Sublingual and buccal administration, commonly delivered through tinctures, oils, or dissolvable strips, provides an intermediate option between inhalation and oral ingestion. Cannabinoids absorbed through the oral mucosa enter systemic circulation more gradually than inhaled products but more predictably than edibles. Onset typically occurs within 15 to 45 minutes, with effects lasting several hours. This route supports flexible titration and is frequently utilized in clinical practice for patients seeking steady symptom control without rapid intoxication. Nurses often recommend sublingual products for patients new to cannabis or those managing chronic conditions such as pain, anxiety, or sleep disturbances (Bruni et al., 2018).

Oral ingestion, including capsules, edibles, and swallowed oils, produces the slowest onset of effects but the longest duration. After ingestion, cannabinoids are absorbed through the gastrointestinal tract and undergo first-pass metabolism in the liver, where THC is converted to 11-hydroxy-THC, a metabolite that is more potent and longer-lasting than THC itself. This metabolic process contributes to delayed onset, often one to three hours, and increases the risk of unintentional overconsumption, particularly among inexperienced users. While oral products may be effective for sustained symptom management, nurses must emphasize conservative dosing, appropriate redosing intervals, and careful monitoring for adverse effects (Bruni et al., 2018).

Topical and transdermal preparations represent additional routes with distinct clinical applications. Topical products, such as creams and balms, are designed for localized relief and generally do not produce systemic psychoactive effects, making them appropriate for musculoskeletal pain, anti-inflammatory support, or dermatologic conditions. Transdermal patches, in contrast, are formulated to deliver cannabinoids across the skin barrier into systemic circulation over extended periods, offering more consistent plasma levels. These delivery systems may be particularly useful for patients who require sustained symptom control and cannot tolerate oral or inhaled routes, although availability and regulation vary by jurisdiction (Bridgeman & Abazia, 2017).

Rectal and vaginal suppositories provide alternative routes that avoid first-pass metabolism and may offer localized or systemic benefits, particularly in palliative care, gynecologic pain, or conditions associated with gastrointestinal intolerance. While clinical research on these routes remains limited, patient-reported outcomes suggest potential value in select populations when guided by knowledgeable clinicians. Nursing education should emphasize careful patient selection, informed consent, and ongoing assessment when these less common routes are utilized (Bruni et al., 2018).

Across all routes of administration, variability in onset, duration, and bioavailability reinforces the importance of patient education and shared decision-making. Nurses are uniquely positioned to help patients align product selection with symptom patterns, daily routines, and safety considerations. Given the variability in individual response and product formulation, clinical guidance should remain flexible and evidence informed. By framing routes of administration as clinical tools rather than consumer preferences, nursing practice can support safer use, improved outcomes, and reduced risk of adverse events (Mack, 2020).

Pharmacokinetics and Pharmacodynamics of Cannabinoids

Understanding the pharmacokinetics (PK) and pharmacodynamics (PD) of cannabinoids is essential for safe clinical guidance, particularly given the variability in patient responses to cannabis-based products. Pharmacokinetics describes how cannabinoids are absorbed, distributed, metabolized, and eliminated by the body, while pharmacodynamics refers to how these compounds exert their effects at receptor and cellular levels (Bridgeman & Abazia, 2017; Lucas et al., 2018). For nursing practice, PK and PD knowledge supports anticipatory guidance, dose titration, monitoring for adverse effects, and patient education across diverse routes of administration.

Absorption of cannabinoids varies significantly by route of administration. Inhaled cannabinoids are rapidly absorbed through the pulmonary alveoli, leading to measurable plasma concentrations within minutes and relatively predictable onset of effects. In contrast, orally ingested cannabinoids undergo slower and more variable absorption due to gastrointestinal transit time and individual differences in digestion and hepatic function. Sublingual and mucosal routes fall between these extremes, offering more gradual absorption while partially bypassing first-pass metabolism. These differences account for much of the variability observed in clinical response and underscore the importance of route selection in individualized care planning (Bruni et al., 2018).

Following absorption, cannabinoids are widely distributed throughout the body due to their lipophilic nature. THC and other cannabinoids readily cross the blood-brain barrier and accumulate in fatty tissues, where they may be slowly released back into circulation over time. This tissue accumulation contributes to prolonged effects, delayed elimination, and the potential for cumulative exposure with repeated dosing. For nurses, this distribution pattern helps explain why cannabinoids may exert lingering effects even after acute intoxication has resolved and why older adults or individuals with higher body fat percentages may experience prolonged or intensified responses (Bridgeman & Abazia, 2017).

Metabolism of cannabinoids occurs primarily in the liver via cytochrome P450 (CYP450) enzymes, most notably CYP2C9, CYP2C19, and CYP3A4. THC is metabolized into 11-hydroxy-THC, an active metabolite that is more potent and longer lasting than THC itself. This metabolite is produced in greater quantities following oral ingestion, contributing to the delayed onset and heightened psychoactive effects associated with edibles and capsules. CBD is also extensively metabolized by CYP450 enzymes and may inhibit or induce these pathways, increasing the potential for drug–drug interactions with commonly prescribed medications such as anticoagulants, anticonvulsants, and certain antidepressants (Bruni et al., 2018; Lucas et al., 2018).

Elimination of cannabinoids occurs slowly and primarily through fecal excretion, with smaller amounts eliminated in urine. Due to fat storage and enterohepatic recirculation, THC metabolites may remain detectable in the body for days or weeks following use, depending on frequency, dose, and individual metabolism. While the presence of metabolites does not equate to ongoing impairment, prolonged elimination has implications for workplace drug testing, patient counseling, and legal considerations, areas in which nurses are frequently asked to provide guidance (Bridgeman & Abazia, 2017).

From a pharmacodynamic perspective, cannabinoids exert their effects through both receptor-mediated and non-receptor-mediated mechanisms. THC acts primarily as a partial agonist at CB1 and CB2 receptors, producing dose-dependent effects on pain perception, mood, appetite, and cognition. CBD demonstrates more complex pharmacodynamics, functioning as a modulator of ECS activity rather than a direct receptor agonist. It influences multiple signaling pathways, including serotonin receptors, transient receptor potential channels, and inflammatory cascades, contributing to its broad therapeutic profile and favorable safety margin (Bruni et al., 2018).

A clinically significant feature of cannabinoid pharmacodynamics is the biphasic dose-response relationship, particularly with THC. Lower doses may produce anxiolytic, analgesic, or antiemetic effects, while higher doses may precipitate anxiety, dysphoria, or cognitive impairment. Tolerance develops with repeated exposure, particularly to THC, resulting in diminished psychoactive effects over time. Importantly, while tolerance may expand the safety window by reducing acute adverse reactions, it does not necessarily enhance therapeutic efficacy and may increase the risk of dependence if dosing escalates without clinical reassessment. Nurses play a critical role in helping patients distinguish between tolerance, effectiveness, and overuse (MacCallum & Russo, 2018).

The pharmacokinetic and pharmacodynamic properties of cannabinoids demonstrate why dosing cannot be easily standardized and underscore the importance of personalized titration. Given significant interindividual variability, comprehensive assessment and individualized selection of cannabinoid type, dose, and route of administration are essential. Nurses are uniquely positioned and increasingly expected to guide this process. By integrating PK and PD concepts into patient education and ongoing monitoring, nurses can promote safer cannabis use, reduce adverse effects, and support patients in achieving realistic therapeutic outcomes.

Laboratory Testing and Certificates of Analysis

Laboratory testing plays a critical role in the safe clinical use of cannabis-based products by providing objective verification of product composition, potency, and contaminant screening. Certificates of Analysis (COAs) summarize laboratory findings for a specific product batch and serve as a primary mechanism for transparency and quality assurance within regulated cannabis markets. For nursing practice, COA literacy supports informed patient counseling, risk reduction, and alignment of therapeutic intent with actual product content (NIST, 2025).

Clinically relevant COAs report quantitative cannabinoid content, including THC, CBD, and other cannabinoids present in the formulation. Accurate potency data is essential for dose calculation, titration planning, and monitoring therapeutic response, particularly given the dose-dependent effects and narrow therapeutic window associated with THC. Terpene profiles may also be included and can help contextualize patient-reported effects related to sedation, alertness, mood, or pain modulation. While terpene data should not be interpreted deterministically, its inclusion contributes to a more complete understanding of product variability and consistency (Woodbridge et al., 2024).

Equally important is contaminant screening, which may include testing for pesticides, heavy metals, residual solvents, microbial contaminants, and mycotoxins. These factors are especially relevant for immunocompromised patients, older adults, and individuals with chronic illness, where exposure may pose significant health risks. Variability in testing standards across jurisdictions underscores the importance of nurse awareness of local regulatory requirements and laboratory accreditation practices (NIST, 2025).

From a nursing perspective, COAs function as clinical safety documents rather than purely technical laboratory reports. Nurses are not expected to interpret raw analytical data; however, foundational literacy, including verification of batch matching, interpretation of cannabinoid ratios, and recognition of contamination risk, strengthens patient education and supports safer product selection. Nurses are increasingly expected to incorporate COA review into patient counseling, particularly as product diversity and access continue to expand.

As cannabis products continue to evolve across medical and consumer markets, familiarity with COAs supports shared decision-making and reinforces evidence-informed, patient-centered care. Whenever available, patients should be encouraged to select products that include accessible and verifiable COAs, regardless of purchase source (Woodbridge et al., 2024).

Evidence Base for Cannabis Therapeutics

The contemporary evidence base for cannabis therapeutics reflects both meaningful clinical potential and persistent research limitations. The most comprehensive synthesis to date, *The Health Effects of Cannabis and Cannabinoids* published by the National Academies of Sciences, Engineering, and Medicine (NASEM), provides a foundational framework for evaluating the strength of evidence across multiple health conditions. Rather than positioning cannabis as a universal intervention, the NASEM report emphasizes condition-specific outcomes and differentiates between substantial, moderate, limited, and insufficient evidence of efficacy (National Academies of Sciences, Engineering, and Medicine, 2017).

According to NASEM, there is substantial evidence supporting the use of cannabis or cannabinoids for the treatment of chronic pain in adults, chemotherapy-induced nausea and vomiting, and patient-reported spasticity symptoms in multiple sclerosis. Moderate evidence exists for sleep disturbances associated with obstructive sleep apnea, fibromyalgia, chronic pain, and multiple sclerosis. These findings align with symptom clusters frequently encountered in nursing practice, particularly among patients managing chronic illness, cancer, neurologic conditions, and palliative care needs (National Academies of Sciences, Engineering, and Medicine, 2017).

In oncology settings, evidence summarized by the National Cancer Institute's PDQ highlights the role of cannabinoids in managing cancer-related symptoms such as pain, nausea, vomiting, appetite loss, and anxiety. While cannabinoids are not recommended as primary anticancer agents, their adjunctive use for symptom control is increasingly recognized, particularly when conventional therapies are insufficient or poorly tolerated. This distinction reinforces the importance of realistic goal setting and clear patient education, both of which are central to nursing practice in supportive and palliative care (National Cancer Institute, n.d.).

Despite these areas of demonstrated benefit, the evidence base remains inconsistent. Many studies are limited by small sample sizes, short study durations, product variability, and ongoing regulatory constraints that affect research design. Differences in cannabinoid ratios, routes of administration, and outcome measures further complicate comparison across studies. As a result, high-quality randomized controlled trials are less prevalent than observational and patient-reported outcome studies, particularly for whole-plant cannabis products. These limitations underscore why clinical decision-making in cannabis care often requires integration of available evidence, patient experience, and clinical judgment (National Academies of Sciences, Engineering, and Medicine, 2017).

For nursing practice, this evolving evidence base highlights the importance of comprehensive assessment and longitudinal monitoring. Nurses are often the clinicians most closely observing symptom patterns, functional changes, adverse effects, and patient-reported outcomes over time. In the context of cannabis therapeutics, this perspective enables identification of both benefits and risks that may not be captured in short-term clinical trials. Nursing documentation, patient education, and outcome tracking therefore function not only as clinical tools but also as contributions to practice-based evidence (Mack, 2020).

As cannabis policy and research infrastructure continue to evolve, the evidence base is expected to expand in both scope and rigor. Until then, nurses are uniquely positioned and increasingly expected to navigate this complexity with clinical judgment, transparency, and ethical clarity. By grounding care in authoritative reviews such as NASEM, integrating condition-specific guidance from oncology and specialty sources, and emphasizing individualized assessment, nurses can provide safe, evidence-informed, and patient-centered care while remaining aligned with current scientific understanding.

Pharmacology Conclusion

Emerging evidence suggests that endocannabinoid system (ECS) tone is influenced by a constellation of lifestyle, biological, and environmental factors, including sleep quality, stress exposure, physical activity, nutrition, and aging. Chronic stress, poor sleep, sedentary behavior, unhealthy diets, toxin exposure, and genetic variability may contribute to diminished endocannabinoid signaling, a phenomenon described as clinical endocannabinoid deficiency (CECD). Although direct measurement of endocannabinoids such as anandamide remains limited to cerebrospinal fluid analysis, symptom patterns observed in conditions such as chronic pain, migraine, irritable bowel syndrome, and mood disorders suggest potential clinical relevance (Russo, 2016).

Nurses play a central role in contextualizing CECD within a biopsychosocial framework, supporting patient education, and guiding interventions that may promote ECS balance through lifestyle optimization and cautious phytocannabinoid use. Di Marzo's framework, often summarized as "eat, sleep, relax, forget, protect," offers a clinically accessible model for understanding the pleiotropic effects of cannabinoids across appetite regulation, circadian rhythm, stress modulation, emotional processing, immune function, and neuroprotection (Di Marzo, 2014). Within this framework, cannabinoid pharmacology requires careful attention to therapeutic windows, tolerance development, and patient safety.

While CBD demonstrates a broad safety margin, THC requires individualized titration due to its biphasic effects and potential for tolerance through CB1 receptor downregulation. Although tolerance may widen the safety window and reduce acute adverse effects, it does not necessarily improve therapeutic outcomes and may contribute to unintended effects if dosing escalates without reassessment (Russo, 2019). Education focused on conservative dosing, product rotation, and periodic tolerance breaks may support efficacy while minimizing risk.

Importantly, no lethal dose of cannabis has been identified, and cannabinoid receptors are not present in brainstem centers responsible for respiratory and cardiovascular control. As a result, most adverse effects are dose-dependent and reversible with appropriate clinical guidance (National Academies of Sciences, Engineering, and Medicine, 2017).

Collectively, cannabinoid pharmacology represents a complex but clinically essential domain for modern nursing practice. By integrating knowledge of phytocannabinoids, terpene interactions, routes of administration, pharmacokinetics and pharmacodynamics, laboratory testing, CECD, and therapeutic safety principles, nurses are uniquely positioned and increasingly expected to deliver individualized, evidence-informed cannabis care. These competencies form the foundation for responsible patient education, clinical monitoring, and stigma reduction, reinforcing the nurse's role as a leader in the ethical integration of cannabinoid therapeutics into contemporary healthcare.

ASSESSMENT AND CARE PLANNING IN CANNABIS NURSING

Comprehensive assessment is foundational to safe and effective cannabis nursing practice. Given that many patients self-administer cannabis for symptom relief, nurses must be prepared to evaluate existing use, determine therapeutic intent, and identify appropriate candidates for cannabinoid-based therapies.

Initial assessment should include a detailed medical history, review of systems, current symptom burden, prior experiences with cannabis, concurrent use of alcohol or other psychoactive substances, and a complete medication profile. This process enables identification of potential drug–drug interactions, particularly those mediated by hepatic enzyme pathways, and supports determination of whether cannabis use can be safely integrated into the patient's care plan (Kitdumrongthum & Trachootham, 2023).

Holistic assessment extends beyond biomedical indicators to include psychosocial, behavioral, and lifestyle factors that influence both endocannabinoid system (ECS) function and therapeutic outcomes. Nursing assessment should explore sleep quality, stress exposure, physical activity, nutrition, emotional well being, social support, and sources of meaning or spiritual resilience. These domains align with whole-person nursing models and reflect the multidimensional ways in which cannabinoids influence health. Framing assessment across these five domains supports both students and clinicians in moving beyond symptom suppression toward understanding cannabis as a modulator of balance across interconnected physiological and psychosocial systems.

Risk assessment is an essential component of cannabis nursing and should be conducted for all patients, regardless of prior experience. Particular caution is warranted in individuals with a history of psychosis or severe mood disorders, as THC exposure may exacerbate psychiatric symptoms in vulnerable populations (Volkow et al., 2014). Additional considerations include pregnancy and lactation, unstable cardiovascular disease, and conditions associated with impaired cognition or fall risk. In these contexts, nurses may guide patients toward non-intoxicating options such as CBD or recommend deferring cannabis use. Risk-reduction strategies include education on conservative dosing, avoidance of high-potency products, delayed redosing, particularly with oral formulations, and selection of delivery methods aligned with patient safety and functional goals (Bridgeman & Abazia, 2017).

Distinguishing therapeutic use from misuse requires nuanced clinical judgment rather than rigid thresholds. Therapeutic cannabis use is defined as the use of cannabis products for medicinal, wellness, or healing purposes (American Cannabis Nurses Association & American Nurses Association, 2024). It may be considered therapeutic when it supports physical, mental, emotional, social, or spiritual well-being without causing harm across any of the other domains. Therapeutic use is characterized by intentional dosing aligned with symptom targets, functional improvement, and minimal interference with daily responsibilities. In contrast, misuse may involve dose escalation without benefit, reliance on cannabis as a primary coping strategy in the absence of other supportive care or continued use despite negative consequences. Understanding the biphasic effects of cannabinoids, particularly THC, helps nurses contextualize patient responses and guide dose adjustments when paradoxical effects such as increased anxiety or sleep disruption occur (CannaKeys, 2024).

Care planning in cannabis nursing is individualized and iterative. Nurses collaborate with patients to establish realistic goals, select appropriate cannabinoid profiles and routes of administration, and develop titration strategies based on symptom response and tolerability. Education should emphasize initiating treatment with the lowest effective dose, allowing adequate time between adjustments, and avoiding rapid escalation, principles commonly summarized as "start low and go slow" (Bell et al., 2023). As tolerance to THC develops through repeated exposure and CB1 receptor downregulation, nurses help patients distinguish between reduced psychoactive effects and true therapeutic benefit, preventing unnecessary dose escalation and supporting long-term safety (Bhaskar et al., 2021).

Patient education is central to effective cannabis care planning. Nurses play a critical role in teaching patients about cannabinoid differences, delivery methods, onset and duration of effects, and realistic expectations for symptom management. Clear, accessible education supports active patient participation while reducing stigma and misinformation surrounding cannabis use (Mack, 2020). Education should also incorporate lifestyle practices that support ECS function, including movement, whole-food nutrition, restorative sleep, and meaningful social connection.

Documentation remains a critical but historically underutilized component of cannabis nursing practice. Fear of judgment, legal ambiguity, and institutional bias have contributed to underreporting of cannabis use in clinical records. Nurses can address this gap by initiating nonjudgmental conversations, documenting cannabis use with the same rigor applied to other therapies, and tracking outcomes related to symptom relief, adverse effects, and functional status. Consistent documentation supports continuity of care, facilitates interdisciplinary collaboration, and contributes to the growing body of practice-based evidence in cannabis therapeutics.

Together, comprehensive assessment, holistic care planning, risk-reduction strategies, patient education, and documentation form the foundation of responsible cannabis nursing practice. By integrating these elements within a multidimensional framework, nurses are uniquely positioned and increasingly expected to guide safe, individualized, and evidence-informed cannabis care across diverse clinical settings.

DOSING AND PRODUCT LITERACY IN CANNABIS NURSING

Cannabis dosing is inherently individualized and influenced by multiple variables, including age, genetics, metabolic rate, prior exposure, symptom profile, and concurrent use of pharmaceuticals. Unlike standardized pharmaceutical dosing, cannabinoids exhibit significant interindividual variability, requiring nurses to guide patients through a process of careful titration rather than fixed-dose regimens. Older adults, in particular, metabolize cannabinoids more slowly, increasing sensitivity to both therapeutic and adverse effects and underscoring the need for conservative dosing strategies in geriatric populations (Kitdumrongthum & Trachootham, 2023).

Prior experience with cannabis and other psychoactive substances also influences patient response. Cannabis-naive individuals are more susceptible to anxiety, dizziness, and dysphoria, particularly with THC-containing products, whereas experienced users may demonstrate tolerance to psychoactive effects. Psychological expectations and fear of intoxication may further shape perceived outcomes, highlighting the importance of anticipatory guidance and reassurance during initial dosing phases (Volkow et al., 2014).

Product literacy is central to safe dosing. Cannabinoid composition, potency, and delivery method all affect onset, duration, and intensity of effects. THC and CBD remain the most clinically relevant cannabinoids, although minor cannabinoids and terpenes contribute to therapeutic variability. Nurses must help patients understand that milligram content alone does not determine clinical response; formulation, route of administration, and individual physiology play equally important roles (Bridgeman & Abazia, 2017).

For patients new to cannabis, initiating therapy with CBD or Chemotype III products may support endocannabinoid system engagement while minimizing psychoactive effects. Evidence supports conservative titration schedules that allow the ECS to adapt prior to the introduction of THC or Chemotype I products, which may reduce adverse effects and improve tolerability (Bell et al., 2023). This approach aligns with the widely accepted principle of "start low and go slow," particularly when oral or long-acting formulations are used.

The concept of the minimum effective dose (MED) is central to cannabis dosing and emphasizes achieving symptom relief without unnecessary escalation. Cannabinoids, especially THC, demonstrate biphasic dose-response effects, in which lower doses may be therapeutic while higher doses may produce diminished benefit or paradoxical outcomes such as anxiety or sleep disruption. Understanding these effects enables nurses to guide dose adjustments based on symptom response rather than the assumption that higher doses produce greater benefit (CannaKeys, 2024).

Patients often use multiple product forms concurrently to manage symptoms with differing onset and duration profiles, a practice sometimes referred to as "stacking." When guided appropriately, combining short-acting and long-acting formulations may support symptom control while preserving dose flexibility. Nurses are uniquely positioned to guide this approach, ensuring cumulative dosing remains appropriate and aligned with therapeutic goals (Mack, 2020).

Safety, Contraindications, and Monitoring

Cannabis is generally well tolerated when used conservatively; however, safety considerations must be integrated throughout assessment, dosing, and ongoing monitoring. Variability in patient response, product composition, and dosing underscores the need for structured clinical oversight. Adverse effects are typically dose-dependent and transient, resolving as cannabinoids are metabolized. THC-related effects may include tachycardia, dizziness, impaired coordination, anxiety, cognitive changes, and orthostatic hypotension. CBD may be associated with sedation, gastrointestinal discomfort, or appetite changes in some individuals (Bridgeman & Abazia, 2017).

THC and CBD: Side Effects, Risks, and Clinical Monitoring

The therapeutic and psychoactive effects of delta-9-tetrahydrocannabinol (THC) arise primarily through activation of CB1 receptors in the central nervous system. At low doses, THC may produce analgesic, anxiolytic, and appetite-stimulating effects; however, higher doses are associated with increased risk of acute adverse reactions and destabilizing symptoms. Common THC-related side effects include tachycardia and palpitations, fluctuations in blood pressure with possible orthostatic hypotension, dizziness, lightheadedness, sedation, impaired balance and coordination, and cognitive changes such as short-term memory lapses. Anxiety, paranoia, and, at higher doses or with concentrated products, hallucinations and excessive euphoria may also occur. Additional effects may include dry mouth and eyes, increased appetite, slowed gastrointestinal motility, reduced urinary frequency, headache, and bronchodilation, which may deepen breathing but irritate airways in some individuals (MacCallum & Russo, 2018; Lee, 2023; Bridgeman & Abazia, 2017).

Clinical interpretation of these effects requires attention to dose, formulation, and individual patient characteristics. In cannabis-naive individuals, adverse effects are less likely at doses below approximately 1 to 5 mg of THC when titration is gradual and conservative. High-potency concentrates increase the likelihood of adverse reactions and potential dependency. Repeated exposure to high doses of THC may result in cognitive impairment that is typically reversible within several weeks of abstinence. Older adults are particularly susceptible to exaggerated effects due to age-related changes in metabolism, hepatic clearance, and renal function, reinforcing the need for cautious dosing and close monitoring in geriatric populations (MacCallum & Russo, 2018).

Cannabidiol (CBD), while non-intoxicating and generally well tolerated, is not entirely free of side effects. Reported reactions include lightheadedness or dizziness at higher doses, paradoxical activation or jitteriness at lower doses, sedation at higher doses, alterations in heart rate, typically slowing, decreased appetite, and gastrointestinal upset such as diarrhea. In some cases, these effects may be related to carrier oils rather than CBD itself. Rarely, palpitations or anxiety may occur (MacCallum & Russo, 2018; Lee, 2023; Bridgeman & Abazia, 2017). Of particular clinical importance is CBD's interaction with cytochrome P450 enzymes, which may amplify or alter the effects of medications including selective serotonin reuptake inhibitors, benzodiazepines, antiepileptics, and anticoagulants. Careful monitoring is therefore essential in patients with polypharmacy and in older adults.

When THC overuse results in distressing effects, nurses can recommend supportive and non-pharmacologic interventions. These include hydration, light snacks or administering cannabinoids with food, resting in a calm and familiar environment, reassurance and grounding techniques, use of lubricating eye drops, exposure to fresh air or mild cooling, and time for metabolism and clearance. Some patients report relief with lemon water, black peppercorns, or the addition of CBD to buffer THC's psychoactive effects; however, these strategies should be framed as supportive rather than definitive (Lee, 2023). Commercial products marketed to counteract THC effects are also available, though evidence supporting their mechanism of action remains limited.

For patients experiencing adverse effects, therapy can often be refined through targeted adjustments rather than discontinued. Strategies may include reducing THC dose, increasing the proportion of CBD, changing the route of administration, selecting alternative chemovars or terpene profiles, modifying timing or setting of use, and slowing titration. These adjustments support patient goals while reinforcing safety and therapeutic intent, recognizing that most patients seek symptom relief rather than escalation (Mack, 2020).

Cannabinoid hyperemesis syndrome (CHS) represents a rare but increasingly recognized condition, most commonly observed in individuals with frequent, high-dose THC use, particularly via inhalation of high-potency products. CHS is characterized by severe abdominal cramping, cyclic vomiting, nausea unresponsive to standard antiemetics, and temporary relief with hot bathing or showers. Management requires cessation of THC, hydration, supportive care, and patient education regarding potency and frequency of use. Nurses should maintain a high index of suspicion in patients presenting with recurrent, unexplained vomiting, especially when cannabis use is minimized or underreported due to stigma (MacCallum & Russo, 2018).

Whole-plant cannabis formulations, which contain multiple cannabinoids, terpenes, flavonoids, and other compounds, may improve tolerability through synergistic interactions. Compared with isolated cannabinoids, whole-plant CBD products may be less sedating, balanced CBD to THC ratios may attenuate psychoactive effects, and terpenes such as linalool, limonene, pinene, and beta-caryophyllene may favorably influence mood, cognition, and inflammation. While evidence remains variable, these interactions may contribute to broader symptom relief and improved patient experience when aligned with clinical goals (MacCallum & Russo, 2018).

During early stages of cannabis care, maintaining existing pharmaceutical regimens while introducing cannabinoids can support symptom stability and continuity during titration. As therapeutic effects become clearer, clinicians may collaboratively reduce sedatives, taper pain medications, adjust antidepressants, or reassess antispasmodics and antiemetics. Drug-drug interactions remain an important consideration, as CBD's inhibition of CYP450 enzymes may alter medication effects, and THC may increase sedation or cognitive impairment when combined with other central nervous system depressants. Close collaboration among nurses, prescribers, and the broader healthcare team supports safe deprescribing and integration of cannabis into comprehensive care planning (National Academies of Sciences, Engineering, and Medicine, 2017).

Certain patient populations require heightened caution. Individuals with a history of psychosis or severe mood disorders may experience symptom exacerbation with THC exposure, making thorough psychiatric screening essential prior to initiation (Volkow et al., 2014). Cannabis use is generally discouraged during pregnancy and lactation due to potential neurodevelopmental risks. Patients with unstable cardiovascular disease, cognitive impairment, or high fall risk also warrant careful consideration and monitoring. Youth should be discouraged from cannabis use due to risks related to brain development, mental health, addiction, and safety (SAMHSA, n.d.).

Tolerance development, particularly with THC, occurs through downregulation of CB1 receptors following repeated exposure. While tolerance may reduce acute adverse effects and widen the safety window, it does not inherently improve therapeutic efficacy and may lead to escalating doses if not addressed clinically. Nurses are uniquely positioned to help patients distinguish between diminished psychoactive effects and meaningful symptom relief, preventing unnecessary dose escalation and associated risks (Bhaskar et al., 2021).

Monitoring is a dynamic and ongoing process that includes evaluation of symptom response, functional outcomes, adverse effects, and patterns of use over time. Patients should be encouraged to track dosing, timing, product type, and perceived effects to support shared decision-making and dose refinement. Monitoring also allows early identification of misuse patterns, including escalating THC use without clinical benefit or reliance on cannabis to manage distress in the absence of other coping strategies.

Importantly, no lethal dose of cannabis has been identified, as cannabinoid receptors are not present in brainstem regions controlling respiration and cardiovascular function. Most adverse events are reversible with dose reduction, supportive care, and time. Nurses should emphasize that cannabis safety depends on informed use, conservative titration, and alignment with individual health status rather than assumptions of inherent harmlessness (National Academies of Sciences, Engineering, and Medicine, 2017).

Lower-Risk Cannabis Use Guidelines (LRCUG)

An international panel comprising representatives from multiple countries with medical and adult-use cannabis programs convened to establish public health guidelines aimed at improving outcomes and minimizing adverse risks. These efforts focused on synthesizing available evidence, identifying best practices, and evaluating effectiveness, particularly in populations at increased risk, including youth, older adults, pregnant individuals, and those with comorbid conditions.

Current evidence suggests that individuals can reduce the risk of adverse health outcomes by delaying cannabis use until after adolescence, avoiding high-potency THC products, and minimizing both frequency and intensity of use. Avoidance of smoking is also recommended due to associated respiratory risks. While youth remain particularly vulnerable to cannabis-related harms, other populations, including pregnant individuals, drivers, older adults, and those with comorbidities, also require careful consideration of use-related risks. Whenever possible, patients should be guided toward legal, regulated, and laboratory-tested cannabis products rather than unregulated or untested sources (Fischer et al., 2022).

Cannabis use may be associated with adverse health outcomes, particularly among high-risk populations. Reducing modifiable risk factors can help mitigate potential harms. The LRCUG provides an evidence-informed framework for public health strategies related to cannabis use, emphasizing targeted education, risk reduction, and ongoing evaluation of outcomes (Fischer et al., 2022).

For nursing practice, these guidelines offer a practical foundation for patient education and risk mitigation. Nurses are uniquely positioned to translate public health guidance into individualized clinical recommendations, reinforcing safer patterns of use and supporting informed decision-making. The guiding principle remains consistent: in cannabinoid therapy, careful dosing and moderation support optimal outcomes.

LEGAL & ETHICAL LITERACY IN CANNABIS NURSING

Legal and ethical literacy is foundational to safe and responsible cannabis nursing practice. Although cannabis has been used therapeutically for millennia, its integration into modern healthcare remains shaped by a fragmented legal framework that influences patient access, clinician education, research infrastructure, and ethical responsibilities. Nurses must understand these dynamics to provide accurate guidance, reduce stigma, and advocate for equitable, patient-centered care within evolving regulatory systems.

Historical and Federal Policy Context

Cannabis was a common component of the United States pharmacopeia until the passage of the Marijuana Tax Act of 1937, which effectively criminalized possession and restricted medical use. This trajectory culminated in the Controlled Substances Act of 1970, which classified cannabis as a Schedule I substance, defined as having no accepted medical use and a high potential for abuse, alongside substances such as heroin and lysergic acid diethylamide (Drug Enforcement Administration, n.d.).

This classification continues to shape significant barriers to clinician education, limit federal research funding for therapeutic applications, impose criminal penalties in prohibition states, and restrict employment in federally regulated industries. As a result, cannabis therapeutics has been largely excluded from medical and nursing curricula, requiring clinicians and patients to rely on self-education rather than standardized, evidence-based guidance (Alcohol Policy Information System, n.d.).

Federal Rescheduling Efforts and Emerging Dual Regulatory Pathways

In May 2024, the U.S. Department of Justice, in coordination with the Department of Health and Human Services and the Food and Drug Administration, endorsed a proposal to reclassify cannabis from Schedule I to Schedule III. While this change would not legalize adult-use cannabis or eliminate federal oversight, a Schedule III designation would formally recognize medical utility, expand research opportunities, reduce regulatory barriers, and improve communication between patients and healthcare providers.

Momentum accelerated on December 18, 2025, when President Trump issued an executive order directing federal agencies to expedite rescheduling and expand research into medical marijuana and cannabidiol (The White House, 2025). If finalized, rescheduling is expected to create dual regulatory pathways: one governing FDA-approved cannabinoid pharmaceuticals within traditional prescribing frameworks and another maintaining state-regulated botanical cannabis programs.

For nursing practice, this evolving regulatory landscape underscores the need to understand both pharmaceutical and botanical models of care, as well as the ethical implications of unequal access influenced by insurance coverage, geographic location, and employment-related constraints.

State-Level Expansion and Persistent Access Inequities

The contemporary reform era began with California's Compassionate Use Act of 1996, which permitted medical cannabis use for serious conditions including cancer and HIV/AIDS. Over subsequent decades, patient advocacy and shifting public sentiment contributed to rapid expansion of state-level medical and adult-use programs. As of early 2026, forty states authorize medical cannabis and twenty-four permit adult-use sales, with dispensaries operating openly in many metropolitan regions.

Despite this expansion, continued federal prohibition has resulted in a fragmented system in which cannabis may be legal, tolerated, or criminalized depending on jurisdiction (Griffith et al., 2025). These inconsistencies contribute to significant inequities in symptom management, employment protections, criminal justice exposure, and overall quality of life for patients.

Hemp-Derived CBD and Emerging Medicare Considerations

Following the 2018 Farm Bill, full-spectrum hemp-derived CBD products became widely accessible nationwide, including in prohibition states. However, federal restrictions enacted on November 12, 2025, limit hemp products to no more than 0.4 mg of THC per container, effectively removing most full-spectrum CBD products from the national market and leaving primarily isolate-based formulations available (Sliwoski, 2025). This regulatory shift reflects congressional concern regarding unintended intoxicant exposure while introducing significant implications for patient access and the hemp industry.

The December 2025 executive order further emphasized federal interest in researching non-intoxicating cannabinoids, including cannabidiol, for potential cost-saving applications within federal health programs. Preliminary policy discussions have explored whether limited CBD coverage could reduce prescription expenditures and healthcare utilization among Medicare beneficiaries, suggesting a possible pathway toward evidence-informed reimbursement models pending further research (Jaeger, 2025b).

For nursing practice, these developments underscore the importance of distinguishing regulatory status from clinical evidence while preparing for evolving changes in coverage, policy, and patient access.

Ethical Responsibilities, Disclosure, and Clinical Silence

Federal restrictions on education and research have left many patients without access to formal clinical guidance when entering medical cannabis programs. As a result, patients often rely on dispensary staff with variable training, online forums, peer advice, or trial and error experimentation. Fewer than half of patients disclose cannabis use to their healthcare providers due to concerns related to stigma, judgment, or legal repercussions, creating safety risks associated with drug–drug interactions, diagnostic accuracy, and care coordination (Griffith et al., 2025).

Ethical nursing practice requires proactive, nonjudgmental inquiry into cannabis use and normalization of disclosure as part of comprehensive assessment. This approach is consistent with professional guidance from the National Council of State Boards of Nursing (2018) and supports safer, more coordinated patient care.

Toward Integrated Policy Reform and Compassionate Care Models

Meaningful cannabis policy reform requires coordinated engagement among federal and state governments, public health agencies, agricultural regulators, research institutions, testing laboratories, clinicians, educators, industry stakeholders, and patient communities. At present, these systems often function in silos, resulting in inconsistent safety standards, limited data collection, and persistent educational gaps (Griffith et al., 2025).

Promising developments include the expansion of continuing education, integration of endocannabinoid system science into health curricula, establishment of national training standards for dispensary staff, and the development of a federally funded cannabis patient research registry at Johns Hopkins University (Cannabis and Health Research Initiative, 2025).

A compelling example of compassionate, evidence-informed policy is California's Senate Bill 311, commonly known as Ryan's Law. Enacted in 2021, the law permits hospitalized hospice patients to continue using non-smokable cannabis-based medicines, including tinctures, oils, edibles, patches, and topical formulations. Implementation at the University of California, Los Angeles (UCLA) between 2022 and 2024 demonstrated safe integration, high nurse satisfaction, and meaningful symptom relief without reported safety incidents. These outcomes illustrate how thoughtful policy can translate into ethical, patient-centered clinical practice (Americans for Safe Access, 2025; McKaig et al., 2025).

TEACHING AND EVALUATION

Successful integration of medical cannabis education into nursing curricula requires intentional instructional design, clearly scaffolded learning outcomes, robust evaluation strategies, and dedicated faculty development. Because cannabis therapeutics intersect pharmacology, patient assessment, ethics, clinical reasoning, and patient education, nursing faculty benefit from a structured approach that integrates didactic instruction with case-based learning, simulation, and competency-based evaluation.

This approach aligns with contemporary nursing education frameworks and reinforces the expectations outlined in **Cannabis Nursing: Scope and Standards of Practice** (American Cannabis Nurses Association & American Nurses Association, 2024). Competency-based education (CBE) is particularly well suited to cannabis nursing, as it ensures that students can translate cannabinoid science into safe clinical application rather than demonstrating knowledge alone (Thoma et al., 2023; Harden et al., 1975).

Curriculum Design Framework

A cannabis nursing curriculum may be implemented in several formats depending on institutional goals and program constraints. Programs may offer cannabis education as a stand-alone elective, embed micro-modules across core nursing courses, or develop an advanced certificate pathway for graduate learners or continuing education. Regardless of format, outcome-based curriculum design is recommended to ensure alignment among learning objectives, instructional activities, and assessment methods, thereby strengthening learning transfer and supporting competency development (Biggs & Tang, 2011).

Ten-Week Module Map as an Instructional Template

A structured ten-week model provides a practical and adaptable template for faculty, offering a clear progression from foundational knowledge to clinical application and competency demonstration. This model is designed to support outcome-based and competency-based education across ADN, BSN, and APRN programs, with flexibility for integration into standalone courses, modular curricula, or continuing education formats. Each week builds upon prior content, reinforcing knowledge acquisition, clinical reasoning, and application to patient care.

Week 1 introduces the foundations of cannabis nursing, including a brief history of cannabis in medicine, core legal and ethical principles, and an overview of the endocannabinoid system (ECS). Learning activities may include assigned readings, guided discussion, and introductory lecture content. A baseline quiz assessing ECS concepts and legal frameworks establishes initial competency and identifies knowledge gaps (American Cannabis Nurses Association & American Nurses Association, 2024; National Council of State Boards of Nursing, 2018).

Week 2 expands ECS content through detailed exploration of anandamide and 2-arachidonoylglycerol (2-AG), CB1 and CB2 receptor distribution, and enzymatic regulation. Concepts of ECS tone and clinical endocannabinoid deficiency (CECD) are introduced. Di Marzo's framework, "eat, sleep, relax, forget, protect," serves as a clinical anchor. Experiential learning activities, such as guided visualization, mapping exercises, or reflective journaling, may be incorporated to support retention and integration of complex concepts (National Council of State Boards of Nursing, 2018).

Week 3 focuses on cannabinoid pharmacology, including major phytocannabinoids, selected minor cannabinoids, terpenes, chemotypes, and distinctions between chemotype classification and strain nomenclature. Foundational pharmacokinetics and pharmacodynamics are introduced. A practical assignment, such as developing a patient-friendly cannabinoid reference chart, supports translation of scientific concepts into clinical education tools (Pertwee, 2015).

Week 4 addresses routes of administration and product literacy, emphasizing differences in onset, duration, and bioavailability across inhaled, mucosal, oral, topical, transdermal, and suppository routes. A certificate of analysis (COA) interpretation workshop may be incorporated to strengthen product evaluation and safety literacy, reinforcing alignment between therapeutic intent and product composition (NIST, 2021; Stella et al., 2021).

Week 5 transitions to nursing assessment and care planning, including comprehensive intake, risk screening, contraindications, and patient-centered goal setting. Structured activities such as mock patient interviews and SOAP note documentation exercises allow students to demonstrate clinical reasoning, communication skills, and application of cannabis-specific assessment frameworks (American Cannabis Nurses Association & American Nurses Association, 2024).

Week 6 focuses on dosing strategies and titration principles, including start low and go slow frameworks, CBD-first approaches, biphasic dose-response effects, and the use of product stacking to manage symptom variability. Assessment may include dosing vignettes, case-based problem solving, or short clinical reasoning exercises that require individualized decision-making (Stella et al., 2021).

Week 7 emphasizes safety, adverse effects, monitoring, cannabis use disorder (CUD), cannabinoid hyperemesis syndrome (CHS), and drug–drug interactions. Instruction may combine evidence-based content with case discussion and clinical scenario analysis to reinforce risk assessment and patient safety considerations (National Academies of Sciences, Engineering, and Medicine, 2017).

Week 8 focuses on special populations and high-risk clinical contexts, including geriatric, pediatric, psychiatric, neurologic, rheumatologic, oncologic, palliative care, and chronic pain populations. Learning activities may include population-specific case studies that emphasize individualized care planning, safety considerations, and ethical decision-making (Vinette et al., 2022).

Week 9 supports clinical integration through simulation and case-based synthesis. Faculty may implement objective structured clinical examination (OSCE) scenarios, such as counseling a cannabis-naive patient, conducting a comprehensive assessment, or developing a dosing and monitoring plan. These activities reinforce applied competence and clinical communication skills (Harden et al., 1975; Cowperthwaite, 2020; Jackson et al., 2024).

Week 10 concludes with capstone evaluation, which may include a comprehensive case synthesis paper, development of a patient education plan, or integration of assessment, dosing, and monitoring into a complete care plan. A final examination and program evaluation survey support competency validation and ongoing curricular quality improvement (Oermann & Gaberson, 2024).

Across all ten weeks, alignment between learning objectives, instructional strategies, and evaluation methods ensures that students not only acquire knowledge but also demonstrate the ability to apply cannabinoid science safely and effectively in clinical practice. This structured progression supports the development of clinical competence, critical thinking, and patient-centered care within the emerging field of cannabis nursing.

Competency Framework and Learning Outcomes

This curriculum model aligns with the six essential areas of knowledge identified by the National Council of State Boards of Nursing (2018) and the professional expectations articulated in *Cannabis Nursing: Scope and Standards of Practice* (American Cannabis Nurses Association & American Nurses Association, 2024). Competencies are organized across three integrated domains to support progressive development from foundational knowledge to clinical application and professional practice.

First, curriculum competencies focus on foundational knowledge, including understanding endocannabinoid system physiology, cannabinoid pharmacology, core pharmacokinetic and pharmacodynamic principles, and the ability to interpret certificates of analysis. These competencies ensure that learners develop a scientifically grounded understanding of cannabinoid therapeutics.

Second, clinical competencies emphasize application in patient care. These include conducting cannabis-informed assessments, developing individualized care plans, delivering safety and harm-reduction counseling, and monitoring patient outcomes over time. These competencies support clinical reasoning, patient education, and safe integration of cannabis into care planning.

Third, professional competencies address the broader responsibilities of nursing practice. These include practicing within legal and ethical frameworks, reducing stigma, supporting patient disclosure, and collaborating effectively within interprofessional care environments (Schauer et al., 2021; Philpot et al., 2019).

Cannabis therapeutics intersect with five domains of health: physical, mental, emotional, social, and spiritual. Integrating competencies across these domains supports a whole-person approach to care, allowing students to understand how cannabinoid therapies influence multiple dimensions of health simultaneously. This framework reinforces nursing's holistic model and supports the development of comprehensive, patient-centered care.

Learning outcomes derived from these competencies should be measurable, practice-oriented, and aligned with competency-based education principles. Students are expected not only to demonstrate knowledge acquisition but also to apply cannabinoid science in clinical scenarios, communicate effectively with patients, and integrate safety considerations into decision-making. This competency-based structure ensures that graduates are prepared to deliver safe, evidence-informed, and ethically grounded cannabis care in diverse clinical settings.

OSCE Design for Cannabis Nursing Competency

Objective structured clinical examinations (OSCEs) are widely recognized as a validated method for assessing clinical competence in health professions education, particularly in the evaluation of communication, clinical reasoning, and applied skills (Harden et al., 1975; Oermann & Gaberson, 2024). In cannabis nursing education, OSCEs can be structured as a progressive series of encounters that reflect real-world clinical practice.

An initial OSCE may focus on cannabis-informed intake and risk screening. Students are expected to obtain a comprehensive history, review current medications, identify potential contraindications or red flags such as psychiatric vulnerability or cardiovascular instability, and clarify patient goals. This station emphasizes foundational assessment skills and clinical judgment (Cowperthwaite, 2020; Jackson et al., 2024).

A second OSCE may assess patient counseling and dosing planning. Scenarios may include anxiety and sleep disturbance, chronic pain, cancer symptom management, or geriatric polypharmacy. Students should demonstrate the ability to explain cannabinoid and terpene selection, recommend appropriate routes of administration, outline a start low and go slow titration strategy, review safety precautions, and interpret a certificate of analysis in a patient-centered manner (Jackson et al., 2024).

A third OSCE may evaluate monitoring and clinical troubleshooting. Students are expected to identify adverse effects, adjust dosing, cannabinoid ratios, or routes of administration, recommend supportive measures, and document the encounter appropriately. Standardized patient scenarios may include common challenges such as oral overconsumption, THC-related anxiety, gastrointestinal discomfort associated with CBD, elevated tolerance, or insufficient symptom response. These scenarios reinforce clinical adaptability and safe decision-making in dynamic care contexts (Lapkin et al., 2010).

Rubrics and Standardized Evaluation

Rubrics support fair, objective, and consistent evaluation across OSCEs, written assignments, care plans, and simulation activities. In nursing education, commonly assessed domains include accuracy of knowledge, clinical reasoning, communication and patient education skills, safety and risk identification, professionalism and ethics, and quality of documentation.

Performance is typically assessed using tiered criteria such as exceeds expectations, meets expectations, and needs improvement. This structure supports both formative feedback and summative evaluation, allowing learners to identify strengths and areas for development while ensuring consistency in grading.

Rubrics may be adapted for use across OSCE stations, intake documentation, dosing plans, and patient education assignments. Standardized evaluation tools promote alignment among faculty and clinical instructors, strengthen inter-rater reliability, and reinforce competency-based learning outcomes within cannabis nursing education (Oermann & Gaberson, 2024).

Quiz Bank, Exams, and Program Evaluation Tools

Competency-aligned assessment strategies may include multiple-choice questions, short-answer prompts, clinical scenario interpretation, and certificate of analysis (COA) evaluation activities. These tools should reinforce outcome-based learning principles and assess students' ability to apply cannabis-related knowledge in patient care contexts rather than relying on recall alone (Biggs & Tang, 2011).

Quiz content may include endocannabinoid system function, cannabinoid pharmacokinetics and pharmacodynamics, route-dependent onset and duration, biphasic dose-response effects, drug-drug interactions, adverse effects, assessment and risk screening, and legal and ethical considerations.

A comprehensive final examination may include 50 to 75 questions with a defined minimum competency threshold. For advanced learners, assessment may be supplemented with a brief case defense or structured clinical reasoning activity to further evaluate application of knowledge and decision-making skills (Vinette et al., 2022).

Program evaluation tools, such as student feedback surveys, course evaluations, and competency tracking measures, support ongoing curricular refinement and quality improvement. These tools enable faculty to assess instructional effectiveness, identify gaps in learning, and ensure alignment with evolving clinical standards in cannabis nursing education.

Faculty Development and Instructional Support

Because most nursing faculty have not received formal education in endocannabinoid system physiology or cannabinoid pharmacology, faculty development is essential to ensure consistent, evidence-informed instruction. Research continues to identify knowledge gaps among clinicians and educators, reinforcing the need for structured faculty preparation and ongoing support (Schauer et al., 2021; Philpot et al., 2019).

Programs can reduce educator burden and improve instructional fidelity by providing continuing education opportunities, standardized teaching toolkits such as slide decks, instructional scripts, and OSCE checklists, curated evidence libraries, interprofessional workshops, and partnerships with experienced cannabis clinicians and researchers.

Faculty development supports both educational quality and program sustainability, strengthening the capacity of nursing programs to remain current as evidence, clinical practice, and policy continue to evolve (American Cannabis Nurses Association & American Nurses Association, 2024).

QUALITY ASSURANCE AND SUSTAINABILITY

Ensuring the long-term effectiveness, credibility, and safety of a medical cannabis curriculum requires a structured quality assurance framework paired with a sustainable implementation strategy. Because cannabis science, regulatory policy, and product innovation continue to evolve rapidly, nursing education programs must adopt an adaptive model that supports continuous updating while preserving instructional consistency and clinical rigor. Quality assurance in cannabis nursing education is therefore an ongoing commitment to accuracy, faculty preparedness, and evidence-informed practice.

A foundational component of quality assurance is regular curriculum review. Course content should undergo comprehensive annual evaluation to incorporate new scientific findings, emerging clinical guidelines, changes in state and federal law, evolving safety data, and advancements in product formulation and delivery systems. This process aligns with the professional expectations outlined in **Cannabis Nursing: Scope and Standards of Practice** and the National Council of State Boards of Nursing knowledge domains for medical marijuana education (American Cannabis Nurses Association & American Nurses Association, 2024; National Council of State Boards of Nursing, 2018). Faculty review should extend beyond didactic materials to include OSCE scenarios, simulation cases, care-planning templates, and dosing frameworks, ensuring continued alignment with current evidence and clinical practice standards.

Faculty preparedness represents another critical pillar of quality assurance. Most nursing educators have not received formal training in endocannabinoid system physiology or cannabinoid therapeutics, creating an instructional gap that must be addressed through ongoing professional development (Philpot et al., 2019). Programs should support faculty through continuing education opportunities, simulation training, standardized teaching guides, and interprofessional collaboration with experienced cannabis clinicians. Periodic faculty calibration sessions further promote instructional consistency, reduce variability in student learning experiences, and ensure alignment of competency interpretation across instructors (Schauer et al., 2021).

Standardization of instructional resources strengthens both quality and equity in cannabis education delivery. The use of shared slide decks, case banks, OSCE checklists, and grading rubrics helps ensure that all students receive comparable instruction regardless of faculty assignment or course modality. Regular review of instructional materials and assessment tools supports alignment with stated learning objectives and reinforces accountability within the curriculum (Oermann & Gaberson, 2024).

Student performance monitoring provides essential feedback on program effectiveness and should include both knowledge-based and skills-based indicators, such as pre- and post-course assessments, OSCE outcomes, care-planning assignments, communication evaluations, and safety screening competencies (Harden et al., 1975). Longitudinal follow-up of graduates' confidence and competence in cannabis-related patient encounters can further inform curriculum refinement and program development.

Sustainability of cannabis nursing education requires institutional commitment and thoughtful integration within existing academic structures. Administrative support, legal consultation, and clearly articulated policies regarding cannabis instruction are essential for long-term viability. Strategic partnerships with accredited testing laboratories, community dispensaries, clinical preceptors, and research institutions, including federally supported cannabis patient registry initiatives, can enhance experiential learning opportunities while supporting faculty scholarship and student engagement (Cannabis and Health Research Initiative, 2025).

Financial sustainability may be supported through continuing education program revenue, academic grants, philanthropic contributions, and ethically structured research collaborations. Safeguards must be maintained to ensure educational independence and prevent undue industry influence. Equity and access considerations must remain central to program design, supporting inclusive participation, reducing stigma, and fostering open dialogue among students and faculty. Aligning cannabis nursing education with public health and social justice frameworks strengthens its relevance and ethical foundation (Griffith et al., 2025).

Together, these quality assurance and sustainability strategies create a continuous improvement cycle in which cannabis nursing curricula are regularly reviewed, refined, and reaffirmed. This model aligns with established accreditation processes in nursing education and supports the delivery of cannabis education that remains current, clinically sound, and responsive to both patient and professional needs.

FUTURE DIRECTIONS FOR CANNABIS NURSING EDUCATION

As medical cannabis continues to transition from the margins of healthcare into more formalized clinical and regulatory frameworks, nursing education must evolve in parallel. The expansion of state-level programs, emerging federal rescheduling efforts, and increasing patient demand for evidence-informed guidance underscore the need for continued research, curricular refinement, and workforce development in cannabis nursing.

Future research should prioritize outcomes-based evaluation of cannabis education within nursing programs, including measures of student confidence, clinical competence, and patient safety outcomes following graduation. Comparative studies examining different curricular delivery models, such as integrated micro-modules, stand-alone electives, and post-licensure certificate programs, may help identify effective and scalable approaches across diverse academic settings. Additional research is needed to examine how cannabis education influences interprofessional collaboration, patient disclosure rates, and harm-reduction counseling in clinical practice.

The evolving federal landscape presents new opportunities for rigorous clinical research. As cannabis is reclassified as a Schedule III substance, expanded access to federally funded research may support studies related to dosing, drug–drug interactions, special populations, and long-term outcomes. Nurses are uniquely positioned to contribute to this evidence base through practice-based research, quality improvement initiatives, and patient registries that capture real-world data across care settings.

Educational priorities must also include faculty development and institutional readiness. As cannabis science advances, nursing programs require mechanisms to ensure that educators remain current, supported, and confident in teaching this content. Partnerships with research institutions, professional nursing organizations, and accredited testing laboratories may help strengthen connections between academic preparation, clinical practice, and emerging evidence.

Future directions in cannabis nursing education must remain grounded in ethical practice, equity, and patient-centered care. Addressing stigma, supporting informed disclosure, and advocating for equitable access to evidence-based education are essential components of preparing nurses to meet the needs of diverse patient populations. Continued investment in research, curriculum innovation, and professional development will support nursing education in shaping the responsible integration of cannabinoid therapeutics into contemporary healthcare.

CONCLUSION

This chapter establishes a structured, evidence-informed framework for integrating cannabis therapeutics into nursing education and clinical practice. By synthesizing endocannabinoid system science, cannabinoid pharmacology, safety considerations, legal and ethical literacy, and competency-based instructional design, it provides a comprehensive model for preparing nurses to engage with cannabis as a legitimate component of contemporary healthcare.

As cannabis continues to intersect with clinical care, education, and public policy, the absence of standardized nursing education in this domain represents a critical gap in patient safety and care quality. Nurses are uniquely positioned and increasingly expected to address this gap through informed assessment, patient education, risk reduction, and interdisciplinary collaboration.

The integration of cannabis nursing competencies into academic curricula is not an elective enhancement but an essential evolution of nursing education. Without structured preparation, patients will continue to rely on inconsistent, non-clinical sources of information, increasing the risk of adverse outcomes, missed therapeutic opportunities, and fragmented care.

Advancing cannabis nursing education requires sustained commitment to research, faculty development, curriculum standardization, and policy engagement. Through these efforts, nursing can play a central role in shaping safe, ethical, and equitable models of cannabinoid-based care. In doing so, the profession affirms its responsibility to meet patients where they are, respond to emerging therapeutic landscapes, and lead with both scientific rigor and compassionate care.

REFERENCES

Aizpurua-Olaizola, O., Elezgarai, I., Rico-Barrio, I., Zarandona, I., Etxebarria, N., & Usobiaga, A. (2017). Targeting the endocannabinoid system: Future therapeutic strategies. *Drug Discovery Today*, *22*(1), 105–110. https://www.sciencedirect.com/science/article/abs/pii/S1359644616302926. DOI: 10.1016/j.drudis.2016.08.005 PMID: 27554802

Alcohol Policy Information System. (n.d.). *About cannabis policy.* https://alcoholpolicy.niaaa.nih.gov/about/about-cannabis-policy

Alger, B. (2013). Getting high on the endocannabinoid system. *Cerebrum.* https://www.ncbi.nlm.nih.gov/pmc/articles/PMC3997295/

American Cannabis Nurses Association & American Nurses Association. (2024). *Cannabis nursing: Scope and standards of practice (2nd ed.).* American Nurses Association. https://www.nursingworld.org/nurses-books/cannabis-nursing-scope-and-standards-of-practice/

American Nurses Association. (2016). *Therapeutic use of marijuana and related cannabinoids* [Position statement]. American Nurses Association. https://www.nursingworld.org/~49a8c8/globalassets/practiceandpolicy/ethics/therapeutic-use-of-marijuana-and-related-cannabinoids-position-statement.pdf

American Nurses Association. (2023). *ANA officially recognizes cannabis nursing as a specialty nursing practice* [News release]. American Nurses Association. https://www.nursingworld.org/news/news-releases/2023/ana-officially-recognizes-cannabis-nursing-as-a-specialty-nursing-practice/

Americans for Safe Access. (2025). *Healthcare facility guide to implementing Ryan's Law.* https://www.safeaccessnow.org/ryanslaw_facilityresources

Bell, A. D., MacCallum, C., Margolese, S., Walsh, Z., Wright, P., Daeninck, P. J., Mandarino, E., Lacasse, G., Deol, J. K., De Freitas, L., St Pierre, M., Belle-Isle, L., Gagnon, M., Bevan, S., Sanchez, T., Arlt, S., Monahan-Ellison, M., O'Hara, J., Boivin, M., & Balneaves, L. (2023). Clinical practice guidelines for cannabis and cannabinoid-based medicines in the management of chronic pain and co-occurring conditions. *Cannabis and Cannabinoid Research*, *8*(1). Advance online publication. DOI: 10.1089/can.2021.0156 PMID: 36971587

Bhaskar, A., Bell, A., Boivin, M., Briques, W., Brown, M., Clarke, H., Cyr, C., Eisenberg, E., De Oliveira Silva, R. F., Frohlich, E., Georgius, P., Hogg, M., Horsted, T. I., MacCallum, C. A., Müller-Vahl, K. R., O'Connell, C., Sealey, R., Seibolt, M., Sihota, A., & Moulin, D. E. (2021). Consensus recommendations on dosing and administration of medical cannabis to treat chronic pain: Results of a modified Delphi process. *Journal of Cannabis Research*, *3*(1), 22. Advance online publication. DOI: 10.1186/s42238-021-00073-1 PMID: 34215346

Biggs, J., & Tang, C. (2011). Teaching for quality learning at university (4th ed.). Open University Press. https://www.scirp.org/reference/referencespapers?referenceid=1856033

Bridgeman, M. B., & Abazia, D. T. (2017). Medicinal cannabis: History, pharmacology, and implications for the acute care setting. *P&T : a Peer-Reviewed Journal for Formulary Management*, *42*(3), 180–188. https://www.ncbi.nlm.nih.gov/pmc/articles/PMC5312634/ PMID: 28250701

Bruni, N., Della Pepa, C., Oliaro-Bosso, S., Pessione, E., Gastaldi, D., & Dosio, F. (2018). Cannabinoid delivery systems for pain and inflammation treatment. *Molecules (Basel, Switzerland)*, *23*(10), 2478. DOI: 10.3390/molecules23102478 PMID: 30262735

Cannabis and Health Research Initiative. (2025). *The National Cannabis Study*. https://www.cannabisandhealth.org/national-cannabis-study/

CannaKeys. (2020). *Cannabis chemotypes*. https://cannakeys.com/cannabis-chemotypes/

CannaKeys. (2024). *Endocannabinoid tone*. https://cannakeys.com/endocannabinoid-tone

Cowperthwaite, A. (2020). NLN/Jeffries Simulation Framework for simulated participant methodology. *Clinical Simulation in Nursing*, *42*, 12–21. https://www.nursingsimulation.org/article/S1876-1399(20)30005-0/fulltext. DOI: 10.1016/j.ecns.2019.12.009

Crocq, M. A. (2020). History of cannabis and the endocannabinoid system. *Dialogues in Clinical Neuroscience*, *22*(3), 223–228. https://www.ncbi.nlm.nih.gov/pmc/articles/PMC7605027/. DOI: 10.31887/DCNS.2020.22.3/mcrocq PMID: 33162765

Di Marzo, V. (2014). The endocannabinoid system: Its general strategy of action, tools for its pharmacological manipulation and potential therapeutic exploitation. *Pharmacological Research*, *86*, 1–14. https://www.ncbi.nlm.nih.gov/pmc/articles/PMC3951193/ PMID: 19559360

Drug Enforcement Administration. (n.d.). *Drug scheduling*. https://www.dea.gov/drug-information/drug-scheduling

Fischer, B., Robinson, T., Bullen, C., Curran, V., Jutras-Aswad, D., Medina-Mora, M. E., Pacula, R. L., Rehm, J., Room, R., Van Den Brink, W., & Hall, W. (2022). Lower-risk cannabis use guidelines (LRCUG) for reducing health harms from non-medical cannabis use: A comprehensive evidence and recommendations update. *The International Journal on Drug Policy*, *99*, 103381. https://pubmed.ncbi.nlm.nih.gov/34465496. DOI: 10.1016/j.drugpo.2021.103381 PMID: 34465496

Gertsch, J., Pertwee, R. G., & Di Marzo, V. (2010). Phytocannabinoids beyond the cannabis plant—Do they exist? *British Journal of Pharmacology*, *160*(3), 523–529. DOI: 10.1111/j.1476-5381.2010.00745.x PMID: 20590562

Griffith, S., Kreider, R., & Leung, J. (2025). A coordinated approach to cannabis policy and product safety. *Issues in Science and Technology*. https://issues.org/coordinated-approach-cannabis-policy-safety-griffith-kreider-leung

Harden, R. M., Stevenson, M., Downie, W. W., & Wilson, G. M. (1975). Assessment of clinical competence using objective structured examination. *British Medical Journal*, *1*(5955), 447–451. DOI: 10.1136/bmj.1.5955.447 PMID: 1115966

Jackson, M., McTier, L., Brooks, L. A., & Wynne, R. (2024). Impact of simulation design elements on undergraduate nursing education: A systematic review. *Clinical Simulation in Nursing*, *78*, 1–10. https://www.nursingsimulation.org/article/S1876-1399(24)00011-2/fulltext. DOI: 10.1016/j.ecns.2024.101519

Jaeger, K. (2025b). Federal health programs will cover up to $500 worth of CBD for certain patients by April, Trump official Dr. Oz says. *Marijuana Moment*. https://www.marijuanamoment.net/federal-health-programs-will-cover-up-to-500-worth-of-cbd-for-certain-patients-by-april-trump-official-dr-oz-says/

Kitdumrongthum, S., & Trachootham, D. (2023). Individuality of response to cannabinoids: Challenges in safety and efficacy of cannabis products. *Molecules (Basel, Switzerland)*, *28*(6), 2791. DOI: 10.3390/molecules28062791 PMID: 36985763

Lapkin, S., Levett-Jones, T., Bellchambers, H., & Fernandez, R. (2010). Effectiveness of patient simulation manikins in teaching clinical reasoning skills to undergraduate nursing students: A systematic review. *Clinical Simulation in Nursing*, *6*(6), e207–e222. https://www.sciencedirect.com/science/article/abs/pii/S1876139910001325. DOI: 10.1016/j.ecns.2010.05.005 PMID: 27820553

Lee, M. (2023). *CBD vs. THC*. Project CBD. https://projectcbd.org/what-is-cbd/cbd-vs-thc/

Lucas, C. J., Galettis, P., & Schneider, J. (2018). The Pharmacokinetics and the Pharmacodynamics of Cannabinoids. *British Journal of Clinical Pharmacology*, *84*(11), 2477–2483. DOI: 10.1111/bcp.13710 PMID: 30001569

MacCallum, C. A., & Russo, E. B. (2018). Practical considerations in medical cannabis administration and dosing. *European Journal of Internal Medicine*, *49*, 12–19. https://pubmed.ncbi.nlm.nih.gov/29307505/. DOI: 10.1016/j.ejim.2018.01.004 PMID: 29307505

Mack, E. A. (2020). *Cannabis for health: Become a coach*. AuthorHouse. https://www.authorhouse.com/en/bookstore/bookdetails/812353-cannabis-for-health-become-a-coach

Mackie, K. (2008). Cannabinoid receptors: Where they are and what they do. *Journal of Neuroendocrinology*, *20*(1), 10–14. DOI: 10.1111/j.1365-2826.2008.01671.x PMID: 18426493

McKaig, A., Ridad, A. R. V., Bell, A., McParlane, R., & Quirch, M. (2025). Implementing Ryan's law on an inpatient medical oncology unit. *Clinical Journal of Oncology Nursing*, *29*(1), 86–90. DOI: 10.1188/25.CJON.86-90 PMID: 39933092

Mechoulam, R., & Hanus, L. (2000). A historical overview of chemical research on cannabinoids. *Chemistry and Physics of Lipids*, *108*(1), 1–13. https://www.sciencedirect.com/science/article/abs/pii/S0009308400001845. DOI: 10.1016/S0009-3084(00)00184-5 PMID: 11106779

Moritz College of Law, Ohio State University (OSU). (2025). *Federal marijuana rescheduling: Process and impact*. https://moritzlaw.osu.edu/faculty-and-research/drug-enforcement-and-policy-center/research-and-grants/policy-and-data-analyses/federal-marijuana-rescheduling

National Academies of Sciences, Engineering, and Medicine. (2017). *The health effects of cannabis and cannabinoids: The current state of evidence and recommendations for research*. The National Academies Press. DOI: 10.17226/24625

National Cancer Institute. (n.d.). *Cannabis and cannabinoids (PDQ®)–Health professional version*. https://www.cancer.gov/about-cancer/treatment/cam/hp/cannabis-pdq

National Council of State Boards of Nursing. (2018). The NCSBN national nursing guidelines for medical marijuana. *Journal of Nursing Regulation*, *9*(2), 19–26. DOI: 10.1016/S2155-8256(18)30094-2

National Institute of Standards and Technology. (2025). *NIST tools for cannabis laboratory quality assurance*. https://www.nist.gov/programs-projects/nist-tools-cannabis-laboratory-quality-assurance

Oermann, M. H., & Gaberson, K. B. (2024). *Evaluation and testing in nursing education*. Springer Publishing. https://connect.springerpub.com/content/book/978-0-8261-9489-3

Pertwee, R. G. (2007). The diverse CB1 and CB2 receptor pharmacology of three plant cannabinoids: Δ9-tetrahydrocannabinol, cannabidiol, and Δ9-tetrahydrocannabivarin. *British Journal of Pharmacology*, *153*(2), 199–215. https://www.ncbi.nlm.nih.gov/pmc/articles/PMC2219532/. DOI: 10.1038/sj.bjp.0707442 PMID: 17828291

Pertwee, R. G. (2015). Endocannabinoids and their pharmacological actions. *Handbook of Experimental Pharmacology*, *231*, 1–37. DOI: 10.1007/978-3-319-20825-1_1 PMID: 26408156

Philpot, L. M., Ebbert, J. O., & Hurt, R. T. (2019). A survey of the attitudes, beliefs, and knowledge about medical cannabis among primary care providers. *BMC Family Practice*, *20*(1), 17. DOI: 10.1186/s12875-019-0906-y PMID: 30669979

Pisanti, S., Malfitano, A. M., Ciaglia, E., Lamberti, A., Ranieri, R., Cuomo, G., Abate, M., Faggiana, G., Proto, M. C., Fiore, D., Laezza, C., & Bifulco, M. (2017). Cannabidiol: State of the art and new challenges for therapeutic applications. *Pharmacology & Therapeutics*, *175*, 133–150. DOI: 10.1016/j.pharmthera.2017.02.041 PMID: 28232276

Reimann-Philipp, U., Speck, M., Orser, C., Johnson, S., Hilyard, A., Turner, H., Stokes, A. J., & Small-Howard, A. L. (2019). Cannabis chemovar nomenclature misrepresents chemical and genetic diversity: Survey of variations in chemical profiles and genetic markers in Nevada medical cannabis samples. *Cannabis and Cannabinoid Research*, *5*(3), 215–230. DOI: 10.1089/can.2018.0063 PMID: 32923659

Russo, E. B. (2016). Clinical endocannabinoid deficiency reconsidered: Current research supports the theory in migraine, fibromyalgia, irritable bowel, and other treatment-resistant syndromes. *Cannabis and Cannabinoid Research*, *1*(1), 154–165. DOI: 10.1089/can.2016.0009 PMID: 28861491

Russo, E. B. (2019). The case for the entourage effect and conventional breeding of clinical cannabis: No "strain," no gain. *Frontiers in Plant Science*, *9*, 1969. DOI: 10.3389/fpls.2018.01969 PMID: 30687364

Russo, E. B., & Marcu, J. (2017). Cannabis pharmacology: The usual suspects and a few promising leads. *Advances in Pharmacology*, *80*, 67–134. DOI: 10.1016/bs.apha.2017.03.004 PMID: 28826544

Schauer, G. L., Njai, R., & Grant, A. M. (2021). Clinician beliefs and practices related to cannabis. *Cannabis and Cannabinoid Research*, *7*(4), 508–515. DOI: 10.1089/can.2020.0165 PMID: 33998899

Sliwoski, V. (2025). *Notes on the federal prohibition of intoxicating hemp*. Harris Sliwoski LLP. https://harris-sliwoski.com/cannalawblog/notes-on-the-federal-prohibition-of-intoxicating-hemp/

Statista. (2025). *Number of Americans who used marijuana in the past year (2009–2024)*. https://www.statista.com/statistics/611714/marijuana-use-during-past-year-in-the-us/

Stella, B., Baratta, F., Della Pepa, C., Arpicco, S., Gastaldi, D., & Dosio, F. (2021). Cannabinoid formulations and delivery systems: Current and future options to treat pain. *Drugs*, *81*(13), 1513–1557. DOI: 10.1007/s40265-021-01579-x PMID: 34480749

Substance Abuse and Mental Health Services Administration (SAMHSA). (n.d.). *Marijuana: The risks are real.* https://www.samhsa.gov/substance-use/learn/marijuana/risks

The White House. (2025). *Increasing medical marijuana and cannabidiol research.* https://www.whitehouse.gov/presidential-actions/2025/12/increasing-medical-marijuana-and-cannabidiol-research/

Thoma, B., Abbott, C., & Snell, L. (2023). The future of the CanMEDS physician competency framework. *Canadian Medical Education Journal, 14*(1), 1–3. https://pmc.ncbi.nlm.nih.gov/articles/PMC10042786/. DOI: 10.36834/cmej.77098 PMID: 36998483

Vinette, B., Côté, J., El-Akhras, A., Mrad, H., Chicoine, G., & Bilodeau, K. (2022). Routes of administration, reasons for use, and approved indications of medical cannabis in oncology: A scoping review. *BMC Cancer, 22*(1), 937. Advance online publication. DOI: 10.1186/s12885-022-09378-7 PMID: 35331185

Volkow, N. D., Baler, R. D., Compton, W. M., & Weiss, S. R. B. (2014). Adverse health effects of marijuana use. *The New England Journal of Medicine, 370*(23), 2219–2227. https://www.ncbi.nlm.nih.gov/pmc/articles/PMC4827335/. DOI: 10.1056/NEJMra1402309 PMID: 24897085

Woodbridge, M., Sarma, N., & Vaillencourt, D. (2024). *Cannabis quality: The need for science-based global harmonization of standards.* U.S. Pharmacopeia. https://www.usp.org/sites/default/files/usp/document/our-work/DS/uspastm-cannabis-quality-recommendations.pdf

Zolotov, Y. (2025). Developing medical cannabis competencies: A consensus statement. *JAMA Network Open.* https://jamanetwork.com/journals/jamanetworkopen/fullarticle/2839750

Zolotov, Y., Grinstein Cohen, O., Findley, P. A., Reznik, A., Isralowitz, R., & Willard, S. (2021). Attitudes and knowledge about medical cannabis among Israeli and American nursing students. *Nurse Education Today, 102*, 104929. https://www.sciencedirect.com/science/article/abs/pii/S0260691721000460. DOI: 10.1016/j.nedt.2021.104789 PMID: 33571928

KEY TERMS AND DEFINITIONS

Biphasic Dose-Response: A pharmacological phenomenon in which cannabinoids, particularly THC, produce different or opposing effects at low versus high doses, with lower doses often therapeutic and higher doses potentially leading to diminished benefit or adverse outcomes.

Cannabis Nursing: A specialty area of nursing practice focused on the assessment, education, risk reduction, and clinical integration of cannabis and cannabinoid-based therapies within ethical, legal, and evidence-informed frameworks.

Certificate of Analysis (COA): A laboratory-issued document that verifies cannabinoid content, terpene profile, and contaminant screening results for a specific product batch, supporting quality assurance, dosing accuracy, and patient safety.

Chemotype: A classification system that categorizes cannabis plants based on their dominant cannabinoid profile rather than strain name, commonly including Chemotype I (THC-dominant), Chemotype II (balanced THC:CBD), and Chemotype III (CBD-dominant).

Endocannabinoid System (ECS): A physiological regulatory network composed of cannabinoid receptors, endogenous cannabinoids, and metabolic enzymes that supports homeostasis across neurological, immune, endocrine, and gastrointestinal systems.

Harm Reduction: A patient-centered approach that prioritizes safety, risk mitigation, and informed decision-making by reducing adverse outcomes associated with substance use rather than requiring abstinence.

Minimum Effective Dose (MED): The lowest dose of a cannabinoid or cannabis-based product that produces the desired therapeutic effect while minimizing adverse effects, serving as a guiding principle for safe and individualized dosing.

Pharmacodynamics: The study of how cannabinoids interact with receptors, enzymes, and signaling pathways to produce therapeutic and adverse effects.

Pharmacokinetics: The study of how cannabinoids are absorbed, distributed, metabolized, and eliminated, influencing onset, duration, and intensity of effects.

Phytocannabinoids: Biologically active compounds produced by the Cannabis sativa plant that interact with the endocannabinoid system and other molecular targets to influence physiological processes.

Routes of Administration: The methods by which cannabis-based products are delivered into the body, including inhalation, oral ingestion, sublingual, topical, transdermal, and suppository routes, each with distinct clinical implications.

Terpenes: Aromatic compounds found in cannabis and other plants that contribute to scent and flavor and may modulate cannabinoid effects through synergistic pharmacological interactions.

Chapter 14
The Cannabis Nurse:
A Dawn of a New Age

Llewellyn Dawn Smith
http://orcid.org/0009-0000-1217-6992
American Cannabis Nurses Association, USA

ABSTRACT

The emergence of cannabis nursing as a recognized specialty reflects a pivotal shift in healthcare policy and practice across the World. As more localities legalize cannabis for medicinal and adult use, nurses are expected to support patients who incorporate cannabis into their health and wellness choices. This chapter examines the evolving role of the cannabis nurse considering the American Nurses Association's (ANA) recognition of cannabis nursing as a specialty practice and the publication of the Cannabis Nursing Scope and Standards by the American Cannabis Nurses Association (ACNA). It emphasizes the urgent need to integrate cannabis education into academic curricula, guided by the National Council of State Boards of Nursing (NCSBN) National Guidelines for Medical Marijuana. With individuals consuming cannabis for a range of reasons, healthcare professionals must be equipped with foundational knowledge of the endocannabinoid neuromodulator system, and the clinical implications of cannabis consumption to provide safe, ethical, and evidence-informed care.

OBJECTIVES

1. Describe the legal and regulatory changes that have contributed to the emergence of cannabis nursing as a specialty.
2. Review the NCSBN Medical Marijuana Guidelines and their relevance to nursing practice and licensure.
3. Highlight the significance of the American Nurses Association's recognition and the Cannabis Nursing Scope and Standards authored by the American Cannabis Nurses Association.
4. Advocate for the inclusion of cannabis-related content in undergraduate and graduate nursing curricula.
5. Explain the importance of understanding the endocannabinoid system in relation to patient safety, pharmacology, and symptom management.

DOI: 10.4018/979-8-3373-7287-7.ch014

6. Identify the responsibilities of nurses in caring individuals who use cannabis for medicinal and adult use purposes.

INTRODUCTION

Cannabis nursing has emerged as a vital specialty amid evolving healthcare policies and widespread legalization of cannabis across the World. Nurses increasingly encounter patients using cannabis for medicinal and wellness purposes, necessitating specialized knowledge and competencies. This chapter explores the development of cannabis nursing as a recognized specialty, emphasizing the American Nurses Association's (ANA) formal recognition and the *American Cannabis Nurses Association's (ACNA) Cannabis Nursing Scope and Standards*. It highlights the critical need to incorporate cannabis education into nursing and medical curricula, guided by the *National Council of State Boards of Nursing (NCSBN) National Nursing Guidelines for Medical Marijuana*. While many advocacy and professional groups contribute to the wider cannabis health landscape, this chapter focuses specifically on the nursing organizations responsible for establishing standards, guiding regulation, and shaping the professional identity of cannabis nursing. Understanding the endocannabinoid system (ECS) and its clinical implications is essential for nurses to provide safe, ethical, and evidence-informed care in this emerging practice. This chapter examines six core objectives, drawn from the NCSBN (2018) Guidelines, that define the specialty, including legal and regulatory literacy, foundational knowledge of the ECS and cannabis pharmacology, comprehensive assessment of patient needs and risks, nonjudgmental patient education, monitor for therapeutic and adverse effects, and accurate documentation and communication. Together, these objectives set the stage for a detailed examination of legal frameworks, educational guidelines, clinical responsibilities, and ethical considerations shaping the new age of cannabis nursing.

BACKGROUND

Cannabis nursing has emerged from a convergence of scientific discovery, shifting public healthcare policy, and evolving patient behavior across the World. As more jurisdictions adopt medicinal and adult use cannabis laws, nurses increasingly encounter health care consumers who incorporate cannabis into their health and wellness decisions. This trend has highlighted longstanding gaps in professional preparation, particularly the absence of foundational education on the endocannabinoid neuromodulator system and the clinical implications of cannabis consumption (Malka, 2022; NCSBN, 2018; Parmelee R. A., 2022). Early nursing scholarship emphasized harm reduction, health care consumer advocacy, and the importance of understanding cannabis within broader frameworks of wellness, physiology, symptom management, and social context (American Cannabis Nurses Association, 2017; Maynard, 2025). These early contributions established the groundwork for a more formalized specialty, later advanced through the development of the Cannabis Nursing Scope and Standards and the ANA's recognition of cannabis nursing as a specialty practice (American Cannabis Nurses Association, 2017; American Cannabis Nurses Association & American Nurses Association, 2024).

Professional organizations have since advanced this foundation through structured guidance and competency development. The National Council of State Boards of Nursing issued the *National Nursing Guidelines for Medical Marijuana in 2018*, establishing minimum expectations for all nurses who care for individuals using cannabis. Building on this regulatory groundwork, the American Cannabis Nurses Association (ACNA) initiated the first *Cannabis Nursing: Scope and Standards of Practice* in 2017 under Dr. Carey Clark's leadership, providing the earliest formal articulation of cannabis-specific nursing competencies. This document was revised in 2019 to include the advanced practice registered nurse (APRN) role, reflecting the expanding clinical responsibilities within the specialty. In 2023, under the leadership of Llewellyn Dawn Smith, Dr. Deanna Sommers and dedicated members of the ACNA Credentialing Committee, the American Nurses Association (ANA) formally recognized cannabis nursing as a specialty practice, an acknowledgment that preceded the full joint publication of the *Cannabis Nursing: Scope and Standards of Practice* by ANA and ACNA in 2024. This progression marked a pivotal moment in the profession, signaling that cannabis nursing requires distinct knowledge, skills, and ethical considerations beyond those traditionally included in nursing curricula.

Regardless of these advances, significant cannabis knowledge gaps remain among practicing nurses across the world. Many faculty and clinicians completed their education before cannabis or the endocannabinoid system (ECS) were addressed in academic programs, leaving them without essential knowledge of cannabinoid pharmacology, product variability, potential drug interactions, and the influence of the ECS on human physiology (NCSBN, 2018; Malka, 2022; Parmelee R. A., 2022). Nurses frequently report uncertainty when discussing cannabis with health care consumers, particularly when asked about safe product selection, dosing considerations, or the differences between medicinal and adult-use markets (King D., 2021; Parmelee R. A., 2022). These gaps are intensified by rapidly evolving regulations, inconsistent terminology, and the wide range of cannabis products available in global markets. Additionally, many nurses and medical professionals carry inherited biases shaped by decades of prohibition, which must be intentionally unlearned and replaced with tolerance, understanding, and a commitment to nonjudgmental practice (American Cannabis Nurses Association, 2017; American Cannabis Nurses Association, 2019; American Cannabis Nurses Association & American Nurses Association, 2024). Without structured continuing education, nurses often rely on informal or non-evidence-based sources of information, which may not reflect current science or regulatory guidance (Maynard, 2025; Russo E., 2025).

Together, these developments illustrate the need for a clear and comprehensive framework that supports nurses in providing safe, ethical, and evidence informed care to health care consumers who use cannabis. They also establish the conditions that make the specialty's core objectives essential to contemporary nursing practice. The following section examines these objectives in depth and situates them within the broader landscape of global health transformation and the responsibilities of nurses in a rapidly evolving therapeutic environment.

Objective 1: Legal and Regulatory Changes Shaping Cannabis Nursing

Cannabis nursing has emerged in response to sweeping legal and regulatory shifts that have transformed access to cannabis across the world. These changes have reshaped health care consumer behavior, influenced institutional policy, and created new expectations for nursing practice. Understanding this evolving landscape is essential for nurses who support individuals using cannabis for wellness and symptom management.

Across the United States, cannabis laws have evolved rapidly, with most states now operating comprehensive medical cannabis programs and nearly half authorizing adult-use markets. Despite this broad expansion, significant variation persists across jurisdictions, creating a fragmented national policy landscape that directly affects nursing practice. This patchwork system requires nurses to remain informed about state-specific regulations, federal restrictions, and institutional policies that influence clinical decision-making. As access has expanded, the likelihood that nurses will encounter health care consumers who use cannabis has increased substantially, making legal literacy a foundational component of safe and ethical practice (NCSBN, 2018). National data underscore this reality: approximately one in five U.S. adults report using cannabis within the past year, highlighting the importance of nursing competence in this area (Substance Abuse and Mental Health Services Administration, 2023).

To understand the current regulatory environment, it is important to consider the historical forces that shaped cannabis policy. Cannabis products were widely used in Western medicine throughout the nineteenth century and was listed in the *U.S. Pharmacopeia* from 1850 to 1942 (Lee, 2012). Its therapeutic applications were well documented, and nurses and physicians used cannabis preparations to manage pain, promote sleep, and support gastrointestinal health. Florence Nightingale's embrace of compassionate botanical remedies offers a powerful historical bridge to the values that now guide modern cannabis nursing. See Spotlight 1 for her views on compassionate cannabis care. Globally, cannabis held a prominent place in traditional healing systems, including Ayurvedic medicine, Chinese herbal practice, and African and Middle Eastern health traditions. These uses reflected long-standing knowledge systems that recognized cannabis as a tool for physical and spiritual well-being (Lee, 2012).

Spotlight 1. Florence Nightingale and Compassionate Cannabis Care

Florence Nightingale practiced during a period when cannabis was an accepted component of Western and traditional medicine. Historical accounts indicate that she was familiar with Indian preparations such as bhang, which were used to ease digestive discomfort, pain, and sleep disturbances. Nightingale reportedly supported its use to relieve her sister's chronic symptoms, reflecting her commitment to individualized, compassionate care (Smith, 2021). Her openness to botanical medicine stresses an important truth for contemporary nurses. Long before cannabis became entangled in political agendas, it was recognized as a legitimate therapeutic tool. Nightingale's legacy invites modern nurses to approach cannabis with curiosity, humility, and a willingness to engage evidence rather than stigma.

This historical acceptance shifted dramatically in the twentieth century. Early regulatory actions, such as the 1906 Pure Food and Drug Act, introduced federal labeling requirements for cannabis-containing medicines but did not restrict access (Congress, 1906). By the 1910s and 1920s, several U.S. states enacted prohibitions influenced by xenophobic and racialized narratives that associated cannabis use with Mexican and other immigrant communities (Lee, 2012; Mills, 2003; O'Leary-Randall, 2014). These fears were amplified by sensationalist media campaigns and federal messaging led by the Federal Bureau of Narcotics under Commissioner Harry Anslinger and later became known as 'Reefer Madness'. Propaganda of the Prohibition era transformed these policy shifts into a moral panic that reshaped public perception and cast a long shadow over nursing practice (Alexander, 2010; Sloman, 1998). The 1937 Marihuana Tax Act effectively criminalized cannabis at the federal level, and in 1942 cannabis was removed from the U.S. Pharmacopeia, severing its formal connection to medical practice (Bonnie, 1974; Lee, 2012; O'Leary-Randall, 2014).

Sidebar 1. Reefer Madness and Its Lasting Impact on Nursing Practice

Harry Anslinger, the first commissioner of the Federal Bureau of Narcotics, shaped much of the twentieth-century narrative surrounding cannabis. His campaign, later known as the *Reefer Madness* era, relied on sensationalized claims, racialized messaging, and strategic alliances with media figures such as William Randolph Hearst. These efforts reframed cannabis as a social threat rather than a therapeutic agent, even though cannabis has its long history of medicinal use (Alexander, 2010; Lee, 2012). The resulting fear-based messaging influenced public perception for generations and laid the groundwork for punitive drug policies that disproportionately targeted marginalized communities.

Anslinger's influence extended far beyond U.S. borders. His advocacy contributed to the inclusion of cannabis in the 1961 United Nations Single Convention on Narcotic Drugs (United Nations, 1961), embedding prohibitionist frameworks into global policy and pressuring countries with longstanding medicinal traditions to adopt restrictive laws (Mills, 2003). These policies disrupted traditional healing practices, criminalized communities, and silenced scientific inquiries, creating a ripple effect that shaped international health systems for decades.

For nurses, traces of the prohibition era (Clark, 2021; Sloman, 1998) persist in modern nursing attitudes and practices. Decades of stigma contributed to the exclusion of cannabis from nursing curricula, limited opportunities for research, and reinforced biases that continue to affect health care consumers and professionals (American Cannabis Nurses Association, 2017; King D. G., 2024; Maynard, 2025; Parmelee R. A., 2022). Nurses often enter practice without foundational knowledge of cannabinoid pharmacology, the endocannabinoid neuromodulator system, or the therapeutic potential of cannabis. This historical silence has created persistent gaps in clinical confidence and ethical clarity. Understanding the origins of these narratives is essential for nurses committed to evidence informed, equitable, and nonjudgmental care. By recognizing how prohibition shaped professional education and public perception, nurses can more effectively unlearn inherited biases and support health care consumers with compassion and integrity.

"Before cannabis became a political symbol, it was a tool of comfort, dignity, and healing" – Llewellyn 2026

Internationally, prohibition gained momentum through treaties such as the 1925 International Opium Convention (United Nations, 1925) and the 1961 United Nations Single Convention on Narcotic Drugs (United Nations, 1961), which classified cannabis as a Schedule I substance. These policies pressured countries with long-standing medicinal and spiritual cannabis traditions to adopt restrictive laws, contributing to global criminalization and the suppression of traditional healing practices. These international agreements transformed localized restrictions into a coordinated global regime that accelerated the spread of cannabis prohibition across continents, see Table 1 for a Cannabis Prohibition Timeline.

Table 1. Cannabis prohibition timeline (1800-1970s)

Cannabis Prohibition Timeline (1800-1970s)		
Year	**Event**	**Description**
1830	Brazil bans cannabis	First national prohibition, targeting slaves for cultural uses.
1840-1860	Colonial bans in Mauritius, Sri Lanka, Egypt	European powers restrict cannabis in colonies, citing moral and racial concerns.
1906	U.S. Pure Food and Drug Act	First federal regulation requiring labeling of cannabis in medicines.
1910-1920s	Statewide level bans in U.S.	Driven by anti-Mexican sentiment post-Mexican Revolution

continued on following page

Table 1. Continued

Cannabis Prohibition Timeline (1800-1970s)		
Year	**Event**	**Description**
1930s	Federal Bureau of Narcotics established	First established to enforce alcohol prohibition and later cannabis prohibition. Led by Harry Anslinger, who spearheaded the anti-cannabis campaign known as Reefer Madness.
1937	Marihuana Tax Act	Effectively criminalizes cannabis in the U.S. using taxation and penalties.
1942	Cannabis removed from the U.S. Pharmacopeia	No longer recognized as a formal medical treatment.
1961	United Nations Single Convention on Narcotic Drugs	Global classification of cannabis as a Schedule I narcotic based on Anslinger's influence internationally.
1970	U.S. Controlled Substances Act	Cannabis designated as a substance with high abuse potential and "no medical use"
1972	Protocol Amending the 1961 Convention	Reinforces global prohibition framework and restricts medical research.
2026	Executive Order by President Trump to move cannabis to Schedule III	First major federal reversal of prohibition policy since 1970! The rescheduling process remains ongoing, pending regulatory review.

(Clarke, 2013; Lee, 2012; Mills, 2003; Smith, 2021)

The modern resurgence of cannabis in health care began with scientific discovery rather than legislation in the mid 1900s, researchers identified the endocannabinoid neuromodulator system, revealing a complex network of receptors and endogenous compounds that regulate pain, mood, appetite, immune function, and homeostasis. This discovery provided a biological foundation for understanding cannabis's therapeutic potential. Despite its significance, the endocannabinoid system remains largely absent from nursing and medical education, perpetuating outdated stigma and limiting evidence informed care (Malka, 2022; Russo E., 2025).

Legal reform accelerated in 1996 when California passed Proposition 215, becoming the first U.S. state to legalize medical cannabis (Lee, 2012). This policy milestone was driven by health care consumers living with HIV/AIDS, cancer, and chronic pain, who witnessed the therapeutic impact firsthand, often supporting consumers informally while lacking institutional guidance or legal protections. Proposition 215 marked a turning point that reframed cannabis as a legitimate therapeutic option and opened pathways for broader reform (Maynard, 2025).

Following California's lead, states across the country developed medical cannabis programs with varying regulatory structures. This expansion created opportunities for improved access but also introduced inconsistencies that complicated nursing practice. Although nurses serve as the most trusted point of contact for health care consumers seeking guidance, they often lack formal education in cannabinoid pharmacology, product variability, and potential drug interactions (Parmelee R. A., 2022). The continued absence of standardized training contributed to uncertainty and limited the ability of nurses to provide evidence informed recommendations.

Globally, countries have adopted diverse regulatory models that offer valuable insights into nursing practice. Canada legalized medical cannabis nationally in 2001 and adult use in 2018, integrating nursing roles into clinical guidance (Health Canada, 2018). Israel developed a research-driven program grounded in scientific discovery (Aviram, 2025). Germany implemented a pharmacy-based model with insurance reimbursement, and Thailand introduced a system that integrates traditional medicine with community-based care (Chokwanich, 2022; Federal Institute for Drugs and Medical Devices, 2020).

These international approaches highlight the importance of regulatory clarity, standardized education, and culturally responsive practice (Aviram, 2025; Chokwanich, 2022; Health Canada, 2018).

As legal reforms continue to expand, nurses must navigate complex intersections of policy, ethics, and professional responsibility. They must understand how cannabis laws influence scope of practice, licensure, workplace policy, and consumer advocacy. They must also unlearn inherited biases shaped by decades of prohibition and replace them with tolerance, understanding, and a commitment to non-judgmental care. Legal literacy, ethical reflection, and evidence informed education are essential for supporting health care consumers who use cannabis within the bounds of the law.

Objective 2: Review the NCSBN Medical Marijuana Guidelines and Their Relevance to Nursing Practice and Licensure

The National Council of State Boards of Nursing (NCSBN) published the *National Nursing Guidelines for Medical Marijuana* in 2018, marking the first comprehensive regulatory document to formally address the intersection of cannabis care and nursing licensure. Released during a period of rapid state-level legalization and ongoing federal prohibition, the guidelines provided clarity for nurses navigating an emerging and often contradictory practice environment. By situating cannabis within a professional and regulatory framework, the NCSBN established both protection and responsibility for nurses as they engage with this evolving area of care.

The NCSBN guidelines are organized into two major components:

- Legislation, literature review, and nursing implications
- Nursing guidelines for medical marijuana consumers

Together, these sections articulate a foundational framework for safe, ethical, and evidence-informed nursing practice. Central to the document are six essential areas of knowledge that all licensed nurses must understand (NCSBN, 2018, p. S19):

1. The nurse shall have a working knowledge of the current state of legalization of medical and recreational cannabis use.
2. The nurse shall have a working knowledge of the jurisdiction's MMP.
3. The nurse shall have an understanding of the endocannabinoid system, cannabinoid receptors, cannabinoids, and the interactions between them.
4. The nurse shall have an understanding of cannabis pharmacology and the research associated with the medical use of cannabis.
5. The nurse shall be able to identify the safety considerations for patient use of cannabis.
6. The nurse shall approach the patient without judgment regarding the patient's choice of treatment or preferences in managing pain and other distressing symptoms.

These competencies extend beyond technical skills. They reflect a professional commitment to licensure protection, patient advocacy, and the ethical delivery of care. The guidelines emphasize mastery of the endocannabinoid system, cannabis pharmacology, drug interactions, patient education, documentation, and professional boundaries, establishing a practice framework that empowers nurses to support consumers confidently and safely. By defining these expectations at the regulatory level, the NCSBN Guidelines anchor cannabis nursing practice in a framework that protects licensure while elevating professional accountability, see sidebar, The Regulatory Significance of the NCSBN MMJ Guidelines (2018).

Sidebar 2. The Regulatory Significance of the NCSBN MMJ Guidelines (2018)

The 2018 *National Nursing Guidelines for Medical Marijuana* represent the first formal acknowledgment by a U.S. nursing regulatory body that cannabis care intersects directly with licensure, scope of practice, and professional accountability. Developed during a period of rapid state-level legalization and persistent federal prohibition, the guidelines provided clarity for nurses navigating an emerging and often contradictory practice environment. Key regulatory contributions include:

- Establishing licensure-aligned expectations for all levels of nursing personnel
- Defining six essential knowledge domains required for safe cannabis care
- Affirming the need for cannabis education in nursing curricula
- Providing a transferable framework adaptable to international health systems
- Reinforcing professional boundaries and the nurse's duty to protect safety

The NCSBN (2018) also highlights the need for ongoing professional development and the integration of cannabis education into nursing curricula. This call to action highlights the widening gap between rapidly changing cannabis policies and the slower evolution of nursing education. For practicing nurses, the guidelines serve as both compass and catalyst: a reminder that staying informed, adaptable, and evidence-driven is essential in a shifting legal and clinical landscape.

Almost a decade old and in need of updates to reflect new research, consumption methods, and policy developments, the NCSBN (2018) guidelines remain the most comprehensive regulatory foundation available. Their relevance extends beyond nursing into academia and other health professions, offering a model for how regulatory clarity can support patient safety, licensure protection, and interprofessional collaboration.

"Cannabis care is nursing care, and the NCSBN MMJ Guidelines remain the profession's clearest compass for safe, ethical, and licensure-protected practice." – Llewellyn 2026

While rooted in the U.S. regulatory environment, the NCSBN (2018) guidelines offer a transferable framework for international nursing practice. Countries with emerging cannabis policies can adapt these competencies to their own legal, cultural, and educational contexts.

- Canada, where cannabis is federally legalized, reinforces nursing accountability through the Lower-Risk Cannabis Use Guidelines (Fischer, 2017) and provincial standards such as Cannabis for Medical Purposes: Standards for Nurse Practitioners (College of Registered Nurses of Alberta (CRNA), 2022).
- European nations experimenting with medical cannabis programs and regulatory pilots draw on similar principles to guide licensure standards and curriculum development (Hoch, 2025).
- Low-and middle-income countries (LMICs), where nurses are often the first point of contact for patients, can use the guidelines to integrate cannabis care into sensitive frameworks that bridge traditional and modern therapeutic practices (World Health Organization, 2025).

Across these diverse systems, the underlying principle remains consistent: all licensed nursing personnel must integrate cannabis-related competencies appropriate to their role to ensure safe, ethical, and evidence-informed care. Persistent misunderstandings about the NCSBN Guidelines continue to shape nursing practice, making it essential to dispel myths that obscure their true regulatory intent, see the Myth-Buster Box 1, Common Misconceptions About the NCSBN MMJ Guidelines.

Myth-Busting Box 1. Common Misconceptions About the NCSBN MMJ Guidelines

Myth 1: "The NCSBN guidelines authorize nurses to recommend or prescribe cannabis."
Fact: They do not. Cannabis is a Schedule I substance and cannot be prescribed, and any authority to recommend it is determined solely by state law, not by NCSBN. The guidelines outline nursing competencies; they do not expand scope of practice.
Myth 2: "Only APRNs need to understand cannabis pharmacology."
Fact: All licensed nursing personnel require foundational knowledge to ensure safe care.
Myth 3: "Cannabis care is optional unless a nurse works in a specialty area."
Fact: Cannabis use is widespread; every nurse may encounter medical and adult-use cannabis health care consumers.
Myth 4: "Documentation is only necessary for medically authorized cannabis consumers."
Fact: Nurses must document all cannabis use, both medical and adult-use.
Myth 5: "The 2018 guidelines are outdated and irrelevant."
Fact: While updates are needed, they remain the most comprehensive regulatory framework available.

The Six Essentials

The NCSBN (2018) identifies six essential areas of competence that guide safe, ethical, and evidence-informed nursing care related to medical cannabis. These Essentials are presented in Table 2 using the exact wording from pp. S19–S20. Briefly, they encompass legal literacy, pharmacologic understanding, patient assessment, education, monitoring, and documentation/communication.

Table 2. The six essentials at a glance

Exact NCSBN Wording (pp. S19-S20)	Relevance to Licensure & Practice
1.The nurse shall have a working knowledge of the current state of legalization of medical and recreational cannabis use.	Understanding legalization status protects nurses from practicing outside the law, ensures compliance with jurisdictional requirements, and prevents licensure risk related to misunderstanding federal vs. state authority.
2.The nurse shall have a working knowledge of the jurisdiction's MMP.	Knowledge of the state's medical marijuana program ensures nurses follow correct procedures, documentation requirements, and scope-specific responsibilities, reducing liability and supporting safe patient guidance.
3. The nurse shall have an understanding of the endocannabinoid system, cannabinoid receptors, cannabinoids, and the interactions between them.	ECS literacy enables nurses to provide evidence-informed education, anticipate therapeutic responses, and recognize adverse effects, all of which support safe practice and professional accountability.
4. The nurse shall have an understanding of cannabis pharmacology and the research associated with the medical use of cannabis.	Pharmacologic knowledge helps nurses identify risks, drug interactions, and contraindications, ensuring safe patient care and aligning practice with evidence-based standards expected by regulatory bodies.

continued on following page

Table 2. Continued

Exact NCSBN Wording (pp. S19-S20)	Relevance to Licensure & Practice
5. The nurse shall be able to identify the safety considerations for patient use of cannabis.	Recognizing safety considerations protects patients from harm and shields nurses from liability by ensuring they can identify red flags, misuse, impairment, and situations requiring escalation or intervention.
6. The nurse shall approach the patient without judgment regarding the patient's choice of treatment or preferences in managing pain and other distressing symptoms.	A nonjudgmental approach upholds ethical standards, supports therapeutic communication, and aligns with regulatory expectations for unbiased, patient-centered care—critical for maintaining trust and professional integrity.

(NCSBN, 2018)

Together, the six essentials outlined in the NCSBN Medical Marijuana Guidelines form a comprehensive framework for nursing practice in cannabis care. They embody the professional values of safety, ethics, and evidence-informed clinical judgment. The guidelines also establish a holistic competency model that protects licensure while advancing consumer safety. These essentials highlight nursing's dual responsibility: to empower health care consumers with knowledge and advocacy, and to safeguard the integrity of nursing practice within evolving healthcare systems. Even as cannabis policies and research continue to evolve, the six essentials remain a foundational compass for nurses worldwide, guiding practice with clarity, accountability, and compassion (NCSBN, 2018)

Objective 3: Recognition of Cannabis Nursing as a Specialty

The American Cannabis Nurses Association (ACNA) and the American Nurses Association (ANA) now stand at the forefront of a pivotal shift in nursing practice. Their collaborative efforts have created the structural foundation for cannabis nursing as an emerging specialty while preparing the profession for a new age of evidence-informed education and clinical guidance. ACNA's development of the *Cannabis Nursing: Scope and Standards of Practice* (American Cannabis Nurses Association & American Nurses Association, 2024) represents the first comprehensive framework that defines the roles, responsibilities, and competencies required for safe and ethical cannabis care. This document establishes essential knowledge domains, including the endocannabinoid system, assessment, and symptom management, and it emphasizes the importance of research, advocacy, and professional accountability.

"Cannabis nursing is entering a new age defined by clarity, collaboration, and global relevance." – Llewellyn 2026

ANA's 2024 recognition of cannabis nursing practice as a specialty marks a transformative milestone. This endorsement affirms the distinct expertise of cannabis nurses and acknowledges the growing need for clinicians who are prepared to support health care consumers using cannabinoid-based therapies. ANA's recognition has accelerated the development of educational pathways, strengthened the profession's commitment to evidence-informed practice, and signaled to institutions and policymakers that cannabis nursing is an essential component of contemporary health care. As part of this evolving landscape, ACNA and ANA are engaged in ongoing collaboration to address the profession's knowledge gaps and to support nurses who seek reliable, structured education in this emerging specialty practice. These developments position ACNA to expand its global influence and to guide international nursing organizations as they respond to increasing cannabis use among health care consumers. ANA's recognition serves as a catalytic force, redefining cannabis nursing as a specialty poised to shape institutional priorities, professional development, and international collaboration, see Sidebar 3, Why ANA's Recognition Matters.

Sidebar 3. Why ANA's Recognition Matters

- Validates cannabis nursing as a specialty
- Signals national professional legitimacy
- Supports educational and competency development
- Encourages institutional acceptance
- Strengthens public trust
- Creates a foundation for global expansion

As state-based medical cannabis programs expanded and demand increased, nurses became primary points of contact for health care consumers seeking guidance. Often nurses were educating, advocating, and supporting people in the absence of formal training or institutional direction. In 2010, during the Patients Out of Time (POT) Conference, a group of nurses established the American Cannabis Nurses Association (ACNA). Founding members included Mary Lynn Mathre, Bryan Krumb, Melanie Dreher, and Julia Glick (later Ed Glick). Each brought clinical expertise, research experience, and a shared commitment to advancing safe and ethical cannabis care (Smith, 2021).

ACNA's founding marked an important moment in nursing history. It created a professional home for nurses who had long worked in legal and ethical uncertainty. The organization provided a platform for clinical standards, research dissemination, and policy engagement. Early efforts focused on defining core competencies, hosting educational conferences, and connecting scientific evidence with nursing practice. ACNA challenged stigma by reframing cannabis as a therapeutic option grounded in compassion, autonomy, and clinical relevance. ACNA's founding wove individual acts of nursing courage into a collective legacy, laying the groundwork for a specialty rooted in evidence, ethics, and patient autonomy, see Table 3, Founders of the American Cannabis Nurses Association (ACNA).

Table 3. Founders of the American Cannabis Nurses Association (ACNA)

Founder	Credentials	Contribution
Mary Lynn Mathre	RN, MSN, CARN	Early advocate, co-founded POT; "Mother of Cannabis Nursing"
Bryan Krumb	APRN	Early advocate, clinical insight; educational support
Melanie Dreher	PHD, RN, FAAN	Researcher; contributed scientific depth
Julia (Ed) Glick	RN	Ethics and advocacy; linked policy and practice

(Smith, 2021)

As cannabis nursing gained visibility, ACNA recognized the need for a formal document that aligned the specialty with national expectations for nursing practice. The organization initiated a structured development process to meet the criteria established by ANA and the American Nurses Credentialing Center (ANCC). This work required a coordinated effort among credentialing-committee members, ACNA leadership, and ANA support staff. The National Council of State Boards of Nursing's 2018 guidelines further emphasized the urgency of this work by identifying essential areas of knowledge required for nurses who support health care consumers using cannabis. See the Development Process for the Cannabis Nursing Scope & Standards.

Development Process for the Cannabis Nursing Scope & Standards

1. Review of existing ACNA and ANA documents
2. Alignment with ANA's *Nursing: Scope and Standards of Practice*
3. Integration of NCSBN's six essential principles
4. Evidence reviews and synthesis
5. Drafting and internal committee review
6. Posting drafts for member feedback
7. Revision and refinement
8. Final preparation for ANA submission

As the ACNA credentialing-committee advanced its work, it relied on the guidance provided in the ANA 3SC booklet, which outlines the criteria for recognition of a nursing specialty and the approval of a specialty scope and standards document. The 3SC framework required ACNA to demonstrate that cannabis nursing is clearly defined, grounded in the profession of nursing, supported by a distinct knowledge base, and practiced by a growing community of nurses (American Nurses Credentialing Center, 2017). ACNA's status as an ANA Organizational Affiliate further strengthened this work by ensuring alignment with national professional expectations. Together, these efforts reveal how ANA and ANCC guidance shaped the specialty's development while charting a clear historical pathway for ACNA's growth and influence, see Highlight 1, ANA and ANCC: supporting the emerging specialty.

Highlight 1. ANA and ANCC: Supporting the Emerging Specialty

- Provided structural guidance
- Ensured Alignment with national expectations
- Clarified 3SC requirements
- Reinforced ethical and professional standards
- Strengthening ACNA's application for recognition

The completion and approval of the *Cannabis Nursing: Scope and Standards of Practice* marked a pivotal moment in the formalization of cannabis nursing as a recognized specialty. This document now serves as the foundational resource for nurses who support health care consumers who use cannabis, reflecting the collective expertise and regulatory alignment achieved through ACNA's multi-year development process. Recent federal actions, including Executive Orders issued under both the Biden and Trump administrations directing federal agencies to evaluate whether cannabis should be moved to Schedule III (National Organization for the Reform of Marijuana Laws, 2025; National Organization for the Reform of Marijuana Laws, 2025). This signals a gradual shift in federal posture rather than a definitive policy change. These directives do not alter cannabis's legal status on their own, and progress toward rescheduling remains slow due to ongoing administrative processes and pending legal challenges. At the same time, some states are reconsidering or rolling back adult-use programs, emphasizing the uneven transition from a prohibition era into a more complex regulatory era. This evolving landscape highlights the importance of the Scope and Standards as a professional framework that equips nurses to navigate shifting policies with clarity, safety, and accountability.

The development of this specialty document demonstrates ACNA's sustained commitment to advancing safe evidence-informed nursing practice in an emerging field. Through the work of a dedicated standing credentialing-committee, ACNA engaged in a rigorous process that included evidence review, member input, and adherence to ANA's 3SC criteria (American Nurses Credentialing Center, 2017). The mentorship provided by ANA and ANCC strengthened this work by offering clarity on expectations related to structure, content, and alignment with the *ANA Code of Ethics for Nurses*. This process ensured that the specialty document met the standards required for national recognition and reflected the needs of health care consumers

> "The recognition of cannabis nursing marks the beginning of a global shift in how nurses support health care consumers who use cannabis products" – Llewellyn 2026

Together, these efforts established the foundation for national recognition of cannabis nursing as an evolving specialty practice. Objective three highlights the significance of this achievement and emphasizes the importance of a unified professional framework that guides nurses who support health care consumers who use cannabis products. The development of the cannabis nursing specialty document carries global implications, since it offers an evidence-informed model that can support international nursing organizations as they consider how to address the growing use of cannabis products among health care consumers.

Objective 4: Advocate for the Inclusion of Cannabis-Related Content in Undergraduate and Graduate Nursing Curricula

Cannabis use is increasingly common among health care consumers worldwide, yet most nursing and medical programs continue to provide little to no formal education on cannabis therapeutics. This persistent gap leaves future clinicians underprepared to deliver safe, ethical, and evidence-informed care. Scholars have long emphasized that without foundational knowledge of the endocannabinoid system, pharmacology, clinical applications, and legal considerations, nurses cannot adequately assess, educate, or advocate for individuals who consume cannabis products. The recent executive orders signal a potential federal reclassification of cannabis to Schedule III and represent a significant policy shift that might expand research opportunities and influence future regulatory and licensure expectations meanwhile prohibitionist efforts continue to resist policy change, creating ongoing variability in state laws that nurses must navigate carefully to protect licensure and ensure safe practice. These developments reinforce the urgency of integrating cannabis-related content into undergraduate and graduate nursing curricula so that professional preparation aligns with contemporary health care needs and emerging standards of practice. The need is amplified by rising adult use, the routine presence of cannabis in clinical encounters (Substance Abuse and Mental Health Services Administration, 2023; Centers for Disease Control, 2025), as well as the absence of robust public health education on cannabis, a gap highlighted in national reviews of clinician preparedness (American Nurses Association, 2021; National Academies of Sciences, Engineering, and Medicine, 2017).

The significance of curriculum inclusion is grounded in established regulatory frameworks. The National Council of State Boards of Nursing (NCSBN) issued clear guidelines in 2018, and the American Cannabis Nurses Association (ACNA) with the American Nurses Association (ANA), further defined cannabis nursing as a recognized specialty through the *Cannabis Nursing: Scope and Standards of*

Practice (2023). Although these standards are recognized, cannabis care remains largely absent from licensure examinations such as the NCLEX-RN and NCLEX-PN, which are administered in the United States, Canada, and Australia and recognized globally as the benchmark for entry-level nursing competence (Australia, 2025; Health Canada, 2018; NCSBN, 2026). Because licensure examinations drive curricular priorities, the absence of cannabis-related content perpetuates gaps in professional readiness and undermines alignment with established standards of care. This challenge is further compounded by the role of accreditation: if accrediting bodies do not explicitly value or require cannabis-related competencies, nursing programs have little structural incentive to integrate this content, regardless of evolving clinical needs or regulatory expectations. Accreditation agencies such as the Commission on Collegiate Nursing Education (CCNE) and the Accreditation Commission for Education in Nursing (ACEN) strongly influence curricular design, and without explicit expectations related to cannabis competencies, programs are unlikely to incorporate this content even when regulatory standards and clinical practice realities indicate a clear need (American Association of Colleges of Nursing, n.d.; Accreditation Commission for Education in Nursing, n.d.).

"If cannabis care isn't tested, it isn't taught – and worldwide, that is a regulatory failure for nurses and health care consumers!" – Llewellyn 2026

This challenge extends beyond the United States. Globally, licensure examinations, including the United Kingdom's Nursing and Midwifery Council Computer-Based Test and OSCE (NMC, 2025), as well as region-specific exams across the Middle East (Saudi Commission for Health Specialties, 2022) and other regions, shape the structure and priorities of nursing programs. Accreditation, institutional reputation, and student progression depend on strong pass rates, compelling nursing schools to align curricula with exam content (Odom-Maryon, 2018). As international nurse mobility expands, gaps in one country influence practice across borders, emphasizing the global urgency of integrating cannabis education into prelicensure and advanced nursing programs. The eventual inclusion of cannabis nursing practice on licensure examinations worldwide would require academic programs to incorporate cannabis care just as prior exam changes have reshaped educational emphasis in other domains. This global convergence of regulatory expectations and workforce mobility makes cannabis education an essential component of every nursing curriculum, see Spotlight 2, Why Cannabis Education Belongs in Every Nursing Program.

Spotlight 2. Why Cannabis Education Belongs in Every Nursing Program

Key Point: Cannabis nursing is already a recognized specialty with established standards of practice.

- **Regulatory Alignment:** NCSBN (2018) and ACNA/ANA (2023) have defined expectations for safe, evidence-informed cannabis care
- **Licensure Influence:** As examinations evolve, curricula must adapt to ensure student success and professional readiness.
- **Global Mobility:** Nurses practice across borders; gaps in one country affect care everywhere.
- **Equity in Care:** Without cannabis education, health care consumers face inconsistent, biased, or uninformed care.

Bottom Line: integrating cannabis content is not optional-it is essential for preparing competent, ethical, and globally relevant nurses.

Systemic barriers continue to impede curriculum integration. The patchwork of cannabis laws across states and nations creates uncertainty for educators who must navigate consistent regulatory environments. Traditionally, health care providers were previously taught explicit bias against cannabis consumption, a legacy of stigma that continues to influence professional attitudes and must be addressed through evidenced-base instruction and faculty development (King D. G., 2024). Although faculty often report a lack of peer-reviewed, standardized academic materials, the challenge increasingly reflects limited awareness of the resources that do exist, such as the Clark textbook (2021), *Cannabis: A Handbook for Nurses* and the *ACNA Cannabis Nursing: Scope and Standards of Practice* (2024) which together provide a sufficient foundation for specialty-level instruction. This text, *Comprehensive Approaches to Cannabis Nursing*, further expands the resources available to faculty developing cannabis-related curriculum. While earlier literature documented a scarcity of peer-reviewed materials (Parmelee R., 2025; Szydlowski, 2020), the more pressing barrier today is ensuring that faculty recognize, access, and confidently use the resources now available. These legal, attitudinal, and knowledge-based barriers collectively limit alignment with established standards of practice and contribute to ongoing inequities in safe, equitable, and evidence-informed care for the health care consumer, see Myth-Buster 2.

Myth-Buster 2. Common Myths About Cannabis in Nursing Education

Myth 1: “Cannabis isn’t relevant to most nursing practice.”
Reality: Cannabis use is widespread across populations and clinical settings. Nurses encounter cannabis-related questions and care needs across all specialty nursing areas.
Myth 2: “We can’t teach cannabis content because laws vary too much.”
Reality: Regulatory variability underscores the need for education. Nurses must understand legal frameworks to practice safely and ethically within any jurisdiction. Nursing students should be empowered to understand legal variabilities across states as nursing practice is mobile.
Myth 3: “There aren’t enough credible resources to teach this content.”
Reality: Foundational standards already exist through NCSBN (2018) and the ACNA/ANA Scope and Standards (2023) and the textbook *Cannabis: A Handbook for Nurses* (2021). Evidence-informed materials continue to expand as research grows.
Myth 4: “Cannabis education is a political issue, not a clinical one.”
Reality: Cannabis care is grounded in patient safety, professional competence, and regulatory expectations, even as cannabis policy remains politically contested in many states. Ongoing efforts to restrict or repeal adult-use programs highlight the political context, but they do not diminish the need for accurate, evidence-informed education for nurses.

Integrating cannabis care into nursing curricula and professional development is not an academic preference but a professional necessity. Established regulatory frameworks—including the NCSBN Guidelines and the *ACNA Cannabis Nursing: Scope and Standards of Practice*—already define cannabis nursing as a legitimate domain of practice, and anticipated federal rescheduling is likely to influence future licensure and regulatory expectations. As global licensure examinations continue to shape curriculum and nurse mobility expands across borders, embedding cannabis content within nursing programs becomes essential to ensuring safe, evidence-informed, and equitable care across diverse clinical and legal contexts.

Objective 5: Explain the importance of understanding the endocannabinoid system in relations to health care consumer safety, pharmacology, and symptom management

Health care consumers use cannabis products for a variety of reasons including pain relief, anxiety reduction, and symptom control in chronic conditions (American Cannabis Nurses Association & American Nurses Association, 2024). Nurses must prepare for practice within a more clearly regulated medical framework. Central to this preparation is a thorough understanding of the endocannabinoid system, which regulates key physiological processes and mediates the effects of cannabis (NCSBN, 2018). Endocannabinoid system literacy enables nurses to anticipate potential benefits and risks, recognize adverse reactions, and tailor interventions to individual needs. As federal scheduling and related policies evolve, nurses will need to apply controlled substance protocols, monitor for misuse, and integrate emerging evidence from clinical research. This section examines the clinical implications of health care consumer cannabis use and highlights the importance of endocannabinoid system education in nursing practice.

The endocannabinoid system regulates physiological processes including pain, mood, appetite, memory, sleep, and immune response. It consists of endogenous cannabinoids, cannabinoid receptors such as CB1 And CB2, and enzymes that synthesize and break down these compounds (Russo E. B., 2016). CB1 receptors are concentrated in the central nervous system, while CB2 receptors are found in immune and peripheral tissues. Enzymes such as FAAH and MAGL regulate cannabinoid levels and shape both therapeutic effects and side-effect profiles (Harvard Health Publishing, 2021).

The system is composed of endogenous lipid-based retrograde neurotransmitters that bind to cannabinoid receptors expressed throughout the vertebrate central and peripheral nervous systems. It influences physiological and cognitive processes including fertility, pregnancy, pre- and postnatal development, appetite, pain sensation, mood, and memory (Harvard Health Publishing, 2021).

Understanding these mechanisms helps nurses interpret how exogenous cannabinoids such as THC and CBD interact with receptor pathways and influence health outcomes. This literacy supports accurate assessment, safe guidance, and integration of emerging clinical evidence as cannabis consumption becomes more medically regulated.

Cannabis and hemp originate from the same botanical species, yet they follow distinctly different regulatory pathways (Congressional Research Service, 2019). Because cannabis regulation remains primarily state-driven, nurses must navigate a patchwork of laws that vary widely across jurisdictions and directly influence clinical practice. Although President Trump's Executive Order directing federal agencies to evaluate cannabis for potential placement in Schedule III signals possible future change, its impact remains uncertain due to ongoing legal and administrative challenges. For now, the most immediate and consequential regulatory considerations for nurses continue to arise from state-level policies, which shape patient access, clinical guidance, and the expectations for safe, evidence-informed care.

Hemp, by contrast, remains regulated under existing U.S. Food and Drug Administration (FDA) frameworks for food, supplements, and cosmetics (Congress, 1906). Hemp is legally defined as containing less than 0.3 percent THC and is cultivated to grow tall with minimal resin production, typically harvested before flowering. Cannabis grown for medical or adult consumption is cultivated to maximize resin-rich flowers with higher concentrations of cannabinoids (Congressional Research Service, 2019)

In practice, hemp products fall under established FDA oversight, while cannabis remains under federal scheduling review for medical and research purposes. Nurses must understand these distinctions to provide accurate education and support informed decision-making. As policy evolves, nurses must remain attentive to these regulatory differences to guide health care consumers safely and effectively. Ongoing federal discussions surrounding the 2026 Farm Bill (Congressional Research Service, 2025), including proposals to tighten oversight of hemp-derived cannabinoids and clarify the legal status of intoxicating hemp products, signal that hemp regulation may undergo significant changes in the coming years (Cannabis Business Times, 2026; Congressional Research Service, 2019). These regulatory distinctions, and the potential shifts ahead, are rooted in fundamental botanical and cultivation differences, as outlined in Table 4, Botanical and Cultivation Differences Between Cannabis and Hemp.

Table 4. Botanical and cultivation differences between cannabis and hemp

Characteristic	**Hemp**	**Cannabis (Medical or Adult Use)**
Botanical Species	Cannabis sativa L.	Cannabis sativa L.
Primary Cultivation Goal	Fiber, seed, industrial biomass, herbal supplement	Resin-rich flowers for cannabinoid concentration
Plant Structure	Tall, slender stalks; minimal branching	Shorter, bushier female plants with dense flowering sites
Resin Production	Minimal resin; low trichome density	High resin production; abundant trichomes
Harvest Timing	Harvested before flowering	Harvested during peak flowering
THC Concentration	<0.3% THC	Typically higher than 0.3% THC
Common Uses	Textiles, rope, paper, building materials, seed oil, supplements	Medical formulations, adult-use products, symptom management
Regulatory Oversight (U.S.)	FDA frameworks	Transitional federal review; state-regulated systems
Cultivar Selection	Height, fiber strength, seed yield	Cannabinoid profile, femineity, terpene expression, resin density

(Adapted from Congressional Research Service, 2019)

Endocannabinoid system literacy supports effective symptom management for health care consumers who use cannabis products. The system regulates processes such as pain perception, mood, appetite, sleep, and immune response, making it central to understanding how cannabis may influence symptoms in chronic conditions. Health care consumers may increasingly access cannabis through regulated medical channels under professional guidance rather than relying solely on self-directed use. This shift requires nurses to collaborate with prescribers, monitor outcomes, and tailor interventions to individual needs.

Endocannabinoid system knowledge also supports harm-reduction strategies for health care consumers who use cannabis for adult purposes. Many individuals titrate their dose to achieve a desired effect while minimizing the likelihood of unpleasant reactions. By recognizing receptor distribution, signaling pathways, and individual variability in response, nurses can provide balanced education that enhances health care consumer trust and supports safe, evidence-based symptom management (American Cannabis Nurses Association & American Nurses Association, 2024). Because misconceptions about cannabis products and symptom relief remain widespread, correcting these myths is critical to supporting safe, evidence-informed adult-use guidance, see Myth-Buster 3: Symptom Management and Cannabis Use.

Myth-Buster 3. Symptom Management and Cannabis Use

Myth: A higher dose provides stronger symptom relief.

Fact: Higher doses often increase the likelihood of unpleasant reactions such as somnolence, impaired coordination, or cardiovascular changes. Health care consumers may achieve better symptom control with lower or gradually titrated doses that align with individual tolerance and receptor sensitivity.
Myth: All cannabis products work the same way.
Fact: Product effects vary based on cannabinoid composition, terpene profile, route of administration, and individual physiology.
Myth: Cannabis is always helpful for sleep.
Fact: Some formulations may aid sleep onset, whereas others may alter sleep architecture, cause next-day fatigue, or gradually downregulate ECS function.
Myth: Hemp products can be used interchangeably with cannabis for symptom control.
Fact: Hemp and cannabis follow different regulatory pathways and contain different cannabinoid concentrations.

Upregulation of the endocannabinoid system refers to engaging in health-promoting activities, such as exercise, meditation, yoga, breathwork, restorative sleep, good nutrition, and other forms of intentional self-care that enhance endogenous cannabinoid tone and support overall physiological balance (Clark, 2021; Knox, 2018). A core component of the cannabis nurse's holistic role is supporting this upregulation, helping individuals potentiate their health and use the least amount of cannabis necessary for the greatest therapeutic benefit. Dr. Carey Clark (now Cadieux) emphasizes this principle throughout *Cannabis: A Handbook for Nurses*, noting that ECS health is foundational to symptom management and that nurses play a key role in guiding consumers toward practices that strengthen endogenous regulation (Clark, 2021). This approach reinforces the importance of ECS-centered wellness and aligns with harm-reduction principles that prioritize safety, autonomy, and informed decision-making.

As cannabis regulation continues to evolve, nurses must integrate endocannabinoid system literacy with controlled substance protocols to ensure safe and effective care (NCSBN, 2018; NCSBN, 2026). Scientific understanding of cannabinoid receptors, signaling pathways, and therapeutic applications is expanding, supported by emerging clinical research and increasing standardization across state-level medical frameworks. Within this shifting landscape, nurses play a critical role in providing balanced, evidence-informed guidance that supports symptom management, promotes patient safety, and upholds professional standards.

International regulatory developments offer additional insight into how cannabis may be incorporated into clinical practice. Canada's national medical cannabis program, administered through Health Canada, provides a unified federal framework for product quality, dosing consistency, and clinician oversight (Health Canada, 2018). Germany's medical cannabis system, regulated through the Federal Institute for Drugs and Medical Devices (BfArM), integrates justification (Federal Institute for Drugs and Medical Devices, 2020). These examples demonstrate how other nations have established structured pathways for medical cannabis access, product regulation, and professional accountability. As the United States shifts from prohibition to regulation, these international frameworks offer practical guidance for shaping policies that better support nursing practice, patient education, and evidence-informed care.

Objective 6: Identify the responsibilities of nurses in caring for individuals who use cannabis for medicinal and adult use purposes

The rapid expansion of medicinal and adult use cannabis laws across the United States and in many countries has reshaped the clinical environment in which nurses practice. As more individuals incorporate cannabis into their symptom management strategies, wellness routines, or adult use choices, nurses are increasingly expected to provide informed, ethical, and patient centered care. This evolving landscape requires nurses to understand the therapeutic potential of cannabis, recognize possible risks, and navigate regulatory variations that influence access and clinical decision-making across jurisdictions. These developments reinforce the importance of ongoing education so nurses can respond confidently to patient questions, support safe use practices, and address emerging clinical needs with accuracy and professionalism.

Nurses practice within a complex framework of federal, state, and institutional policies that shape expectations for both patient care and personal conduct. State laws vary widely in their definitions of medical use, product access, and health care consumer protections, and international regulatory approaches add further variation to how cannabis is classified and managed across health systems (World Health Organization, 2019). Federal scheduling changes, including the potential movement of certain cannabis products to Schedule III, may influence research access, prescribing frameworks, and workplace expectations.

Guidance from regulatory bodies such as the National Council of State Boards of Nursing provides direction on recognizing impairment, supporting safe practice, and addressing substance use in a manner that promotes recovery and fairness (NCSBN, 2018). Institutions also carry responsibility for creating clear and consistent policies that distinguish impairment from lawful off duty consumption.

In some settings, cannabis products may be included in controlled substance counts to ensure accountability and prevent diversion, which aligns with the expectation that nurses safeguard all medications under their care. Impairment recognition should not rely on urine drug screening for tetrahydrocannabinol, since these tests detect metabolites that remain in the body for extended periods due to their storage in fat cells and may remain detectable for up to ninety days depending on consumption patterns (National Academies of Sciences, Engineering, and Medicine, 2017). This approach does not measure impairment and raises concerns about fairness and employee rights. More reliable and scientifically valid methods for assessing impairment exist and should be applied consistently across institutions to support both patient safety and professional integrity.

Nurses have an essential responsibility to distinguish between medicinal and adult-use cannabis consumption, since each pattern of use carries different implications for health, wellness, and clinical decision making. Medicinal use is often guided by symptom-management goals, while adult use may be motivated by relaxation, sleep, creativity, social engagement, or general well-being. At the same time, cannabis activist Dennis Peron famously argued that "all use is medicinal," (Lee, 2012) a perspective that invites nurses to consider how many forms of adult use may reflect underlying needs for rest, emotional ease, or stress relief. Lee Martin (2012) expands on this interpretation, noting that Peron's philosophy challenges clinicians to recognize the wellness-oriented motivations embedded in adult-use patterns while still maintaining clear clinical distinctions for assessment and safety. The NCSBN essentials offer a strong foundation for assessing medicinal use, yet they do not fully address the ways adult use influences health behaviors, safety considerations, or the potential for overconsumption (NCSBN, 2018). Nurses assume these responsibilities because health care consumers frequently confide their cannabis use during admission histories, assessments, and medication reconciliation. By exploring reasons for use, frequency, product selection, and perceived effects, nurses expand upon existing guidelines to support individualized care that aligns with each person's goals and safety needs. These persistent myths underscore why clarifying the realities of cannabis consumption is vital for nurses striving to deliver safe, ethical, and informed practice, see Table 5, Common misconceptions about cannabis use and nursing practice.

Table 5. Common misconceptions about cannabis use and nursing practice

Misconception	Reality
A positive THC urine test means impairment.	THC metabolites indicate past exposure, not impairment. They can remain detectable for weeks to months.
Adult-use cannabis has no relevance to nursing care.	Adult-use motivations often overlap with wellness goals; understanding them supports nonjudgmental, harm-reduction-focused care.
All cannabis products are the same.	Potency, formulation, terpene profiles, and delivery methods vary widely across markets and regions.
Smoking is the primary route of use.	Often adults use vaporization, oral products, tinctures, and other methods with different benefit and risk profiles.
Nurses cannot use cannabis under any circumstances.	Nurses may lawfully use cannabis when not impaired at work and when compliant with institutional policy.
Adult-use cannabis is inherently irresponsible.	Intentional, informed adult use can support stress reduction, emotional ease, and overall well-being.
Cannabis is a gateway drug.	Evidence shows cannabis may serve as an exit strategy for reducing or discontinuing more harmful substances.

Nurses play a central role in harm reduction by helping consumers understand safer methods of cannabis use. Many individuals rely on smoking as their primary route of administration, yet inhaling combusted plant material can irritate the respiratory system (National Academies of Sciences, Engineering, and Medicine, 2017). Nurses can guide consumers toward safer alternatives such as vaporizing dry herbal flower, which eliminates exposure to combustion byproducts while preserving the benefits of whole plant medicine.

Whole plant products contain a diverse array of cannabinoids and terpenes that may work synergistically to enhance therapeutic effects, a phenomenon often described as the entourage effect (Russo E. B., 2016). This aligns with recommendations from the American Cannabis Nurses Association, which emphasizes the therapeutic value of whole plant products and encourages approaches that minimize harm (American Cannabis Nurses Association, 2025). Medicinal guidelines provide a useful framework for understanding cannabis in clinical settings, yet they do not fully address adult use patterns, which are often motivated by enjoyment, relaxation, or the pursuit of euphoria.

Euphoria itself is not a harmful or undesirable state; it is a natural expression of well-being that societies have embraced for centuries. When adults seek cannabis for the purpose of feeling good, they are engaging in a long-standing human practice of pursuing comfort, pleasure, and emotional ease. Peron argued that pleasure, comfort, and emotional ease are themselves forms of healing, and that adult-use motivations often reflect unmet needs for rest, connection, or relief from daily stressors (Lee, 2012). These motivations are consistent across global context and have been present within traditional cultural, spiritual, and social practices for centuries prior to prohibition, reinforcing Peron's assertion that "all use is medicinal". Historical and traditional continuities reveal euphoria as a natural facet of well-being, inviting a more compassionate and informed understanding of adult cannabis consumption, see Figure 1, Euphoria – a natural expression of well-being.

Figure 1. Euphoria – A natural expression of well-being

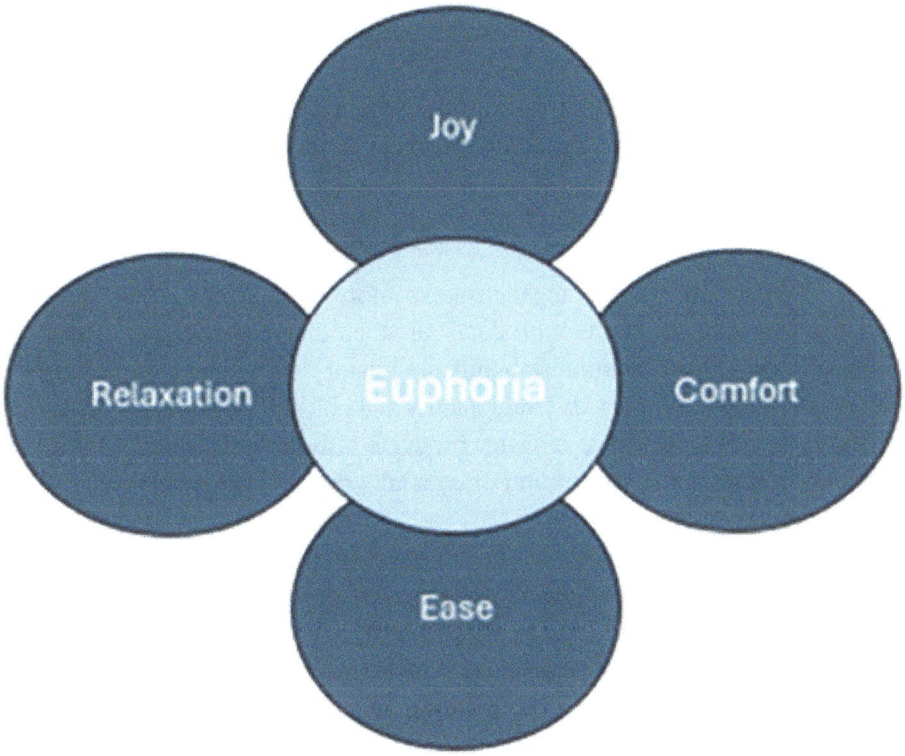

Euphoria emerges at the intersection of joy, comfort, relaxation, and emotional ease. Rather than signaling misuse, euphoria often reflects relief, restoration, or a return to balance (Knox, 2018). Across time and place, people have sought uplifting experiences through music, movement, ceremony, and plant medicines (Lee, 2012), and cannabis-related euphoria fits within this continuum. When adults seek cannabis to feel lighter, calmer, or more connected, they are engaging in a long-standing human practice of pursuing well-being. Dr. Julie Holland, in *The Pot Book: A Complete Guide to Cannabis*, emphasizes that pleasure and emotional ease are normal aspects of human functioning and may represent meaningful shifts toward balance rather than pathology, reinforcing that euphoria can be a legitimate wellness outcome (Knox, 2018; Holland, 2010). Recognizing euphoria as a natural, intentional experience allows nurses to provide nonjudgmental, evidence informed guidance that respects autonomy and supports safer use.

"There's nothing wrong with a little euphoria." – Llewellyn 2026

Harm-reduction frameworks recognize that cannabis is a far safer alternative to other Scheduled substances and high-risk drugs. Cannabis products have been used as an exit strategy for individuals seeking to reduce or discontinue their use of more harmful substances, including alcohol and cigarettes. This idea has appeared in mainstream media as well; during a 2017 appearance on Fox & Friends, Dr.

Mehmet Oz challenged the "gateway drug" narrative by suggesting that cannabis may instead serve as an "exit drug" from the narcotic epidemic (Oz, 2017). While such media statements helped shift public perception, the scientific evidence is even more definitive. The National Academies of Sciences, Engineering, and Medicine (NASEM, 2017) concluded that there is no substantial evidence supporting the claim that cannabis use leads to the use of harder substances, effectively debunking the gateway theory. Additional research further suggests that alcohol—not cannabis—is more strongly associated with progression to other drug use, reinforcing the need for evidence-informed harm-reduction guidance.

In these settings, nurses help consumers approach adult use with intension and awareness, reinforcing the principle to 'manage your party, don't let your party manage you'. Adults already understand the need to use certain substances responsibly, and cannabis is not different. By recognizing how individuals incorporate cannabis into their daily lives, nurses can offer timely, nonjudgmental education that supports safer choices, reduces the likelihood of overconsumption, and aligns with each person's goals and lived experience.

Nurses support adult consumers by helping them make informed decisions about the cannabis products they choose and how they incorporate those products into their daily lives. Product variability is further shaped by global differences in cultivation standards, regulatory oversight, and labeling requirements, meaning that adults may encounter very different quality and potency profiles depending on where they live or travel. Legal markets and cottage industry products offer a wide range of options that vary in potency, formulation, and intended effects, and often adults rely on budtenders or THC concentration rather than evidence informed guidance.

In some states, budtenders enter the cannabis industry with prior pharmacy technician experience, particularly in medically oriented or boutique-style dispensaries where familiarity with controlled substances and product handling is valued. Michael Moskowitz 2017 describes this trend within boutique dispensary models, noting that staff often come from pharmacy or customer-service backgrounds and receive extensive product-focused training, though not clinical preparation (Moskowitz, 2017). In the Commonwealth of Virginia, this structure is formalized: all medical cannabis dispensaries must be operated by a licensed pharmacist and employ registered pharmacy technicians who often function in budtender roles, as required by the Virginia Board of Pharmacy's pharmaceutical processor regulations (Virginia Board of Pharmacy, 2023). While this model enhances regulatory compliance and product-handling standards, pharmacy technicians are not trained in physiology, clinical assessment, or disease-specific symptomology. Because nurses bring expertise in these areas, dispensaries would benefit from incorporating cannabis nurse specialists as consultants who can strengthen consumer education, enhance harm-reduction practices, and support safer, more informed product use. Given the public health implications of expanding cannabis access, nurses should be calling for regulatory models that include cannabis nurse specialists as part of the dispensary health care team and advocating for broader public health education to ensure that consumers receive the safest, most clinically grounded guidance possible.

Nurses are not expected to recommend specific products, yet they do have a responsibility to help health care consumers recognize factors that influence safer use, such as understanding potency ranges, avoiding products with unclear sourcing, and selecting forms that align with their goals and tolerance. Self-titration is a best practice that includes encouraging consumers to start with lower potency options, avoid overreliance on high concentration products, and be mindful of how different products may shape their overall consumption patterns (American Cannabis Nurses Association & American Nurses Association, 2024).

As adult use cannabis becomes increasingly normalized across diverse global settings, nurses play a vital role in supporting health care consumers with balanced, evidence informed guidance that promotes safer use for both medicinal and adult use consumers. Their responsibility is not to direct individuals toward or away from cannabis products, but to help consumers make thoughtful decisions that reflect their goals, health status, and personal circumstances. By offering clear information, reducing stigma, and encouraging intentional consumption patterns, nurses strengthen harm reduction efforts and foster environments where adults can engage with cannabis more safely and confidently.

This same framework applies to nurses themselves, who also deserve access to responsible, stigma free self-care practices, including lawful adult cannabis use that supports their well-being and resilience. Nurses, like all members of the public, have the right to use cannabis legally and responsibly for their own well-being, whether their consumption is medicinal or adult use. The demands of nursing are intense and often expose clinicians to burnout, post-traumatic stress, moral distress, and the cumulative emotional and physical toll of caring for others. The American Nurses Association emphasizes that nurses must prioritize their own mental health and recognize early signs of exhaustion, compassion fatigue, and chronic stress. ANA's Healthy Nurse Healthy Nation initiative identifies burnout as a significant threat to the workforce and encourages evidence informed strategies for self-care and resilience (American Nurses Association, 2024).

Within this context, responsible adult-use consumption may serve as one strategy that supports emotional restoration and helps mitigate symptoms of burnout, provided the individual maintains control of their use by 'managing their party rather than letting their party manage them'. Dr. Carey Clark (now Cadieux) reinforces this perspective by noting that nurses have lost jobs or had their licenses threatened because of their cannabis advocacy, and she emphasizes that nurses should be supported in their own healing journey, which may include cannabis use (Clark, 2021). These insights affirm that personal wellness is essential to safe and competent practice and reinforce the need for supportive environments that respect lawful self-care choices while upholding professional standards.

"Manage your party, don't let your party manage you!" – Llewellyn 2026

CONCLUSION

Cannabis nursing stands at the threshold of a transformative era. As scientific understanding deepens and global regulatory landscapes evolve, nurses are emerging as essential guides in helping individuals, families, and communities navigate the therapeutic potential of cannabis with clarity, safety, and dignity. The six objectives explored in this chapter collectively demonstrate that cannabis nursing is not merely an emerging specialty, it is a paradigm shift rooted in the core values of the profession: advocacy, harm reduction, cultural humility, global awareness, and a commitment to evidence-informed practice.

This new age calls for leadership capable of shaping the future of health care at scale. The American Cannabis Nurses Association (ACNA) is uniquely positioned to steward this evolution. Together with ANA, these organizations are laying the structural, educational, and ethical foundation for a specialty that will influence nursing practice across borders. Their collaboration signals a profound shift: cannabis nursing is moving from the margins of clinical curiosity to the center of professional legitimacy, competency development, and global health discourse.

Notably, the International Council of Nurses (ICN) has not issued guidance on cannabis or cannabinoid therapeutics, leaving global nursing without unified international direction and further emphasizing the significance of ACNA and ANA's leadership in defining this emerging specialty. As global discourse evolves, ICN could play a pivotal role by developing international guidance that supports nurses in delivering safe, socially responsive, and evidence-informed care to cannabis health care consumers worldwide. Looking ahead, ICN could strengthen global nursing capacity by collaborating with ANA and ACNA to develop internationally aligned guidance that supports nurses and cannabis health care consumers across various regulatory environments.

As nations reconsider cannabis policy and patients seek guidance grounded in science rather than stigma, the nursing profession has unprecedented opportunity to lead. ACNA and ANA's emerging partnership offers a model for how professional organizations can respond to rapidly changing therapeutic landscapes-by elevating standards, supporting clinicians, and ensuring that patient care remains grounded in compassion, safety, and human dignity. Their work will not only shape practice within the United States but will also inform international frameworks as countries look to nursing for guidance in integrating cannabis therapeutics responsibly and equitably.

A Vision for the Dawn of a New Age

The concepts presented in this chapter are not competencies themselves; they are the philosophical scaffolding that strengthens and reinforces the formal competencies articulated by ACNA, ANA, and the NCSBN. They invite nurses to imagine what cannabis care can become when grounded in ethical clarity, scientific rigor, and cultural humility. As the *ACNA Cannabis Nursing: Scope & Standards of Practice* charts the profession's expectations, this chapter offers the horizon line-the vision that animates those standards and calls nurses to step into their role as global leaders in this emerging specialty.

In this dawn of a new age, cannabis nurses are not simply responding to change; they are shaping it. They are reclaiming accurate language, challenging outdated narratives, and illuminating pathways toward equitable, person-centered care. Yet the horizon extends far beyond the borders of any single state or nation. As global attitudes toward cannabis continue to shift, nurses are uniquely positioned to guide public understanding, influence policy development, and champion international standards that reflect contemporary science, including the essential role of endocannabinoid system (ECS) upregulation in promoting health and resilience.

The future of cannabis nursing practice will be defined by those who embrace this moment with courage, curiosity, and a commitment to advancing health for all. Nurses have long served as trusted educators, advocates, and innovators; in the emerging global cannabis landscape, these roles take on new urgency. Whether shaping public health messaging, informing regulatory frameworks, or contributing to international dialogues on safety, equity, and access, cannabis nurses will help ensure that policy decisions are grounded in evidence, compassion, and a deep understanding of human physiology.

As ACNA and ANA continue to guide the profession forward, nurses everywhere are invited to rise with them, carrying the ACNA mission to advance excellence in cannabis nursing practice through advocacy, collaboration, education, research, and policy development (American Cannabis Nurses Association & American Nurses Association, 2024). The next era of cannabis nursing will not be defined solely by what cannabis is, but by what nurses choose to do with this knowledge on the global stage: elevate public understanding, promote ECS-supportive health strategies, and lead with integrity as the world reimagines what health and healing can be.

"When the world finally recognizes the endocannabinoid system as a foundation of health, it will be because nurses led the way." - Llewellyn 2026

ACKNOWLEDGMENT

I am profoundly grateful to the American Cannabis Nurses Association (ACNA) for offering the brave nurturing space where I could grow into the nurse, scholar, and leader I am today. When I joined ACNA in 2016, I carried a passion for cannabis nursing care that was often dismissed or misunderstood in traditional nursing environments. ACNA not only welcomed that passion, but it also honored it, challenged it, and helped me refine it. Serving as ACNA's Credentialing Committee Co-Chairman with Dr. Sommers and the entire committee was one of the most meaningful experiences of my career, giving me the opportunity to contribute to a specialty that shaped me as much as I helped shape it. In this community, I found the safety to advocate for a controversial topic, the mentorship to deepen my expertise, and the courage to stand firmly in my convictions. ACNA's trust and support allowed me to become the subject matter expert I am today where I played an essential role in the development of cannabis nursing as a recognized specialty practice.

This chapter received no specific grant from any funding agency in the public, commercial, or not-for-profit sectors.

The author has no conflict of interest regarding the content of this paper.

ARTIFICIAL INTELLIGENCE

This statement is to disclose that artificial intelligence (AI) tools were used solely for text-based support during the preparation of this chapter, including narrative refinement, grammar and structural editing, organizational guidance, citation formatting, and summarization of publicly available, properly cited sources. No AI tools were used to generate tables, figures, graphs, diagrams, images, or any other visual or data-driven elements prohibited by IGI Global's policy. All scholarly content, interpretations, and final decisions reflect my own academic judgment, and all sources were independently verified and cited according to IGI Global and APA guidelines. This disclosure is provided in the interest of transparency and compliance with IGI Global's requirements for responsible AI use.

REFERENCES

Accreditation Commission for Education in Nursing. (n.d.). *ACEN About Us*. https://www.acenursing.org/about

Alexander, M. (2010). *The new Jim Crow: Mass incarceration in the age of colorblindness*. The New Press.

American Association of Colleges of Nursing. (n.d.). *About AACN*. Retrieved April 10, 2026, from American Assoicaiation of Colleges of Nursing: https://www.aacnnursing.org/about-aacn

American Cannabis Nurses Association. (2017). *Cannabis Nursing Scope and Standards of Practice* (1st ed.). American Cannabis Nurses Association.

American Cannabis Nurses Association. (2019). *Cannabis Nursing Scope and Standards of Practice* (2nd ed.). American Cannabis Nurses Association.

American Cannabis Nurses Association. (2025, November 20). *Use and regulation of synthetic cannabinoids and hemp-derived substances and semi-synthetic cannabinoid receptor agonists.* http://cannabisnurses.org

American Cannabis Nurses Association & American Nurses Association. (2024). *Cannabis nursing: Scope and standards of practice*. American Nurses Association.

American Nurses Association. (2021). *Therapeutic use of marijuana and related cannabinoids.* ANA Center for Ethics and Human Rights. https://www.nursingworld.org/globalassets/practiceandpolicy/nursing-excellence/ana-position-statements/therapeutic-use-of-marijuana-and-related-cannabinoids-position-statement-final-2021.pdf?utm_source=copilot.com

American Nurses Association. (2024). *Healthy Nurse Healthy Nation.* Silver Spring, MD: American Nurse Journal. https://www.nursingworld.org/ana/about-ana/

American Nurses Credentialing Center. (2017). *American Nurses Association recognition of a nursing specialty, approval of specialty nursing scope and practice statement, acknowledgment of specialty nursing standards of practice, and affirmation of focused practice competencies*. American Nurses Association.

Australia, N. a. (2025). *Registration Standards.* Retrieved December 15, 2025, from Australian Health Practitioner Regulation Agency: https://www.nursingmidwiferyboard.gov.au/registration-standards.aspx

Aviram, J. (2025, November 13). Medical cannabis in Israel: A comprehensive review of trends and regulations. *Journal of Cannabis Research*, *7*(1), 90. Advance online publication. DOI: 10.1186/s42238-025-00344-1 PMID: 41233935

Bonnie, R. W. (1974). *The marijuana conviction: A history of marijuana prohibition in the United States*. University Press of Virginia.

Cannabis Business Times. (2026, March 5). *Proposed hemp regulations in the 2026 Farm Bill and implications for the cannabis industry*. Retrieved April 11, 2026, from Cannabis Business Times: https://www.cannabisbusinesstimes.com/hemp/news/15818903/intoxicating-hemp-ban-unchanged-in-2026-farm-bills-advancement

Centers for Disease Control. (2025, March 7). *Cannabis facts and stats*. Retrieved April 10, 2026, from Cannabis and public health: https://www.cdc.gov/cannabis/data-research/facts-stats/index.html

Chokwanich, N. e. (2022). Traditional medicine and cannabis integration in Thailand's public health system. *Journal of Ethhnopharmacology*.

Clark, C. (2021). The nurses's role: Providing cannabis care. In Clark, C. F., & Clark, C. (Eds.), *Cannabis: A handbook for nurses* (1st ed., p. 272). Wolters Kluwer.

Clarke, R. M. (2013). History of cannabis use for fiber. In Clarke, R. M. (Ed.), *Cannabis: Evolution and Ethnobotany* (p. 172). University of California Press.

College of Registered Nurses of Alberta (CRNA). (2022). Cannabis for medical purposes: standards for Nurse Practitioners. Alberta: College of Registered Nurses of Alberta (CRNA).

Congress, U. S. (1906, June 30). *Pure Food and Drug Act of 1906*. Retrieved January 5, 2026, from Schaffer Drug Library History 1900s: https://www.druglibrary.org/schaffer/History/e1900/pfda.htm

Congressional Research Service. (2019). *Defining hemp: A fact sheet.* U. S. Government. Washington DC: Library of Congress. https://crsreports.congress.gov/product/pdf/R/R44742

Congressional Research Service. (2025). *Hemp regulation and federal considerations under the forthcoming Farm Bill*. CRS.

Federal Institute for Drugs and Medical Devices. (2020). *Medical cannabis in Germany: Regulatory overview*. Government of Germany.

Fischer, B. R., Russell, C., Sabioni, P., van den Brink, W., Le Foll, B., Hall, W., Rehm, J., & Room, R. (2017). Lower-risk cannabis use guidelines (LRCUG): A comprehensive update of evidence and recommendations. *American Journal of Public Health, 107*(8), 1277. Advance online publication. DOI: 10.2105/AJPH.2017.303818a PMID: 28644037

Harvard Health Publishing. (2021, August 11). *The endocannabinoid system: Essential and mysterious.* (P. Grinspoon, Editor) https://www.health.harvard.edu/blog/the-endocannabinoid-system-essential-and-mysterious-202108112569

Health Canada. (2018). *Cannabis legalization and regulation.* Government of Canada.

Hoch, E. H., Hall, W., & Feingold, D. (2025, February 14). Cannabis use in Europe. *European Archives of Psychiatry and Clinical Neuroscience, 277-279*(2), 277–279. Advance online publication. DOI: 10.1007/s00406-025-01972-7 PMID: 39951121

Holland, J. (2010). The Pot Book: A complete guide to cannabis: Its role in medicine, politics, science, and culture. In Holland, J. (Ed.), *The Pot Book: A complete guide to cannabis: Its role in medicine, politics, science, and culture* (p. 246). Park Street Press.

King, D. (2021). Anesthesia for patients who self report cannabis (marijuana) use before esophogogastrodoudenoscopy: A retrospective review. *American Associatin of Nurse Anesthesiology*, 205-212.

King, D. G., Gill, C. J., Cadieux, C. S., & Singh, N. (2024). The role of stigma in cannabis use disclosure: An exploratory study. *Harm Reduction Journal, 21*(21), 1–13. DOI: 10.1186/s12954-024-00929-8 PMID: 38273362

Knox, R. (Producer). (2018). *The endocannabinoid system and the revolution of one* [Motion Picture]. https://www.youtube.com/watch?v=oJbOQ9P2NYQ

Lee, M. A. (2012). *Smoke signals: A social history of marijuana-medical, recreational, and scientific.* Simon & Schuster, Inc.

Malka, D. (2022). *Medicinal Cannabis.* CRC Press.

Maynard, F. (2025, April). Cannabis and healthcare: Complicated policies and laws. (L. Gelinas, Ed.) *American Nurse, 20*(4), 14-18. https://www.myamericannurse.com/wp-content/uploads/2025/03/an4-Cannabis-321.pdf

Mills, J. (2003). *Cannabis Britannica: empire, trade and prohibition 1800-1928.* Oxford University Press. DOI: 10.1093/oso/9780199249381.001.0001

Moskowitz, M. H. (2017). Dispensaries. In Moskowitz, M. H. (Ed.), *Medical cannabis: A guide for patients, practitioners, and caregivers* (pp. 138–139). Koehlerbooks.

National Academies of Sciences, Engineering, and Medicine. (2017). *The health effects of cannabis and cannabinoids: The current state of evidence and recommendations for research.* Washington, DC: National Academies Press. DOI: 10.17226/24625

National Organization for the Reform of Marijuana Laws. (2025, August 14). *A brief history of cannabis rescheduling petitions in the United States.* https://norml.org/news/2025/08/14/trump-says-cannabis-rescheduling-decision-is-forthcoming/

National Organization for the Reform of Marijuana Laws. (2025, December 18). *President Trump takes executive action to federally reschedule marijuana.* https://norml.org/blog/2025/12/18/president-trump-takes-executive-action-to-federally-reschedule-marijuana/

NCSBN. (2018, July). The NCSBN national nursing guidelines for medical marijuana. *Journal of Nursing Regulation: Advancing nursing excellence for public protection, 9*(2), S1-S60.

NCSBN. (2026). *Global regulatory atlas.* Retrieved January 20, 2026, from NCSBN Leading Regulatory Excellence: https://www.regulatoryatlas.com/

NMC. (2025). *Test of Competence.* Retrieved December 15, 2025, from Nursing & Midwifery Council: https://www.nmc.org.uk/registration/joining-the-register/toc/

O'Leary-Randall, A. (2014). *Medical marijuana in America: Memoir of a Pioneer.*

Odom-Maryon, T. B., Bailey, L. A., & Amiri, S. (2018). The influences of nursing school characteristics on NCLEX-RN pass rates: A national study. *Journal of Nursing Regulation, 9*(3), 59–69. DOI: 10.1016/S2155-8256(18)30154-6

Oz, M. (2017, September 15). Cannabis as an exit drug strategy. *Fox and Friends* . New York, NY.

Parmelee, R. (2025). Nurse educators' experiences with medical cannabis education (Doctoral dissertation, Walden University). Walden University ScholarWorks. https://scholarworks.waldenu.edu/dissertations/17290/

Parmelee, R. A., & Clark, C. S. (2022). Nursing students knowledge, skills, and attitudes regarding medicinal cannabis care. *Journal of Nursing Regulation, 13*(3), 13–23. DOI: 10.1016/S2155-8256(22)00082-5

Russo, E. (2025, October 9). Critical gaps in cannabis and endocannabinoid system education. *Deficiencies in medical training and necessary curriculm reform for future clinicians.* USA.

Russo, E. B. (2016). *Cannabis and Cannabinoids: Pharmacology, Toxicology, and Therapeutic Potential.* Routledge.

Saudi Commission for Health Specialties. (2022). *Saudi Nursing Licensing Exam.* Specialties, Saudi Commission for Health. Saudi Arabia: SCFHS. https://scfhs.org.sa/sites/default/files/2022-06/SNLE%20Applicant%20Guide%20-%20March%202022.pdf

Sloman, L. (1998). *Reefer Madness: A history of marijuana* (3rd ed.). St. Martin's Press.

Smith, L. (2021). History of cannabis and prohibition. In Clark, C. (Ed.), *Cannabis: A handbook for nurses* (pp. 3–6). Wolters Kluwer.

Substance Abuse and Mental Health Services Administration. (2023). *Key substance use and mental health indicators in the United States: Results from the 2023 National Survey on Drug Use and Health.* SAMHSA, Center for Behavioral Health Statistics and Quality, Substance Abuse and Mental Health Administration. HHS Publication No. PEP24-07-021, NSDUH Series H-59). Retrieved from https://www.samhsa.gov/data/report/2023-nsduh-annual-national-report

Szydlowski, S. A. (2020). Medical cannabis knowledge and practice: A survey of healthcare providers. *Journal of Cannabis Research*, *2*, 1–9.

United Nations. (1925). League of Nations Treaty Series. *International Opium Convention. 81*, p. 319. Geneva: United Nations. Retrieved January 24, 2025, from https://treaties.un.org/pages/ViewDetails.aspx?src=TREATY&mtdsg_no=VI-6-a&chapter=6&clang=_en

United Nations. (1961). United Nations Treaty Series. [New York, Geneva, Switzerland: United Nations Office on Drugs and Crime.]. *Single Convention on Narcotic Drugs.*, *520*, 151.

Virginia Board of Pharmacy. (2023, July 17). *Regulations governing pharmaceutical processors.* https://register.dls.virginia.gov/details.aspx?id=10719

World Health Organization. (2019). *WHO review of cannabis and cannabis related substances.* https://www.who.int/teams/health-product-and-policy-standards/controlled-substances/who-review-of-cannabis-and-cannabis-related-substances

World Health Organization. (2025). *State of the world's nursing 2025: investing in education, jobs, leadership and service delivery.* Geneva: World Health Organization. https://iris.who.int/server/api/core/bitstreams/a4173924-a18f-49b6-8bd1-9c2a4a098980/content

KEYWORDS AND DEFINITIONS

American Cannabis Nurses Association (ACNA): The specialty nursing organization that advances cannabis nursing through education, advocacy, and the development of professional standards and research, serving as the organizational steward of cannabis care nursing.

American Nurses Association (ANA): The national professional organization that established standards for nursing practice and formally recognizes nursing specialties, including cannabis nursing in 2024. Partners with ACNA to fill in educational gaps related to cannabis care nursing.

Cannabis Nursing: Scope and Standards of Practice: The foundational professional publication developed by the ACNA and recognized by the ANA, defining the specialty of cannabis care nursing through its scope, standards, competencies, and expectations for safe, ethical, and evidence-informed practice.

Cannabis Nursing Specialty Recognition: The formal acknowledgment by the ANA that cannabis nursing constitutes a distinct area of professional practice supported by a defined scope, standards, and body of knowledge.

Cannabis Cultivar: A cultivated variety of the cannabis plant selected and maintained for specific genetic, chemical or agricultural characteristics. Replaces inappropriate use of the word "strain", which is a bacteria or virus, not a botanical plant.

Cannabis Care Nursing: A specialty practice focused on evidence-informed assessment, education, and care of health care consumers who use cannabis products.

Euphoria: a natural state of well-being or pleasure characterized by feelings of comfort, ease, relaxation, or uplifted mood.

Global Health Workforce Mobility: The movement of nurses across international borders for education, licensure, and employment, influencing how nursing competencies, curricula, and regulatory expectations evolve worldwide.

International Nursing Regulation: The systems, policies, and standards established by global or national regulatory bodies that shape licensure, scope of practice, and educational requirements for nurses across countries.

National Council of State Boards of Nursing (NCSBN): The organization that supports nursing regulation through licensure examinations, policy guidance, and model rules that influence educational standards and safe nursing practices.

Chapter 15
The Cannabis Nurse Entrepreneur:
Integrating Clinical Insight, Business Innovation, and Policy Leadership in a Growing Industry

Drudys Ledbetter
http://orcid.org/0009-0009-7122-0039
American Cannabis Nurses Association, USA

ABSTRACT

This chapter examines the cannabis nurse entrepreneur as a multidisciplinary leader addressing misalignment between patient behavior, clinical practice, and regulatory frameworks within an evolving therapeutic landscape. As more patients use cannabis for symptom management and wellness, gaps in clinical integration, documentation, and professional oversight have become increasingly visible. This chapter outlines core competencies in regulatory navigation, operational design, quality assurance, and patient-centered education. It synthesizes evidence on documentation gaps, including that fewer than 5 percent of patients reporting medical cannabis use have this documented in the electronic health record, alongside variability in outcomes and clinician preparedness. Case studies demonstrate how nurse-informed models address gaps in retail education, health equity, and data integrity, while consultation models, harm reduction, and interprofessional collaboration are presented as pathways for more accountable cannabis care systems.

1. INTRODUCTION

1.1 The Rise of the Cannabis Nurse Entrepreneur

The rapid expansion of the legal cannabis industry has created increasingly complex intersections among healthcare delivery, business innovation, and public policy. As regulatory frameworks evolve and patient access expands, the demand for clinically grounded, ethically informed leadership within this emerging sector has intensified. Contemporary scholarship positions cannabis not as an isolated

DOI: 10.4018/979-8-3373-7287-7.ch015

commercial product, but as a component of broader health and wellness systems requiring structured clinical oversight (Balbuena, 2024). This framing underscores the need for leadership capable of translating therapeutic potential into safe, accountable, and evidence-informed practice.

At a broader level, this moment reflects earlier inflection points in nursing history. Care was widely delivered but inconsistently structured, with variable educational preparation, limited documentation, and outcomes often accepted rather than systematically evaluated. Progress emerged through the development of standards, formal education, data collection, and policy engagement. Nursing became legible to institutions through the articulation of measurable outcomes, operational design, and professional responsibility rather than moral authority alone (Dock & Stewart, 1938; Reverby, 1987).

A comparable dynamic is now evident in cannabis care. Use across both medical and adult-use contexts has become increasingly prevalent, with approximately 18 to 20 percent of U.S. adults reporting past-year use (Substance Abuse and Mental Health Services Administration [SAMHSA], 2023). Patients report taking cannabis as part of symptom management, quality-of-life support, and general wellness across conditions including chronic pain, sleep disturbance, anxiety, and cancer-related symptoms (Whiting et al., 2015; Hill, 2015). Yet increased utilization has not been accompanied by parallel development of standardized education, documentation protocols, or safety frameworks, producing a gap between widespread behavioral adoption and the professional structures needed to support it safely.

These structural limitations carry measurable consequences. Patient education varies widely, risk stratification remains underutilized, and adverse effects including drug-drug interactions and overconsumption may go undocumented or unrecognized (National Council of State Boards of Nursing [NCSBN], 2018). Responsibility is frequently shifted to patients without sufficient professional support, redistributing risk from structured care environments to individuals navigating complex decisions without adequate guidance.

A significant and underexamined dimension of this gap involves how stigma shapes communication between patients and providers. Patients routinely assess the interpersonal risk of disclosure before sharing their cannabis use or the fact that they are taking cannabis with a clinician, and anticipated stigma—the expectation of judgment or devaluation if a stigmatized behavior is revealed—functions as a measurable barrier to that communication (King et al., 2024). Even as social normalization of cannabis use increases, concerns about provider bias, legal ambiguity, and perceived clinical irrelevance continue to suppress disclosure. The result is a pattern in which cannabis-related discussions are often patient-initiated and, in many encounters, absent altogether, reflecting both patient hesitation and provider-level knowledge gaps including limited training in cannabinoid therapeutics, uncertainty regarding dosing and safety, and inconsistent regulatory understanding (Baral et al., 2025).

The consequences of this communication failure are not abstract. Incomplete cannabis histories limit accurate medication reconciliation, increase the risk of drug-drug interactions, and compromise treatment planning. Patients who take cannabis in place of prescribed medications without provider awareness introduce additional risk that clinicians cannot manage without disclosure (Boehnke et al., 2021). The inverse is equally instructive. When disclosure occurs and clinicians engage knowledgeably with patients who are taking cannabis as part of their care, patients report more effective symptom management, more appropriate product selection, and improved outcomes overall (Clobes et al., 2025). Professional oncology guidelines now explicitly address the need for open, nonjudgmental clinician communication regarding cannabis use, recommending that providers initiate these conversations proactively and avoid unsupported self-directed use among patients (Braun et al., 2024). The central problem is not cannabis use itself. It is the absence of the professional infrastructure needed to incorporate that use safely into care.

International experience reinforces this point. In Canada, federal legalization formalized healthcare provider involvement in medical authorization and created defined documentation pathways, yet variability in clinician education and inconsistent care integration persist. In the Netherlands, pharmacist involvement in regulated cannabis dispensing introduced professional oversight absent in retail-only models, yet provider training gaps remain documented. Across both contexts, a consistent pattern emerges: legalization establishes access, but without deliberate investment in professional education, documentation standards, and interprofessional coordination, clinical integration lags behind availability. This divergence strengthens the case for healthcare-led infrastructure as a prerequisite for safe and equitable cannabis care, regardless of the regulatory model in place.

The cannabis nurse entrepreneur emerges in response to this structural limitation. This role is not defined by product sales, prescribing authority, or scope expansion beyond licensure. It is defined by the application of nursing standards to environments where care-related decisions are already occurring without sufficient professional structure. The nurse entrepreneur functions as a translator between patient experience and clinical language, a designer of education and competency frameworks, and a steward of ethical, scope-appropriate practice within highly regulated environments (American Nurses Association [ANA], 2021).

1.2 Nursing Leadership in Cannabis Systems

Nurses, as the largest and most trusted group of healthcare professionals, are uniquely positioned to address the clinical and ethical demands emerging as more patients begin taking cannabis as part of symptom management and self-directed care. Core competencies in patient assessment, education, care coordination, and quality assurance provide a foundation for guiding cannabis-related services in ways that prioritize safety, equity, and evidence-informed care. This positioning aligns with longstanding national recommendations emphasizing nursing leadership in population health, system redesign, and care coordination (Institute of Medicine, 2011).

Within this landscape, the cannabis nurse entrepreneur has emerged as a distinct professional pathway situated at the intersection of clinical practice, operational leadership, and regulatory navigation. This function extends beyond traditional roles to include business formation, compliance infrastructure, workflow design, and policy engagement within a highly regulated and commercially active environment. In practice, nurse entrepreneurs translate professional standards into operational models, ensuring that patient education, documentation, and risk mitigation processes are embedded within service delivery across settings including dispensaries, consulting practices, and interdisciplinary care environments.

This professional pathway is further differentiated from adjacent nonclinical actors operating within cannabis environments. While dispensary personnel, consultants, and advocates may facilitate access or provide experiential guidance, they do not function within licensure-based accountability structures or ethical frameworks grounded in patient safety. Nurses conduct assessment, deliver education, support documentation, and advocate for safe use within defined professional boundaries, introducing a level of reliability and responsibility that remains inconsistently established across the industry (National Council of State Boards of Nursing, 2018).

Concerns related to commercialization of care, conflicts of interest, and preservation of professional independence warrant careful consideration within this model. These concerns require explicit governance structures, transparency in financial relationships, and clearly defined ethical boundaries. Excluding nurses from cannabis environments, however, does not address these risks. It removes professionally trained practitioners from spaces where individuals are already seeking guidance, limiting opportunities for risk assessment, education, and harm reduction. In this context, professional absence constrains the development of safe and accountable care rather than protecting it.

The measurable case for nursing engagement is compelling. While more than one quarter of patients report medical cannabis use, many are actively taking cannabis for therapeutic purposes, yet fewer than 5 percent have this documented in structured clinical records (Lapham et al., 2022). Evidence from substance use care models further demonstrates that nurse-driven approaches produce measurable impact: in a cluster randomized clinical trial, nurse care management significantly expanded medication treatment for opioid use disorder across primary care settings, demonstrating replicable, operationally feasible results (Wartko et al., 2023). What is not documented cannot be managed, and what is not managed cannot be evaluated for safety, efficacy, or equity. Cannabis care environments present the same unmet need and the same opportunity for professional leadership to make a measurable difference.

1.3 Chapter Objectives and Scope

For the purposes of this chapter, the cannabis nurse entrepreneur is defined as a licensed nurse who integrates clinical expertise, ethical accountability, and entrepreneurial strategy within cannabis-related enterprises.

The objectives of this chapter are to:

1. define the role and scope of the cannabis nurse entrepreneur;
2. identify the core competencies and operational considerations required for effective practice in this role; and
3. examine emerging opportunities for innovation that advance patient safety, public trust, and professional accountability within the cannabis industry.

This chapter adopts an interdisciplinary perspective to examine how nursing knowledge and professional standards can be operationalized within cannabis-related enterprises. It positions the cannabis nurse entrepreneur as a critical bridge between healthcare and industry, emphasizing the role of professional oversight, patient education, and ethical stewardship across both medical and adult-use contexts.

2. BACKGROUND

2.1 Regulatory and Practice Landscape of Cannabis Care

The legalization and commercialization of cannabis across multiple jurisdictions have introduced complex and evolving intersections among healthcare delivery, regulatory structures, and public access. Once confined to illicit markets and narrowly defined medical contexts, cannabis now occupies a rapidly expanding legal industry that includes medical treatment, adult-use consumption, wellness products, and ancillary services. This expansion has occurred alongside a growing but uneven body of scientific evidence related to therapeutic applications, potential risks, and population-level health outcomes. As a result, clinical guidance, ethical oversight, and regulatory compliance remain inconsistently aligned across practice environments (Hill, 2015; Whiting et al., 2015).

Unlike most therapeutic modalities encountered in nursing practice, cannabis exists within a fragmented legal and regulatory architecture that directly shapes how education is delivered, how risk is identified, and how professional responsibility is enforced. Regulatory literacy is therefore a prerequisite for nurses entering this space, informing ethical participation, licensure protection, and risk mitigation (National Council of State Boards of Nursing, 2018).

A significant and ongoing development in federal cannabis policy involves the potential rescheduling of marijuana under the Controlled Substances Act. For decades, cannabis was classified as a Schedule I substance, defined as having no accepted medical use and a high potential for abuse, a designation that constrained federally sanctioned research and limited clinical investigation (Controlled Substances Act, 1970). In May 2024, the U.S. Department of Justice published a proposed rule to transfer marijuana to Schedule III, reflecting a recommendation from the Department of Health and Human Services that cannabis has recognized medical use and a lower abuse potential than substances remaining in Schedule I (U.S. Department of Justice, 2024; U.S. Department of Health and Human Services, 2024). Schedule III classification, consistent with substances such as ketamine and buprenorphine, would reduce barriers to research, evidence development, and broader clinical engagement. In December 2025, Executive Order No. 14370 directed the Attorney General to expedite the rulemaking process required to complete this reclassification (Executive Office of the President, 2025). This process remains active at the time of writing and carries significant implications for research infrastructure, evidence generation, regulatory clarity, and the evolving role of nurses within cannabis-related care and practice environments.

2.2 Lack of Standardized Clinical Practice Frameworks

Despite increasing prevalence of cannabis use, including patients taking cannabis as part of their care for therapeutic purposes, standardized practice frameworks remain limited. Unlike prescription medications, cannabis products frequently lack consistent dosing guidance, uniform labeling standards, and comprehensive pharmacovigilance systems. Variability in potency, formulation, and route of administration complicates patient education, assessment, and risk stratification across care settings.

Professional guidance reflects this ambiguity. The National Council of State Boards of Nursing notes that nurses may engage in patient education and harm reduction related to cannabis use but must avoid recommending or prescribing cannabis, which falls outside nursing scope of practice (National Council of State Boards of Nursing, 2018). In the absence of institutional policies or national guidelines, nurses are often required to navigate these conversations independently, contributing to variability in documentation and patient education quality.

Cannabis use may also be underreported or omitted from health records entirely, increasing the risk of unrecognized adverse effects, drug-drug interactions, and incomplete clinical histories (Hill, 2015). These gaps constrain continuity of care and place disproportionate responsibility on individual clinicians to manage risk within incomplete informational environments.

2.3 Retail Environments as De Facto Sites of Education

In the absence of widespread clinical incorporation, retail dispensaries have become primary sites of education and access for individuals taking cannabis as part of wellness or symptom-related care decisions. While dispensary staff often complete state-mandated training, these programs typically emphasize regulatory compliance and product knowledge rather than assessment or patient safety. Dispensary personnel are not licensed healthcare professionals and do not operate within healthcare ethical frameworks or documentation standards.

This shift carries structural consequences. Education traditionally delivered within clinical settings is now occurring in commercial environments shaped by sales incentives and operational priorities. Without licensure-based professional responsibility, it becomes difficult to standardize risk screening, identify vulnerable populations, or maintain continuity across healthcare encounters.

Addressing this gap does not mean converting retail environments into clinical settings. It means introducing healthcare literacy into how cannabis education is designed and delivered, through structured frameworks, safety protocols, referral awareness, and clearly defined boundaries that support informed decision-making and reduce preventable harm (American Nurses Association, 2015; National Council of State Boards of Nursing, 2018).

2.4 Evolution of the Nursing Role in Cannabis and Emerging Markets

Nursing scholarship has long emphasized the profession's role in health promotion, patient advocacy, harm reduction, and ethical decision-making within emerging and contested areas of practice (American Nurses Association, 2015). As cannabis has entered mainstream healthcare and consumer markets, calls for greater involvement of licensed healthcare professionals have grown, driven by documented concerns around patient safety, education quality, and evidence-informed engagement. However, incorporation of nursing expertise into cannabis-related enterprises remains inconsistent, with many operations functioning without clinical leadership or established professional frameworks.

This absence contributes to concerns related to misinformation, variability in product quality, inequitable access, and ethical tensions between commercial incentives and patient-centered care. Regulatory analyses further underscore the importance of professional oversight in addressing risks associated with dosing variability, drug-drug interactions, and vulnerable populations (Hill, 2015; National Council of State Boards of Nursing, 2018).

Patient-centered narratives reflect the consequences of limited research infrastructure and inconsistent guidance. As Manalo-Morgan (2022) observes, "until we open up pathways to research, dosing will remain a significant concern for today's cannabis market" (p. 144). This uncertainty reinforces the need for grounded clinical leadership capable of supporting education, risk mitigation, and the development of structured care models.

Entrepreneurship within nursing has gained increasing attention as healthcare evolves and nurses pursue roles beyond traditional employment. Nurses who move into entrepreneurial practice apply professional expertise, integrative thinking, and patient-centered values to address unmet needs while contributing to economic sustainability and workforce diversification (Institute of Medicine, 2011). Within cannabis-related environments, these pathways create opportunities to shape service delivery, education, product development, and policy engagement, while also introducing novel ethical and regulatory considerations.

Taken together, these conditions produce a predictable gap. Cannabis use is widespread, yet the supporting infrastructure for safe health behavior, including consistent education, documentation norms, and risk mitigation processes, remains uneven. When a health behavior expands more rapidly than the professional structures built to support it, the result is not neutral. It produces role ambiguity, fragmented responsibility, and inconsistent quality across settings.

The following section examines the most persistent misalignments shaping cannabis care and identifies where nursing leadership can reduce preventable risk through clearer frameworks and stronger operational standards.

3. CRITICAL MISALIGNMENTS, CONTESTED ROLES, AND MISSED OPPORTUNITIES

The challenges and opportunities shaping cannabis care can be meaningfully distinguished between persistent structural problems that characterize the current landscape and emerging trends that are beginning to reshape it. The former include regulatory fragmentation, limited professional integration, inconsistent education, and underrepresentation of licensed healthcare professionals across cannabis environments. The latter include the emergence of clinically grounded practice models, federal policy movement toward rescheduling, increasing interprofessional engagement, and the development of data-informed infrastructure for disclosure and documentation. This section addresses the most significant current misalignments. Future directions and emerging opportunities are addressed in subsequent sections.

3.1 Structural and Regulatory Misalignments in Cannabis Care

The legalization and commercialization of cannabis across multiple jurisdictions have unfolded without parallel development of coherent professional frameworks, producing persistent challenges at the intersection of clinical practice, regulation, and commerce. Chief among these is the misalignment between widespread consumer access to cannabis products and the limited involvement of licensed healthcare professionals in cannabis-related service delivery. In many jurisdictions, cannabis operations function with minimal professional oversight, relying on nonclinical staff to guide consumers and patients despite well-documented risks related to adverse effects, drug-drug interactions, and misuse among medically vulnerable populations (Hill, 2015). This gap reflects not a lack of need for clinical expertise, but an underdeveloped infrastructure for incorporating it, raising concerns related to patient safety, informed decision-making, and ethical responsibility.

Regulatory fragmentation further complicates professional participation within the cannabis sector. Although state and regional policies increasingly authorize both medical and adult-use markets, standards governing education, scope of practice, and professional responsibility remain highly variable. Nurses seeking to engage in cannabis-related work often encounter ambiguous, restrictive, or outdated regulations that fail to reflect their competencies in patient assessment, education, risk mitigation, and quality assurance (National Council of State Boards of Nursing, 2018). In the absence of clearly articulated professional pathways, nonclinical models of cannabis commerce have become the default, frequently emphasizing sales performance and market growth over evidence-informed care. This reflects a broader tension between public health objectives and commercial imperatives that nurses are uniquely positioned to help resolve.

3.2 Ethical Tensions and Missed Opportunities for Clinical Leadership

Ethical tensions emerge within this landscape as nurses navigate entrepreneurial opportunities in a market shaped by profit incentives and evolving social norms. Questions have been raised about whether participation in cannabis enterprises risks compromising professional boundaries or undermining nursing's ethical commitments. These concerns are real and must be addressed through governance, transparency, and role clarity. However, exclusion is not a protective strategy. When nurses are absent from cannabis environments, clinical voice is removed from spaces where patients and consumers are already seeking guidance, and the gap is filled by less accountable alternatives.

From a professional standpoint, continued marginalization of nurses from leadership and decision-making roles represents a missed opportunity to align cannabis services with the principles of beneficence, nonmaleficence, and patient-centered care that are foundational to nursing practice (American Nurses Association, 2015). When nurses are present, operations gain structure: consistent education, disciplined risk screening, documentation awareness, and ethical guardrails. When nurses are absent, guidance becomes variable and is often driven by nonclinical incentives.

Current approaches to cannabis education and service delivery frequently rely on informal training, variable standards, and experiential knowledge rather than professionally grounded frameworks. This stands in contrast to emerging models that integrate nursing expertise into dispensary operations, product development, quality assurance, and patient consultation. These models emphasize structured education, documentation, risk assessment, and interprofessional collaboration, illustrating how established nursing competencies can directly address persistent gaps in safety, accountability, and public trust.

4. PROFESSIONAL ROLE CLARITY: SCOPE, ETHICS, AND BOUNDARIES

4.1 Scope of Practice Considerations

Scope of practice defines the activities that nurses are legally and professionally authorized to perform based on licensure, education, and regulatory standards. Cannabis use does not alter these boundaries, and clarity about what falls within and outside those boundaries is essential for nurses working in any cannabis-adjacent environment.

For registered nurses, practice in cannabis-related settings remains centered on education, assessment, documentation, and advocacy (National Council of State Boards of Nursing, 2018). Nurses may discuss routes of administration, onset and duration, impairment risk, general safety considerations, and known interaction concerns within a harm-reduction context. They may assess patient understanding, identify areas of concern, and encourage open communication with prescribing clinicians or primary care teams. These activities are consistent with core nursing competencies and do not constitute product recommendation.

Where advanced practice nurses hold state-specific authority to certify patients for medical cannabis programs, that authority remains distinct from prescribing and is governed by state law and institutional policy. Regardless of setting or role structure, precise role language matters. It protects patients who deserve accurate information, protects licensure from ambiguity, and protects public trust in the profession.

4.2 Ethical Obligations and Professional Accountability

Ethical practice in nursing is governed by the ANA Code of Ethics, with its emphasis on patient safety, informed decision-making, integrity, and professional responsibility (American Nurses Association,

2015). These obligations apply regardless of practice setting, including cannabis businesses, consulting arrangements, educational platforms, and policy-adjacent work.

Ethical challenges in cannabis environments most commonly arise at the intersection of commercial incentives and education. Nurses must maintain a clear distinction between providing education and endorsing products or outcomes. Transparency regarding role, compensation structure, and the limits of professional authority is not optional. It is the foundation on which patient trust and professional credibility rest.

The principle of nonmaleficence carries particular weight in this context. Product variability, incomplete evidence, and evolving regulatory standards mean that uncertainty is a persistent feature of cannabis care. Responsible practice requires acknowledging that uncertainty directly, refraining from overstating benefits, and avoiding minimization of documented risks (Hill, 2015; U.S. Food and Drug Administration [FDA], 2016). Honest communication about the limits of current evidence is itself an ethical act.

4.3 Boundaries in Commercial and Retail Environments

Retail dispensaries serve a commercial function, and nurses who consult within these environments must maintain clear boundaries that reflect both professional standards and patient safety obligations. Role delineation should be explicit and communicated consistently, covering the scope of the nurse's function, the activities that fall outside that scope, and how consumers should interpret the educational information they receive.

Educational materials developed or delivered by nurses in these settings should be evidence-informed, clearly attributed, and consistent with nursing scope and ethical standards. Documentation practices, where applicable, must respect privacy, confidentiality, and applicable data protection requirements. Professional responsibility follows the nurse into every setting, and the commercial nature of a given environment does not modify that obligation (National Council of State Boards of Nursing, 2018).

4.4 Managing Conflicts of Interest

Conflicts of interest arise when secondary interests, including financial gain or business affiliation, have the potential to influence professional judgment. In cannabis environments, these risks may be heightened by market volatility, rapid commercialization, and the blurring of educational and promotional functions.

Nurses must proactively identify and disclose potential conflicts, maintain separation between clinical and commercial roles where necessary, and adhere to established ethical guidelines. Compensation structures tied directly to product volume or consumer purchasing behavior are particularly inconsistent with professional standards and should be avoided. When financial arrangements create incentives that could compromise the integrity of education or assessment, those arrangements require restructuring or disclosure. Sustainable professional engagement in cannabis environments depends on prioritizing patient welfare and practice integrity over short-term commercial advantage, not as an aspirational standard, but as a nonnegotiable operational baseline (American Nurses Association, 2015).

4.5 Legal Risk, Licensure Protection, and Professional Liability

Nurses operating within cannabis environments face professional, civil, and in some jurisdictions criminal liability considerations that require deliberate and ongoing risk management. These exposures do not diminish in the absence of a formal clinical employment relationship. Professional responsibility follows the nurse regardless of setting, and cannabis-adjacent work is not exempt from the oversight of state boards of nursing (National Council of State Boards of Nursing, 2018).

Licensure protection is a primary consideration. State boards retain authority to investigate and discipline nurses whose conduct is deemed inconsistent with professional standards, including conduct occurring outside traditional healthcare settings. Nurses providing cannabis-related education, consultation, or operational leadership must ensure their activities remain within defined scope, do not constitute product endorsement beyond educational boundaries, and are documented in ways that reflect professional accountability. Vague or undocumented roles create ambiguity that complicates board proceedings and weakens professional defensibility.

Professional liability exposure is shaped by the nature of the nurse's activities and the clarity of their defined role within a given enterprise. Nurses conducting assessments, providing individualized guidance, or functioning in advisory capacities that influence patient or consumer decisions should carry professional liability coverage that explicitly includes cannabis-related practice. Standard malpractice policies may exclude roles operating outside traditional clinical settings or involving substances with unresolved federal legal status. Reviewing policy language carefully and securing appropriate coverage before engaging in cannabis-adjacent work is a necessary precaution, not an afterthought.

Contractual clarity provides an additional layer of protection. Written agreements defining role scope, compensation structure, and limits of professional authority reduce boundary violation risk and provide documentation in the event of dispute. Nurses should decline arrangements that tie compensation to sales volume or outcomes misaligned with patient safety. Federal legal status adds a further dimension: cannabis remains federally controlled, and nurses contracting with cannabis enterprises may face exposure in federal jurisdictions or regulated environments under federal oversight. Current legal counsel, maintained as an ongoing resource, is essential to sustainable participation in this space.

5. THE CANNABIS NURSE ENTREPRENEUR AS A SYSTEMS ROLE

5.1 Systems Thinking in Emerging Care Environments

The cannabis nurse entrepreneur is best understood not as an individual practitioner, but as a systems role, one centered on designing, stabilizing, and sustaining the operational conditions that support safe, ethical, and evidence-informed engagement with cannabis across healthcare-adjacent environments.

Systems thinking involves understanding how components within a complex environment interact and influence outcomes. In cannabis-related contexts, these components include regulatory frameworks, retail operations, consumer education, clinical workflows, documentation practices, and public health oversight. Weakness in any single component can compromise safety and equity across the whole. Applying this lens shifts focus away from individual product decisions and toward structural questions: how information is delivered, how risk is identified, how outcomes are tracked, and how professional responsibility is maintained.

Nursing has a long history of contributing to care in precisely this way, from infection prevention to medication safety to quality measurement. Cannabis care presents a comparable opportunity. Use is widespread, access is expanding, and the professional infrastructure needed to support safe engagement remains inconsistent across settings and populations (Institute of Medicine, 2011). The question is not whether nurses belong in these environments. It is what they build when they are there.

5.2 Translating Nursing Competencies Into Operational Infrastructure

Core nursing competencies translate directly into operational contributions that cannabis environments currently lack. Assessment skills inform the development of risk screening tools and consumer education frameworks that introduce clinical discipline into settings where decisions are otherwise unguided. Documentation expertise supports the creation of data capture processes that improve continuity, enable pattern recognition, and strengthen safety monitoring over time. Quality improvement methodologies guide the evaluation of outcomes and the identification of breakdowns before they become entrenched.

Education design is among the most transferable contributions. Standardized educational content ensures consistent messaging, emphasizes harm reduction, and establishes clear guidance on when referral to a licensed provider is appropriate. In environments where education has historically been shaped by product knowledge rather than patient safety, this shift is consequential.

Nurses also serve as effective connectors among regulators, operators, clinicians, and community stakeholders. This bridging function strengthens alignment between public health priorities and operational realities, particularly in settings where healthcare obligations and commercial pressures coexist. Implementation of nurse care management in a cluster randomized clinical trial produced measurable increases in access to treatment for opioid use disorder across primary care settings, demonstrating that structured nursing involvement improves outcomes in ways that are replicable across contexts (Abram et al., 2024; Wartko ct al., 2023). Cannabis care environments stand to benefit from the same disciplined approach.

5.3 Quality, Safety, Sustainability, and Replicability

Quality and safety are foundational to healthcare practice, yet formal quality structures within cannabis environments remain largely underdeveloped. Professionally grounded operational leadership introduces the mechanisms that make consistent, defensible care possible: standardized education protocols, incident awareness processes, documentation standards, and outcome monitoring practices that reduce reliance on individual discretion and informal judgment.

Equally important are the conditions that allow these structures to endure. A defining characteristic of effective operational models is their ability to function beyond the involvement of any single individual. Sustainability requires alignment with regulatory realities, ethical standards, and economic constraints. Practices grounded in clear governance, defined roles, and repeatable processes are far more resilient than those built around informal knowledge or the continued presence of a founding practitioner. When a nurse entrepreneur builds infrastructure rather than dependency, the work continues after they step back.

Replicability extends this principle further. Models that are documented, transferable, and adaptable across settings contribute more to the field than those that remain context-specific. In cannabis care, where inconsistency is itself the central problem, replicating a functional, ethical, professionally grounded model is not a secondary consideration. It is a measure of whether the work has succeeded, and it distinguishes professional operational leadership from participation alone.

6. APPLIED CASE STUDIES: NURSE-INFORMED AND HEALTHCARE-CENTERED MODELS IN PRACTICE

The following case studies illustrate applied responses to the structural, ethical, and regulatory misalignments described above. Each demonstrates how healthcare literacy, nursing values, and operational thinking can be translated into real-world cannabis enterprises, advocacy organizations, and public health initiatives. Together, they show how professionally grounded leadership can move clinical integrity from concept into practice across retail, community, and data governance environments. A comparative summary of all three cases is provided at the conclusion of this section (see Table 1).

6.1 Case Study 1: Integrating Healthcare Literacy and Data-Informed Strategy Into Cannabis Retail Development

Problem Type: Consumer safety and information asymmetry
System Level: Retail as a pre-clinical decision layer
Primary Risk: Uninformed use in the absence of structured guidance
Intervention Type: AI-enabled conversational intake and guided decision-making

Context

Following the legalization of adult-use cannabis in New York State, extended delays in retail licensure created a gap between policy reform and regulated consumer access. During this period, many consumers, particularly those in historically marginalized communities, continued to rely on unregulated markets, increasing exposure to unsafe products, misinformation, and inconsistent guidance. This period revealed a broader limitation: market expansion occurring without parallel development of healthcare-informed education, consumer protections, or structured service models aligned with public health principles.

Operational Challenge

Entrepreneurs operating in this environment faced a consequential decision: whether to adopt conventional retail models focused on product selection and transaction efficiency, or to design engagement models that prioritize informed decision-making and consumer safety. Traditional retail tools present product options and attributes but do not assess user context, intent, or risk. A healthcare-informed approach requires engagement, assessment, and guided decision support. Without this structure, a trust deficit develops, repeat engagement suffers, and the likelihood of uninformed or inconsistent use increases.

Nursing Lens Applied

The Dope Connection, a technology-enabled platform co-founded by biochemist Jessica Naissant, addressed this challenge by designing an AI-enabled conversational interface that prioritizes engagement before recommendation. Rather than presenting static product menus, the platform initiates dialogue, asking users about intended use, prior experience, tolerance, and wellness goals. This approach mirrors clinical intake processes in which assessment precedes intervention. The platform creates space for individuals to articulate their patterns in how individuals take cannabis and intentions, enabling recommendations that are context-aware rather than product-driven. From a nursing perspective, this model reflects core competencies in assessment, patient education, and harm reduction, introducing structure into environments where decisions are otherwise unassessed and unstandardized.

Derived Model: Retail as a Conversational Pre-Clinical Decision Support Layer

This case demonstrates that cannabis retail environments, such as Renaissañt Dispensary, can function as an early-stage decision support layer when structured engagement replaces passive product selection. The model moves from user-reported intent, prior use, tolerance, and context through a process of conversational intake and guided recommendation, producing informed selection and a clearer use strategy. The downstream effect is improved alignment between use and intent, increased consumer trust, and reduced preventable risk. Unlike conventional retail approaches that optimize for transaction volume, this model optimizes for decision quality and user understanding.

Outcome and Insight

Following implementation of New York's Conditional Adult-Use Retail Dispensary program, these principles were translated into physical retail through the launch of Renaissant NYC, a licensed dispensary emphasizing concierge-style engagement and culturally responsive education. This case illustrates a broader insight: legalization without infrastructure produces access on paper but inequity in practice. In the absence of structured engagement, individuals navigate complex decisions without guidance, reinforcing variability in outcomes. For nurses considering entrepreneurial practice, this case demonstrates that competencies in assessment, education, and risk mitigation translate directly into enterprise design, creating trust-based operations that improve both safety and sustainability.

6.2 Case Study 2: Equity-Centered Advocacy and Policy Navigation in Cannabis Systems

Problem Type: Health equity and access disparity
System Level: Policy, community, and clinical interface
Primary Risk: Unequal access to safe, informed cannabis use
Intervention Type: Community-based education, access facilitation, and policy navigation

Context

Minorities for Medical Marijuana (M4MM), founded by Roz McCarthy, is a national nonprofit organization addressing inequities in cannabis access, education, and industry participation. The organization serves Black, Brown, LatinX, veteran, and other historically marginalized populations disproportionately affected by criminalization and systemic exclusion from both healthcare and cannabis environments.

M4MM operates across community education, policy advocacy, workforce development, and healthcare navigation, positioning health equity as a structural rather than symbolic objective.

Systemic Challenge

Cannabis policy expansion has not translated uniformly into equitable access. Regulatory decisions are frequently shaped by competing economic, political, and institutional interests that may not reflect patient-level realities. As a result, access is defined legally but remains constrained operationally. Documented barriers include the cost of medical cannabis registration, limited transportation access, absence of culturally responsive education, provider knowledge deficits, and the persistent influence of stigma on disclosure behavior. These conditions produce measurable disparities in access, engagement, and safety outcomes across populations.

Organizational Decision and Strategy

M4MM made a deliberate choice to move beyond advocacy alone and intervene directly in access pathways. Rather than relying solely on policy change, the organization implemented community-centered strategies that address barriers in real time, including subsidizing the cost of medical cannabis registration for underserved individuals, conducting direct community outreach and education, creating culturally aligned messaging through trusted communication channels, and guiding individuals through complex regulatory processes. This approach reframes access as a multidimensional challenge that encompasses financial, informational, and navigational components, each of which requires intentional intervention.

Nursing Lens Applied

Nursing competencies are reflected throughout M4MM's operational model, particularly in its emphasis on education, advocacy, harm reduction, and patient-centered framing of cannabis use. Nurses contributed by translating policy into practical guidance, reframing cannabis as a health-related behavior rather than a moral or legal issue, and introducing professional structure into environments shaped by stigma and misinformation. This reframing is consequential. It shifts the conversation from access to products toward access to safe, informed, and clinically contextualized use, enabling more consistent and safety-oriented engagement across communities that have historically been underserved by both healthcare and regulatory systems.

Derived Model: Equity as an Access, Literacy, and Navigation Infrastructure

This case demonstrates that health equity is not achieved through legalization alone. It requires coordinated intervention across three interdependent domains. Access encompasses the financial and physical ability to obtain safe products and participate in regulated systems. Literacy encompasses understanding of use, dosing, risk, and the ability to make informed decisions. Navigation encompasses the capacity to move through regulatory, healthcare, and commercial systems without prohibitive barriers. When any one of these domains is underdeveloped, the others are undermined. Equity-centered design requires active, ongoing intervention at the community level rather than passive reliance on policy change.

Outcome and Insight

This case reinforces a central principle: legal access does not guarantee equitable access. Without intentional infrastructure, disparities persist across both health outcomes and industry participation. For nurses in entrepreneurial practice, M4MM illustrates that equity is measurable and operational, shaped by concrete decisions about access design, education quality, and navigation support rather than abstract commitment. It also demonstrates that nursing competencies translate meaningfully into advocacy and community health contexts, not only clinical ones.

6.3 Case Study 3: Project Destigmatize Healthcare -- Reconstructing Clinical Truth Through Nurse-Led Data Integrity Systems

Problem Type: Stigma-driven disclosure suppression and data distortion
System Level: Clinical documentation, intake design, and population health data
Primary Risk: Structurally compromised health records producing downstream harm
Intervention Type: Nurse-led disclosure-supportive intake design and structured data capture

Context

Every day, patients make a calculation before they speak. They assess whether their provider can be trusted, whether disclosure will change how they are treated, and whether honesty is worth the risk. For patients who are taking cannabis, often as part of how they manage symptoms or wellbeing, that calculation is frequently resolved in favor of silence. Not because they do not want accurate care, but because the conditions under which they are asked to disclose do not feel safe enough to answer honestly. Project Destigmatize Healthcare begins with that moment, because that is where the problem actually lives.

Problem Definition

When a patient withholds that they are taking cannabis from their provider, the clinical record becomes incomplete. That incompleteness does not stay contained to a single encounter. It moves downstream into medication reconciliation, treatment planning, quality measurement, population health datasets, and ultimately the policy narratives that determine where resources are directed and which populations are seen as having clinical need. Over time, patterns of nondisclosure are misread as absence of use rather than evidence of suppression, creating a self-reinforcing cycle in which the populations most affected by stigma become the least visible in the data used to serve them.

Project Destigmatize Healthcare frames this not as a cultural problem or an individual failure, but as a measurable operational breakdown with direct consequences for patient safety, data integrity, and health equity. Stigma, in this context, functions as a data distortion mechanism. Addressing it requires intervening not after the data is collected, but at the conditions under which disclosure occurs in the first place.

Why a Nurse-Led Model

Nurses occupy the precise intersection where this problem plays out. Intake conversations, medication reconciliation, patient education encounters, care transitions: these are the moments where stigma most predictably disrupts honest communication, and they are the moments nurses most consistently inhabit. From that position, nurses observe how the language of a question shapes the answer it receives, how documentation practices reflect and reinforce bias, and how incomplete information propagates into systems that appear objective but are structurally shaped by what patients chose not to say.

This observational vantage point is not incidental. It is the professional foundation for the project's design, which centers on psychologically safer survey structures, neutral and clinically relevant language, and structured data capture aligned with future integration into clinical workflows and quality improvement frameworks.

Clinical and Ethical Framework

The project is grounded in nursing standards of ethical advocacy, harm reduction, unbiased documentation, and continuous quality improvement (American Nurses Association, 2015; American Nurses Association, 2021). Data is treated as a clinical asset rather than an advocacy instrument, with protections that include voluntary participation, transparency regarding data use, minimal and purpose-driven collection, and the deliberate avoidance of identifiable, punitive, or surveillance-oriented data structures. These safeguards extend nursing ethics into data governance, ensuring that the act of collecting information does not itself reproduce the harm the project is designed to address.

Implementation and Early Outcomes

Preliminary findings from initial data collection, while limited in scale, reveal consistent and directional patterns. Disclosure is not absent; it is conditional. Participants demonstrate willingness to share cannabis use when language is neutral, nonjudgmental, and clinically relevant, indicating that intake design is itself a determinant of data quality. Patients frequently report self-directing how they take cannabis, including decisions about dosing, formulation, and use, without clinical input, and even when disclosure occurs, many express uncertainty about whether their provider has the knowledge to act on what they share. Trust, in these findings, precedes accuracy. When participants perceive the interaction as safe and aligned with their wellbeing rather than their evaluation, disclosure increases.

These early signals do not establish causal relationships, but they consistently indicate that disclosure behavior is responsive to environmental conditions and can be improved through intentional design. The outputs produced by this project, including standardized intake language, disclosure-supportive question structures, and adaptable data fields, are designed for translation into clinical workflows, dispensary-based education touchpoints, and public health surveillance efforts. The objective is not a single dataset but a replicable method that improves disclosure reliability while producing structured, ethically collected information capable of informing training programs, quality improvement initiatives, and policy discussion. If scaled, this approach offers a pathway for strengthening documentation integrity and rebuilding trust across multiple stigmatized domains of care, including substance use history, sexual health, mental health, and chronic pain, wherever patients have learned to protect themselves by withholding what they know.

6.4 Synthesis

These cases demonstrate that integrating clinical knowledge, ethical responsibility, and entrepreneurial strategy is not a departure from nursing practice. It is an extension of nursing's established role in building structures that protect patients when formal systems fail to keep pace with real-world behavior. Across retail development, community advocacy, and data governance, professionally grounded approaches introduce discipline into environments where variability, fragmentation, and informal decision-making have become normalized.

A consistent pattern emerges across all three cases. Each identifies a gap and responds by introducing structure at a different point along the continuum of care: structured retail engagement improves decision quality before use occurs, direct community intervention transforms legal eligibility into practical accessibility, and disclosure-supportive design improves clinical information reliability at the point of origin. This pattern reinforces a broader insight. Legalization without infrastructure produces access on paper but inequity in practice. Professionally informed models counter this dynamic by embedding assessment, education, documentation, and ethical oversight into operational design, transforming loosely defined interactions into repeatable processes.

Across cases, nursing contributes three consistent functions: the introduction of assessment where none previously existed, the establishment of ethical boundaries within commercially or politically influenced environments, and the insistence on outcomes that can be measured and improved over time. The central challenge is not cannabis expansion itself, but the absence of coordinated professional infrastructure capable of translating that use into clinically meaningful, measurable, and equitable practice. The role of the nurse entrepreneur is not only to participate in these environments, but to design the conditions that make them safer, more coherent, and more aligned with the standards patients deserve.

The three cases are compared across problem type, intervention strategy, and measurable outcome indicators below (see Table 1).

Table 1. Nurse-informed cannabis system models: Problem type, intervention strategy, and measurable outcome indicators across three applied case studies

Case	System-Level Problem	Nurse-Informed Intervention	Measurable Outcome Indicators
Case 1: The Dope Connection / Renaissant NYC	Consumer safety and information asymmetry in retail environments	AI-enabled conversational intake; assessment-before-recommendation model	Decision support utilization; recommendation alignment; consumer comprehension; customer retention
Case 2: Minorities for Medical Marijuana (M4MM)	Health equity and access disparity across marginalized populations	Community education; financial access support; policy navigation	Educational access rates; reduction in registration cost barriers; navigation efficiency; market participation equity
Case 3: Project Destigmatize Healthcare	Stigma-driven disclosure suppression compromising data integrity	Disclosure-supportive intake design; neutral clinical language; structured data capture	Disclosure rates by language condition; documentation completeness; provider knowledge gap identification

Note. Each case operates at a distinct point along the cannabis care continuum. Case 1 addresses retail decision support, Case 2 addresses community access and health equity, and Case 3 addresses clinical data integrity and disclosure-supportive design. Together they reflect the breadth of environments in which nursing competencies can reduce variability and strengthen professional accountability.

7. SOLUTIONS AND RECOMMENDATIONS

7.1 Integrating Nursing Expertise Into Cannabis Systems

Addressing challenges within cannabis systems requires deliberate incorporation of clinical expertise, ethical governance, and operational architecture capable of supporting safe, informed use. One foundational strategy is the formal inclusion of nurses as clinical leaders, consultants, and decision-makers within cannabis-related enterprises. By embedding competencies such as assessment, education, quality assurance, and risk mitigation into operational models, organizations can better align commercial activity with public health priorities and regulatory expectations (Institute of Medicine, 2011).

Integration does not require transforming cannabis businesses into healthcare facilities. It requires introducing healthcare literacy into how these environments are built and run, through structured education, consistent safety messaging, defined boundaries, referral awareness, and processes that support continuity across care encounters. When these elements are embedded, operations shift from informal, variable interactions toward repeatable, measurable processes that support both safety and sustainability.

7.2 Regulatory, Educational, and Organizational Pathways for Change

Educational preparation represents a primary intervention point. Standardized curricula and continuing professional development focused on cannabis science, pharmacology, regulatory literacy, and ethical practice are necessary to support responsible engagement. Such training should emphasize interdisciplinary collaboration, cultural competence, and applied decision-making to ensure services are responsive to diverse populations and real-world contexts. Clear educational standards also strengthen professional legitimacy and distinguish clinically grounded roles from the informal training models currently prevalent across the industry.

Regulatory and policy alignment is equally critical. Policymakers and professional organizations are encouraged to establish clearer guidance regarding scope of practice, documentation expectations, and professional responsibility structures for nurses working in cannabis-related environments. Where possible, harmonization across jurisdictions may reduce ambiguity, support compliance, and promote consistent standards of care. Nurses can contribute to these processes by bringing clinical perspective into regulatory design and by modeling ethically grounded, compliant operational practices.

Organizational implementation requires translation of these principles into practice. Care models built on standardized intake questions, disclosure-supportive communication, structured documentation, and follow-up awareness contrast with transaction-driven approaches by prioritizing long-term trust, safety, and outcome consistency over short-term efficiency, creating operations that are not only functional but designed to endure.

Collectively, these strategies position the cannabis nurse entrepreneur as a catalyst for broader improvement across cannabis environments. By combining clinical expertise with entrepreneurial strategy, nurses contribute to the development of more coherent, credible, and ethically grounded cannabis markets.

7.3 Interprofessional Collaboration as a Structural Requirement

Effective cannabis care does not occur in professional isolation. Safe practice requires coordinated engagement across disciplines, including medicine, pharmacy, social work, public health, and behavioral health. Interprofessional collaboration is a structural requirement for managing the complexity that cannabis use introduces across clinical workflows, not an optional enhancement.

Physicians and advanced practice providers play an essential role in authorizing participation in medical cannabis programs, adjusting pharmaceutical regimens in response to cannabis use, and establishing documented clinical rationale for therapeutic applications. Without physician engagement, medication reconciliation that accounts for cannabis remains incomplete and drug-drug interaction risk is inadequately managed. In cannabis-adjacent environments, nurses serve as a critical communication bridge, flagging disclosure patterns, initiating referral pathways, and ensuring that cannabis-related information reaches the prescribing clinician as part of a complete clinical picture.

Pharmacists contribute essential expertise in cannabinoid pharmacology, interaction profiling, and product-level safety evaluation. As cannabis products become increasingly varied in formulation and delivery, pharmacist collaboration supports more precise guidance around dosing, onset, duration, and contraindications, reducing reliance on informal or commercially driven product recommendations.

Public health professionals and community health workers extend clinical reach into populations where formal engagement is limited by access, stigma, or systemic barriers. Their involvement supports health equity goals by embedding cannabis safety education into community settings and ensuring that harm reduction frameworks reach individuals who may not engage regularly with healthcare systems.

Building these collaborative structures requires intentional planning. Nurses can lead the development of referral protocols, shared documentation frameworks, and cross-disciplinary communication standards that formalize the relationship between cannabis environments and broader healthcare networks. These structures do not require full institutional integration at the outset. They can be introduced incrementally through consultation agreements, shared intake tools, and defined escalation pathways that connect cannabis-adjacent environments to licensed clinical oversight.

7.4 Business Sustainability and Economic Feasibility of Cannabis Nurse Enterprises

Cannabis nurse enterprises operate within a distinct financial landscape shaped by regulatory constraints, reimbursement limitations, and market variability. Understanding this economic context is essential to building practice models that are clinically sound and operationally durable over time.

A significant financial constraint involves federal tax limitations that prevent cannabis businesses from deducting standard operating expenses, substantially increasing their effective tax burden compared to businesses in other industries (Internal Revenue Service, 2022). As federal rescheduling progresses this constraint may ease, but nurses entering cannabis business ownership should engage qualified legal and financial counsel to navigate current obligations and structure operations in ways that protect both viability and professional licensure.

Reimbursement presents a parallel challenge. Cannabis products and cannabis-related consultations are not currently covered by federal insurance programs or most private insurers. As a result, consultation models in this space typically operate on a direct-pay or fee-for-service basis. Emerging approaches have explored subscription-based wellness consulting, employer wellness partnerships, and consultation integrated within existing licensed healthcare settings as pathways toward more stable revenue.

Despite these constraints, clinically grounded enterprises carry structural advantages that support long-term viability. Professional credibility reduces reputational and compliance risk, translating into stronger relationships with regulators and institutional partners. Standardized education and documentation infrastructure reduces staff training costs and operational variability. Trust-based engagement tends to produce stronger client retention over time, reducing the sustained cost of building a consistent practice.

As federal rescheduling progresses, the financial landscape may shift materially, opening pathways for insurance coverage exploration, research partnerships, and expanded institutional collaboration. Financial sustainability ultimately depends on building practices that extend beyond individual involvement, structured for regulatory adaptation and grounded in models that produce measurable, defensible outcomes, qualities that align directly with the operational leadership approach that defines effective cannabis nurse entrepreneurship.

8. IMPLICATIONS FOR PRACTICE AND POLICY

8.1 Implications for Nursing Practice and Professional Preparation

The integration of nurses into leadership and entrepreneurial roles within cannabis systems expands practice into nontraditional environments while maintaining alignment with core professional competencies. Assessment, education, ethical reasoning, and quality assurance remain central, applied now within operational, community, and commercially influenced settings that require disciplined boundary management (American Nurses Association, 2021).

In practice, this includes the normalization of consultation within community-based environments, where clinically informed guidance can reduce harm, improve decision-making, and support patient autonomy. In these spaces, nurses serve as clinical interpreters, clarifying uncertainty, identifying risk patterns, and supporting informed engagement without displacing individual choice.

From an educational and workforce perspective, these developments signal a growing need for training pathways that prepare nurses for roles in highly regulated, nontraditional industries. Incorporation of cannabis science, regulatory literacy, interprofessional collaboration, and foundational business competencies into nursing education supports both individual career development and broader professional legitimacy within this space.

8.2 Implications for Health Policy and Regulatory Frameworks

Policy implications are equally consequential. As cannabis systems continue to evolve, decisions regarding licensure, scope of practice, and clinical oversight will shape both safety and access. Inclusion of nurses in policy development ensures that public health considerations remain central to how these environments are governed. Clear regulatory guidance recognizing nursing competencies in cannabis-related roles may reduce ambiguity, strengthen compliance, and support ethically grounded operational models (American Nurses Association, 2015).

Clinically grounded enterprises also provide practical examples of how healthcare standards can be incorporated into nonclinical environments, offering insight into how education, documentation, and safety processes can be embedded into settings where use is already occurring but professional structure remains limited (National Council of State Boards of Nursing, 2018).

Current evidence underscores the urgency of this work. While a substantial proportion of patients report medical cannabis use, fewer than 5 percent have this use documented in the electronic health record, reflecting a persistent gap between real-world behavior and clinical practice (Lapham et al.,

2022). This gap directly limits the ability to assess risk, reconcile medications, and incorporate cannabis use into care planning. Nurses are uniquely positioned to close it, not only through direct practice, but by building the intake frameworks, documentation standards, and referral structures that make clinical integration possible at scale (American Nurses Association, 2021; National Council of State Boards of Nursing, 2018; Institute of Medicine, 2011).

9. FUTURE RESEARCH DIRECTIONS

The structural gaps and practice models described throughout this chapter point toward a clear and pressing research agenda. Systematic investigation of outcomes across education, consultation, and quality practice is essential to advancing both professional standards and public health objectives as this field matures.

Priority areas include empirical evaluation of cannabis consultation models built on nursing competencies, with particular attention to patient safety indicators, harm reduction outcomes, documentation completeness, and the quality of clinical decision-making when cannabis use is disclosed and incorporated into care. Research across diverse populations and regulatory environments will be necessary to determine whether these models produce consistent, equitable outcomes or whether their benefits remain concentrated in contexts with existing clinical infrastructure.

Educational research represents an equally important domain. The competencies required for nurses pursuing entrepreneurial roles in cannabis environments are not yet well defined in the literature, and available training pathways remain inconsistent. Studies evaluating credentialing frameworks, continuing education designs, and competency-based curricula can inform the development of standardized preparation aligned with both professional expectations and real-world practice demands.

Policy-focused investigation should examine regulatory frameworks governing cannabis and nursing practice across jurisdictions, identifying barriers to participation and opportunities for alignment with public health goals. Research documenting nursing involvement in compliance oversight, regulatory design, and implementation can further establish the value of clinical expertise in shaping emerging therapeutic industries.

Finally, there is a need for interdisciplinary work integrating nursing, public health, business, and legal perspectives to examine how healthcare professionals contribute to the governance of highly regulated industries more broadly. Cannabis provides a timely and well-defined context for this investigation, but the questions it raises about clinical integration, professional boundaries, and practice infrastructure extend well beyond a single substance or sector. Addressing them rigorously will strengthen the evidence base for nursing leadership in emerging industries and the professional foundations of cannabis practice itself.

10. CONCLUSION

The emergence of the cannabis nurse entrepreneur reflects a broader transformation at the intersection of healthcare, entrepreneurship, and public policy. As legal cannabis markets expand, the central challenge is no longer access alone, but the absence of coordinated infrastructure capable of translating real-world behavior into clinically actionable and measurable systems. This chapter has demonstrated that nursing expertise, grounded in assessment, education, ethical practice, and systems thinking, offers a structured approach to addressing this gap within cannabis-related environments.

Across regulatory complexity, operational variability, and evolving market conditions, prevailing nonclinical models have often relied on informal education, inconsistent guidance, and fragmented oversight. These approaches introduce preventable risk by placing decision-making responsibility on individuals without sufficient structure or support. In contrast, nurse-informed models introduce discipline into system design through structured engagement, standardized education, and disclosure-supportive communication, directly influencing whether cannabis use—and more specifically, whether patients are taking cannabis as part of their care—is documented, reconciled with medications, and incorporated into clinical decision-making.

Current evidence reinforces this structural limitation. Despite widespread prevalence of patients taking cannabis across both medical and wellness contexts, documentation of that use within the electronic health record remains critically low, underscoring the persistent gap between real-world behavior and clinical integration. This gap directly limits clinicians' ability to assess risk, reconcile medications, and incorporate cannabis use into care planning.

Entrepreneurial engagement, when grounded in professional standards, represents a legitimate extension of nursing practice into emerging domains. It enables the application of clinical competencies within environments where health-related decisions are already occurring, but where formal care structures remain underdeveloped. In this context, the nurse entrepreneur functions not only as a participant, but as a system designer, translating clinical knowledge into operational models that improve safety, consistency, and trust.

The analyses presented in this chapter, including enterprise innovation, equity-centered advocacy, and data-informed system design, demonstrate that the integration of nursing into cannabis systems is both feasible and necessary. These approaches establish pathways for aligning business operations with public health objectives while maintaining clear ethical boundaries between healthcare and commerce.

As cannabis systems continue to evolve, the role of nursing leadership will extend beyond participation into the design of infrastructure that supports safe disclosure, consistent documentation, and clinically grounded education. These functions are foundational to ensuring that expanding access translates into meaningful safety and health equity across populations. The future of cannabis systems will not be determined by access alone, but by the growing inclusion of consumer voices in the research that shapes those systems, by the standards that govern how cannabis is clinically understood and applied, and by the degree to which that understanding is translated into practice that is informed, equitable, and built to protect the people it serves.

REFERENCES

Abram, M. D., Marzano, M., Caniano, L., & Searby, A. (2024). Nurse-led models of care for outpatient substance use disorder treatment: A scoping review. *Journal of Clinical Nursing*, *33*(11), 4280–4296. Advance online publication. DOI: 10.1111/jocn.17377 PMID: 39020508

American Nurses Association. (2015). Code of ethics for nurses with interpretive statements. https://www.nursingworld.org/coe-view-only

American Nurses Association. (2021). Nursing: Scope and standards of practice (4th ed.). https://www.nursingworld.org

Balbuena, J. M. (2024). *Green renaissance: Unveiling the historical influence of the cannabis plant on wellness, lifestyle, and culture*. Self-published.

Baral, A., Diggs, B.-N. A., Greengold, J., Foronda, C., Anglade, D., Camacho-Rivera, M., Islam, J. Y., & Vidot, D. C. (2025). State of the science: Health care provider communication of cannabis use among adults living with cancer. *Journal of Cancer Education*, *40*(3), 329–347. DOI: 10.1007/s13187-024-02484-z PMID: 39160419

Boehnke, K. F., Litinas, E., Worthing, B., Conine, L., Kruger, D. J., & Clauw, D. J. (2021). Communication between healthcare providers and medical cannabis patients regarding referral and medication substitution. *Journal of Cannabis Research*, *3*(1), 2. Advance online publication. DOI: 10.1186/s42238-021-00058-0 PMID: 33526140

Braun, I. M., Blinder, V. S., Freedman-Cass, D. A., Bhatt, D. L., Blanke, C. D., Cleary, J. F., Cyr, D., Danaher, B. G., Davis, M. P., Enright, K. M., Goldstein, D. A., Gralow, J. R., Henry, D. H., Hershman, D. L., Kaur, S., Ligibel, J. A., Moy, B., Mustian, K. M., Patt, D. A., & Loprinzi, C. L. (2024). Cannabis and cannabinoids in adults with cancer: ASCO guideline. *Journal of Clinical Oncology*, *42*(16), 1774–1803. DOI: 10.1200/JCO.23.02501 PMID: 38478773

Clobes, T. A., Mee, M. M., Jimenez, J. M., Maldonado, J., & Song, J. R. (2025). Impact of healthcare provider awareness and guidance on the medical cannabis experience. *Medical Cannabis and Cannabinoids*, *8*(1), 47–57. DOI: 10.1159/000544125 PMID: 40104431

Controlled Substances Act, 21 U.S.C. § 801 et seq. (1970).

Dock, L. L., & Stewart, I. M. (1938). *A short history of nursing: From the earliest times to the present*. G. P. Putnam's Sons.

Executive Office of the President. (2025, December 18). Increasing medical marijuana and cannabidiol research, Exec. Order No. 14370. https://www.whitehouse.gov

Hill, K. P. (2015). Medical marijuana for treatment of chronic pain and other medical and psychiatric problems. *Journal of the American Medical Association*, *313*(24), 2474–2483. DOI: 10.1001/jama.2015.6199 PMID: 26103031

Institute of Medicine. (2011). *The future of nursing: Leading change, advancing health*. The National Academies Press., DOI: 10.17226/12956

Internal Revenue Service. (2022). Internal Revenue Code § 280E. https://www.irs.gov

Lapham, G. T., Matson, T. E., Carrell, D. S., Bobb, J. F., Luce, C., Oliver, M. M., Ghitza, U. E., Hsu, C., Browne, K. C., Binswanger, I. A., Campbell, C. I., Saxon, A. J., Vandrey, R., Schauer, G. L., Pacula, R. L., Horberg, M. A., Bailey, S. R., McClure, E. A., & Bradley, K. A. (2022). Comparison of medical cannabis use reported on a confidential survey vs documented in the electronic health record among primary care patients. *JAMA Network Open*, *5*(5), e2211677. DOI: 10.1001/jamanetworkopen.2022.11677 PMID: 35604691

Manalo-Morgan, A. (2022). *Mighty flower: How cannabis saved my son*. Forbes Books.

National Council of State Boards of Nursing. (2018). The NCSBN national nursing guidelines for medical marijuana. https://www.ncsbn.org

Reverby, S. M. (1987). *Ordered to care: The dilemma of American nursing, 1850-1945*. Cambridge University Press.

Substance Abuse and Mental Health Services Administration. (2023). *Results from the 2022 National Survey on Drug Use and Health*. U.S. Department of Health and Human Services.

U.S. Department of Health and Human Services. (2024). Medical and scientific analysis of marijuana. https://www.hhs.gov

U.S. Department of Justice, Drug Enforcement Administration. (2024). Schedules of controlled substances: Rescheduling of marijuana (Proposed rule). *Federal Register*, *89*(168), 44597–44616. https://www.federalregister.gov

U.S. Food and Drug Administration. (2016). FDA and marijuana: Questions and answers. https://www.fda.gov

Wartko, P. D., Bobb, J. F., Boudreau, D. M., Matthews, A. G., McCormack, J., Lee, A. K., Qiu, H., Yu, O., Hyun, N., Idu, A. E., Campbell, C. I., Saxon, A. J., Liu, D. S., Altschuler, A., Samet, J. H., Labelle, C. T., Zare-Mehrjerdi, M., Stotts, A. L., Braciszewski, J. M., & Bradley, K. A. (2023). Nurse care management for opioid use disorder treatment: The PROUD cluster randomized clinical trial. *JAMA Internal Medicine*, *183*(12), 1343–1354. DOI: 10.1001/jamainternmed.2023.5701 PMID: 37902748

Whiting, P. F., Wolff, R. F., Deshpande, S., Di Nisio, M., Duffy, S., Hernandez, A. V., Keurentjes, J. C., Lang, S., Misso, K., Ryder, S., Schmidlkofer, S., Westphal, M., & Kleijnen, J. (2015). Cannabinoids for medical use: A systematic review and meta-analysis. *Journal of the American Medical Association*, *313*(24), 2456–2473. DOI: 10.1001/jama.2015.6358 PMID: 26103030

KEY TERMS AND DEFINITIONS

Anticipated Stigma: The expectation of judgment, discrimination, or devaluation if a stigmatized behavior or condition is disclosed. In cannabis-related care, it functions as a barrier to communication, contributing to nondisclosure and incomplete clinical histories.

Cannabis Nurse Entrepreneur: A licensed nurse who integrates clinical expertise, ethical accountability, and entrepreneurial strategy within cannabis-related enterprises, applying nursing standards to patient education, operational design, regulatory navigation, and quality assurance.

Clinical Integration of Cannabis: The incorporation of cannabis-related behaviors into healthcare workflows, including screening, documentation, medication reconciliation, and care planning.

Data Integrity: The accuracy, completeness, and reliability of data used in clinical care, research, and policy. In cannabis-related contexts, it is often compromised by nondisclosure and inconsistent documentation.

Dispensary-Based Care: A healthcare-adjacent model in which education, screening, and safety guidance occur within or alongside cannabis dispensary operations, introducing clinical literacy through structured education and defined professional boundaries.

Harm Reduction: An approach that focuses on reducing risk and preventing harm without requiring abstinence, including education on product variability, impairment, and drug interactions.

Interprofessional Collaboration: A coordinated model in which multiple disciplines work together to support patient safety, medication reconciliation, and effective care planning in cannabis-related environments.

Regulatory Literacy: The ability to interpret and apply cannabis-related laws, regulations, and compliance requirements within clinical and operational practice.

Scope of Practice: The legally and professionally defined boundaries of nursing practice that guide permissible activities such as assessment, education, documentation, and advocacy.

Systems Thinking: An approach that examines how components within complex environments interact to influence outcomes, emphasizing infrastructure, process reliability, and accountability.

Compilation of References

Abram, M. D., Marzano, M., Caniano, L., & Searby, A. (2024). Nurse-led models of care for outpatient substance use disorder treatment: A scoping review. *Journal of Clinical Nursing*, *33*(11), 4280–4296. Advance online publication. DOI: 10.1111/jocn.17377 PMID: 39020508

Abu Baker, D., Cruz Rivera, P. N., Narasimhan, R., Nguyen, N., Tibiriçá, L., Kepner, W. E., O'Malley, P., Nguyen, A. L., & Moore, A. A. (2024). Older adults' use of cannabis and attitudes around disclosing medical cannabis use to their healthcare providers in California: A mixed methods study. *Drugs - Real World Outcomes*, *11*(4), 647–658. DOI: 10.1007/s40801-024-00451-0 PMID: 39294485

Abuhasira, R., Shbiro, L., & Landschaft, Y. (2018). Medical use of cannabis and cannabinoids containing products: Regulations in Europe and North America. *European Journal of Internal Medicine*, *49*, 2–6. DOI: 10.1016/j.ejim.2018.01.001 PMID: 29329891

Accreditation Commission for Education in Nursing. (n.d.). *ACEN About Us*. https://www.acenursing.org/about

Act, C. S. 21 U.S.C. §§ 801–971 (1970). https://www.govinfo.gov/content/pkg/USCODE-2023-title21/pdf/USCODE-2023-title21-chap13.pdf

Adam, K. C. S., Doss, M. K., Pabon, E., Vogel, E. K., & de Wit, H. (2020). Δ9-Tetrahydrocannabinol (THC) impairs visual working memory performance: A randomized crossover trial. *Neuropsychopharmacology : Official Publication of the American College of Neuropsychopharmacology*, *45*(11), 1807–1816. DOI: 10.1038/s41386-020-0690-3 PMID: 32386395

Adams, I. B., & Martin, B. R. (1996). Cannabis: Pharmacology and toxicology in animals and humans. *Addiction (Abingdon, England)*, *91*(11), 1585–1614. DOI: 10.1046/j.1360-0443.1996.911115852.x PMID: 8972919

Agriculture Improvement Act of 2018, Pub. L. No. 115-334, 132 Stat. 4490 (2018). https://www.congress.gov/115/plaws/publ334/PLAW-115publ334.pdf

Agriculture Improvement Act of 2018, S.3042, 115th Cong. (2018). Congress.gov. June 18, 2018. https://www.congress.gov/bill/115th-congress/senate-bill/3042?q=%7B%22search%22%3A%22farm+bill%22%7D&s=3&r=1

Ahuja, A. S. (2019). Should RCTs be used as the gold standard for evidence-based medicine? *Integrative Medicine Research*, *8*(1), 31–32. DOI: 10.1016/j.imr.2019.01.001 PMID: 30805294

Aizpurua-Olaizola, O., Elezgarai, I., Rico-Barrio, I., Zarandona, I., Etxebarria, N., & Usobiaga, A. (2017). Targeting the endocannabinoid system: Future therapeutic strategies. *Drug Discovery Today, 22*(1), 105–110. https://www.sciencedirect.com/science/article/abs/pii/S1359644616302926. DOI: 10.1016/j.drudis.2016.08.005 PMID: 27554802

Ajzen, I. (1991). The theory of planned behavior. *Organizational Behavior and Human Decision Processes, 50*(2), 179–211. DOI: 10.1016/0749-5978(91)90020-T

Alcohol Policy Information System. (n.d.). *About cannabis policy.* https://alcoholpolicy.niaaa.nih.gov/about/about-cannabis-policy

Alcohol Policy Information System. (n.d.). *About cannabis policy.* National Institute on Alcohol Abuse and Alcoholism. https://alcoholpolicy.niaaa.nih.gov/about/about-cannabis-policy

Alexander, M. (2010). *The new Jim Crow: Mass incarceration in the age of colorblindness.* The New Press.

Alexander, S. P. (2020). Barriers to the wider adoption of medicinal Cannabis. *British Journal of Pain, 14*(2), 122–132. DOI: 10.1177/2049463720922884 PMID: 32537151

Alger, B. (2013). Getting high on the endocannabinoid system. *Cerebrum.* https://www.ncbi.nlm.nih.gov/pmc/articles/PMC3997295/

American Association of Colleges of Nursing. (2021). *The Essentials: Core competencies for professional nursing education.* Retrieved January 30, 2026, from American Association of Colleges of Nursing: https://www.aacnnursing.org/Portals/0/PDFs/Publications/Essentials-2021.pdf

American Association of Colleges of Nursing. (n.d.). *About AACN.* Retrieved April 10, 2026, from American Assoicaiation of Colleges of Nursing: https://www.aacnnursing.org/about-aacn

American Bar Association. (2024). *Rescheduling cannabis: Implications for health law, research, and regulation. The Health Lawyer, 36*(3). https://www.americanbar.org/groups/health_law/resources/health-lawyer/2024-february/rescheduling-cannabis/

American Cannabis Nurse Association. (2025). Clinical Cannabis Policies in Compassionate Care Position Paper. https://cannabisnurses.org/statements

American Cannabis Nurses Association & American Nurses Association. (2024). *Cannabis nursing: Scope and standards of practice* (2nd ed.). American Nurses Association. https://www.nursingworld.org/nurses-books/cannabis-nursing-scope-and-standards-of-practice

American Cannabis Nurses Association & American Nurses Association. (2024). Cannabis nursing: Scope and standards of practice (2nd ed.). American Nurses Association. https://www.nursingworld.org/nurses-books/cannabis-nursing-scope-and-standards-of-practice/

American Cannabis Nurses Association & American Nurses Association. (2024). *Cannabis nursing: Scope and standards of practice.* American Nurses Association.

American Cannabis Nurses Association, & American Nurses Association. (2024). *Cannabis nursing: Scope and standards of practice* (2nd ed.). American Nurses Association.

American Cannabis Nurses Association. (2021). *About ACNA.* https://cannabisnurses.org/about-the-acna

American Cannabis Nurses Association. (2023). *Cannabis nursing scope and standards of practice*. ACNA.

American Cannabis Nurses Association. (2025). American Cannabis Nurses Association Position on Cannabis Rescheduling: Advocating for Schedule VI Position & Policy Statement of the American Cannabis Nurses Association. ACNA.https://cannabisnurses.org/statements

American Cannabis Nurses Association. (2025, November 20). *Use and regulation of synthetic cannabinoids and hemp-derived substances and semi-synthetic cannabinoid receptor agonists.* http://cannabisnurses.org

American Cannabis Nurses Association. (n.d.). Lobbying/Advocacy with 501 (c) (3) status. https://docs.google.com/document/d/132J3taSi4QnXMR_JFW3hnemQcusZaEdF/edit?usp=sharing&ouid=107587315507364884473&rtpof=true&sd=true

American Civil Liberties Union. (2020). *A tale of two countries: Racially targeted arrests in the era of marijuana reform.* https://www.aclu.org

American Holistic Nurses Association. (n.d.). *What is holistic nursing?* https://www.ahna.org/About-Us/What-is-Holistic-Nursing

American Nurses Association & American Cannabis Nurses Association. (2021). Cannabis Nursing: Scope and standards of practice. American Nurses Association.

American Nurses Association and American Cannabis Nurses Association. (2024). *Cannabis Nursing Scope and Standards of Practice* (1st ed.).

American Nurses Association Center for Ethics and Human Rights. (2016). Therapeutic Use of Marijuana and Related Cannabinoids. ANA Silver Spring.https://www.nursingworld.org/globalassets/docs/ana/therapeutic-use-of-marijuna-and-related-cannabinoids.pdf

American Nurses Association Center for Ethics and Human Rights. (2021). Therapeutic Use of Marijuana and Related Cannabinoids Position Statement. ANA.https://www.nursingworld.org/globalassets/practiceandpolicy/nursing-excellence/ana-position-statements/therapeutic-use-of-marijuana-and-related-cannabinoids-position-statement-final-2021.pdf#:~:text=Position%20Statement%3A%20Providing%20patients%20safe,marijuana%2Fcannabis.&text=Code%20of%20ethics%20for%20nurses,interpretive%20statements.%20Silver%20Spring%2C%20MD%3A

American Nurses Association Position Statement: Nurses' professional responsibility to promote ethical practice environments. (January 23, 2023) . OJIN: The *Online Journal of Issues in Nursing 28(1).* https://ojin.nursingworld.org/table-of-contents/volume-28-2023/number-1-january-2023/responsibility-to-promote-ethical-practice-environments/

American Nurses Association Position Statement: Therapeutic use of marijuana and related cannabinoids. (2022). *OJIN: The Online Journal of Issues in Nursing, 27*(1). https://doi.org/10.3912/OJIN.Vol27No01PoSCol01

American Nurses Association. (1994, December 8). Drug Testing for Health Care Workers. https://www.nursingworld.org/practice-policy/nursingexcellence/official-position-statements/id/drug-testing-forhealth-care-workers

American Nurses Association. (2015). Code of ethics for nurses with interpretive statements. https://www.nursingworld.org/coe-view-only

American Nurses Association. (2015). *Nursing: Scope and standards of practice* (3rd ed.).

American Nurses Association. (2015/2021). *Code of ethics for nurses with interpretive statements*. American Nurses Association.

American Nurses Association. (2016). Nursing Administration: Scope and Standards of Practice, 2nd Edition eBook. Nursesbooks. https://api.pageplace.de/preview/DT0400.9781558106444_A30487125/preview-9781558106444_A30487125.pdf

American Nurses Association. (2016). Therapeutic use of marijuana and related cannabinoids [Position statement]. American Nurses Association. https://www.nursingworld.org/~49a8c8/globalassets/practiceandpolicy/ethics/therapeutic-use-of-marijuana-and-related-cannabinoids-position-statement.pdf

American Nurses Association. (2016). *Therapeutic use of marijuana and related cannabinoids* [Position statement]. https://www.nursingworld.org/practice-policy/nursing-excellence/official-position-statements/id/therapeutic-use-of-marijuana-and-related-cannabinoids/

American Nurses Association. (2021). *Nursing: Scope and standards of practice* (4th ed.). American Nurses Association.

American Nurses Association. (2021). Nursing: Scope and standards of practice (4th ed.). https://www.nursingworld.org

American Nurses Association. (2021). *Therapeutic use of marijuana and related cannabinoids*. ANA Center for Ethics and Human Rights. https://www.nursingworld.org/globalassets/practiceandpolicy/nursing-excellence/ana-position-statements/therapeutic-use-of-marijuana-and-related-cannabinoids-position-statement-final-2021.pdf?utm_source=copilot.com

American Nurses Association. (2023). *ANA Enterprise impact report 2023; Imagining the Enterprise into 2040.* Silver Springs, MD: American Nurse Enterprise. Retrieved from https://www.nursingworld.org/ana/about-ana/annual-reports/

American Nurses Association. (2023). ANA officially recognizes cannabis nursing as a specialty nursing practice [News release]. American Nurses Association. https://www.nursingworld.org/news/news-releases/2023/ana-officially-recognizes-cannabis-nursing-as-a-specialty-nursing-practice/

American Nurses Association. (2023). *ANA officially recognizes cannabis nursing as a specialty nursing practice* [News release]. https://www.nursingworld.org/news/news-releases/2023/ana-officially-recognizes-cannabis-nursing-as-a-specialty-nursing-practice/

American Nurses Association. (2023). *Cannabis nursing: Scope and standards of practice*. American Nurses Association. https://www.nursingworld.org/nurses-books/cannabis-nursing-scope-and-standards-of-practice/

American Nurses Association. (2023). *Recognition of cannabis nursing as a specialty practice*. ANA.

American Nurses Association. (2023, July 10). *ANA officially recognizes cannabis nursing as a specialty nursing practice.* https://www.nursingworld.org/news/news-releases/2023/ana-officially-recognizes-cannabis-nursing-as-a-specialty-nursing-practice/

American Nurses Association. (2023, September 27). *ANA officially recognises cannabis nursing as a specialty nursing practice.* https://www.nursingworld.org/news/news-releases/2023/ana-officially-recognizes-cannabis-nursing-as-a-specialty-nursing-practice/

American Nurses Association. (2024). *Healthy Nurse Healthy Nation.* Silver Spring, MD: American Nurse Journal. https://www.nursingworld.org/ana/about-ana/

American Nurses Association. (2024). *Nursing Leadership: Scope and Standards of Practice* (3rd ed.). American Nurses Association.

American Nurses Association. (2024). Re: Schedules of Controlled Substances: Rescheduling of Marijuana [DEA–1362; A.G. Order No. 5931– 2024]. Letter to Attorney General Garland: Submitted electronically at www.regulations.gov https://www.nursingworld.org/globalassets/docs/ana/comment-letters/ana-cannbbis-eschedule-comments-final-2024-07-17.pdf

American Nurses Association. (2025). *Code of ethics for nurses with interpretive statements: Provisions 1-9.* ANA.

American Nurses Association. (2025). Code of ethics for nurses. American Nurses Association.https://codeofethics.ana.org/home

American Nurses Association. (2025). Code of ethics for nurses. In A. N. Association.

American Nurses Credentialing Center. (2017). *American Nurses Association recognition of a nursing specialty, approval of specialty nursing scope and practice statement, acknowledgment of specialty nursing standards of practice, and affirmation of focused practice competencies.* American Nurses Association.

American Society for Quality. (n.d.). Retrieved February 4, 2026, from What is Six Sigma?: https://asq.org/quality-resources/six-sigma

Americans for Safe Access. (2025). California healthcare facility implementation guide for the compassionate access to Medical Cannabis Act Ryan's Law SB 311(2021), SB 988 (2022), SB 302 (2023). https://www.safeaccessnow.org/ryanslaw_facilityresources#gsc.tab=0

Americans for Safe Access. (2025). *Healthcare facility guide to implementing Ryan's Law.* https://www.safeaccessnow.org/ryanslaw_facilityresources

Amin, M. R., & Ali, D. W. (2019). Pharmacology of medical cannabis. *Recent advances in cannabinoid physiology and pathology. Advances in Experimental Medicine and Biology, 1162*, 151–165. DOI: 10.1007/978-3-030-21737-2_8 PMID: 31332738

Ananth, P., Ma, C., Al-Sayegh, H., Kroon, L., Klein, V., Wharton, C., Hallez, E., Braun, I., Michelson, K., Rosenberg, A. R., London, W., & Wolfe, J. (2018). Provider perspectives on use of medical marijuana in children with cancer. *Pediatrics, 141*(1), e20170559. DOI: 10.1542/peds.2017-0559 PMID: 29233937

Anderson, D. M., & Rees, D. I. (2023). The public health effects of legalizing marijuana. Journal of Economic Literature, 61(1), 86–143. doi:10.1257/jel.20211635

Anscombe, G. E. M. (1963). *Intention* (2nd ed.). Basil Blackwell. (Original work published 1957)

Arkell, R., Kevin, R. C., Stuart, J., Lintzeris, N., Haber, P. S., Ramaekers, J. G., & McGregor, I. S. (2019). Detection of Δ(9) THC in oral fluid following vaporized cannabis with varied cannabidiol (CBD) content: An evaluation of two point-of-collection testing devices. *Drug Testing and Analysis*, *11*(10), 1486–1497. DOI: 10.1002/dta.2687 PMID: 31442003

Arkell, T. R., Downey, L. A., Hayley, A. C., & Roth, S. (2023). Assessment of medical cannabis and health-related quality of life. *JAMA Network Open*, *6*(5), e2312522. DOI: 10.1001/jamanetworkopen.2023.12522 PMID: 37159196

Armentano, P.A. (2021, September 13). *California: Lawmakers advance legislation providing for medical cannabis use in hospitals,* NORML. https://norml.org/blog/2021/09/13/california-lawmakers-advance-legislation-permitting-medical-cannabis-use-in-hospitals/

Aroskar, M. (1998, December 31). Administrative Ethics: Perspectives on Patients and Community-Based Care. *Online Journal of Issues in Nursing*, *3*(3). Advance online publication. https://doi.org/10.3912/OJIN.Vol3No03Man04DOI: 10.3912/OJIN.Vol3No03Man04

Ashare, R. L., Turay, E., Worster, B., Wetherill, R. R., Bidwell, L. C., Doucette, A., & Meghani, S. H. (2023). Social determinants of health associated with how cannabis is obtained and used in patients with cancer receiving care at a cancer treatment center in Pennsylvania. *Cannabis (Research Society on Marijuana)*, *6*(2), 1–12. DOI: 10.26828/cannabis/2023/000151 PMID: 37484056

Ashton, C. H. (2001). Pharmacology and effects of cannabis: A brief review. *The British Journal of Psychiatry*, *178*(2), 101–106. DOI: 10.1192/bjp.178.2.101 PMID: 11157422

Australia, N. a. (2025). *Registration Standards*. Retrieved December 15, 2025, from Australian Health Practitioner Regulation Agency: https://www.nursingmidwiferyboard.gov.au/registration-standards.aspx

Aviram, J. (2025, November 13). Medical cannabis in Israel: A comprehensive review of trends and regulations. *Journal of Cannabis Research*, *7*(1), 90. Advance online publication. DOI: 10.1186/s42238-025-00344-1 PMID: 41233935

Balachandran, P., Elsohly, M., & Hill, K. P. (2021). Cannabidiol interactions with medications, illicit substances, and alcohol: A comprehensive review. *Journal of General Internal Medicine*, *36*(7), 2074–2084. DOI: 10.1007/s11606-020-06504-8 PMID: 33515191

Balbuena, J. M. (2024). *Green renaissance: Unveiling the historical influence of the cannabis plant on wellness, lifestyle, and culture*. Self-published.

Balneaves, G., Alraja, A. A., Thompson, G., Penner, J. L., John, P. S., Scerbo, D., & van Dyck, J. (2024). Cannabis use in a Canadian long-term care facility: A case study. *BMC Geriatrics*, *24*(1), 467. DOI: 10.1186/s12877-024-05074-2 PMID: 38811895

Balneaves, L. B., & Alraja, A. A. (2019). "Guarding their practice": A descriptive study of Canadian nursing policies and education related to medical cannabis. *BMC Nursing*, *18*(1), 1–10. DOI: 10.1186/s12912-019-0390-7 PMID: 31827392

Balneaves, L. G. (2018). Medical cannabis education: The Canadian experience. *Journal of Nursing Regulation*, *9*(2), 22–29.

Balneaves, L. G., Alraja, A., Ziemianski, D., McCuaig, F., & Ware, M. (2018). A national needs assessment of Canadian nurse practitioners regarding cannabis for therapeutic purposes. *Cannabis and Cannabinoid Research*, *3*(1), 66–73. DOI: 10.1089/can.2018.0002 PMID: 29588917

Balneaves, L. G., Watling, C. Z., Strus, J. A., Boscow, M., Davis, L., Graveline, K., Harrigan, T., Henriquez, N., Mitchell, K., & Thompson, G. (2023). Baccalaureate nursing students' knowledge, attitudes, educational needs, and use of medical and non-medical cannabis at five institutions in Manitoba, Canada: A cross-sectional analysis. *Nurse Education Today*, *130*, 105955. Advance online publication. DOI: 10.1016/j.nedt.2023.105955 PMID: 37677985

Banerjee, R., Erridge, S., Salazar, O., Mangal, N., Couch, D., Pacchetti, B., & Sodergren, M. H. (2022). Real-world evidence in medical cannabis research. *Therapeutic Innovation & Regulatory Science*, *56*(1), 8–14. DOI: 10.1007/s43441-021-00346-0 PMID: 34748204

Baral, A., Diggs, B.-N. A., Greengold, J., Foronda, C., Anglade, D., Camacho-Rivera, M., Islam, J. Y., & Vidot, D. C. (2025). State of the science: Health care provider communication of cannabis use among adults living with cancer. *Journal of Cancer Education*, *40*(3), 329–347. DOI: 10.1007/s13187-024-02484-z PMID: 39160419

Bar-Lev Schleider, L., Mechoulam, R., Sikorin, I., Naftali, T., & Novack, V. (2022). Adherence, safety, and effectiveness of medical cannabis and epidemiological characteristics of the patient population: A prospective study. *Frontiers in Medicine*, *9*, 827849. DOI: 10.3389/fmed.2022.827849 PMID: 35223923

Barry, R. A., & Glantz, S. (2016). A public health framework for legalized retail marijuana based on the US experience: Avoiding a new tobacco industry. *PLoS Medicine*, *13*(9), e1002131. DOI: 10.1371/journal.pmed.1002131 PMID: 27676176

Bass, B. M. (2006). *Transformational leadership*. Psychology Press. DOI: 10.4324/9781410617095

Bassi, G. M., Giorgi, V., Lazzarin, M., Meanti, R., Omeljaniuk, R. J., Sarzi-Puttini, P., & Torsello, A. (2025). Symptom management, adherence to therapy, and filling the gaps of medical cannabis therapy: A qualitative study on the importance of nursing consultations for fibromyalgia patients. *Journal of Cannabis Research*, *7*(1), 84. Advance online publication. DOI: 10.1186/s42238-025-00346-z PMID: 41163201

Batalla, A., Bhattacharyya, S., Yücel, M., Fusar-Poli, P., Crippa, J. A., Nogué, S., Torrens, M., Pujol, J., Farré, M., & Martin-Santos, R. (2013). Structural and functional imaging studies in chronic cannabis users: A systematic review of adolescent and adult findings. *PLoS One*, *8*(2), e55821. DOI: 10.1371/journal.pone.0055821 PMID: 23390554

Baumbusch, J., & Yip, I. S. (2022). Older adults' experiences of using recreational cannabis for medicinal purposes following legalization. *The International Journal on Drug Policy*, *108*, 103812. DOI: 10.1016/j.drugpo.2022.103812 PMID: 35930902

Becker, M. P., Collins, P. F., & Luciana, M. (2014). Neurocognition in college-aged daily marijuana users. *Journal of Clinical and Experimental Neuropsychology*, *36*(4), 379–398. DOI: 10.1080/13803395.2014.893996 PMID: 24620756

Begley, A. M. (2006). Facilitating the development of moral insight in practice: Teaching ethics and teaching virtue. *Nursing Philosophy*, *7*(4), 257–265. DOI: 10.1111/j.1466-769X.2006.00284.x PMID: 16965307

Behling-Hess, C., Simonson, G., Salz, T., Feuerstein, N., & Zullig, L. L. (2025). The impact of cannabis on immune checkpoint inhibitor therapy: A systematic review of immunomodulatory effects of cannabis in patients with and without cancer. *Supportive Care in Cancer*, *33*(3), 166. Advance online publication. DOI: 10.1007/s00520-025-09218-x PMID: 39921765

Bell, A. D., MacCallum, C. A., Margolese, S., Walsh, Z., Wright, P., Daeninck, P. J., Mandarino, E., Lacasse, G., Deol, J. K., de Freitas, L., St. Pierre, M., Belle-Isle, L., Gagnon, M., Bevan, S., Sanchez, T., Arlt, S., Monahan-Ellison, M., O'Hara, J., Boivin, M., & Costiniuk, C. (2024). Clinical practice guidelines for cannabis and cannabinoid-based medicines in the management of chronic pain and co-occurring conditions. *Cannabis and Cannabinoid Research*, *9*(2), 669–687. DOI: 10.1089/can.2021.0156 PMID: 36971587

Benca, R. M., Bertisch, S. M., Ahuja, A., Mandelbaum, R., & Krystal, A. D. (2023). Wake up America: National survey of patients' and physicians' views and attitudes on insomnia care. *Journal of Clinical Medicine*, *12*(7), 2498. Advance online publication. DOI: 10.3390/jcm12072498 PMID: 37048582

Bennett, M. I., Rayment, C., Hjermstad, M., Aass, N., Caraceni, A., & Kaasa, S. (2012). Prevalence and aetiology of neuropathic pain in cancer patients: A systematic review. *Pain*, *153*(2), 359–365. DOI: 10.1016/j.pain.2011.10.028 PMID: 22115921

Bergamaschi, M. M., Queiroz, R. H. C., Chagas, M. H. N., de Oliveira, D. C. G., De Martinis, B. S., Kapczinski, F., Quevedo, J., Roesler, R., Schröder, N., Nardi, A. E., Martín-Santos, R., Hallak, J. E. C., Zuardi, A. W., & Crippa, J. A. S. (2011). Cannabidiol reduces the anxiety induced by simulated public speaking in treatment-naïve social phobia patients. *Neuropsychopharmacology : Official Publication of the American College of Neuropsychopharmacology*, *36*(6), 1219–1226. DOI: 10.1038/npp.2011.6 PMID: 21307846

Bhaskar, A., Bell, A., Boivin, M., Briques, W., Brown, M., Clarke, H., Cyr, C., Eisenberg, E., de Oliveira Silva, R. F., Frohlich, E., Georgius, P., Hogg, M., Horsted, T. I., MacCallum, C. A., Müller-Vahl, K. R., O'Connell, C., Sealey, R., Seibolt, M., Sihota, A., & Moulin, D. E. (2021). Consensus recommendations on dosing and administration of medical cannabis to treat chronic pain: Results of a modified Delphi process. *Journal of Cannabis Research*, *3*(1), 22. DOI: 10.1186/s42238-021-00073-1 PMID: 34215346

Biggs, J., & Tang, C. (2011). Teaching for quality learning at university (4th ed.). Open University Press. https://www.scirp.org/reference/referencespapers?referenceid=1856033

Bimonte, S., Nocerino, D., Schiavo, D., Crisci, M., Cascella, M., & Cuomo, A. (2024). Cannabinoids for cancer-related pain management: An update on therapeutic applications and future perspectives. *Anticancer Research*, *44*(3), 895–900. DOI: 10.21873/anticanres.16883 PMID: 38423660

Birken, S.A., Lee, S.D., & Weiner, B.J. (2012). Uncovering middle managers' role in healthcare innovation implementation. *Implementation Science, 7*(1), 28. doi.org/10.1186/1748-5908-7-28

Birkhead, S., Edwards, P., Nettleton, M., Oppenlander, J., & Stapleton, M. (2022). Roles and Skills for Effective Academic Nurse Leaders. *Journal of the American Nurses Association.*, *3*(1), 22–32.https://doi.org/10.47988/janany.28237684.3.1

Black, N. (2013). Patient-reported outcome measures could help transform healthcare. *BMJ (Clinical Research Ed.)*, *346*(jan28 1), f167. DOI: 10.1136/bmj.f167 PMID: 23358487

Black, N., Stockings, E., Campbell, G., Tran, L. T., Zagic, D., Hall, W. D., & Farrell, M. (2019). Cannabinoids for the treatment of mental health disorders: A systematic review and meta-analysis. *The Lancet. Psychiatry*, *6*, 995–1010. DOI: 10.1016/S2215-0366(19)30401-8 PMID: 31672337

Blesching, U. (2022). *The cannabis health index: Mind, body, spirit guide to a healthy endocannabinoid system* (3rd ed.). North Atlantic Books.

Board-certified case manager | Commission for Case Manager Certification (CCMC). (2024). Ccmcertification.org. https://ccmcertification.org/about-commissiontm/differences-between-certified-case-managers-and-case-managers/board-certified

Boehning, A. P., & Haddad, L. M. (2023). Nursing Practice Act. [Updated 2023 Jul 17]. In: StatPearls [Internet]. Treasure Island (FL): StatPearls Publishing; 2026 Jan-. Available from: https://www.ncbi.nlm.nih.gov/books/NBK559012/

Boehnke, K. F., Bowyer, G., McAfee, J., Smith, T., Klida, C., Kurtz, V., Litinas, E., Purohit, P., Arewasikporn, A., Horowitz, D., Thomas, L., Eckersley, J., Railing, M., Williams, D. A., Clauw, D. J., Kidwell, K. M., Bohnert, A. S. B., & Bergmans, R. S. (2025). Feasibility pilot of a novel coaching intervention to optimize cannabis use for chronic pain management among veterans. *Journal of Cannabis Research*, *7*(1), 7. Advance online publication. DOI: 10.1186/s42238-025-00265-z PMID: 39856785

Boehnke, K. F., Litinas, E., & Clauw, D. J. (2016). Medical cannabis use is associated with decreased opiate medication use in a retrospective cross-sectional survey of patients with chronic pain. *The Journal of Pain*, *17*(6), 739–744. DOI: 10.1016/j.jpain.2016.03.002 PMID: 27001005

Boehnke, K. F., Litinas, E., Worthing, B., Conine, L., Kruger, D. J., & Clauw, D. J. (2021). Communication between healthcare providers and medical cannabis patients regarding referral and medication substitution. *Journal of Cannabis Research*, *3*(1), 2. Advance online publication. DOI: 10.1186/s42238-021-00058-0 PMID: 33526140

Boehnke, K. F., Scott, J. R., Litinas, E., & Clauw, D. J. (2019). Cannabis use for medical conditions: Patterns and outcomes. *Journal of Psychoactive Drugs*, *51*, 425–435.

Boehnke, K. F., Scott, J. R., Litinas, E., Sisley, S., Clauw, D. J., Goesling, J., & Williams, D. A. (2019). Cannabis use preferences and decision-making among medical cannabis patients with chronic pain. *The Journal of Pain*, *20*(11), 1362–1372. DOI: 10.1016/j.jpain.2019.05.009 PMID: 31132510

Boehnke, K. F., Scott, J. R., Martel, M. O., Smith, T., Bergmans, R. S., Kruger, D. J., Williams, D. A., & Fitzcharles, M. A. (2024). Substituting medical cannabis for medications among patients with rheumatic conditions in the United States and Canada. *ACR Open Rheumatology*, *6*(12), 826–835. DOI: 10.1002/acr2.11717 PMID: 39236308

Bonanni, P., Ragona, F., Fusco, C., Gambardella, A., Operto, F. F., Parmeggiani, L., Sartori, S., & Specchio, N. (2023). Cannabidiol use in patients with Dravet syndrome and Lennox–Gastaut syndrome: Experts' opinions using a nominal group technique approach. *Expert Opinion on Pharmacotherapy*, *24*(5), 655–663. DOI: 10.1080/14656566.2023.2187697 PMID: 37021712

Bonnie, R. W. (1974). *The marijuana conviction: A history of marijuana prohibition in the United States*. University Press of Virginia.

Borrego-Ruiz, A., & Borrego, J. J. (2025). A holistic review of cannabis and its potential risks and benefits in mental health. *Psychiatry International*, *6*(3), 92. DOI: 10.3390/psychiatryint6030092

Borrell-Carrió, F., Suchman, A. L., & Epstein, R. M. (2004). The biopsychosocial model 25 years later: Principles, practice, and scientific inquiry. *Annals of Family Medicine*, *2*(6), 576–582. DOI: 10.1370/afm.245 PMID: 15576544

Bosley, H. G., Peña, J. M., Penn, A. D., Sorensen, J. L., Tierney, M., & Flentje, A. (2023). A Pragmatic, Person-Centered View of Cannabis in the United States: Pursuing Care That Transcends Beliefs. *Substance Abuse*, *44*(4), 337–347.https://doi.org/10.1177/08897077231202836

Bratman, M. E. (1987). *Intention, plans, and practical reason*. Harvard University Press.

Braun, R.L. (1991). Uniform Controlled Substances Act of 1990. Campbell Law Review Volume 13 Issue 3 Summer Article 5 Uniform Controlled Substances Act of 1990. Retrieved January 6, 2026, from https://scholarship.law.campbell.edu/cgi/viewcontent.cgi?article=1222&context=clr#:~:text=The%201990%20Uniform%20Controlled%20Substances%20Act%20also%20provides%20for%20emergency,analogs%20or%20other%20dangerous%20substances.&text=prohibiting%20a%20substance%20becomes%20necessary,be%20scheduled%20without%20any%20delay

Braun, I. M., Blinder, V. S., Freedman-Cass, D. A., Bhatt, D. L., Blanke, C. D., Cleary, J. F., Cyr, D., Danaher, B. G., Davis, M. P., Enright, K. M., Goldstein, D. A., Gralow, J. R., Henry, D. H., Hershman, D. L., Kaur, S., Ligibel, J. A., Moy, B., Mustian, K. M., Patt, D. A., & Loprinzi, C. L. (2024). Cannabis and cannabinoids in adults with cancer: ASCO guideline. *Journal of Clinical Oncology*, *42*(16), 1774–1803. DOI: 10.1200/JCO.23.02501 PMID: 38478773

Braun, I. M.-J. (2023). Medical cannabis use in oncology: A review of clincal care models and patient-centered approaches. *Journal of Clinical Oncology*, *41*(2), 123–130. PMID: 38048518

Braun, V., & Clarke, V. (2006, January 1). Using Thematic Analysis in Psychology. *Qualitative Research in Psychology*, *3*(2), 77–101. DOI: 10.1191/1478088706qp063oa

Breuning, M., Nie, J., Schlesinger, M., Smith, L., Lavie-Ajayi, M., Babinski, S., & Law, S. (2026). The persistence of stigma and other challenges experienced by medical cannabis users: A thematic synthesis of qualitative studies. *Medical Cannabis and Cannabinoids*, •••, 1–36. DOI: 10.1159/000551584

Bridgeman, M. B., & Abazia, D. T. (2017). Medicinal cannabis: History, pharmacology, and implications for the acute care setting. *P&T : a Peer-Reviewed Journal for Formulary Management*, *42*(3), 180–188. https://www.ncbi.nlm.nih.gov/pmc/articles/PMC5312634/ PMID: 28250701

Brown, J. D., & Winterstein, A. G. (2020). Potential adverse drug events and drug–drug interactions with medical cannabis. *Journal of Clinical Medicine*, *9*, 989. DOI: 10.3390/jcm9040919

Brown, T. M. (2016). Working with the panthers to transform health care for poor black communities. *American Journal of Public Health*, *106*(10), 1756–1757. DOI: 10.2105/AJPH.2016.303402 PMID: 27552281

Broyd, S. J., van Hell, H. H., Beale, C., Yücel, M., & Solowij, N. (2016). Acute and chronic effects of cannabinoids on human cognition: A systematic review. *Biological Psychiatry*, *79*(7), 557–567. DOI: 10.1016/j.biopsych.2015.12.002 PMID: 26858214

Bruce, D., Brady, J. P., Foster, E., & Shattell, M. (2018). Preferences for medical marijuana over prescription medications among persons living with chronic conditions. *Journal of Alternative and Complementary Medicine (New York, N.Y.)*, *24*(2), 146–153. DOI: 10.1089/acm.2017.0184 PMID: 28945457

Bruni, N., Della Pepa, C., Oliaro-Bosso, S., Pessione, E., Gastaldi, D., & Dosio, F. (2018). Cannabinoid delivery systems for pain and inflammation treatment. *Molecules (Basel, Switzerland)*, *23*(10), 2478. DOI: 10.3390/molecules23102478 PMID: 30262735

Bryan, K. (2024). Cannabis Overview 2025 by the National Conference of State Legislatures. https://www.ncsl.org/civil-and-criminal-justice/cannabis-overview

Bryan, K. (2024). *Cannabis overview*. National Conference of State Legislators. https://www.ncsl.org/civil-and-criminal-justice/cannabis-overview

Cadieux, C. S., Garrett, J., & Ewen, H. (2025). Unpublished pilot study data: Nursing students' medical cannabis knowledge, attitudes, and skills (unpublished, raw data). Binghamton University, Decker College of Nursing and Health Sciences.

Cadmus, E., Dempsey, C., Boston-Leary, K., & Bates, M. (2024).. . *Nursing Leadership Scope and Standards and Pathway to Excellence Nursing Management*, *55*(6), 7–12.https://doi.org/10.1097/nmg.0000000000000139

Campbell, G., Hall, W., Peacock, A., Lintzeris, N., Bruno, R., Larance, B., Nielsen, S., Cohen, M., Chan, G., Mattick, R., Blyth, F., Shanahan, M., & Degenhardt, L. (2018). Effect of cannabis use in people with chronic non-cancer pain prescribed opioids: Findings from a 4-year prospective cohort study. *The Lancet. Public Health*, *3*(7), e341–e350. DOI: 10.1016/S2468-2667(18)30110-5 PMID: 29976328

Canadian Nurses Association. (2017). Cannabis for medical purposes: Legal implications for nurses. *The Canadian Nurse*, *113*(1), 16–18. PMID: 29236416

Cannabis academic research grants—Department of Cannabis Control. (n.d.). Retrieved January 6, 2026, from https://www.cannabis.ca.gov/about-us/grant-funding/cannabis-academic-research-grants/

Cannabis and Health Research Initiative. (2025). The National Cannabis Study.

Cannabis and Health Research Initiative. (2025). *The National Cannabis Study*. https://www.cannabisandhealth.org/national-cannabis-study/

Cannabis Business Times. (2026, March 5). *Proposed hemp regulations in the 2026 Farm Bill and implications for the cannabis industry*. Retrieved April 11, 2026, from Cannabis Business Times: https://www.cannabisbusinesstimes.com/hemp/news/15818903/intoxicating-hemp-ban-unchanged-in-2026-farm-bills-advancement

Cannabis Nurses Network. (n.d.). *Ryan's Law Action Center: Guidance for nurses and health care professionals on California Senate Bill 311*. https://www.cannabisnursesnetwork.com/ryans-law-action-center/

Cannabis Nurses of Color. (n.d.). 1*st 'Day at the Capital': Health policy summit*. https://cannabisnursesofcolor.com/capitalday/

Cannabis use in hospice and palliative care – Compassionate Oregon. (n.d.). Retrieved January 6, 2026, from https://compassionateoregon.org/cannabis-use-in-hospice-and-palliative-care/

CannaKeys. (2020). *Cannabis chemotypes*. https://cannakeys.com/cannabis-chemotypes/

CannaKeys. (2024). Cannabis and cancer: Research summary. https://cannakeys.com/thc-cbd-for-cancer/#top-dboard

CannaKeys. (2024). *Endocannabinoid tone*. https://cannakeys.com/endocannabinoid-tone

Capitani, L. (2026, February 20). *Supporting terminally ill patients in Connecticut health care facilities to use cannabis (HB 5242)* [Testimony]. Connecticut General Assembly Public Health Committee. https://www.d4dpr.org/post/expert-testimony-terminally-ill-cannabis-use-hb-5242

Carla Monti, M. (2022). Analysis of Synthetic and Natural Cannabinoids in the Forensic Field Applying High-Resolution. *Mass Spectrometry (Tokyo, Japan)*.

Carliner, H., Mauro, P. M., Brown, Q. L., Shmulewitz, D., Rahim-Juwel, R., Sarvet, A. L., Wall, M. M., & Hasin, D. S. (2017). The widening gender gap in marijuana use prevalence in the United States during a period of economic change. *JAMA Psychiatry*, *74*, 567–575.

Carlini, B. H., Garrett, S. B., & Carter, G. T. (2017). Medicinal cannabis: A survey among health care providers in Washington State. *The American Journal of Hospice & Palliative Care*, *34*(1), 85–91. DOI: 10.1177/1049909115604669 PMID: 26377551

Carter, N., Valaitis, R. K., Lam, A., Feather, J., Nicholl, J., & Cleghorn, L. (2018). Navigation delivery models and roles of navigators in primary care: A scoping literature review. *BMC Health Services Research*, *18*(1), 96. Advance online publication. DOI: 10.1186/s12913-018-2889-0 PMID: 29422057

Cashin, A. G., Furlong, B. M., Kamper, S. J., De Carvalho, D., Machado, L. A. C., Davidson, S. R. E., Bursey, K. K., Abdel Shaheed, C., & Hall, A. M. (2025). Analgesic effects of non-surgical and non-interventional treatments for low back pain: A systematic review and meta-analysis of placebo-controlled randomized trials. *BMJ Evidence-Based Medicine*, bmjebm-2024-112974. Advance online publication. DOI: 10.1136/bmjebm-2024-112974 PMID: 40101974

Castle, R. D., Marzolf, J., Morris, M., & Bushell, W. C. (2025). Meta-analysis of medical cannabis outcomes and associations with cancer. *Frontiers in Oncology, 15*, 1490621. Advance online publication. DOI: 10.3389/fonc.2025.1490621 PMID: 40303989

Cawthorn, A. (2024, November 19). *The role of technology in modern nursing: From telehealth to AI.* Retrieved January 30, 2026, from Healthcare: https://www.indwes.edu/articles/2024/11/the-role-of-technology-in-modern-nursing-from-telehealth-to-ai

Cella, D., Riley, W., Stone, A., Rothrock, N., Reeve, B., Yount, S., Amtmann, D., Bode, R., Buysse, D., Choi, S., Cook, K., DeVellis, R., DeWalt, D., Fries, J. F., Gershon, R., Hahn, E. A., Lai, J.-S., Pilkonis, P., Revicki, D., & Hays, R. (2010). The Patient-Reported Outcomes Measurement Information System (PROMIS): Development and testing of adult self-reported health outcome item banks, 2005–2008. *Journal of Clinical Epidemiology, 63*(11), 1179–1194. DOI: 10.1016/j.jclinepi.2010.04.011 PMID: 20685078

Center for Disease Control and Prevention. (2025). Cannabis and Public Health. CDC. https://www.cdc.gov/cannabis/data-research/facts-stats/index.html

Centers for Disease Control and Prevention (CDC). (2025, March 7). *Cannabis and public health.* Retrieved January 30th, 2026, from Centers for Disease Control and Prevention: https://www.cdc.gov/cannabis/about/what-cdc-is-doing.html

Centers for Disease Control and Prevention. (2022). *Cannabis and public health.* CDC.

Centers for Disease Control and Prevention. (n.d.). *Well-being concepts.* https://archive.cdc.gov/www_cdc_gov/hrqol/wellbeing.htm

Centers for Disease Control. (2025, March 7). *Cannabis facts and stats.* Retrieved April 10, 2026, from Cannabis and public health: https://www.cdc.gov/cannabis/data-research/facts-stats/index.html

Certification principles | Commission for Case Manager Certification (CCMC). (n.d.). Ccmcertification.org. https://ccmcertification.org/about-ccmc/about-case-management/certification-principles

Charani, E., & Holmes, A. H. (2013). Antimicrobial stewardship programmes: The need for wider engagement. *BMJ Quality & Safety, 22*(11), 885–887. DOI: 10.1136/bmjqs-2013-002444 PMID: 24046440

Chávez-Valenzuela, P., Kappes, M., Sambuceti, C. E., & Díaz-Guio, D. A. (2025). Challenges in the implementation of inter-professional education programs with clinical simulation for health care students: A scoping review. *Nurse Education Today, 146*, 106548. DOI: 10.1016/j.nedt.2024.106548 PMID: 39740591

Chayasirisobhon, S. (2021). Mechanisms of action and pharmacokinetics of cannabis. *The Permanente Journal, 25*, 19–200. PMID: 33635755

Chen, R. (2025, April 15). Evaluation of Nurses' Performance: Key Metrics to Track Bucketlist Blog https://bucketlistrewards.com/blog/evaluation-nurses-performance/#:~:text=By%20assessing%2vvarious%20aspects%20of%20a%20nurse's,to%20transform%20your%20healthcare%20organization%20%C2%B7%20Performance

Chokwanich, N. e. (2022). Traditional medicine and cannabis integration in Thailand's public health system. *Journal of Ethhnopharmacology.*

Chou, R., Ahmed, A. Y., Dana, T., Morasco, B. J., Bougatsos, C., Fu, R., & Williams, L. (2025). *Living systematic review on cannabis and other plant-based treatments for chronic pain: 2025 update*. Agency for Healthcare Research and Quality. DOI: 10.23970/AHRQEPCCER250UPDATE2025

Christidis, M., Al-Moraissi, E. A., Miah, T., Mihasi, L., Razavian, A., Christidis, N., & De la Torre Canales, G. (2025). Living with pain: A systematic review on patients' subjective experiences. *Systematic Reviews, 14*(1), 188. Advance online publication. DOI: 10.1186/s13643-025-02953-6 PMID: 41053837

Chuang, E., Jason, K., & Morgan, J. C. (2011). Factors influencing middle manager support. *Health Care Management Review, 36*(4), 369–379.https://doi.org/10.1097/HMR.0b013e3182100cc2

Chye, Y., Christensen, E., Solowij, N., & Yücel, M. (2019). The endocannabinoid system and cannabidiol's promise for the treatment of substance use disorder. *Frontiers in Psychiatry, 10*, 63. DOI: 10.3389/fpsyt.2019.00063 PMID: 30837904

Clark, C. (2021). *Cannabis: A handbook for nurses* (1st, North American ed.). Lippincott Williams & Wilkins.

Clark, C. S. (2019 a). *Evaluating the evidence: Cannabis and psychosis, Part I.* https://nursemanifest.com/2019/03/21/evaluating-the-evidence-cannabis-and-psychosis-part-i/

Clark, C. S. (2019b). *Evaluating the evidence: Cannabis and psychodid, Part II.* https://nursemanifest.com/2019/03/26/evaluating-the-evidence-cannabis-and-psychosis-part-ii/

Clark, C. S. (2021). Cannabis Science Education: Meeting the Need for Cannabis Care Competencies. American Association of Colleges of Nursing.https://www.aacnnursing.org/portals/0/pdfs/conferences-webinars/presentations/2021/Clark_Carey.pdf

Clark, C. S. (2022). Three questions about the nurse's role and medical cannabis. Blogpost.Nursing-center.comhttps://www.nursingcenter.com/blogs-plus/blogs/blogs-post?identifier=the-Nurses-Role-and-Medical-Cannabis#/post/the-Nurses-Role-and-Medical-Cannabis

Clark, C.S. (2018). Medical cannabis: The oncology nurse's role in patient education about the effects of marijuana on cancer palliation. *Clinical Journal of Oncology Nursing*, 22(1), E-1E-6. https://doi.org/. CJON.E1-E6DOI: 10.1188/18

Clark, C. (2021). The nurses's role: Providing cannabis care. In Clark, C. F., & Clark, C. (Eds.), *Cannabis: A handbook for nurses* (1st ed., p. 272). Wolters Kluwer.

Clark, C. M. (2019). *Fostering civility in nursing education* (2nd ed.). Sigma Theta Tau International.

Clark, C. S. (2019). High-potency cannabis and incident psychosis: Correcting the causal assumption. *The Lancet. Psychiatry, 6*(6), e14. DOI: 10.1016/S2215-0366(19)30178-6 PMID: 31122483

Clark, C. S. (2021). *Legal, ethical, and advocacy concerns: Cannabis from the federal to the state level. Cannabis: A handbook for nurses* (1st ed.). Wolters Kluwer.

Clarke, R. M. (2013). History of cannabis use for fiber. In Clarke, R. M. (Ed.), *Cannabis: Evolution and Ethnobotany* (p. 172). University of California Press.

Clobes, T. A., Himebaugh, S., Gamez, S. A., & Torres, M. (2025). Relationship between cannabis dispensary density, proximity, and attitudes toward medical cannabis: A cross-sectional study. *Health Science Reports*, *8*(4), e70685. DOI: 10.1002/hsr2.70685 PMID: 40260030

Clobes, T. A., Mee, M. M., Jimenez, J. M., Maldonado, J., & Song, J. R. (2025). Impact of healthcare provider awareness and guidance on the medical cannabis experience. *Medical Cannabis and Cannabinoids*, *8*(1), 47–57. DOI: 10.1159/000544125 PMID: 40104431

Code of professional conduct | Commission for Case Manager Certification (CCMC). (2024). Ccmcertification.org. https://ccmcertification.org/about-commissiontm/code-professional-conduct

College of Nurses of Ontario. (2018). *Practice standard: Medical cannabis*. https://www.cno.org/en/learn-about-standards-guidelines/educational-tools/ask-practice/medical-marijuana/

College of Registered Nurses of Alberta (CRNA). (2022). Cannabis for medical purposes: standards for Nurse Practitioners. Alberta: College of Registered Nurses of Alberta (CRNA).

Commonwealth Project. (2025). Policy briefs on cannabinoid integration in value-based care. https://commonwealthproject.org

Comprehensive Drug Abuse Prevention and Control Act of 1970, Pub. L. 91–513, 84 Stat. 1236 (1970)

Comprehensive Pain Management. (n.d.). Understanding Ethical and Regulatory Issues in Prescribing Medical Cannabis: A Comprehensive Overview. Comprehensive Pain Management Associates.https://www.cpmany.org/understanding-ethical-and-regulatory-issues-in-prescribing-medical-cannabis-a-comprehensive-overview/

Compton, W. M., Han, B., Jones, C. M., Blanco, C., & Hughes, A. (2016). Marijuana use and use disorders in adults in the USA, 2002–14: Analysis of annual cross-sectional surveys. *The Lancet. Psychiatry*, *3*(10), 954–964. DOI: 10.1016/S2215-0366(16)30208-5 PMID: 27592339

Conant v Walters, 309 F. 3d 629, 636 (9th Cir 2002).

Congress, U. S. (1906, June 30). *Pure Food and Drug Act of 1906*. Retrieved January 5, 2026, from Schaffer Drug Library History 1900s: https://www.druglibrary.org/schaffer/History/e1900/pfda.htm

Congressional Research Service. (2019). *Defining hemp: A fact sheet*. U. S. Government. Washington DC: Library of Congress. https://crsreports.congress.gov/product/pdf/R/R44742

Congressional Research Service. (2023). *The Controlled Substances Act (CSA): A legal overview for the 118th Congress* (LSB11105). https://crsreports.congress.gov

Congressional Research Service. (2024). *Federal marijuana policy: Rescheduling and implications* (R48048). https://crsreports.congress.gov

Congressional Research Service. (2025). *Hemp regulation and federal considerations under the forthcoming Farm Bill*. CRS.

Congressional Research Service. (2025, December 3). *Change to federal definition of hemp and implications for federal enforcement* (CRS Insight No. IN12620). https://www.congress.gov/crs-product/IN12620

Connor, P., Stjepanović, D., Budney, A. J., Le Foll, B., & Hall, W. D. (2022). Clinical management of cannabis withdrawal. *Addiction (Abingdon, England)*, *117*(7), 2075–2095. DOI: 10.1111/add.15743 PMID: 34791767

Controlled Substances Act, 21 U.S.C. § 801 et seq. (1970).

Cooper, Z. D., Abrams, D. I., Gust, S., Salicrup, A., & Throckmorton, D. C. (2021). Challenges for clinical cannabis and cannabinoid research in the United States. *Journal of the National Cancer Institute. Monographs*, *2021*(58), 114–122. DOI: 10.1093/jncimonographs/lgab009 PMID: 34850896

Costantino, R. C., Felten, N., Todd, M., Maxwell, T., & McPherson, M. L. (2019). A survey of hospice professionals regarding medical cannabis practices. *Journal of Palliative Medicine*, *22*(10), 1208–1212. DOI: 10.1089/jpm.2018.0535 PMID: 31094609

Costiniuk, C. T., MacCallum, C. A., Boivin, M., Rueda, S., Lacasse, G., Walsh, Z., Daeninck, P. J., Margolese, S., Mandarino, E., Jagpaul Kaur Deol, Sanchez, T., & Bell, A. D. (2023). *Why a distinct medical stream is necessary to support patients using cannabis for medical purposes.* *5*(1), 25–25. https://doi.org/10.1186/s42238-023-00195-8

Cowperthwaite, A. (2020). NLN/Jeffries Simulation Framework for simulated participant methodology. *Clinical Simulation in Nursing*, *42*, 12–21. https://www.nursingsimulation.org/article/S1876-1399(20)30005-0/fulltext. DOI: 10.1016/j.ecns.2019.12.009

Crocker, E., Carter, A. J. E., Emsley, J. G., Magee, K., Atkinson, P., & Tibbo, P. G. (2021). When Cannabis Use Goes Wrong: Mental Health Side Effects of Cannabis Use That Present to Emergency Services. *Frontiers in Psychiatry*, *12*, 640222. DOI: 10.3389/fpsyt.2021.640222 PMID: 33658953

Crocq, M. A. (2020). History of cannabis and the endocannabinoid system. *Dialogues in Clinical Neuroscience*, *22*(3), 223–228. DOI: 10.31887/DCNS.2020.22.3/mcrocq PMID: 33162765

Cronin, S.P., Cruz, J., Cameron, E., Azemar, S., Dudley, S., Largent-Milnes, T.M., Brady, B.R., Wallace, J.S., Arnett, M.R., Dahmer, S.M., Ibrahim, M.M., Padilla, A.R., Vanderah, T.W., & De La Rosa, J.S. (2025). "It's legal, now what?" development, implementation, and evaluation of interdisciplinary cannabis education for healthcare trainees. *Journal of Cannabis Research;7*(1),68. https://doi.org/10.1186/s42238-025-00321-8

Crowell, B., Seamon, M., Buckley, T., & Gildner, J. (2021). Nurses' knowledge, perceptions and clinical experiences with medical cannabis. *Journal of Clinical Nursing*, *30*, 3530–3540.

Cummings, H., Ul Haq, M. Z., Dargham, A., Shakeel, N., Busse, J. W., Darzi, A. J., & Alvarez, E. (2024). Individuals' values and preferences regarding medical cannabis for chronic pain: A descriptive qualitative study. *Journal of Pain Research*, *17*, 21–34. DOI: 10.2147/JPR.S432823 PMID: 38192366

Curran, H. V., Freeman, T. P., Mokrysz, C., Lewis, D. A., Morgan, C. J., & Parsons, L. H. (2016). Keep off the grass? Cannabis, cognition and addiction. *Nature Reviews. Neuroscience*, *17*(5), 293–306. DOI: 10.1038/nrn.2016.28 PMID: 27052382

Cuttler, C., Spradlin, A., Cleveland, M. J., & Craft, R. M. (2018). Short- and long-term effects of cannabis on symptoms of post-traumatic stress disorder. *Journal of Affective Disorders*, *227*, 298–304. DOI: 10.1016/j.jad.2017.10.049 PMID: 32469819

D'Anna, T., Puntarello, M., Cannella, G., Scalzo, G., Buscemi, R., Zerbo, S., & Argo, A. (2023). The Chain of Custody in the Era of Modern Forensics: From the Classic Procedures for Gathering Evidence to the New Challenges Related to Digital Data. *Health Care*, *11*(5), 634. PMID: 36900637

Dahlke, S., Butler, J. I., Hunter, K. F., Toubiana, M., Kalogirou, M. R., Shrestha, S., Devkota, R., Law, J., & Scheuerman, M. (2024). The effects of stigma: Older persons and medicinal cannabis. *Qualitative Health Research*, *34*(8-9), 717–731. DOI: 10.1177/10497323241227419 PMID: 38305270

Damkier, P., Lassen, D., Christensen, M. M. H., Madsen, K. G., Hellfritzsch, M., & Pottegård, A. (2019). Interaction between warfarin and cannabis. *Basic & Clinical Pharmacology & Toxicology*, *124*(1), 28–31. DOI: 10.1111/bcpt.13152 PMID: 30326170

Das, A., Hendershot, C. S., Husain, M. I., Knyahnytska, Y., Elsaid, S., Le Foll, B., & Kloiber, S. (2024). Perceptions, experiences and patterns of cannabis use in individuals with mood and anxiety disorders in the context of cannabis legalization and medical cannabis programme in Canada: A qualitative study. *Pharmacopsychiatry*, *57*(3), 141–151. DOI: 10.1055/a-2264-1047 PMID: 38467156

de Bode, N., Kroon, E., Sznitman, S. R., & Cousijn, J. (2025). The differential effects of medicinal cannabis on mental health: A systematic review. *Clinical Psychology Review*, *118*, 102581. DOI: 10.1016/j.cpr.2025.102581 PMID: 40186931

de Brito Sena, M. A., Moreira-Almeida, A., Koenig, H. G., Vallada, H., & Lucchetti, G. (2021). Defining spirituality in healthcare: A systematic review and concept analysis. *Frontiers in Psychology*, *12*, 756080. DOI: 10.3389/fpsyg.2021.756080 PMID: 34867654

De Petrocellis, L., & Di Marzo, V. (2009). An introduction to the endocannabinoid system: From the early to the latest concepts. *Best Practice & Research. Clinical Endocrinology & Metabolism*, *23*(1), 1–15. DOI: 10.1016/j.beem.2008.10.013 PMID: 19285257

de Roon-Cassini, T. A., Stollenwerk, T. M., Beatka, M., & Hillard, C. J. (2020). Meet your stress management professionals: The endocannabinoids. *Trends in Molecular Medicine*, *26*(10), 953–968. DOI: 10.1016/j.molmed.2020.07.002 PMID: 32868170

Delatte, G. (2024, May 29). Why is cannabis not allowed on college campuses? Campus rules vs. State freedom. *Eminent*. https://www.eminentconsultingfirm.com/why-cant-you-bring-cannabis-to-college-campuses/

Devinsky, O., Cross, J. H., Laux, L., Marsh, E., Miller, I., Nabbout, R., Scheffer, I. E., Thiele, E. A., & Wright, S. (2017). Trial of cannabidiol for drug-resistant seizures in the Dravet syndrome. *The New England Journal of Medicine*, *376*(21), 2011–2020. DOI: 10.1056/NEJMoa1611618 PMID: 28538134

Di Forti, M., Quattrone, D., Freeman, T. P., Tripoli, G., Gayer-Anderson, C., Quigley, H., Rodriguez, V., Jongsma, H. E., Ferraro, L., La Cascia, C., La Barbera, D., Tarricone, I., Berardi, D., Szöke, A., Arango, C., Tortelli, A., Velthorst, E., Bernardo, M., Del Ben, C., & Murray, R. M. (2019). The contribution of cannabis use to variation in the incidence of psychotic disorder across Europe. *The Lancet. Psychiatry*, *6*(5), 427–436. DOI: 10.1016/S2215-0366(19)30048-3 PMID: 30902669

Di Marzo, V. (2014). The endocannabinoid system: Its general strategy of action, tools for its pharmacological manipulation and potential therapeutic exploitation. *Pharmacological Research*, *86*, 1–14. https://www.ncbi.nlm.nih.gov/pmc/articles/PMC3951193/ PMID: 19559360

Di Marzo, V. (2018). New approaches and challenges to targeting the endocannabinoid system. *Nature Reviews. Drug Discovery*, *17*(9), 623–639. DOI: 10.1038/nrd.2018.115 PMID: 30116049

Di Marzo, V. (2018). New approaches and challenges to targeting the endocannabinoid system. *Nature Reviews. Neuroscience*, *19*, 723–738. PMID: 30116049

Di Marzo, V., Melck, D., Bisogno, T., & De Petrocellis, L. (1998). Endocannabinoids: Endogenous cannabinoid receptor ligands with neuromodulatory action. *Trends in Neurosciences*, *21*(12), 521–528. DOI: 10.1016/S0166-2236(98)01283-1 PMID: 9881850

Diagnosed Substance Use Disorders (DSU) - NCQA. (2025, August). NCQA. https://www.ncqa.org/report-cards/health-plans/state-of-health-care-quality-report/diagnosed-substance-use-disorders-dsu

Dickison, P., Haerling, K. A., & Lasater, K. (2019). Integrating the National Council of State Boards of Nursing Clinical Judgment Model into nursing educational frameworks. *The Journal of Nursing Education*, *58*(2), 72–78.https://doi.org/10.3928/01484834-20190122-03

Diener, E., Oishi, S., & Tay, L. (2018). Advances in subjective well-being research. *Nature Human Behaviour*, *2*(4), 253–260. DOI: 10.1038/s41562-018-0307-6 PMID: 30936533

DiGirolamo, E. (2026). Approaching conversations about cannabis use with patients. *Oncology Times*, *48*(5), 17–18. https://journals.lww.com/oncology-times/fulltext/2026/03000/approaching_conversations_about_cannabis_use_with.11.aspx. DOI: 10.1097/01.COT.0000000000000330

Diversion Control Division. (n.d.). United States Department of Justice. Usdoj.gov. Retrieved January 7, 2026, from https://www.deadiversion.usdoj.gov/administrative_actions.html

Djilali, E., Pappalardo, L., Posadino, A. M., Giordo, R., & Pintus, G. (2022). Effects of the storage conditions on the stability of natural and synthetic cannabis in biological matrices for forensic toxicology analysis: An update from the literature. *Metabolites*, *12*(9), 801. DOI: 10.3390/metabo12090801 PMID: 36144208

Dock, L. L., & Stewart, I. M. (1938). *A short history of nursing: From the earliest times to the present*. G. P. Putnam's Sons.

Doctors for Drug Policy Reform. (2023, February 17). *Legislative and administrative guidelines for regulating cannabis use in healthcare facilities* [White paper]. https://www.d4dpr.org/post/d4dpr-publishes-white-paper-on-legislating-cannabis-use-in-healthcare-facilities

Donahue, D. M., Metzger, M., Baker, M., & Rosenof, L. (2023). Let's match: Making cannabis policy guided by research. *Clinical Therapeutics*, *45*(6), 515–520. DOI: 10.1016/j.clinthera.2023.03.011 PMID: 37414501

Doody, O. D., & Doody, C. M. (2012). Transformational leadership in nursing practice. *British Journal of Nursing (Mark Allen Publishing)*, *21*(20), 1212–1218. DOI: 10.12968/bjon.2012.21.20.1212 PMID: 23132001

Dossey, B. M., & Keegan, L. (2022). *Holistic nursing: A handbook for practice* (9th ed.). Jones & Bartlett Learning., https://www.jblearning.com/catalog/productdetails/9781284196528

Dowell, D., Ragan, K. R., Jones, C. M., Baldwin, G. T., & Chou, R. (2022). CDC clinical practice guideline for prescribing opioids for pain—United States, 2022. *MMWR. Recommendations and Reports*, *71*(3), 1–95. DOI: 10.15585/mmwr.rr7103a1 PMID: 36327391

Drug Enforcement Administration. (n.d.). *Drug scheduling*. https://www.dea.gov/drug-information/drug-scheduling

Drug Enforcement Administration. (n.d.). *Drug scheduling*. U.S. Department of Justice. https://www.dea.gov/drug-information/drug-scheduling

Drug-Free Workplace Act of 1988, 41 U.S.C. § 8101 et seq. (2018).

Eddy, M. (2010). Medical marijuana: Review and analysis of federal and state policies. Congressional Research Service. https://files.iowamedicalmarijuana.org/imm/RL33211_20100402.pdf

Elphick, M. R. (2012). The evolution and comparative neurobiology of endocannabinoid signalling. *Philosophical Transactions of the Royal Society of London. Series B, Biological Sciences*, *367*(1607), 3201–3215. DOI: 10.1098/rstb.2011.0394 PMID: 23108540

Elwyn, G., Frosch, D., Thomson, R., Joseph-Williams, N., Lloyd, A., Kinnersley, P., Coulter, A., Barry, M., Eden, A., & Rollnick, S. (2012). Shared decision making: A model for clinical practice. *Journal of General Internal Medicine*, *27*(10), 1361–1367. DOI: 10.1007/s11606-012-2077-6 PMID: 22618581

Emerson, J. (2025, April 25). *Insurers not required to cover medical marijuana, federal judge rules.* Becker's Payers Issues, Payer News. https://www.beckerspayer.com/policy-updates/insurers-not-required-to-cover-medical-marijuana-federal-judge-rules/

Employer drug-testing policies must evolve with state law—Troutman Pepper Locke. (2023, July 27). https://www.troutman.com/insights/employer-drug-testing-policies-must-evolve-with-state-law/

Engel, G. L. (1977). The need for a new medical model: A challenge for biomedicine. *Science*, *196*(4286), 129–136. DOI: 10.1126/science.847460 PMID: 847460

Engle, R. L., Lopez, E. R., Gormley, K. E., Chan, J. A., Charns, M. P., & Lukas, C. V. (2017). What roles do middle managers play in implementation of innovative practices? *Health Care Management Review*, *42*(1), 14–27. https://doi.org/10.1097/HMR.0000000000000090

Englund, A., Morrison, P. D., Nottage, J., Hague, D., Kane, F., Bonaccorso, S., Stone, J. M., Reichenberg, A., Brenneisen, R., Holt, D., Feilding, A., Walker, L., Murray, R. M., & Kapur, S. (2013). Cannabidiol inhibits THC-elicited paranoid symptoms and hippocampal-dependent memory impairment. *Journal of Psychopharmacology (Oxford, England)*, *27*(1), 19–27. DOI: 10.1177/0269881112460109 PMID: 23042808

EPIDIOLEX® (cannabidiol). (n.d.). EPIDIOLEX.com. https://www.epidiolex.com/

Erridge, S., Clarke, E., McLachlan, K., Coomber, R., Beri, S., Khan, S., Weatherall, M. W., Platt, M. W., Rucker, J. J., Mediano, P. A. M., & Sodergren, M. H. (2026). Clinical outcomes and patient profiles in the UK medical cannabis registry: A k-means clustering analysis. *Journal of Clinical Pharmacology*, *66*(1), e70151. Advance online publication. DOI: 10.1002/jcph.70151 PMID: 41510842

Ethics- cannabis and case management: Medical marijuana updates | Commission for Case Manager Certification (CCMC). (2023, December 29). Ccmcertification.org. https://ccmcertification.org/courses/ethics-cannabis-and-case-management-medical-marijuana-updates#

European Monitoring Centre for Drugs and Drug Addiction. (2018). *Medical use of cannabis and cannabinoids: Questions and answers for policymaking*. https://doi.org/DOI: 10.2810/979004

Evanoff, A. B., Quan, T., Dufault, C., Awad, M., & Bierut, L. J. (2017). Physicians-in-training are not prepared to prescribe medical marijuana. *Drug and Alcohol Dependence*, *180*, 151–155. DOI: 10.1016/j.drugalcdep.2017.08.010 PMID: 28892720

Evans, D. G. (2013). The economic impacts of marijuana legalization. *The Journal of Global Drug Policy and Practice*, *7*(4), 2–40.

Executive Office of the President. (2025, December 18). Increasing medical marijuana and cannabidiol research, Exec. Order No. 14370. https://www.whitehouse.gov

Falk-Rafael, A. (2005). Advancing nursing theory through theory-guided practice: The emergence of a critical caring perspective. *Advances in Nursing Science*, *28*(1), 38–49. DOI: 10.1097/00012272-200501000-00005 PMID: 15718937

Fanaroff, A. C., Califf, R. M., Windecker, S., Smith, S. C.Jr, & Lopes, R. D. (2019). Levels of evidence supporting American College of Cardiology/American Heart Association and European Society of Cardiology guidelines, 2008–2018. *Journal of the American Medical Association*, *321*(11), 1069–1080. DOI: 10.1001/jama.2019.1122 PMID: 30874755

Federal Institute for Drugs and Medical Devices. (2020). *Medical cannabis in Germany: Regulatory overview*. Government of Germany.

Federal law preempts state coverage rules for medical cannabis. (2025, May 9). Reedsmith.com. https://www.reedsmith.com/articles/federal-law-preempts-state-coverage-rules-for-medical-cannabis/

Federal marijuana rescheduling | Moritz College of Law. (n.d.). The Ohio State University. Retrieved January 6, 2026, from https://moritzlaw.osu.edu/faculty-and-research/drug-enforcement-and-policy-center/research-and-grants/policy-and-data-analyses/federal-marijuana-rescheduling#:~:text=What%20would%20rescheduling%20marijuana%20from,opportunities%20to%20participate%20in%20research

Federal Policies. (n.d.) Marijuana Policy Project. Retrieved January 6, 2026, from https://www.mpp.org/policy/federal/

Figueiredo, P. R., Tolomeo, S., Steele, J. D., & Baldacchino, A. (2020). Neurocognitive consequences of chronic cannabis use: A systematic review and meta-analysis. *Neuroscience and Biobehavioral Reviews, 108*, 358–369. DOI: 10.1016/j.neubiorev.2019.10.014 PMID: 31715191

Fink, D. S., Samples, H., Malte, C. A., Olfson, M., Wall, M. M., Alschuler, D. M., Simpson, T., Mannes, Z., Saxon, A. J., & Hasin, D. S. (2025). Cannabis legalization and increasing cannabis use in the United States: Data from urine toxicology testing in emergency room patients. *The International Journal on Drug Policy, 138*, 104765. DOI: 10.1016/j.drugpo.2025.104765 PMID: 40058102

Fischer, B. R., Russell, C., Sabioni, P., van den Brink, W., Le Foll, B., Hall, W., Rehm, J., & Room, R. (2017). Lower-risk cannabis use guidelines (LRCUG): A comprehensive update of evidence and recommendations. *American Journal of Public Health, 107*(8), 1277. Advance online publication. DOI: 10.2105/AJPH.2017.303818a PMID: 28644037

Fischer, B., Robinson, T., Bullen, C., Curran, V., Jutras-Aswad, D., Medina-Mora, M. E., Pacula, R. L., Rehm, J., Room, R., Brink, W., & Hall, W. (2022). Lower-risk cannabis use guidelines for reducing health harms from non-medical cannabis use: A comprehensive evidence and recommendations update. *The International Journal on Drug Policy, 99*, 103381. DOI: 10.1016/j.drugpo.2021.103381 PMID: 34465496

Fischer, B., Russell, C., Sabioni, P., Van den Brink, W., Le Foll, B., Hall, W., Rehm, J., & Room, R. (2017). Lower-risk cannabis use guidelines: A comprehensive update of evidence and recommendations. *American Journal of Public Health, 107*(8), e1–e12. DOI: 10.2105/AJPH.2017.303818 PMID: 28644037

Fitzgerald, R. L., Umlauf, A., Hubbard, J. A., Hoffman, M. A., Sobolesky, P. M., Ellis, S. E., Grelotti, D. J., Suhandynata, R. T., Huestis, M. A., Grant, I., & Marcotte, T. D. (2023). Driving under the influence of cannabis: Impact of combining toxicology testing with field sobriety tests. *Clinical Chemistry, 69*(7), 724–733. https://doi.org/10.1093/clinchem/hvad054

Fleider, E. (2025, October 6). *Medical Marijuana: Implications for nurses in Ohio.* UC News. https://www.uc.edu/news/articles/2025/10/medical-marijuana--implications-for-nurses-in-ohio.html

Follow-Up After Emergency Department Visit for Substance Use (FUA) - NCQA. (2025, August). NCQA. https://www.ncqa.org/report-cards/health-plans/state-of-health-care-quality-report/follow-up-after-emergency-department-visit-for-substance-use-fua/

for Medicare and Medicaid Services. (2024). *Hospital readmissions reduction program (HRRP).* Www.cms.gov https://www.cms.gov/medicare/payment/prospective-payment-systems/acute-inpatient-pps/hospital-readmissions-reduction-program-hrrp

Foster, K. T., Arterberry, B. J., Zucker, R. A., & Hicks, B. M. (2021). Differences in child and adult biopsychosocial characteristics associated with regular cannabis use in individuals with and without cannabis use disorder. *Drug and Alcohol Dependence, 226*, 108887. DOI: 10.1016/j.drugalcdep.2021.108887 PMID: 34216859

Freeman, H. P., & Rodriguez, R. L. (2011). History and principles of patient navigation. *Cancer, 117*(S15), 3537–3540. DOI: 10.1002/cncr.26262 PMID: 21780088

Free, T., Grossoehme, D. H., Richner, G., Brown, M. F., & Friebert, S. (2025). Characterizing the population of a medical cannabis clinic in a pediatric hospital. *Journal of Palliative Medicine*, *28*(8), 1020–1028. DOI: 10.1089/jpm.2024.0533 PMID: 40180570

Freudenberg, N., & Tsui, E. (2014). Evidence, power, and policy change in community-based participatory research. *American Journal of Public Health*, *104*(1), 11–14. DOI: 10.2105/AJPH.2013.301471 PMID: 24228677

Furman, D., Campisi, J., Verdin, E., Carrera-Bastos, P., Targ, S., Franceschi, C., Ferrucci, L., Gilroy, D. W., Fasano, A., Miller, G. W., Miller, A. H., Mantovani, A., Weyand, C. M., Barzilai, N., Goronzy, J. J., Rando, T. A., Effros, R. B., Lucia, A., Kleinstreuer, N., & Slavich, G. M. (2019). Chronic inflammation in the etiology of disease across the life span. *Nature Medicine*, *25*(12), 1822–1832. DOI: 10.1038/s41591-019-0675-0 PMID: 31806905

Fusar-Poli, P., Crippa, J. A., Bhattacharyya, S., Borgwardt, S., Allen, P., Martin-Santos, R., Seal, M., Surguladze, S. A., O'Carroll, C., Atakan, Z., Zuardi, A. W., McGuire, P. K., & Stone, J. M. (2009). Distinct effects of Δ9-tetrahydrocannabinol and cannabidiol on neural activation during emotional processing. *Archives of General Psychiatry*, *66*(1), 95–105. DOI: 10.1001/archgenpsychiatry.2008.519 PMID: 19124693

Gallagher, A. T. (2010). Educating for ethical leadership. *Nursing Ethics*, *17*(4), 421–432. PMID: 20610575

Gallup Poll. (2026, January 12). *Nurses continue to lead in honesty and ethics ratings*. Retrieved January 30th, 2026, from Gallup: https://news.gallup.com/poll/700736/nurses-continue-lead-honesty-ethics-ratings.aspx

Garcia-Romeu, A., Elmore, J., Mayhugh, R. E., Schlienz, N. J., Martin, E. L., Strickland, J. C., Bonn-Miller, M., Jackson, H., & Vandrey, R. (2022). Online survey of medicinal cannabis users: Qualitative analysis of patient-level data. *Frontiers in Pharmacology*, *13*, 965535. Advance online publication. DOI: 10.3389/fphar.2022.965535 PMID: 36147312

Gardiner, K. M., Singleton, J. A., Sheridan, J., Kyle, G. J., & Nissen, L. M. (2019). Health professional beliefs, knowledge, and concerns surrounding medicinal cannabis: A systematic review. *PLoS One*, *14*(5), e0216556. DOI: 10.1371/journal.pone.0216556 PMID: 31059531

Garmany, A., & Terzic, A. (2024). Global healthspan–lifespan gaps among 183 World Health Organization member states. *JAMA Network Open*, *7*(12), e2450241. Advance online publication. DOI: 10.1001/jamanetworkopen.2024.50241 PMID: 39661386

Gastmans, C. (2013). Dignity-enhancing nursing care: A foundational ethical framework. *Nursing Ethics*, *20*(2), 142–149. DOI: 10.1177/0969733012473772 PMID: 23466947

GBD 2017 Causes of Death Collaborators. (2018). Global, regional, and national age-sex-specific mortality for 282 causes of death in 195 countries and territories, 1980–2017: A systematic analysis for the Global Burden of Disease Study 2017. *The Lancet*, *392*(10159), 1736–1788. https://doi.org/DOI: 10.1016/S0140-6736(18)32203-7

Gertsch, J., Pertwee, R. G., & Di Marzo, V. (2010). Phytocannabinoids beyond the cannabis plant—Do they exist? *British Journal of Pharmacology*, *160*(3), 523–529. DOI: 10.1111/j.1476-5381.2010.00745.x PMID: 20590562

Geurts, J. W., Willems, P. C., Lockwood, C., van Kleef, M., Kleijnen, J., & Dirksen, C. (2017). Patient expectations for management of chronic non-cancer pain: A systematic review. *Health Expectations*, *20*(6), 1201–1217. DOI: 10.1111/hex.12527 PMID: 28009082

Ghelani, A. (2021). Cannabis use among mental health professionals: A qualitative study of cannabis-related risk perceptions. *Journal of Drug Issues*, *51*(4), 679–689. DOI: 10.1177/00220426211032558 PMID: 34511638

Giangregorio, A., Wang, L., Sprague, S., Arbus, M., & Busse, J. W. (2024). Predictors of response to medical cannabis for chronic pain: A retrospective review of real-time observational data. *Cannabis (Research Society on Marijuana)*, *7*(3), 167–176. DOI: 10.26828/cannabis/2024/000259 PMID: 39781554

Giddens, J. (2018). Transformational leadership: What every nursing dean should know. *Journal of Professional Nursing*, *117-121*(2), 117–121. Advance online publication. DOI: 10.1016/j.profnurs.2017.10.004 PMID: 29703313

Giordano, G., Mattia, M., Boracchi, M., Biehler-Gomez, L., Cummaudo, M., Porro, A., Caccianiga, M., Sardanelli, F., Slavazzi, F., Galimberti, P. M., Di Candia, D., & Cattaneo, C. (2023). Forensic toxicological analyses reveal the use of cannabis in Milano (Italy) in the 1600s. *Journal of Archaeological Science*, *160*, 105873. DOI: 10.1016/j.jas.2023.105873

González-García, A., Pinto-Carral, A., Pérez-González, S., & Marqués-Sánchez, P. (2021). Nurse managers' competencies: A scoping review. *Journal of Nursing Management*, *29*(6), 1410–1419.https://doi.org/10.1111/jonm.13380

Government of Canada. (2021, December 15). Cannabis Act (S.C. 2018, c. 16). https://laws-lois.justice.gc.ca/PDF/C-24.5.pdf

Gowen, K., Cahill, M., Russell, K., & Cronquist, R. (2018). Medical Marijuana and Nursing Practice: Legislation, Scientific Literature review, and nursing implications. National Council of State Board of Nursing.https://www.ncsbn.org/public-files/presentations/2018DCM_Medical-Marijuana.pdf

Graham, M., Martin, J. H., Lucas, C. J., Murnion, B., & Schneider, J. (2022). Cannabidiol drug interaction considerations for prescribers and pharmacists. *Expert Review of Clinical Pharmacology*, *15*(12), 1383–1397. DOI: 10.1080/17512433.2022.2142114 PMID: 36317739

Graham, M., Pacula, R. L., Pessar, S. C., Ge, Y., Kritikos, A. F., Hall, W., & Hammond, D. (2025). Understanding medical cannabis use internationally: Why definitions and context matter. *Addiction (Abingdon, England)*, *120*(10), 2141–2146. DOI: 10.1111/add.70117 PMID: 40590488

Gray, S. (2016). *Cannabis spirituality: An explorer's guide to an ancient plant spirit.* Park Street Press.

Grbic, J., Goddard, P., & Ryder, D. (2017). Observations of the role of science in the United States medical cannabis state policies: Lessons learnt. *The International Journal on Drug Policy*, *42*, 109–114. DOI: 10.1016/j.drugpo.2016.12.019 PMID: 28190671

Greenway, M., & Acai, A. (2024). Academic leadership in nursing: A concept analysis. *Nurse Education Today*, *141*, 106338.https://doi.org/10.1016/j.nedt.2024.106338

Griffith, S., Kreider, R., & Leung, J. (2025). *A coordinated approach to cannabis policy and product safety. Issues in Science and Technology*. https://issues.org/coordinated-approach-cannabis-policy-safety-griffith-kreider-leung

Guidance Regarding Marijuana Enforcement. (2013, August 23). U.S. Department of Justice Office of the Deputy Attorney General. https://www.justice.gov/iso/opa/resources/3052013829132756857467.pdf

Gupta, K. (2023). Validity and Reliability of Students' Assessment: Case for Recognition as a Unified Concept of Valid Reliability. *International Journal of Applied & Basic Medical Research*, *13*(3), 129–132. https://doi.org/10.4103/ijabmr.ijabmr_382_23

Hallinan, C. M., Gunn, J. M., & Bonomo, Y. A. (2021). Implementation of medicinal cannabis in Australia: Innovation or upheaval? *BMJ Open*, *11*(10), e054044. DOI: 10.1136/bmjopen-2021-054044 PMID: 34686558

Hall, W., & Degenhardt, L. (2014). The adverse health effects of chronic cannabis use. *Drug Testing and Analysis*, *6*(1–2), 39–45. DOI: 10.1002/dta.1506 PMID: 23836598

Hammond, D., Goodman, S., Wadsworth, E., Rynard, V., Boudreau, C., & Hall, W. (2020). Evaluating the impacts of cannabis legalization: The International Cannabis Policy Study. *The International Journal on Drug Policy*, *77*, 102698. DOI: 10.1016/j.drugpo.2020.102698 PMID: 32113149

Han, B. H., Compton, W. M., Blanco, C., & Jones, C. M. (2023). Trends in cannabis use disorder prevalence among medical and nonmedical cannabis users in the United States. *JAMA Network Open*, *6*(1), e2251621. Advance online publication. DOI: 10.1001/jamanetworkopen.2022.51621 PMID: 36701154

Han, B. H., Yang, K. H., Cleland, C. M., & Palamar, J. J. (2025). Trends in past-month cannabis use among older adults. *JAMA Internal Medicine*, *185*(7), 881–883. DOI: 10.1001/jamainternmed.2025.1156 PMID: 40455425

Harden, R. M., Stevenson, M., Downie, W. W., & Wilson, G. M. (1975). Assessment of clinical competence using objective structured examination. *British Medical Journal*, *1*(5955), 447–451. DOI: 10.1136/bmj.1.5955.447 PMID: 1115966

Hardy, J. R., Greer, R. M., Pelecanos, A. M., Huggett, G. E., Kearney, A. M., Gurgenci, T. H., & Good, P. D. (2025). Medicinal cannabis for symptom control in advanced cancer: A double-blind, placebo-controlled, randomised clinical trial of 1:1 tetrahydrocannabinol and cannabidiol. *Supportive Care in Cancer*, *33*(8), 1–12. DOI: 10.1007/s00520-025-09763-5 PMID: 40705150

Hardy, J., Greer, R., Huggett, G., Kearney, A., Gurgenci, T., & Good, P. (2023). Phase IIb randomised, placebo-controlled, dose-escalating, double-blind study of cannabidiol oil for symptom relief in advanced cancer (MedCan1-CBD). *Journal of Clinical Oncology*, *41*(7), 1444–1452. DOI: 10.1200/JCO.22.01632 PMID: 36409969

Hartenstein, L., & Latkovic, T. (2022). *The secret to great health? Escaping the healthcare matrix.* McKinsey Health Institute. https://www.mckinsey.com/mhi/our-insights/the-secret-to-great-health-escaping-the-healthcare-matrix

Hartley, S., Simon, N., Larabi, A., Vaugier, I., Barbot, F., Quera-Salva, M. A., & Alvarez, J. C. (2019). Effect of smoked cannabis on vigilance and accident risk using simulated driving in occasional and chronic users and the pharmacokinetic–pharmacodynamic relationship. *Clinical Chemistry*, *65*(5), 684–693. DOI: 10.1373/clinchem.2018.299727 PMID: 30872375

Harvard Health Publishing. (2021, August 11). *The endocannabinoid system: Essential and mysterious.* (P. Grinspoon, Editor) https://www.health.harvard.edu/blog/the-endocannabinoid-system-essential-and-mysterious-202108112569

Hasin, D. (2023). Legalization of cannabis for medical and recreational use. *European Psychiatry : the Journal of the Association of European Psychiatrists*, *66*(S1, Suppl 1), S20–S21. DOI: 10.1192/j.eurpsy.2023.83

Hasin, D., & Walsh, C. (2020). Cannabis Use, Cannabis Use Disorder, and Comorbid Psychiatric Illness: A Narrative Review. *Journal of Clinical Medicine*, *10*(1), 15. DOI: 10.3390/jcm10010015 PMID: 33374666

Hathaway, A. D., Mostaghim, A., Erickson, P. G., Kolar, K., & Osborne, G. (2018). A nuanced view of normalisation: Attitudes of cannabis non-users in a study of undergraduate students. *Drugs: Education Prevention & Policy*, *25*(1), 68–77. DOI: 10.1080/09687637.2017.1290780

Haug, N. A., Kieschnick, D., Sottile, J. E., Babson, K. A., Vandrey, R., & Bonn-Miller, M. O. (2016). Training and practices of cannabis dispensary staff. *Cannabis and Cannabinoid Research*, *1*(1), 244–251. DOI: 10.1089/can.2016.0024 PMID: 28861496

Haug, N. A., Padula, C. B., Sottile, J. E., Vandrey, R., Heinz, A. J., & Bonn-Miller, M. O. (2022). Cannabis use patterns and motives: A comparison of younger, middle-aged, and older medical cannabis dispensary patients. *Addictive Behaviors*, *125*, 107–110. DOI: 10.1016/j.addbeh.2021.107110 PMID: 28340421

Hays, R. D., Bjorner, J. B., Revicki, D. A., Spritzer, K. L., & Cella, D. (2009). Development of physical and mental health summary scores from the PROMIS global items. *Quality of Life Research: An International Journal of Quality of Life Aspects of Treatment, Care and Rehabilitation*, *18*(7), 873–880. DOI: 10.1007/s11136-009-9496-9 PMID: 19543809

Health Canada. (2018). *Cannabis legalization and regulation.* Government of Canada.

Health Canada. (2022). *Canadian cannabis survey.* Government of Canada.

Hill, K. P. (2015). Medical marijuana for treatment of chronic pain and other medical and psychiatric problems. *Journal of the American Medical Association*, *313*(24), 2474–2483. DOI: 10.1001/jama.2015.6199 PMID: 26103031

Hoch, E. H., Hall, W., & Feingold, D. (2025, February 14). Cannabis use in Europe. *European Archives of Psychiatry and Clinical Neuroscience*, *277-279*(2), 277–279. Advance online publication. DOI: 10.1007/s00406-025-01972-7 PMID: 39951121

Ho, I. K., Sheldon, T. A., & Botelho, E. (2022). Medical mistrust among women with intersecting marginalized identities: A scoping review. *Ethnicity & Health, 27*(8), 1733–1751. DOI: 10.1080/13557858.2021.1990220 PMID: 34647832

Ho, J. J. Y., Goh, C., Leong, C. S. A., Ng, K. Y., & Bakhtiar, A. (2024). Evaluation of potential drug–drug interactions with medical cannabis. *Clinical and Translational Science, 17*(5), e13812. DOI: 10.1111/cts.13812 PMID: 38720531

Holdman, R., Vigil, D., Robinson, K., Shah, P., & Contreras, A. E. (2022). Safety and efficacy of medical cannabis in autism spectrum disorder compared with commonly used medications. *Cannabis and Cannabinoid Research, 7*(4), 451–463. DOI: 10.1089/can.2020.0154 PMID: 34432543

Holland, J. (2010). The Pot Book: A complete guide to cannabis: Its role in medicine, politics, science, and culture. In Holland, J. (Ed.), *The Pot Book: A complete guide to cannabis: Its role in medicine, politics, science, and culture* (p. 246). Park Street Press.

Hong, G., Sideris, A., Waldman, S., Stauffer, J., & Wu, C. L. (2024). Legal and regulatory aspects of medical cannabis in the United States. *Anesthesia and Analgesia, 138*(1), 31–41. DOI: 10.1213/ANE.0000000000006301 PMID: 38100798

Hossain, M. K., & Chae, H. J. (2024). Medical cannabis: From research breakthroughs to shifting public perceptions and ensuring safe use. *Integrative Medicine Research, 13*(4), 101094. DOI: 10.1016/j.imr.2024.101094 PMID: 39640076

Huerne, K., Ells, C., Grad, R., Filion, B., & Eisenberg, M. J. (2022). Cannabis-Impaired driving: Ethical considerations for the primary care practitioner. *Annals of Medicine, 55*(1), 24–33. DOI: 10.1080/07853890.2022.2151716 PMID: 36444881

Huestis, M. A. (2007). Human cannabinoid pharmacokinetics. *Chemistry & Biodiversity, 4*(8), 1770–1804. DOI: 10.1002/cbdv.200790152 PMID: 17712819

Hulaihel, A., Gliksberg, O., Feingold, D., Brill, S., Amit, B. H., Lev-ran, S., & Sznitman, S. R. (2023). Medical cannabis and stigma: A qualitative study with patients living with chronic pain. *Journal of Clinical Nursing, 32*(7-8), 1103–1114. DOI: 10.1111/jocn.16340 PMID: 35488381

Hunault, C. C., Mensinga, T. T., Böcker, K. B. E., Schipper, C. M. A., Kruidenier, M., Leenders, M. E., de Vries, I., & Meulenbelt, J. (2009). Cognitive and psychomotor effects in males after smoking a combination of tobacco and cannabis containing up to 69 mg delta-9-tetrahydrocannabinol (THC). *Psychopharmacology, 204*(1), 85–94. DOI: 10.1007/s00213-008-1440-0 PMID: 19099294

Hurn, S. (2023). An individual's lived experiences of taking cannabis-based medicinal products to treat anxiety. *International Journal of Environmental Research and Public Health, 20*(18), 6776. DOI: 10.3390/ijerph20186776 PMID: 37754635

Hurst, H., & Bolton, J. (2004). Assessing the clinical significance of change scores recorded on subjective outcome measures. *Journal of Manipulative and Physiological Therapeutics, 27*(1), 26–35. DOI: 10.1016/j.jmpt.2003.11.003 PMID: 14739871

Ibeas Bih, C., Chen, T., Nunn, A. V. W., Bazelot, M., Dallas, M., & Whalley, B. J. (2015). Molecular targets of cannabidiol in neurological disorders. *Neurotherapeutics; the Journal of the American Society for Experimental NeuroTherapeutics*, *12*(4), 699–730. DOI: 10.1007/s13311-015-0377-3 PMID: 26264914

Iffland, K., & Grotenhermen, F. (2017). An update on safety and side effects of cannabidiol: A review of clinical data and relevant animal studies. *Cannabis and Cannabinoid Research*, *2*(1), 139–154. DOI: 10.1089/can.2016.0034 PMID: 28861514

Institute of Medicine. (2001). *Crossing the quality chasm: A new health system for the 21st century*. National Academies Press., DOI: 10.17226/10027

Institute of Medicine. (2011). *The future of nursing: Leading change, advancing health*. The National Academies Press., DOI: 10.17226/12956

Internal Revenue Service. (2022). Internal Revenue Code § 280E. https://www.irs.gov

International Association of Clinical Research Nurses. (2024). *Clinical research nursing: Scope and standards of practice* (2nd ed.). American Nurses Association.

International Council of Nurses. (n.d.). *The global voice of nursing*. Retrieved February 4, 2026, from ICN: https://www.icn.ch/

Ioannidis, J. P. A. (2005). Why most published research findings are false. *PLoS Medicine*, *2*(8), e124. Advance online publication. DOI: 10.1371/journal.pmed.0020124 PMID: 16060722

Jackson, M., McTier, L., Brooks, L. A., & Wynne, R. (2024). Impact of simulation design elements on undergraduate nursing education: A systematic review. *Clinical Simulation in Nursing*, *78*, 1–10. https://www.nursingsimulation.org/article/S1876-1399(24)00011-2/fulltext. DOI: 10.1016/j.ecns.2024.101519

Jaeger, K. (2025b). Federal health programs will cover up to $500 worth of CBD for certain patients by April, Trump official Dr. Oz says. *Marijuana Moment*. https://www.marijuanamoment.net/federal-health-programs-will-cover-up-to-500-worth-of-cbd-for-certain-patients-by-april-trump-official-dr-oz-says/

Jaeger, K. (2026, February 3). Lawmakers in multiple states push to allow medical marijuana use in hospitals by qualifying patients. *Marijuana Moment*. https://www.marijuanamoment.net/lawmakers-in-multiple-states-push-to-allow-medical-marijuana-use-in-hospitals-by-qualifying-patients/

Jaiswal, J. (2019). Whose responsibility is it to dismantle medical mistrust? Future directions for researchers and health care providers. *Behavioral Medicine (Washington, D.C.)*, *45*(2), 188–196. DOI: 10.1080/08964289.2019.1630357 PMID: 31343959

Javeed, M. (2024, February 28). Confronting the Crisis: Exploring the Challenges of Nurse Educator Shortages Today. Top content on LinkedIn. https://www.linkedin.com/pulse/confronting-crisis-exploring-challenges-nurse-edccator-javeed-0eh4f#:~:text=1

Johnson, E. C., Colbert, S. M., Jeffries, P. W., Tillman, R., Bigdeli, T. B., Karcher, N. R., Chan, G., Kuperman, S., Meyers, J. L., Nurnberger, J. I., Plawecki, M. H., Degenhardt, L., Martin, N. G., Kamarajan, C., Schuckit, M. A., Murray, R. M., Dick, D. M., Edenberg, H. J., D'Souza, D. C., & Agrawal, A. (2023). Associations between cannabis use, polygenic liability for schizophrenia, and cannabis-related experiences in a sample of cannabis users. *Schizophrenia Bulletin*, *49*(3), 778–787. DOI: 10.1093/schbul/sbac196 PMID: 36545904

Johnson, J. R., Burnell-Nugent, M., Lossignol, D., Ganae-Motan, E. D., Potts, R., & Fallon, M. T. (2010). Multicentre, double-blind, randomised, placebo-controlled study of nabiximols in patients with opioid-refractory cancer pain. *Journal of Pain and Symptom Management*, *39*, 167–179. DOI: 10.1016/j.jpainsymman.2009.06.008 PMID: 19896326

Johnson, O. E., Miskelly, G. M., & Rindelaub, J. D. (2022). Testing for cannabis intoxication: Current issues and latest advancements. *WIREs Forensic Science*, *4*(4), e1450. DOI: 10.1002/wfs2.1450

Kalant, H. (2001). Medicinal use of cannabis: History and current status. *Pain Research & Management*, *6*(2), 80–91. DOI: 10.1155/2001/469629 PMID: 11854770

Kansagara, D., Morasco, B. J., Iacocca, M. O., Bair, M. J., Hooker, E. R., & Becker, W. C. (2020). Clinician knowledge, attitudes, and practice regarding cannabis: Results from a National Veterans Health Administration survey. *Pain Medicine*, *21*(11), 3180–3186. DOI: 10.1093/pm/pnz322 PMID: 31909803

Kansagara, D., Terry, G. E., Ayers, C. K., & D'Souza, D. C. (2026). Cannabis and mental health: A review. *JAMA Internal Medicine*, *186*(5), 618. Advance online publication. DOI: 10.1001/jamainternmed.2025.8215 PMID: 41801216

Kaplan, L., Klein, T., Wilson, M., & Graves, J. (2020). Knowledge, practices, and attitudes of Washington State health care professionals regarding medical cannabis. *Cannabis and Cannabinoid Research*, *5*(2), 172–182. DOI: 10.1089/can.2019.0051 PMID: 32656349

Karki, P., & Rangaswamy, M. (2023). A review of historical context and current research on cannabis use in India. *Indian Journal of Psychological Medicine*, *45*(2), 105–116. DOI: 10.1177/02537176221109272 PMID: 36925496

Kaskie, B. (2023). The cannabis and older persons study: What we have learned. *Innovation in Aging*, *7*(Suppl 1), 173. DOI: 10.1093/geroni/igad104.0567

Kasturi, S., Szymonifka, J., Burket, J. C., Berman, J. R., Kirou, K. A., Levine, A. B., & Mandl, L. A. (2018). Feasibility, validity, and reliability of the 10-item PROMIS Global Health Short Form in outpatients with systemic lupus erythematosus. *The Journal of Rheumatology*, *45*(3), 397–404. DOI: 10.3899/jrheum.170590 PMID: 29419473

Katerenchuk, J., & Salas, A. S. (2023). An integrative review on the oncology nurse navigator role in the Canadian context. *Canadian Oncology Nursing Journal = Revue Canadienne de Nursing Oncologique*, *33*(4), 385–399. DOI: 10.5737/23688076334385 PMID: 38919590

Kavousi, P., Giamo, T., Arnold, G., Alliende, M., Huynh, E., Lea, J., Lucine, R., Tillett Miller, A., Webre, A., Yee, A., Champagne-Zamora, A., & Taylor, K. (2022). What do we know about opportunities and challenges for localities from Cannabis legalization? *The Review of Policy Research*, *39*(2), 143–169. DOI: 10.1111/ropr.12460

Kellogg, A., Anderson, C., & Michiels, M. (2022, April). A Cannabis Conflict of Law: Federal vs. State Law Business Law Today American Bar Association, https://www.americanbar.org/groups/business_law/resources/business-law-today/2022-april/a-cannabis-conflict-of-law-federal-vs-state-law/#:~:text=As%20we%20examined%20in%20the,substance%20is%20a%20federal%20offense

Khak, M., Ramtin, S., Chung, J., Ilyas, A. M., & Greis, A. (2025). Discontinuation rates and predictors of medical cannabis cessation for chronic musculoskeletal pain. *PLoS One*, *20*(8), e0329897. Advance online publication. DOI: 10.1371/journal.pone.0329897 PMID: 40773423

Khezrian, M., McNeil, C. J., Murray, A. D., & Myint, P. K. (2020). An overview of prevalence, determinants, and health outcomes of polypharmacy. *Therapeutic Advances in Drug Safety*, *11*, 2042098620933741. Advance online publication. DOI: 10.1177/2042098620933741 PMID: 32587680

Kiel, L., Hsu, C., Wartko, D., Albertson-Junkans, L., Ewing, J., & Lapham, G. T. (2022). Perspectives from women who engaged in prenatal and postpartum cannabis use in a U.S. State with legal non-medical use. *Preventive Medicine Reports*, *31*, 102075. DOI: 10.1016/j.pmedr.2022.102075 PMID: 36820379

Kilmer, J. (2018, November 13). Cannabis and the college campus: Considering the impact on students in a changing legal climate. *Higher Education Today*. https://www.higheredtoday.org/2018/11/13/cannabis-college-campus-considering-impact-students-changing-legal-climate/

King, D. (2021). Anesthesia for patients who self report cannabis (marijuana) use before esophogo-gastrodoudenoscopy: A retrospective review. *American Associatin of Nurse Anesthesiology*, 205-212.

King, R. (1972). The drug hang-up: America's fifty-year folly. W.W. Norton.https://www.google.com/url?q=https://www.druglibrary.net/special/king/dhu/dhu28.htm&sa=D&source=docs&ust=1765298703276722&usg=AOvVaw3-RFfIpiJtPV-UD2Ax05Uz

King, D. D., DeCarlo, M., Mylott, L., & Yarossi, M. (2023). Cannabis knowledge gaps in nursing education: Pilot testing cannabis curriculum. *Teaching and Learning in Nursing*, *18*(4), 474–479. DOI: 10.1016/j.teln.2023.06.012

King, D. D., Gill, C. J., Cadieux, C. S., & Singh, N. (2024). The role of stigma in cannabis use disclosure: An exploratory study. *Harm Reduction Journal*, *21*(21), 1–13. DOI: 10.1186/s12954-024-00929-8 PMID: 38273362

King, K. (2024). Cannabis nursing. *AJN. The American Journal of Nursing*, *124*(5), 31. DOI: 10.1097/01.NAJ.0001016368.03202.a8 PMID: 38661699

Kitdumrongthum, S., & Trachootham, D. (2023). Individuality of response to cannabinoids: Challenges in safety and efficacy of cannabis products. *Molecules (Basel, Switzerland)*, *28*(6), 2791. DOI: 10.3390/molecules28062791 PMID: 36985763

Klein, A., & Clark, C. S. (2022). Therapeutic use of cannabis in the US. *The Nurse Practitioner*, *47*(12), 16–25. DOI: 10.1097/01.NPR.0000884880.81603.c5 PMID: 36399143

Kloft, L., Otgaar, H., Blokland, A., Monds, L. A., Toennes, S. W., Loftus, E. F., & Ramaekers, J. G. (2020). Cannabis increases susceptibility to false memory. *Proceedings of the National Academy of Sciences of the United States of America*, *117*(9), 4585–4589. DOI: 10.1073/pnas.1920162117 PMID: 32041881

Knox, R. (Producer). (2018). *The endocannabinoid system and the revolution of one* [Motion Picture]. https://www.youtube.com/watch?v=oJbOQ9P2NYQ

Kocis, P. T., Mallinson, D. J., & Servinsky Jr., T. J. (2024). Cannabinoid Awareness, Reporting Use to Health Care Providers, and Perceptions Regarding Safety – Pennsylvania, March 2023–April 2023. *Medical Cannabis and Cannabinoids,* *7*(1), 119–124. https://doi.org/10.1159/000539956

Köck, P., Badek, A., Meyer, M., Klaassen, A. L., Walter, M., & Kindler, J. (2024). Cannabinoids for treating psychiatric disorders in youth: A systematic review of randomised controlled trials. *Child and Adolescent Psychiatry and Mental Health*, *18*(1), 158. DOI: 10.1186/s13034-024-00846-5 PMID: 39696457

Kogan, M., Temple, L. M., Zolotov, Y., & Isralowitz, R. (2025). 2025 International Congress Abstract Supplement. *Global Advances in Integrative Medicine and Health*, *14*, 27536130251324543. https://doi.org/10.1177/27536130251324543

Kokorelias, K. M., DasGupta, T., & Hitzig, S. L. (2022). Designing the ideal patient navigation program for older adults with complex needs: A qualitative exploration of the preferences of key informants. *Journal of Applied Gerontology*, *41*(4), 1002–1010. DOI: 10.1177/07334648211059056 PMID: 34905440

Kokorelias, K. M., Shiers-Hanley, J. E., Rios, J., Knoepfli, A., & Hitzig, S. L. (2021). Factors influencing the implementation of patient navigation programs for adults with complex needs: A scoping review of the literature. *Health Services Insights*, *14*, 11786329211033267. Advance online publication. DOI: 10.1177/11786329211033267 PMID: 34349519

Kruger, D. J., Mokbel, M. A., Clauw, D. J., & Boehnke, K. F. (2022). Assessing health care providers' knowledge of medical cannabis. *Cannabis and Cannabinoid Research*, *7*(4), 501–507. DOI: 10.1089/can.2021.0032 PMID: 34463161

Kurtzman, E. T., Greene, J., Begley, R., & Drenkard, K. N. (2022). "We want what's best for patients." Nurse leaders' attitudes about medical cannabis: A qualitative study. *International Journal of Nursing Studies Advances*, *4*, 100065. Advance online publication. DOI: 10.1016/j.ijnsa.2022.100065 PMID: 38745605

Kvamme, S. L., Pedersen, M. M., Thomsen, K. R., & Thylstrup, B. (2021). Exploring the use of cannabis as a substitute for prescription drugs in a convenience sample. *Harm Reduction Journal*, *18*(1), 72. Advance online publication. DOI: 10.1186/s12954-021-00520-5 PMID: 34246279

L.M., & BorgeltFranson, K.L. (2017). Considerations for Hospital Policies Regarding Medical Cannabis Use. *Hospital Pharmacy*. *52*(2), 89–90. https://doi:10.1310/hpj5202-89

Lampe, J. R., Sacco, L. N., & Sheikh, H. Z. (2024, May 2). The Federal Status of Marijuana and the Policy Gap with States. LIBRARY OF CONGRESS https://www.congress.gov/crs-product/IF12270

Lange, T. (2025). American Council of Cannabis Medicine unveils major industry initiative to expand medical cannabis access. Cannabis Business Times. https://www.cannabisbusinesstimes.com/business-issues-benchmarks/medical-cannabis-access-and-pricing/news/15769892/american-council-of-cannabis-medicine-unveils-major-industry-initiative-to-expand-medical-cannabis-access

Lange, T. (2025, November 19). US Congresswoman Unveils Bill to Repeal Federal Hemp Product Ban. Cannabis Business Times. https://www.cannabisbusinesstimes.com/hemp/news/15772220/us-congresswoaan-unveils-bill-to-repeal-federal-hemp-product-ban

Langley, P. C. (2019). Tracking and Reporting Outcomes in Medical Marijuana: Establishing Condition-Specific State-Level Registries. *Innovations in Pharmacy*, *10*(2), 4. https://doi.org/10.24926/iip.v10i2.1800

Lapham, G. T., Matson, T. E., Carrell, D. S., Bobb, J. F., Luce, C., Oliver, M. M., Ghitza, U. E., Hsu, C., Browne, K. C., Binswanger, I. A., Campbell, C. I., Saxon, A. J., Vandrey, R., Schauer, G. L., Pacula, R. L., Horberg, M. A., Bailey, S. R., McClure, E. A., & Bradley, K. A. (2022). Comparison of medical cannabis use reported on a confidential survey vs documented in the electronic health record among primary care patients. *JAMA Network Open*, *5*(5), e2211677. DOI: 10.1001/jamanetworkopen.2022.11677 PMID: 35604691

Lapham, G. T., Matson, T. E., Carrell, D. S., Bobb, J. F., Luce, C., Oliver, M. M., Ghitza, U. E., Hsu, C., Browne, K. C., Binswanger, I. A., Campbell, C. I., Saxon, A. J., Vandrey, R., Schauer, G. L., Pacula, R. L., Horberg, M. A., Bailey, S. R., McClure, E. A., & Bradley, K. A. (2022). Comparison of Medical Cannabis Use Reported on a Confidential Survey vs Documented in the Electronic Health Record Among Primary Care Patients. *JAMA Network Open*, *5*(5), e2211677–e2211677. https://doi.org/10.1001/jamanetworkopen.2022.11677

Lapkin, S., Levett-Jones, T., Bellchambers, H., & Fernandez, R. (2010). Effectiveness of patient simulation manikins in teaching clinical reasoning skills to undergraduate nursing students: A systematic review. *Clinical Simulation in Nursing*, *6*(6), e207–e222. https://www.sciencedirect.com/science/article/abs/pii/S1876139910001325. DOI: 10.1016/j.ecns.2010.05.005 PMID: 27820553

Lawler, Z. (2025). Medical Cannabis & Cannabinoid Regulation 2025. Last Updated May 29, 2025. USA https://practiceguides.chambers.com/practice-guides/comparison/1003/17057/25531-25538-25540#:~:text=Under%20federal%20law%2C%20cannabis%20is,Enforcement%20Policies:%20The%20Cole%20Memorandum

Lee, M. (2023). *CBD vs. THC*. Project CBD. https://projectcbd.org/what-is-cbd/cbd-vs-thc/

Lee, M. A. (2012). *Smoke signals: A social history of marijuana-medical, recreational, and scientific*. Simon & Schuster, Inc.

Lefebvre, È., Tawil, N., & Yahia, L. (2024). Transdermal delivery of cannabidiol for the management of acute inflammatory pain: A comprehensive review of the literature. *International Journal of Molecular Sciences*, *25*(11), 5858. Advance online publication. DOI: 10.3390/ijms25115858 PMID: 38892047

Lewis, K. (2025, May 29). The Vital Role of Performance Reviews and Appraisals in Nursing. ACI Training and Consultancy LTD. https://www.acitrainingandconsultancy.co.uk/post/the-vital-role-of-performance-reviews-and-appraisals-in-nursing#:~:text=Foster%20a%20supportive%20environment:%20Focus,support%20nurses%20with%20NMC%20revalidation.

Lewis, N., Broitman, D., & Sznitman, S. R. (2015). Medical cannabis: A framing analysis of Israeli newspaper coverage. *Science Communication*, *37*(6), 675–702. DOI: 10.1177/1075547015608507

Lin, C.-Y., Updegraff, J. A., & Pakpour, A. H. (2016). The relationship between the theory of planned behavior and medication adherence in patients with epilepsy. *Epilepsy & Behavior*, *61*, 231–236. DOI: 10.1016/j.yebeh.2016.05.030 PMID: 27390026

Lopera, V., Rodríguez, A., & Amariles, P. (2022). Clinical relevance of drug interactions with cannabis: A systematic review. *Journal of Clinical Medicine*, *11*(5), 1154. DOI: 10.3390/jcm11051154 PMID: 35268245

Lucas, C. J., Galettis, P., & Schneider, J. (2018). The Pharmacokinetics and the Pharmacodynamics of Cannabinoids. *British Journal of Clinical Pharmacology*, *84*(11), 2477–2483. DOI: 10.1111/bcp.13710 PMID: 30001569

Lucas, P. (2012). It can't hurt to ask: A patient-centered quality of service assessment of Health Canada's medical cannabis policy and program. *Harm Reduction Journal*, *9*(1), 2. DOI: 10.1186/1477-7517-9-2 PMID: 22214382

Lucas, P., & Walsh, Z. (2017). Medical cannabis access, use, and substitution for prescription opioids and other substances: A survey of authorised medical cannabis patients. *Harm Reduction Journal*, *14*, 58. DOI: 10.1186/s12954-017-0183-9 PMID: 28821296

Lu, H. C., & Mackie, K. (2016). An introduction to the endogenous cannabinoid system. *Biological Psychiatry*, *79*(7), 516–525. DOI: 10.1016/j.biopsych.2015.07.028 PMID: 26698193

M, F. (2025, March 31). *Cannabis and healthcare: Complicated policies and laws*. American Nurse. https://www.myamericannurse.com/cannabis-and-healthcare-complicated-policies-and-laws/

MacCallum, C. A., Lo, L. A., Pistawka, C., Christiansen, A., Boivin, M., & Snider-Adler, M. (2022). A Clinical Framework for Assessing Cannabis-Related Impairment Risk. *Frontiers in Psychiatry*, *13*, 883517. DOI: 10.3389/fpsyt.2022.883517 PMID: 35832600

MacCallum, C. A., & Russo, E. B. (2018). Practical considerations in medical cannabis administration and dosing. *European Journal of Internal Medicine*, *49*, 12–19. DOI: 10.1016/j.ejim.2018.01.004 PMID: 29307505

Mack, E. (2020). *Cannabis for health: Become a coach*. AuthorHouse. https://www.authorhouse.com/en/bookstore/bookdetails/805950-cannabis-for-health

Mack, E. A. (2020). Cannabis for health: Become a coach. AuthorHouse. https://www.authorhouse.com/en/bookstore/bookdetails/812353-cannabis-for-health-become-a-coach

Mack, S. (2025). Cannabis nursing: the heart of holistic care. Holistic Caring. https://holisticcaring.com/cannabis-nursing-the-heart-of-holistic-care/

Mack, S. (2026). Coherence in cannabis care. Ask The Green Nurse. https://thegreennurse.substack.com/p/coherence-in-cannabis-care

Mack, S. (2026). Medical, recreational, and wellness: Understanding cannabis use across contexts. Ask The Green Nurse Substack https://thegreennurse.substack.com/p/medical-recreational-and-wellness

Mackie, K. (2020). Cannabinoid receptors: Where they are and what they do. *Journal of Neuroendocrinology*, *32*(1), e12805. DOI: 10.1111/jne.12805 PMID: 18426493

Maldonado, R., Berrendero, F., Ozaita, A., & Robledo, P. (2011). Neurochemical basis of cannabis addiction. *Neuroscience*, *181*, 1–17. DOI: 10.1016/j.neuroscience.2011.02.035 PMID: 21334423

Malka, D. (2022). *Medicinal Cannabis*. CRC Press.

Malpas, S. C. (2010). Sympathetic nervous system overactivity and its role in the development of cardiovascular disease. *Physiological Reviews*, *90*(2), 513–557. DOI: 10.1152/physrev.00007.2009 PMID: 20393193

Management Society of America. (2024, May 31). *The Impact of Case Management on the Healthcare System: A CMSA Perspective*. Cmsa.org. https://cmsa.org/the-impact-of-case-management-on-the-healthcare-system-3/

Manalo-Morgan, A. (2022). *Mighty flower: How cannabis saved my son*. Forbes Books.

Mancia, G., & Grassi, G. (2014). The autonomic nervous system and hypertension. *Circulation Research*, *114*(11), 1804–1814. DOI: 10.1161/CIRCRESAHA.114.302524 PMID: 24855203

Marcotte, T. D., Umlauf, A., Grelotti, D. J., Sones, E. G., Mastropietro, K. F., Suhandynata, R. T., Huestis, M. A., Grant, I., & Fitzgerald, R. L. (2023). Evaluation of field sobriety tests for identifying drivers under the influence of cannabis: A randomized clinical trial. *JAMA Psychiatry*, *80*(9), 914–923.https://doi.org/10.1001/jamapsychiatry.2023.2345

Marie Figueroa-Rivera, I., Estremera-Marcial, R., Sierra-Mercado, M., Gutiérrez-Núñez, J., & Toro, H. (2015). D. (2015). Cannabinoid Hyperemesis Syndrome: A Paradoxical Cannabis Effect. *Case Reports in Gastrointestinal Medicine*, 405238.

Marijuana Policy Project. (2022, February 7). *Medical Cannabis Laws and Anti-Discrimination Provisions*. MMP. Retrieved January 6, 2026, from https://www.mpp.org/issues/medical-marijuana/medical-marijuana-laws-anti-discrimination-provisions/

Marijuana Policy Project. (2024). *Medical marijuana patient numbers*. https://www.mpp.org/issues/medical-marijuana/state-by-state-medical-marijuana-laws/medical-marijuana-patient-numbers/

Marijuana Policy Project. (n.d.) *Medical Cannabis Laws and Employment Protections. MPP.* Retrieved January 6, 2026, from https://www.mpp.org/issues/medical-marijuana/medical-cannabis-laws-and-employment-protections/

Marijuana Policy Project. (n.d.). *DEA moves to reschedule marijuana to Schedule III: questions and answers*. MPP. Retrieved January 6, 2026, from https://www.mpp.org/policy/federal/dea-moves-to-reschedule-marijuana-to-schedule-iii-questions-and-answers/

Martin, E. L., Strickland, J. C., Schlienz, N. J., Munson, J., Bonsu, H., Mueller, A. S., & Vandrey, R. (2021). Antidepressant and anxiolytic effects of medicinal cannabis use in an observational subset of patients with anxiety and depression. *Frontiers in Psychiatry, 12*, 729800. Advance online publication. DOI: 10.3389/fpsyt.2021.729800 PMID: 34566726

Martins, S. S., Segura, L. E., Levy, N. S., Mauro, P. M., Mauro, C. M., Philbin, M. M., & Hasin, D. S. (2021). Racial and ethnic differences in cannabis use following legalization in US states with medical cannabis laws. *JAMA Network Open, 4*(9), e2127002–e2127002. DOI: 10.1001/jamanetworkopen.2021.27002 PMID: 34570205

Martin-Willett, R., Stanger, M., James, W., Bryan, A. D., & Bidwell, L. C. (2023). Effects of historical inequity and institutional power on cannabis research: Moving toward equity and inclusion. *PNAS Nexus, 2*(12), pgad383. Advance online publication. DOI: 10.1093/pnasnexus/pgad383 PMID: 38089600

Maryland General Assembly. (2021). *House Bill 331: Connor's Courage Act.* https://mgaleg.maryland.gov

Maryland General Assembly. (2023). *House Bill 1135 / Senate Bill 587.* https://mgaleg.maryland.gov

Maryland Medical Cannabis Commission. (n.d.). *Medical cannabis use in schools: Physician authorization form.* Maryland Department of Health. https://www.marylandpublicschools.org/about/Documents/DSFSS/SSSP/SHS/SHSGuidelines/StudentMedicalCannabisAuthForm.pdf

Matson, E., Lapham, G. T., Bobb, J. F., Oliver, M., Hallgren, K. A., Williams, E. C., & Bradley, K. A. (2022). Validity of the Single-Item Screen–Cannabis (SIS-C) for Cannabis Use Disorder Screening in Routine Care. *JAMA Network Open, 5*(11), e2239772. DOI: 10.1001/jamanetworkopen.2022.39772 PMID: 36318205

Maynard, F. (2025, April). Cannabis and healthcare: Complicated policies and laws. (L. Gelinas, Ed.) *American Nurse, 20*(4), 14-18. https://www.myamericannurse.com/wp-content/uploads/2025/03/an4-Cannabis-321.pdf

McCance, T., & McCormack, B. (2025). The person-centred nursing framework: A mid-range theory for nursing practice. *Journal of Research in Nursing : JRN, 30*(1), 47–60. DOI: 10.1177/17449871241281428 PMID: 40093819

McCormack, B., & McCance, T. (2017). *Person-centered practice in nursing and health care: Theory and practice* (2nd ed.). Wiley-Blackwell.

McEachan, R. R. C., Conner, M., Taylor, N. J., & Lawton, R. J. (2011). Prospective prediction of health-related behaviours with the theory of planned behaviour: A meta-analysis. *Health Psychology Review, 5*(2), 97–144. DOI: 10.1080/17437199.2010.521684

McIntosh, N., Wilson, N. J., Povalej, P., Hunt, L., & Lewis, P. (2024). An exploration of registered nurses' experiences caring for patients taking medicinal cannabis. *Nursing Open, 11*(10), e70063. DOI: 10.1002/nop2.70063 PMID: 39455290

McIntyre, R. S., Alsuwaidan, M., Baune, B. T., Berk, M., Demyttenaere, K., Goldberg, J. F., Gorwood, P., Ho, R., Kasper, S., Kennedy, S. H., Ly-Uson, J., Mansur, R. B., McAllister-Williams, R. H., Murrough, J. W., Nemeroff, C. B., Nierenberg, A. A., Rosenblat, J. D., Sanacora, G., Schatzberg, A. F., & Maj, M. (2023). Treatment-resistant depression: Definition, prevalence, detection, management, and investigational interventions. *World Psychiatry; Official Journal of the World Psychiatric Association (WPA)*, *22*(3), 394–412. DOI: 10.1002/wps.21120 PMID: 37713549

McKaig, A., Ridad, A., Bell, A., McParlane, R., & Quirch, M. (2025). Implementing Ryan's Law on an Inpatient Medical Oncology Unit, *Clinical Journal of Oncology Nursing 20;29*(1), 86–90. https://doi.org/10.1188/25.CJON.86-90

McKaig, A., Ridad, A. R. V., Bell, A., McParlane, R., & Quirch, M. (2025). Implementing Ryan's Law on an inpatient medical oncology unit. *Clinical Journal of Oncology Nursing*, *29*(1), 86–90. DOI: 10.1188/25.CJON.86-90 PMID: 39933092

McLennan, A., Kerba, M., Subnis, U., Campbell, T., & Carlson, L. E. (2020). Health care provider preferences for, and barriers to, cannabis use in cancer care. *Current Oncology (Toronto, Ont.)*, *27*(2), e199–e205. DOI: 10.3747/co.27.5615 PMID: 32489269

McNichol, W. J. (2025). Pseudoscience and the Detection of Marijuana-Based Impairment: We Can and Must Do Better, 86. *Journal of Studies on Alcohol and Drugs*, *86*(4), 503–509.https://doi.org/10.15288/jsad.24-00307

McPartland, J. M., Guy, G. W., & Di Marzo, V. (2014). Care and feeding of the endocannabinoid system: A systematic review of potential clinical interventions that upregulate the endocannabinoid system. *PLoS One*, *9*(3), e89566. DOI: 10.1371/journal.pone.0089566 PMID: 24622769

Mead, A. (2019). Legal and Regulatory Issues Governing Cannabis and Cannabis-Derived Products in the United States. *Frontiers in Plant Science*, (10), 679.https://doi.org/10.3389/fpls.2019.00697

Mechoulam, R., & Hanus, L. (2000). A historical overview of chemical research on cannabinoids. *Chemistry and Physics of Lipids*, *108*(1), 1–13. https://www.sciencedirect.com/science/article/abs/pii/S0009308400001845. DOI: 10.1016/S0009-3084(00)00184-5 PMID: 11106779

Mechoulam, R., & Parker, L. A. (2013). The endocannabinoid system and the brain. *Annual Review of Psychology*, *64*(1), 21–47. DOI: 10.1146/annurev-psych-113011-143739 PMID: 22804774

Meckes, K. (2025, November 24). *This is an inflection point for hemp. U.S. Hemp Roundtable.* https://hempsupporter.com/news/this-is-an-inflection-point-for-hemp/

Medical Cannabis Glossary. (n.d.) MM411. https://medicalmarijuana411.com/glossary/medical-marijuana-program-mmp/#:~:text=Definition:%20An%20official%20jurisdictional%20resource,medical%20marijuana%20(MMJ)%20card

*Medical Cannabis Insurance Coverage: Are We Getting Closer? (*2025, August 27). MedCard.com https://getmedcard.co/medical-cannabis-insurance-coverage-are-we-getting-closer/#:~:text=Key%20Takeaways,hindered%20by%20its%20federal%20status

Medicare to test coverage of medical marijuana. (n.d.). AARP. Retrieved January 6, 2026, from https://www.aarp.org/medicare/faq/does-medicare-cover-medical-marijuana/

Mee, M., Maldonado, J., Jimenez, J., Villegas, M., & Clobes, T. (2026). Dispensary budtender guidance versus clinician consensus: A comparative study of medical cannabis advice. Clinical Therapeutics. https://www.sciencedirect.com/science/article/pii/S0149291826000470

Meier, M. H., Caspi, A., Ambler, A., Harrington, H., Houts, R., Keefe, R. S. E., McDonald, K., Ward, A., Poulton, R., & Moffitt, T. E. (2012). Persistent cannabis users show neuropsychological decline from childhood to midlife. *Proceedings of the National Academy of Sciences of the United States of America, 109*(40), E2657–E2664. DOI: 10.1073/pnas.1206820109 PMID: 22927402

Meiri, D. e. (2021). Cannabis clinical trials in Israel: A regulatory and scientific overview. *The Israel Medical Association Journal.*

Melnikov, S., Aboav, A., Shalom, E., Phriedman, S., & Khalaila, K. (2021). The effect of attitudes, subjective norms, and stigma on healthcare providers' intention to recommend medicinal cannabis to patients. *International Journal of Nursing Practice, 27*(1), 1–10. DOI: 10.1111/ijn.12836 PMID: 32237017

Melnyk, B. M., & Raderstorf, T. (Eds.). (2024). *Evidence-based leadership, innovation, and entrepreneurship in nursing and healthcare: A practical guide for success* (2nd ed.). Springer Publishing Company. DOI: 10.1891/9780826160720

Mennis, J., Stahler, G. J., & Mason, M. (2016). Risky substance use environments and addiction: A new frontier for environmental justice research. *International Journal of Environmental Research and Public Health, 13*(6), 607. DOI: 10.3390/ijerph13060607 PMID: 27322303

Mercurio, A., Aston, E. R., Claborn, K. R., Waye, K., & Rosen, R. K. (2019). Marijuana as a substitute for prescription medications: A qualitative study. *Substance Use & Misuse, 54*(11), 1894–1902. DOI: 10.1080/10826084.2019.1618336 PMID: 31179810

Merlin, J. S., Merlin, J. S., Althouse, A., Feldman, R., Arnsten, J. H., Bulls, H. W., Liebschutz, J. M., Nugent, S. M., Orris, S. R., Rohac, R., Starrels, J. L., Morasco, B. J., & Kansagara, D. (2021). Analysis of state cannabis laws and dispensary staff recommendations to adults purchasing medical cannabis. *JAMA Network Open, 4*(9), e2124511. DOI: 10.1001/jamanetworkopen.2021.24511 PMID: 34524435

Metha, D. H. (2025). Cannabis education: A professional and moral obligation for physicians. *JAMA Network Open, 8*(10), e2536224. DOI: 10.1001/jamanetworkopen.2025.36224 PMID: 41055911

Mick, G., & Douek, P. (2024). Clinical benefits and safety of medical cannabis products: A narrative review on natural extracts. *Pain and Therapy, 13*(5), 1063–1094. DOI: 10.1007/s40122-024-00643-0 PMID: 39096481

Mills, J. (2003). *Cannabis Britannica: empire, trade and prohibition 1800-1928.* Oxford University Press. DOI: 10.1093/oso/9780199249381.001.0001

Mok, J., Milloy, M. J., Grant, C., Lake, S., DeBeck, K., Hayashi, K., Kerr, T., & Socías, M. E. (2023). Use of cannabis as a harm reduction strategy among people who use drugs: A cohort study. *Cannabis and Cannabinoid Research, 8*(4), 670–678. DOI: 10.1089/can.2021.0229 PMID: 35647886

Moore, E. (2024, July 2). *Connecting the dots with cannabis care.* American Nurse. https://www.myamericannurse.com/connecting-the-dots-with-cannabis-care/

Moore, E. (2024). Connecting the dots with cannabis care. *American Nurse Journal, 19*(7), 30–32. DOI: 10.51256/ANJ072430

Moritz College of Law, Ohio State University (OSU). (2025). *Federal marijuana rescheduling: Process and impact.* https://moritzlaw.osu.edu/faculty-and-research/drug-enforcement-and-policy-center/research-and-grants/policy-and-data-analyses/federal-marijuana-rescheduling

Moritz College of Law, Ohio State University. (2025). *Federal marijuana rescheduling: Process and impact.* Drug Enforcement and Policy Center. https://moritzlaw.osu.edu/faculty-and-research/drug-enforcement-and-policy-center/research-and-grants/policy-and-data-analyses/federal-marijuana-rescheduling

Moskowitz, M. H. (2017). Dispensaries. In Moskowitz, M. H. (Ed.), *Medical cannabis: A guide for patients, practitioners, and caregivers* (pp. 138–139). Koehlerbooks.

Moustaqim-Barrette, A.. (2019). Healthcare provider knowledge, attitudes, and practices related to cannabis. *Cannabis and Cannabinoid Research, 4*(3), 204–212. DOI: 10.1089/can.2018.0054 PMID: 31579835

Murray, R. M., Englund, A., Abi-Dargham, A., Lewis, D. A., Di Forti, M., Davies, C., Sherif, M., McGuire, P., & D'Souza, D. C. (2021). Cannabis-associated psychosis: Neural substrate and clinical impact. *Nature Reviews. Neuroscience, 22*(11), 691–702. DOI: 10.1038/s41583-021-00509-8

Murray, R. M., Quigley, H., Quattrone, D., Englund, A., & Di Forti, M. (2017). Traditional marijuana, high-potency cannabis, and synthetic cannabinoids: Increasing risk for psychosis. *The Lancet. Psychiatry, 4*, 643–653.

Musto, D. F. (1999). *The American disease: Origins of narcotic control* (3rd ed.). Oxford University Press. DOI: 10.1093/oso/9780195125092.001.0001

Muth, C., Blom, J. W., Smith, S. M., Johnell, K., Gonzalez-Gonzalez, A. I., Nguyen, T. S., Brueckle, M. S., Cesari, M., Tinetti, M. E., & Valderas, J. M. (2019). Evidence supporting the best clinical management of patients with multimorbidity and polypharmacy: A systematic guideline review and expert consensus. *Journal of Internal Medicine, 285*(3), 272–288. DOI: 10.1111/joim.12842 PMID: 30357955

Nabil, E. L., Metouekel, A., Serondo, H. U., El Koufi, C., El Amri, H., El Fahime, E., & El Kazzouli, S. (2024). Cannabis unveiled: From history to innovation, exploring the world of cannabis strains, chemistry, industry and economic impact. *Chemical Review and Letters, 7*(5), 827–845.

Nachnani, R., Knehans, A., Neighbors, J. D., Kocis, P. T., Lee, T., Tegeler, K., Trite, T., Raup-Konsavage, W. M., & Vrana, K. E. (2024). Systematic review of drug-drug interactions of delta-9-tetrahydrocannabinol, cannabidiol, and cannabis. *Frontiers in Pharmacology, 15*, 1282831. Advance online publication. DOI: 10.3389/fphar.2024.1282831 PMID: 38868665

Nadzam, D. M. (2009). Nurses' role in communication and patient safety. *Journal of Nursing Care Quality, 24*(3), 184–188. DOI: 10.1097/01.NCQ.0000356905.87452.62 PMID: 19525757

Narouze, S., Hakim, S. M., Kohan, L., Adams, D., & Souza, D. (2020). Medical cannabis attitudes and beliefs among pain physicians. *Regional Anesthesia and Pain Medicine*, *45*(11), 917–919. DOI: 10.1136/rapm-2020-101658 PMID: 32759172

Nasrin, S. J. W., Watson, C. X., Perez-Paramo, Y., & Lazarus, P. (2021). Cannabinoid Metabolites as Inhibitors of Major Hepatic CYP450 Enzymes, with Implications for Cannabis-Drug Interactions. *Drug Metabolism and Disposition: the Biological Fate of Chemicals*, *49*(12), 1070–1080. DOI: 10.1124/dmd.121.000442 PMID: 34493602

NASW Practice Standards & Guidelines. (2025). Socialworkers.org. https://www.socialworkers.org/Practice/NASW-Practice-Standards-Guidelines/SASW-Standards%20for%20Social-Work-Case-Management

Natale-Pereira, A., Enard, K. R., Nevarez, L., & Jones, L. A. (2011). The role of patient navigators in eliminating health disparities. *Cancer*, *117*(S15), 3543–3552. DOI: 10.1002/cncr.26264 PMID: 21780089

National Academies of Science, Engineering, and Medicine. (2017). *The health effects of cannabis and cannabinoids: The current state of evidence and recommendations for research*. National Academies Press.

National Academies of Sciences, Engineering, and Medicine, Health and Medicine Division, & Board on Population Health and Public Health Practice. (2017, January 12). *Challenges and Barriers in Conducting Cannabis Research*. Nih.gov; National Academies Press (US). https://www.ncbi.nlm.nih.gov/books/NBK425757/

National Academies of Sciences, Engineering, and Medicine. (2017). *The health effects of cannabis and cannabinoids*. https://nap.nationalacademies.org/catalog/24625/the-health-effects-of-cannabis-and-cannabinoids-current-state-of-evidence

National Academies of Sciences, Engineering, and Medicine. (2017). *The health effects of cannabis and cannabinoids: The current state of evidence and recommendations for research*. National Academies Press.

National Academies of Sciences, Engineering, and Medicine. (2017). *The health effects of cannabis and cannabinoids: The current state of evidence and recommendations for research*. National Academies Press. https://doi.org/DOI: 10.17226/24625

National Academies of Sciences, Engineering, and Medicine. (2017). *The health effects of cannabis and cannabinoids: The current state of evidence and recommendations for research*. The National Academies Press. DOI: https://doi.org/10.17226/24625

National Academies of Sciences, Engineering, and Medicine; Health and Medicine Division; Board on Population Health and Public Health Practice; Committee on the Public Health Consequences of Changes in the Cannabis Policy Landscape. (2024). *Cannabis policy impacts public health and health equity*. National Academies Press (US). https://www.ncbi.nlm.nih.gov/sites/books/NBK609489/

National Academies Press (US). (2017). Mental health. The Health Effects of Cannabis and Cannabinoids - NCBI Bookshelf. https://www.ncbi.nlm.nih.gov/books/NBK425748/

National Cancer Institute. (2025). Cannabis and cannabinoids (PDQ®)–Health professional version. https://www.cancer.gov/about-cancer/treatment/cam/hp/cannabis-pdq

National Cancer Institute. (2025). *Cannabis and cannabinoids: Health professional version.* https://www.cancer.gov/about-cancer/treatment/cam/hp/cannabis-pdq

National Cancer Institute. (n.d.). *Cannabis and cannabinoids (PDQ®)–Health professional version.* https://www.cancer.gov/about-cancer/treatment/cam/hp/cannabis-pdq

National Conference of State Legislators. (2025). *More* https://www.ncsl.org/health/state-medical-cannabis-laws

National Conference of State Legislatures. (2025). *State medical cannabis laws.* https://www.ncsl.org/health/state-medical-cannabis-laws

National Council of State Boards of Nursing. (2018). The NCSBN national nursing guidelines for medical marijuana. https://www.ncsbn.org

National Council of State Boards of Nursing. (2018). The NCSBN national nursing guidelines for medical marijuana. *Journal of Nursing Regulation*, *9*(2), 19–26. DOI: 10.1016/S2155-8256(18)30094-2

National Council of State Boards of Nursing. (2018). *The NCSBN national nursing guidelines for medical marijuana.* Journal of Nursing Regulation, 9*(2)*. DOI.https://www.ncsbn.org/marijuana-guidelines.htm10.1016/S2155-8256(18)30094-2

National Council of State Boards of Nursing. (2018). The NCSBN nursing guidelines for medical marijuana. *Journal of Nursing Regulation*, *9*(2), S2–S60.

National Council of State Boards of Nursing. (2019, Winter). *Clinical judgment measurement model. Next Generation NCLEX News*. https://www.ncsbn.org/NGN_Winter19.pdf

National Institute for Health and Care Excellence. (2019). *Cannabis-based medicinal products: NICE guideline [NG144].*

National Institute of Standards and Technology. (2025). *NIST tools for cannabis laboratory quality assurance*. https://www.nist.gov/programs-projects/nist-tools-cannabis-laboratory-quality-assurance

National Institute on Drug Abuse. (2020). *Marijuana research report.* NIH.

National Organization for the Reform of Marijuana Laws. (2025, August 14). *A brief history of cannabis rescheduling petitions in the United States.* https://norml.org/news/2025/08/14/trump-says-cannabis-rescheduling-decision-is-forthcoming/

National Organization for the Reform of Marijuana Laws. (2025, December 18). *President Trump takes executive action to federally reschedule marijuana.* https://norml.org/blog/2025/12/18/president-trump-takes-executive-action-to-federally-reschedule-marijuana/

Navarrete, F., Salud García-Gutiérrez, M., Gasparyan, A., Austrich-Olivares, A., Femenía, T., & Manzanares, J. (2020). Cannabis Use in Pregnant and Breastfeeding Women: Behavioral and Neurobiological Consequences. *Frontiers in Psychiatry*, *11*, 586447. DOI: 10.3389/fpsyt.2020.586447 PMID: 33240134

Nayak, M. M., Revette, A., Chai, P. R., Lansang, K., Sannes, T., Tung, S., & Braun, I. M. (2022). Medical cannabis-related stigma: Cancer survivors' perspectives. *Journal of Cancer Survivorship: Research and Practice*, *17*(3), 951–956. DOI: 10.1007/s11764-022-01297-7 PMID: 36435953

NCLEX. (n.d.). Clinical Judgment Measurement Model: A framework to measure clinical judgment & decision making. https://www.nclex.com/clinical-judgment-measurement-model.page

NCSBN. (2018). The NCSBN National Nursing Guidelines for Medical Marijuana. *Journal of Nursing Regulation: Advancing Nursing Excellence for Public Protection*, S 3-S 58.

NCSBN. (2018, July). The NCSBN national nursing guidelines for medical marijuana. *Journal of Nursing Regulation: Advancing nursing excellence for public protection, 9*(2), S1-S60.

NCSBN. (2026). *Global regulatory atlas*. Retrieved January 20, 2026, from NCSBN Leading Regulatory Excellence: https://www.regulatoryatlas.com/

New marijuana laws have companies questioning current drug testing policies. (n.d.). Reference Services. Retrieved January 6, 2026, from https://www.referenceservices.com/new-marijuana-laws-have-companies-questioning-current-drug-testing-policies/

New York City Council passes trailblazing bill to ban all preemployment marijuana testing. (2019). Genova Burns LLC. https://www.genovaburns.com/news/labor-law/2019-04-16-new-york-city-council-passes-trailblazing-bill-to-ban-all-preemployment-marijuana-testing

Newell, S., & Jordan, Z. (2015). The patient experience of patient-centered communication with nurses in the hospital setting: A qualitative systematic review protocol. *JBI Evidence Synthesis*, *13*(1), 76–87. DOI: 10.11124/jbisrir-2015-1072 PMID: 26447009

Nisbet, L. A., DiEmma, G. E., & Scott, K. S. (2023). Drug stability in forensic toxicology. *Wiley Interdisciplinary Reviews: Forensic Science*, *5*(4), e1481.

NMC. (2025). *Test of Competence*. Retrieved December 15, 2025, from Nursing & Midwifery Council: https://www.nmc.org.uk/registration/joining-the-register/toc/

Noble, M. J., Hedberg, K., & Hendrickson, R. G. (2019). Acute cannabis toxicity. *Clinical Toxicology*, *57*(8), 735–742. DOI: 10.1080/15563650.2018.1548708 PMID: 30676820

Ntais, C., Kontodimopoulos, N., & Melanthiou, Y. (2025). Marketing management and policymaking for medical cannabis: Overcoming barriers and shaping strategies. *Cannabis (Research Society on Marijuana).* Advance online publication. DOI: 10.26828/cannabis/2025/000316 PMID: 40909146

Nyblade, L., Stockton, M. A., Giger, K., Bond, V., Ekstrand, M. L., Lean, R. M., Mitchell, E. M., Nelson, L. R. E., Sapag, J. C., Siraprapasiri, T., Turan, J., & Wouters, E. (2019). Stigma in health facilities: Why it matters and how we can change it. *BMC Medicine*, *17*(1), 25. DOI: 10.1186/s12916-019-1256-2 PMID: 30764806

O'Brien, K., Beilby, J., Frans, M., Lynskey, M., Barnes, M., Jayasuriya, M., Athanasiou-Fragkouli, A., Blair, P., & Nutt, D. (2023). Medicinal cannabis for pain: Real-world data on three-month changes in symptoms and quality of life. *Drug Science, Policy and Law*, *9*, 20503245231172535. DOI: 10.1177/20503245231172535

Odom-Maryon, T. B., Bailey, L. A., & Amiri, S. (2018). The influences of nursing school characteristics on NCLEX-RN pass rates: A national study. *Journal of Nursing Regulation*, *9*(3), 59–69. DOI: 10.1016/S2155-8256(18)30154-6

Oermann, M. H., & Gaberson, K. B. (2024). *Evaluation and testing in nursing education.* Springer Publishing. https://connect.springerpub.com/content/book/978-0-8261-9489-3

O'Leary-Randall, A. (2014). *Medical marijuana in America: Memoir of a Pioneer.*

Olfson, M., Wall, M., Liu, S.-M., Schoenbaum, M., & Blanco, C. (2018). Declining health-related quality of life in the United States. *American Journal of Preventive Medicine, 54*(3), 325–333. DOI: 10.1016/j.amepre.2017.11.012 PMID: 29338955

Olson, R. E., Smith, A., Huggett, G., Good, P., Dudley, M., & Hardy, J. (2022). Using a qualitative sub-study to inform the design and delivery of randomised controlled trials on medicinal cannabis for symptom relief in patients with advanced cancer. *Trials, 23*(1), 752. DOI: 10.1186/s13063-022-06691-1 PMID: 36064621

Order, E. Increasing medical marijuana and cannabidiol research. (2025, December 18). The White House. https://www.whitehouse.gov/presidential-actions/2025/12/increasing-medical-marijuana-and-cannabidiol-research/

Orenstein, D. G., & Glantz, S. A. (2020). Cannabis legalization in state legislatures: Public health opportunity and risk. *Marquette Law Review, 103*(4), 1313–1340. PMID: 34376874

Organization of Nurse Executives and American Organization for Nursing Leadership. (2022). AONL Nurse Leader Core Competencies, Chicago, IL; AONE, AONL.

Oz, M. (2017, September 15). Cannabis as an exit drug strategy. *Fox and Friends* . New York, NY.

Pacher, P., & Kunos, G. (2013). Modulating the endocannabinoid system in human health and disease: Successes and failures. *The FEBS Journal, 280*(9), 1918–1943. DOI: 10.1111/febs.12260 PMID: 23551849

Pacula, R. L., & Smart, R. (2017). Medical marijuana and marijuana legalization. *Annual Review of Clinical Psychology, 13*(1), 397–419. DOI: 10.1146/annurev-clinpsy-032816-045128 PMID: 28482686

Paiva, C., Santos, T., Cunha-Oliveira, A., Rosendo, I., & Pita, J. R. (2024). Knowledge, opinions and experiences of nurses and nursing students in Portugal regarding the use of medical cannabis. *BMC Nursing, 23*(1), 788. Advance online publication. DOI: 10.1186/s12912-024-02443-5 PMID: 39468501

Papanagnou, D., Klein, M. R., Zhang, X. C., Cameron, K. A., Doty, A., McCarthy, D. M., Rising, K. L., & Salzman, D. H. (2021). Developing standardized patient-based cases for communication training: Lessons learned from training residents to communicate diagnostic uncertainty. *Advances in Simulation (London, England), 6*(1), 26.https://doi.org/10.1186/s41077-021-00176-y

Parmalee, R. A., & Clark, C. S. (2022). Nursing students' knowledge, skills, and attitudes regarding medical cannabis care: A national study. *Journal of Nursing Regulation, 13*(3), 13–23.https://doi.org/10.1016/S2155-8256(22)00082-5

Parmelee, R. (2025). Nurse educators' experiences with medical cannabis education (Doctoral dissertation, Walden University). Walden University ScholarWorks. https://scholarworks.waldenu.edu/dissertations/17290/

Parmelee, R. (2025). Nurse educators' experiences with medical cannabis education. Walden University, College of Nursing. Walden University., Retrieved December 15, 2025, from.

Parmelee, R. A. (2025). *Nurse Educators' Experiences With Medical Cannabis Education* (Doctoral dissertation, Walden University).

Parmelee, R. A. (2025). *Nurse educators' experiences with medical cannabis education* (Doctoral dissertation, Walden University). Walden University ScholarWorks. https://scholarworks.waldenu.edu/cgi/viewcontent.cgi?article=18960&context=dissertations

Parmelee, R. A., & Clark, C. S. (2022). Nursing students knowledge, skills, and attitudes regarding medicinal cannabis care. *Journal of Nursing Regulation*, *13*(3), 13–23. DOI: 10.1016/S2155-8256(22)00082-5

Partridge, C. (2024). *Cannabis, sacred and profane*. Bloomsbury Academic. DOI: 10.5040/9781350116238

Patel, D. (2022). Cannabis use disorder. In Avery, J. D., & Hankins, D. (Eds.), *Addiction medicine: A case and evidence-based guide*., DOI: 10.1007/978-3-030-86430-9_4

Paulraj, S., Upreti, P., Tamirisa, K., & Batnyam, U. (2025). Arrhythmias and cannabis use: A comprehensive overview. *Heart Rhythm O2*, *6*(1), 78–85. DOI: 10.1016/j.hroo.2024.10.020 PMID: 40224259

Pergam, S. A., Woodfield, M. C., Lee, C. M., Cheng, G. S., Baker, K. K., Marquis, S. R., & Fann, J. R. (2017). Cannabis use among patients at a comprehensive cancer center in a state with legalized medicinal and recreational use. *Cancer*, *123*(22), 4488–4497. DOI: 10.1002/cncr.30879 PMID: 28944449

Perisetti, A., Gajendran, M., Shekhar Dasari, C., Bansal, P., Aziz, M., Inamdar, S., Tharian, B., & Goyal, H. (2020). Cannabis hyperemesis syndrome: An update on the pathophysiology and management. *Annals of Gastroenterology*, *33*(6), 571–578. DOI: 10.20524/aog.2020.0528 PMID: 33162734

Perlman, A. I., McLeod, H. M., Ventresca, E. C., Salinas, M. G., Post, P. J., Schuh, M. J., & Abu Dabrh, A. M. (2021). Medical cannabis state and federal regulations: Implications for United States health care entities. *Mayo Clinic Proceedings*, *96*(10), 2671–2681. DOI: 10.1016/j.mayocp.2021.05.005 PMID: 34607636

Perlman, A. I., McLeod, H. M., Ventresca, E. C., Salinas, M. G., Post, P. J., Schuh, M. J., & Dabrah, A. M. A. (2021). Medical Cannabis State and Federal Regulations: Implications for United States Health Care Entities. *Mayo Clinic Proceedings*, *96*(10), 2671–2681. https://doi.org/10.1016/j.mayocp.2021.05.005

Pertwee, R. G. (2007). The diverse CB1 and CB2 receptor pharmacology of three plant cannabinoids: Δ9-tetrahydrocannabinol, cannabidiol, and Δ9-tetrahydrocannabivarin. *British Journal of Pharmacology*, *153*(2), 199–215. https://www.ncbi.nlm.nih.gov/pmc/articles/PMC2219532/. DOI: 10.1038/sj.bjp.0707442 PMID: 17828291

Pertwee, R. G. (2015). Endocannabinoids and their pharmacological actions. *Handbook of Experimental Pharmacology*, *231*, 1–37. DOI: 10.1007/978-3-319-20825-1_1 PMID: 26408156

Pertwee, R. G., Howlett, A. C., Abood, M. E., Alexander, S. P. H., Di Marzo, V., Elphick, M. R., Greasley, P. J., Hansen, H. S., Kunos, G., Mackie, K., Mechoulam, R., & Ross, R. A. (2010). Cannabinoid receptors and their ligands: Beyond CB1 and CB2. *Pharmacological Reviews*, *62*(4), 588–631. DOI: 10.1124/pr.110.003004 PMID: 21079038

Pew Center for Research. (2024). *Most Americans now live in a legal marijuana state – and most have at least one dispensary in their county.* https://www.pewresearch.org/short-reads/2024/02/29/most-americans-now-live-in-a-legal-marijuana-state-and-most-have-at-least-one-dispensary-in-their-county/

Philpot, L. M., Ebbert, J. O., & Hurt, R. T. (2019). A survey of the attitudes, beliefs, and knowledge about medical cannabis among primary care providers. *BMC Family Practice*, *20*(1), 17. DOI: 10.1186/s12875-019-0906-y PMID: 30669979

Physicians' Guide to Ryan's Law. (2021). *Americans for Safe Access.* https://d3n8a8pro7vhmx.cloudfront.net/americansforsafeaccess/pages/17096/attachments/original/1640099846/Physician's_Guide_to_Ryan's_Law.pdf?1640099846

Physicians, medical marijuana, and the law. (2014). *AMA Journal of Ethics, 16*(9), 732–738. https://doi.org/10.1001/virtualmentor.2014.16.9.hlaw1-1409

Pichette, N. (2024). *Provider review: Evaluating individual criteria to support cannabis use disorder* (Publication No. 1816) [Doctoral dissertation, Salve Regina University]. Sigma Repository. https://www.sigmarepository.org/dissertations/1816

Pichette, N., O'Sullivan, D., Caruso, A., Blair, E., & Pearlson, G. (2025, November 13). *Exploring cannabis patient care: Institute of Living staff experience and knowledge* [Poster presentation]. Trinity Health of New England Annual Research Day, Hartford, CT, United States. https://www.trinityhealthofne.org/sites/default/files/Education%20and%20Research/Research%20Day%202025/34-Exploring-Cannabis-Patient_Care.pdf

Piontek, D., Kraus, L., & Klempova, D. (2008). Short scales to assess cannabis-related problems: A review of psychometric properties. *Substance Abuse Treatment, Prevention, and Policy*, *3*(1), 25. DOI: 10.1186/1747-597X-3-25 PMID: 19055741

Pisanti, S., Malfitano, A. M., Ciaglia, E., Lamberti, A., Ranieri, R., Cuomo, G., Abate, M., Faggiana, G., Proto, M. C., Fiore, D., Laezza, C., & Bifulco, M. (2017). Cannabidiol: State of the art and new challenges for therapeutic applications. *Pharmacology & Therapeutics*, *175*, 133–150. DOI: 10.1016/j.pharmthera.2017.02.041 PMID: 28232276

Porter, J. (2016, November 16). Cannabis and the mission of higher education. *Inside Higher Ed*. https://www.insidehighered.com/views/2016/11/17/dangers-students-regular-marijuana-use-essay

Pravosud, V., Lum, E., Vali, M., Cohen, B. E., Hoggatt, K. J., Byers, A. L., Austin, P. C., Walter, L. C., Hasin, D., Zaman, T., & Keyhani, S. (2025). Cannabis use among older adults. *JAMA Network Open*, *8*(5), e2510173. DOI: 10.1001/jamanetworkopen.2025.10173 PMID: 40366653

Prieto González, J. M., & Vila Silván, C. (2021a). Safety and tolerability of nabiximols oromucosal spray: A review of more than 15 years of accumulated evidence from clinical trials. *Expert Review of Neurotherapeutics*, *21*(7), 755–778. DOI: 10.1080/14737175.2021.1935879 PMID: 34092180

Prieto González, J. M., & Vila Silván, C. (2021b). Safety and tolerability of nabiximols oromucosal spray: A review of real-world experience in observational studies, registries, and case reports. *Expert Review of Neurotherapeutics*, *21*(5), 547–558. DOI: 10.1080/14737175.2021.1904896 PMID: 33749480

Prompahakul, C., Keim-Malpass, J., LeBaron, V., Yan, G., & Epstein, E. G. (2021). Moral distress among nurses: A mixed-methods study. *Nursing Ethics*, *28*(7-8), 1165–1182. DOI: 10.1177/0969733021996028 PMID: 33888021

Pruitt, Z., & Sportsman, S. (2013). The presence and roles of nurse navigators in acute care hospitals. *The Journal of Nursing Administration*, *43*(11), 592–596. DOI: 10.1097/01.NNA.0000434510.74373.40 PMID: 24153201

Pursio, K., Kankkunen, P., Sanner-Stiehr, E., & Kvist, T. (2021). Professional autonomy in nursing: An integrative review. *Journal of Nursing Management*, *29*(6), 1565–1577. DOI: 10.1111/jonm.13282 PMID: 33548098

Putra, A. D. M., & Sandhi, A. (2021). Implementation of nursing case management to improve community access to care: A scoping review. *Belitung Nursing Journal*, *7*(3), 141–150. https://doi.org/10.33546/bnj.1449

QSEN Institute. (2020). *Quality and safety education for nurses: Competencies*. Retrieved January 30, 2026, from Quality and Safety Education for Nurses: https://www.qsen.org/competencies-pre-licensure-ksas

Rabinak, C. A., & Phan, K. L. (2014). Cannabinoid modulation of fear extinction brain circuits: A novel target to advance anxiety treatment. *Current Pharmaceutical Design*, *20*(13), 2212–2217. DOI: 10.2174/13816128113199990437 PMID: 23829364

Ramaekers, J. G., Kauert, G., van Ruitenbeek, P., Theunissen, E. L., Schneider, E., & Moeller, M. R. (2006). High-potency marijuana impairs executive function and inhibitory motor control. *Neuropsychopharmacology : Official Publication of the American College of Neuropsychopharmacology*, *31*(10), 2296–2303. DOI: 10.1038/sj.npp.1301068 PMID: 16572123

Ramaekers, J. G., Vinckenbosch, F., & Gilman, J. M. (2023). High traffic—The quest for a reliable test of cannabis impairment. *JAMA Psychiatry*, *80*(9), 871–872. https://doi.org/10.1001/jamapsychiatry.2023.2309

Rami, F., Thompson, L., & Solis-Cortes, L. (2023). Healthcare disparities: Vulnerable and marginalized populations. In Searight, H. R. (Ed.), *COVID-19: Health disparities and ethical challenges across the globe*. Springer International Publishing., DOI: 10.1007/978-3-031-26200-5_6

Reddy, T. S., Zomer, R., & Mantri, N. (2023). Nanoformulations as a strategy to overcome the delivery limitations of cannabinoids. *Phytotherapy Research*, *37*(4), 1526–1538. DOI: 10.1002/ptr.7742 PMID: 36748949

Reece, A. S. (2009). Chronic toxicology of cannabis. *Clinical Toxicology*, *47*(6), 517–524. DOI: 10.1080/15563650903074507 PMID: 19586351

Reed, M., McCartney, D., & Guttmannova, K. (2020). Marijuana sources in a medical marijuana environment: Dynamics in access and use among a cohort of young adults in Los Angeles, California. *Drugs: Education Prevention & Policy*, *27*(1), 69–78. DOI: 10.1080/09687637.2018.1557595 PMID: 31949332

Rehman, A., Naz, Z., Ali, A., Naz, F., & Siddique, F. (2025). Meta-analysis of nurse-led interventions on medication adherence and clinical outcomes in patients with chronic illnesses. *Insights: Journal of Health and Rehabilitation, 3*(10), 38–47. DOI: 10.71000/w46qy993

Reimann-Philipp, U., Speck, M., Orser, C., Johnson, S., Hilyard, A., Turner, H., Stokes, A. J., & Small-Howard, A. L. (2019). Cannabis chemovar nomenclature misrepresents chemical and genetic diversity: Survey of variations in chemical profiles and genetic markers in Nevada medical cannabis samples. *Cannabis and Cannabinoid Research, 5*(3), 215–230. DOI: 10.1089/can.2018.0063 PMID: 32923659

Respiratory Therapy. (2025). Chronic pain patients stop medical cannabis within 1 year | RT. https://respiratory-therapy.com/public-health/healthcare-policy/general-healthcare/chronic-pain-medical-cannabis/

Reverby, S. M. (1987). *Ordered to care: The dilemma of American nursing, 1850-1945.* Cambridge University Press.

Riba, J., Valle, M., Sampedro, F., Rodríguez-Pujadas, A., Martínez-Horta, S., Kulisevsky, J., & Rodríguez-Fornells, A. (2015). Telling true from false: Cannabis users show increased susceptibility to false memories. *Molecular Psychiatry, 20*(6), 772–777. DOI: 10.1038/mp.2015.36 PMID: 25824306

Rice, J., Hildebrand, A., Waslo, C. S., Cameron, M. H., & Jones, K. D. (2022). Cannabis for medical purposes: A cross-sectional analysis of health care professionals' knowledge. *Journal of the American Association of Nurse Practitioners, 34*(1), 100–106. DOI: 10.1097/JXX.0000000000000590 PMID: 33767121

Rice, L. J., Cannon, L., Dadlani, N., Cheung, M. M. Y., Einfeld, S. L., Efron, D., Dossetor, D. R., & Elliott, E. J. (2024). Efficacy of cannabinoids in neurodevelopmental and neuropsychiatric disorders among children and adolescents: A systematic review. *European Child & Adolescent Psychiatry, 33*(2), 505–526. DOI: 10.1007/s00787-023-02169-w PMID: 36864363

Rimmelzwaan, L. M., Bogerd, M. J. L., Schumacher, B. M. A., Slottje, P., van Hout, H. P. J., & Reinders, M. E. (2020). Multimorbidity in general practice: Unmet care needs from a patient perspective. *Frontiers in Medicine, 7*, 530085. Advance online publication. DOI: 10.3389/fmed.2020.530085 PMID: 33415113

Roberts, B. (2019). Legalized Cannabis in Colorado Emergency Departments: A Cautionary Review of Negative Health and Safety Effects. *The Western Journal of Emergency Medicine, 20*(4), 557–572. DOI: 10.5811/westjem.2019.4.39935 PMID: 31316694

Rogers, M., Stephenson, J., Ali, G., Andrews, C., Curran, S., Gulliksen, E., Kra-Friedman, A., Ali, N., Lamarche, K., Niu, Y., Slater, H., & Pike, J. (2025). Advanced practice nurse perceptions of spirituality: A global quantitative perspective in everyday life and practice settings. *Journal of Holistic Nursing*, 08980101251377815. Advance online publication. DOI: 10.1177/08980101251377815 PMID: 41148204

Romero, D., Mendez, D., Fowler, L. A., Morales, J., & Glantz, S. A. (2025). Medical cannabis utilization across U.S. states with varying legal status. *Preventive Medicine Reports, 39*, 102582. Advance online publication. DOI: 10.1016/j.pmedr.2025.102582

Ronne, S. T., Rosenbaek, F., Pedersen, L. B., Waldorff, F. B., Nielsen, J. B., Riisgaard, H., & Søndergaard, J. (2021). Physicians' experiences, attitudes, and beliefs toward medical cannabis: A systematic literature review. *BMC Family Practice*, *22*(1), 212. Advance online publication. DOI: 10.1186/s12875-021-01559-w PMID: 34674661

Roten, A., Baker, N. L., & Gray, K. M. (2015). Cognitive performance in a placebo-controlled pharmacotherapy trial for youth with marijuana dependence. *Addictive Behaviors*, *45*, 119–123. DOI: 10.1016/j.addbeh.2015.01.013 PMID: 25661990

Ruheel, M. A., Gomes, Z., Usman, S., Homayouni, P., & Ng, J. Y. (2021). Facilitators and barriers to the regulation of medical cannabis: A scoping review of the peer-reviewed literature. *Harm Reduction Journal*, *18*(1), 106. DOI: 10.1186/s12954-021-00547-8 PMID: 34649577

Ruksakulpiwat, S., Pongsuwun, K., Junphongsri, P., Preeprem, C., Nguantad, S., & Samart, B. (2025). Nurse-led interventions to improve health, adherence, and functional outcomes in adults and older adults with multimorbidity: A systematic review of randomized and quasiexperimental studies. *Journal of Nursing Management*, *2025*(1), 6252049. Advance online publication. DOI: 10.1155/jonm/6252049 PMID: 41019866

Russell, K., Cahill, M., Gowen, K., Cronquist, R., Smith, V., Borris-Hale, C., Fischer, H., Heywood, D., Johnston, J., & Sutton-Johnson, S. (2018). The National Council of State Boards of Nursing national nursing guidelines for medical marijuana. *Journal of Nursing Regulation*, *9*(2), S1–S60. https://www.ncsbn.org/public-files/The_NCSBN_National_Nursing_Guidelines_for_Medical_Marijuana_JNR_July_2018.pdf

Russo, E. (2025, October 9). Critical gaps in cannabis and endocannabinoid system education. *Deficiencies in medical training and necessary curriculm reform for future clinicians*. USA.

Russo, E. B. (2007). History of cannabis and its preparations in saga, science, and sobriquet. *Chemistry & Biodiversity*, *4*(8), 1614–1648. DOI: 10.1002/cbdv.200790144 PMID: 17712811

Russo, E. B. (2011). Taming THC: Potential cannabis synergy and phytocannabinoid–terpenoid entourage effects. *British Journal of Pharmacology*, *163*(7), 1344–1364. DOI: 10.1111/j.1476-5381.2011.01238.x PMID: 21749363

Russo, E. B. (2016). *Cannabis and Cannabinoids: Pharmacology, Toxicology, and Therapeutic Potential*. Routledge.

Russo, E. B. (2016). Clinical endocannabinoid deficiency reconsidered: Current research supports the theory in migraine, fibromyalgia, irritable bowel, and other treatment-resistant syndromes. *Cannabis and Cannabinoid Research*, *1*(1), 154–165. DOI: 10.1089/can.2016.0009 PMID: 28861491

Russo, E. B. (2017). History of cannabis as medicine: Nineteenth-century Irish physicians and correlations of their observations to modern research. In Collen, L., & Robson, P. (Eds.), *Cannabinoids in neurologic and mental disease* (pp. 3–20). Academic Press.

Russo, E. B. (2018). Cannabis therapeutics and the future of neurology. *Frontiers in Integrative Neuroscience*, *12*, 51. DOI: 10.3389/fnint.2018.00051 PMID: 30405366

Russo, E. B. (2019). The case for the entourage effect and conventional breeding of clinical cannabis: No "strain," no gain. *Frontiers in Plant Science*, *9*, 1969. DOI: 10.3389/fpls.2018.01969 PMID: 30687364

Russo, E. B., & Marcu, J. (2017). Cannabis pharmacology: The usual suspects and a few promising leads. *Advances in Pharmacology*, *80*, 67–134. DOI: 10.1016/bs.apha.2017.03.004 PMID: 28826544

Russo, E. B., Spooner, C., May, L., Leslie, R., & Whiteley, V. L. (2022). Cannabinoid hyperemesis syndrome survey and genomic investigation. *Cannabis and Cannabinoid Research*, *7*(3), 336–344. DOI: 10.1089/can.2021.0046 PMID: 34227878

Ryan's Law Foundation. (n.d.). Retrieved January 6, 2026, from https://ryanslawfoundation.org/

Ryan, J. E., McCabe, S. E., & Boyd, C. J. (2021). Medicinal Cannabis: Policy, patients, and providers. *Policy, Politics & Nursing Practice*, *22*(2), 126.https://doi.org/10.1177/1527154421989609

Ryan, J. E., McCabe, S. E., & Boyd, C. J. (2021). Medicinal cannabis: Policy, patients, and providers. *Policy, Politics & Nursing Practice*, *22*(2), 126–133. DOI: 10.1177/1527154421989609 PMID: 33567970

Ryan, J., & Sharts-Hopko, N. (2017). The experiences of medical marijuana patients: A scoping review of the qualitative literature. *The Journal of Neuroscience Nursing : Journal of the American Association of Neuroscience Nurses*, *49*(3), 185–190.https://doi.org/10.1097/JNN.0000000000000283

Sacco, L. N. (2024, July 23). Rescheduling Marijuana: Implications for Criminal and Collateral Consequences. *In Focus.* https://www.congress.gov/crs-product/IF12715#:~:text=If%20marijuana%20is%20rescheduled%20to,costs%20of%20selling%20their%20product.&text=As%20with%20other%20controlled%20substances,alcohol%20by%20students%20and%20employees

Sackett, D. L., Rosenberg, W. M. C., Gray, J. A. M., Haynes, R. B., & Richardson, W. S. (1996). Evidence-based medicine: What it is and what it isn't. *BMJ (Clinical Research Ed.)*, *312*(7023), 71–72. DOI: 10.1136/bmj.312.7023.71 PMID: 8555924

Salter, A. R., Cutter, G. R., Tyry, T., Marrie, R. A., & Fox, R. J. (2022). Sources of cannabis information and medical guidance among people with multiple sclerosis. *Neurology. Clinical Practice*, *12*(1), 52–60. DOI: 10.1212/CPJ.0000000000001081 PMID: 35733947

Samuel, A., O'Brien, J., & Pontious, A. (2025). Lawmakers Introduce Bill to Regulate Hemp Products Ahead of an Impending Ban. Husch Blackwell Cannabis Law Now.https://www.cannabislawnow.com/2025/12/lawmakers-introduce-bill-to-regulate-hemp-products-ahead-of-an-impending-ban/?utm_source=Husch+Blackwell+-+Cannabis+Law+Now&utm_campaign=99e716313a-RSS_EMAIL_CAMPAIGN&utm_medium=email&utm_term=0_6a9bb772e1-99e716313a-73179189

Sarathy, L., Chou, J. H., Lerou, P. H., Terplan, M., Mark, K., Dorfman, S., Wilens, T. E., Bernstein, S. N., & Schiff, D. M. (2023). Limited utility of toxicology testing at delivery for perinatal cannabis use. *Hospital Pediatrics*, *13*(4), 317–325. DOI: 10.1542/hpeds.2022-006897 PMID: 36855896

Saudi Commission for Health Specialties. (2022). *Saudi Nursing Licensing Exam.* Specialties, Saudi Commission for Health. Saudi Arabia: SCFHS. https://scfhs.org.sa/sites/default/files/2022-06/SNLE%20Applicant%20Guide%20-%20March%202022.pdf

Schauer, G. L. (2021). Cannabis policy in the United States: Implications for public health. *Journal of the National Cancer Institute. Monographs, 2021*(58), 39–52. DOI: 10.1093/jncimonographs/lgab016 PMID: 34850901

Schauer, G. L. (2024). Improving cannabis policy research at a pivotal time for policy development. *American Journal of Public Health, 114*(S8, Suppl. 8), S635–S638. DOI: 10.2105/AJPH.2024.307799 PMID: 39442025

Schauer, G. L., Njai, R., & Grant, A. M. (2021). Clinician beliefs and practices related to cannabis. *Cannabis and Cannabinoid Research, 7*(4), 508–515. DOI: 10.1089/can.2020.0165 PMID: 33998899

Schep, L. J., Slaughter, R. J., Glue, P., & Gee, P. (2020). The clinical toxicology of cannabis. *The New Zealand Medical Journal (Online), 133*(1523), 96–103. PMID: 33032307

Schermele, Z. (2025, November 11). *Inside the details of the shutdown deal, from new cannabis rules to a Jack Smith jab.* USA TODAY. Retrieved January 6, 2026, from https://www.usatoday.com/story/news/politics/2025/11/11/inside-shutdown-deal-cannabis-charlie-kirk-jack-smith/87214014007/

Schlag, A. K., Zafar, R. R., Lynskey, M. T., Athanasiou-Fragkouli, A., Phillips, L. D., & Nutt, D. J. (2022). The value of real-world evidence: The case of medical cannabis. *Frontiers in Psychiatry, 13*, 1027159. Advance online publication. DOI: 10.3389/fpsyt.2022.1027159 PMID: 36405915

Schmid, S., Lapaire, O., Huang, D., Jürgens, F., & Güth, U. (2018). Cannabinoid hyperemesis syndrome: An underreported entity causing nausea and vomiting of pregnancy. *Archives of Gynecology and Obstetrics, 284*(5), 1095–1097. DOI: 10.1007/s00404-010-1811-8 PMID: 21170540

Schuster, R. M., Gilman, J., Schoenfeld, D., Evenden, J., Hareli, M., Ulysse, C., Nip, E., Hanly, A., Zhang, H., & Evins, A. E. (2018). One month of cannabis abstinence in adolescents and young adults is associated with improved memory. *The Journal of Clinical Psychiatry, 79*(6), 18m12138.

Schuster, R. M., Mermelstein, R., & Gonzalez, R. (2022). Early onset of cannabis use is associated with greater risk of cannabis use disorder in adulthood. *Drug and Alcohol Dependence, 231*, 109245. Advance online publication. DOI: 10.1016/j.drugalcdep.2021.109245

Schweiger, V., Ganz, B., Martini, A., Sarzi-Puttini, P., Bazzichi, L., Bonora, E., Vendramin, P., Nizzero, M., Zamboni, L., Polati, L., Lugoboni, F., Raniero, D., Polati, E., & Del Balzo, G. (2025). Medical cannabis for chronic pain management: Questions and answers between clinical and medico-legal issues. *Clinical and Experimental Rheumatology*. Advance online publication. DOI: 10.55563/clinexprheumatol/o23y55 PMID: 40556619

Sellman, D. (2024). Virtue ethics and nursing practice. In *Key Concepts and Issues in Nursing Ethics* (pp. 135–146). Springer Nature Switzerland. DOI: 10.1007/978-3-031-54108-7_9

Senge, P. M. (2006). *The fifth discipline: The art and practice of learning the organization.* (Rev., Ed.) Doubleday.

Shannon, S., Lewis, N., Lee, H., & Hughes, S. (2019). Cannabidiol in anxiety and sleep: A large case series. *The Permanente Journal, 23*(1), 18–041. DOI: 10.7812/TPP/18-041 PMID: 30624194

Sharma, P., Murthy, P., & Bharath, M. M. (2012, Fall). Chemistry, metabolism, and toxicology of cannabis: Clinical implications. *Iranian Journal of Psychiatry*, *7*(4), 149–156. PMID: 23408483

Sharma, P., Rao, V., Kumar Chand, P., & Murthy, P. (2023). Quantification of Δ9-tetrahydrocannabinol in urine as a marker of cannabis abuse. *The Indian Journal of Medical Research*, *158*(5-6), 535–541. DOI: 10.4103/ijmr.IJMR_3899_20 PMID: 37929356

Shepherd, J. M. (2024). Advancing nursing practice through artificial intelligence: Unlocking its transformative impact. *Online Journal of Issues in Nursing*, *29*(1). Advance online publication. DOI: 10.3912/OJIN.Vol29No01PPT77

Sherman, R. O. (2010). Growing future nurse leaders to build and sustain health work environments. *Nursing Administration Quarterly*, *34*(4), 346–358. PMID: 20838181

Shirey, M. R. (2013). Lewin's theory of planned change as a strategic resource. *The Journal of Nursing Administration*, *43*(2), 69–72. DOI: 10.1097/NNA.0b013e31827f20a9 PMID: 23343723

Shover, C. L., & Humphreys, K. (2019). Six policy lessons relevant to cannabis legalization. *The American Journal of Drug and Alcohol Abuse*, *45*(6), 698–706. DOI: 10.1080/00952990.2019.1569669 PMID: 30870053

Siani-Rose, M., Cox, S., Goldstein, B., Abrams, D., Taylor, M., & Kurek, I. (2023). Cannabis-responsive biomarkers: A pharmacometabolomics-based application to evaluate the impact of medical cannabis treatment on children with autism spectrum disorder. *Cannabis and Cannabinoid Research*, *8*(1), 126–137. DOI: 10.1089/can.2021.0129 PMID: 34874191

Sinclair, J., Parker, M., & Armour, M. (2024). Cultivating understanding: Navigating the complexities associated with medicinal cannabis and implications for nursing practice. *The Australian Journal of Advanced Nursing*, *41*(3), 1–5.

Sitzman, K., & Watson, J. (2018). *Caring science, mindful practice: Implementing Watson's human caring theory* (2nd ed.). Springer Publishing Company. DOI: 10.1891/9780826135568

Skalisky, J., Leickly, E., Oluwoye, O., & McPherson, M. (2017). *S., Srebnik, D., M. Roll, J., K. Ries, R., & G. McDonell, M.* Prevalence and Correlates of Cannabis Use in Outpatients with Serious Mental Illness Receiving Treatment for Alcohol Use Disorders.

Sliwoski, V. (2025). *Notes on the federal prohibition of intoxicating hemp*. Harris Sliwoski LLP. https://harris-sliwoski.com/cannalawblog/notes-on-the-federal-prohibition-of-intoxicating-hemp/

Sloman, L. (1998). *Reefer Madness: A history of marijuana* (3rd ed.). St. Martin's Press.

Smart, R., & Pacula, R. L. (2019). Early evidence of the impact of cannabis legalization on cannabis use, cannabis use disorder, and the use of other substances: Findings from state policy evaluations. *The American Journal of Drug and Alcohol Abuse*, *45*(6), 644–663. DOI: 10.1080/00952990.2019.1669626 PMID: 31603710

Sobel, K. (2023). *Testimony of Ken Sobel, Esq. Exhibit SHHS1069AC submitted to the Nevada Senate Committee on Health and Human Services, 82nd Nevada Legislative Session*. Nevada Legislature. https://archive.leg.state.nv.us/Session/82nd2023/Exhibits/Senate/HHS/SHHS1069AC.pdf

Sommers, D. M. (2023). Cannabis nursing scope and standards of practice: Panel Presentation. *ACNA National Conference* May 20-22, 2023 Denver, Colorado, (pp. 1-21). Denver.

Sorkhou, M., Bedder, R. H., & George, T. P. (2021). The behavioural sequelae of cannabis use in healthy people: A systematic review. *Frontiers in Psychiatry, 12*, 630247. DOI: 10.3389/fpsyt.2021.630247 PMID: 33664685

South, A. M., Babalonis, S. L., Fanucchi, L. C., & Lofwall, M. R. (2025). "Medical Cannabis": Advising patients while navigating medical ethics and limited evidence. *Journal of General Internal Medicine, 1-5*. Advance online publication. DOI: 10.1007/s11606-025-09680-7 PMID: 40624323

Spears, L. (2010). Character and servant leadership: Ten characteristics of effective caring leaders. *The Journal of Virtues and Leadership, 1*(1), 25–30.

Spector, C. B. (2018). Medical marijuana: A national survey of nursing education and practice. *Journal of Nursing Regulation, 9*(2), 36–43.

Srinivasana, G., & Shukla, D. (2024). Cannabis-derived pharmaceutical products: Therapeutic, pharmacokinetic and clinical implications – A comprehensive review. *Indian Drugs, 61*(10).

St. Pierre, M., Matthews, L., & Walsh, Z. (2020). Cannabis education needs assessment among Canadian physicians-in-training. *Complementary Therapies in Medicine, 49*. https://doi-org/DOI: 10.1016/j.ctim.2020.102328

Stacey, D., Légaré, F., Lewis, K., Barry, M. J., Bennett, C. L., Eden, K. B., Holmes-Rovner, M., Llewellyn-Thomas, H., Lyddiatt, A., Thomson, R., & Trevena, L. (2017). Decision aids for people facing health treatment or screening decisions. *Cochrane Database of Systematic Reviews, 4*(4), CD001431. DOI: 10.1002/14651858.CD001431.pub5 PMID: 28402085

Stanford Medicine. (2025). Cannabis and older adults: Five things medical experts want you to know. News Center. https://med.stanford.edu/news/insights/2025/10/cannabis-marijuana-seniors-cautions.html

State Policies. (n.d.). Marijuana Policy Project. Retrieved January 6, 2026, from https://www.mpp.org/states/

Statista. (2025). *Number of Americans who used marijuana in the past year (2009–2024)*. https://www.statista.com/statistics/611714/marijuana-use-during-past-year-in-the-us/

Stella, B., Baratta, F., Della Pepa, C., Arpicco, S., Gastaldi, D., & Dosio, F. (2021). Cannabinoid formulations and delivery systems: Current and future options to treat pain. *Drugs, 81*(13), 1513–1557. DOI: 10.1007/s40265-021-01579-x PMID: 34480749

Substance Abuse and Mental Health Services Administration (SAMHSA). (n.d.). *Marijuana: The risks are real*. https://www.samhsa.gov/substance-use/learn/marijuana/risks

Substance Abuse and Mental Health Services Administration. (2023). *Clinical guidance for treating cannabis use disorder*. SAMHSA.

Substance Abuse and Mental Health Services Administration. (2023). *Key substance use and mental health indicators in the United States: Results from the 2023 National Survey on Drug Use and Health.* SAMHSA, Center for Behavioral Health Statistics and Quality, Substance Abuse and Mental Health Administration. HHS Publication No. PEP24-07-021, NSDUH Series H-59). Retrieved from https://www.samhsa.gov/data/report/2023-nsduh-annual-national-report

Substance Abuse and Mental Health Services Administration. (2023). *Results from the 2022 National Survey on Drug Use and Health.* U.S. Department of Health and Human Services.

Sulak, D. (2021). Handbook of cannabis for clinicians: Principles and practice. https://wwnorton.com/books/9780393714180

Sulak, D. (n.d.). *The inner inventory: A method for finding your optimal cannabis dose.* Healer. https://healer.com/programs/the-inner-inventory/

Supra, J. D. (2025). Taking the LEAD: CMS unveils the new LEAD model, focused on Long-Term Primary Care success. https://www.jdsupra.com/legalnews/taking-the-lead-cms-unveils-the-new-6671061

Szaflarski, M., McGoldrick, P., Currens, L., Blodgett, D., Land, H., Szaflarski, J. P., & Segal, E. (2020). Attitudes and knowledge about cannabis and cannabis-based therapies among US neurologists, nurses, and pharmacists. *Epilepsy & Behavior, 109,* 107102. Advance online publication. DOI: 10.1016/j.yebeh.2020.107102 PMID: 32442891

Szydlowski, S. A. (2020). Medical cannabis knowledge and practice: A survey of healthcare providers. *Journal of Cannabis Research, 2,* 1–9.

Tabaei-Aghdaei, Z., McColl-Kennedy, J. R., & Coote, L. V. (2023). Goal setting and health-related outcomes in chronic diseases: A systematic review and meta-analysis of the literature from 2000 to 2020. *Medical Care Research and Review : MCRR, 80*(2), 145–164. DOI: 10.1177/10775587221113228 PMID: 35904147

Tait, M. A., Costa, D. S. J., Campbell, R., Warne, L. N., Norman, R., Schug, S., & Rutherford, C. (2025). Improvements in health-related quality of life are maintained long-term in patients prescribed medicinal cannabis in Australia: The QUEST initiative 12-month follow-up observational study. *PLoS One, 20*(4), e0320756. Advance online publication. DOI: 10.1371/journal.pone.0320756 PMID: 40173146

Tait, M. A., Costa, D. S., Campbell, R., Norman, R., Warne, L. N., Schug, S., & Rutherford, C. (2023). Health-related quality of life in patients accessing medicinal cannabis in Australia: The QUEST initiative results of a 3-month follow-up observational study. *PLoS One, 18*(9), e0290549. DOI: 10.1371/journal.pone.0290549 PMID: 37672515

Tavabi, N., Raza, M., Singh, M., Golchin, S., Singh, H., Hogue, D., & Kiapour, A. M. (2023). Disparities in cannabis use and documentation in electronic health records among children and young adults. *NPJ Digital Medicine, 6*(1), 138. DOI: 10.1038/s41746-023-00885-w PMID: 37553423

Temple, L.M., Lampert, S.L., & Ewigman, B. (2019). Barriers to Achieving Optimal Success with Medical Cannabis: Opportunities for Quality Improvement. *The Journal of Alternative and Complementary Medicine, 25*(1), 5–7. https://doi.org/10.1089/acm.2018.0250

Thanki, D., Domingo-Salvany, A., Barrio Anta, G., Sánchez Mañez, A., Llorens Aleixandre, N., Maria Suelves, J., Brime Beteta, B., & Vicente, J. (2013). The Choice of Screening Instrument Matters: The Case of Problematic Cannabis Use Screening in Spanish Population of Adolescents. International Scholarly Research Notices, 723131, 13 pages

The Evolution of Marijuana as a Controlled Substance and the Federal-State Policy Gap (Updated April 7, 2022) (R44782). https://www.congress.gov/crs_external_products/R/HTML/R44782.html#:~:text=91%2D513).,for%20purposes%20of%20sanctioned%20research.&text=(A)%20The%20drug%20or%20other,other%20substance%20under%20medical%20supervision.&text=The%20CSA%20was%20enacted%20as,and%20Control%20Act%20of%201970.&text=It%20regulates%20the%20manufacture%2C%20possession,unauthorized%20activities%20involving%20controlled%20substances.&text=whether%20the%20substance%20is%20an%20immediate%20precursor%20of%20an%20already%20scheduled%20substance

The White House. (2025). *Increasing medical marijuana and cannabidiol research.* https://www.whitehouse.gov/presidential-actions/2025/12/increasing-medical-marijuana-and-cannabidiol-research/

The White House. (2025). INCREASING MEDICAL MARIJUANA AND CANNABIDIOL RESEARCH. https://www.whitehouse.gov/presidential-actions/2025/12/increasing-medical-marijuana-and-cannabidiol-research/

Theisen, E. & Konieczny, E. (2019, November 4). Medical cannabis: What nurses need to know. *American Nurse.* American Nurses Association. https://www.myamericannurse.com/medical-cannabis-what-nurses-need-to-know/#:~:text=of%20cannabis%20impossible.-,Cannabis:%206%20essential%20principles,pain%20and%20other%20distressing%20symptoms.

Theisen, E., & Konieczny, E. (2019). Medical cannabis: What nurses need to know. *American Nurse Today*, *14*(11), 6–11. https://www.myamericannurse.com/medical-cannabis-what-nurses-need-to-know/

Thoma, B., Abbott, C., & Snell, L. (2023). The future of the CanMEDS physician competency framework. *Canadian Medical Education Journal*, *14*(1), 1–3. https://pmc.ncbi.nlm.nih.gov/articles/PMC10042786/ . DOI: 10.36834/cmej.77098 PMID: 36998483

Tinetti, M. E., Fried, T. R., & Boyd, C. M. (2012). Designing health care for the most common chronic condition: Multimorbidity. *Journal of the American Medical Association*, *307*(23), 2493–2494. DOI: 10.1001/jama.2012.5265 PMID: 22797447

Tishler, J. (n.d.). *Many patients using cannabis yet medical cannabis systems failing*. Association of Cannabinoid Specialists. https://www.cannaspecialists.org/medical_cannabis_systems_are_failing

Trif, C., Harpaz, D., Eltzov, E., Parcharoen, Y., Pechyen, C., & Marks, S. (2024). Detection of Cannabinoids in Oral Fluid Specimens as the Preferred Biological Matrix for a Point-of-Care Biosensor Diagnostic Device. *Biosensors (Basel)*, *14*(3), 126. DOI: 10.3390/bios14030126 PMID: 38534233

Troyer, J., & Tanco, K. (2024). Review of the use of medicinal cannabis products in palliative care. *Cancers (Basel)*, *16*(7), 1412. DOI: 10.3390/cancers16071412 PMID: 38611090

Trump, D. (2025, December 18). *Increasing medical marijuana and cannabidiol research* (Executive Order 14370). The White House. https://www.whitehouse.gov/presidential-actions/2025/12/increasing-medical-marijuana-and-cannabidiol-research/

U.S. Congress. (1938). *Federal Food, Drug, and Cosmetic Act*, 21 U.S.C. § 301 et seq. https://www.govinfo.gov/content/pkg/USCODE-2023-title21/pdf/USCODE-2023-title21-chap9.pdf

U.S. Department of Health and Human Services. (2023). *Basis for the recommendation to reschedule marijuana from Schedule I to Schedule III.* https://www.hhs.gov

U.S. Department of Health and Human Services. (2023). *Basis for the recommendation to reschedule marijuana under the Controlled Substances Act.* https://www.hhs.gov/about/news/2023/08/30/hhs-recommends-marijuana-rescheduling.html

U.S. Department of Health and Human Services. (2024). Medical and scientific analysis of marijuana. https://www.hhs.gov

U.S. Department of Justice, Drug Enforcement Administration. (2024). Schedules of controlled substances: Rescheduling of marijuana (Proposed rule). *Federal Register*, *89*(168), 44597–44616. https://www.federalregister.gov

U.S. Food and Drug Administration. (2016). FDA and marijuana: Questions and answers. https://www.fda.gov

U.S. Food and Drug Administration. (2020). *FDA regulation of cannabis and cannabis-derived products.*

U.S. Food and Drug Administration. (2023). *FDA and cannabis: Research and drug approval process.* https://www.fda.gov/news-events/public-health-focus/fda-and-cannabis-research-and-drug-approval-process

Unger, J. B. (2022). Regulation of cannabis retailers: Facilitating responsible adult use and promoting health equity while preventing access to minors. *American Journal of Public Health*, *112*(11), 1532–1534. DOI: 10.2105/AJPH.2022.307102 PMID: 36223589

United Nations. (1925). League of Nations Treaty Series. *International Opium Convention. 81*, p. 319. Geneva: United Nations. Retrieved January 24, 2025, from https://treaties.un.org/pages/ViewDetails.aspx?src=TREATY&mtdsg_no=VI-6-a&chapter=6&clang=_en

United Nations. (1961). United Nations Treaty Series. [New York, Geneva, Switzerland: United Nations Office on Drugs and Crime.]. *Single Convention on Narcotic Drugs.*, *520*, 151.

United States Congress. (2025). Agriculture, Rural Development, Food and Drug Administration, and Related Agencies Appropriations Act, 2026, Pub. L. No. 119-37, div. B (2025). https://www.congress.gov/119/plaws/publ37/PLAW-119publ37.pdf

Utah Canna (2025, September 10). The Federal-State Divide: Why Medical Cannabis Remains Complex. https://utahcanna.org/the-federal-state-divide-why-medical-cannabis-remains-complex/

Valente, A. C., Lopes, L. P. N., & Matheus, M. E. (2024). Medical cannabis use in oncology and associated outcomes: A scoping review. *Journal of Oncology Pharmacy Practice*, *30*(4), 737–751. DOI: 10.1177/10781552241239006 PMID: 38477532

Vázquez, M., García-Carnelli, C., Maldonado, C., & Fagiolino, P. (2021). Clinical pharmacokinetics of cannabinoids and potential drug–drug interactions. In *Cannabinoids and sleep: Molecular, functional and clinical aspects* (pp. 27–42). Springer International Publishing. DOI: 10.1007/978-3-030-61663-2_3

Vederhus, J.-K., Rørendal, M., Skårdal, M., Næss, M. O., Clausen, T., & Kristensen, Ø. (2022). Successful outcomes with low–threshold intervention for cannabis use disorders in Norway - an observational study. *PLOS ONE, 17*(6), e0269988. https://doi.org/10.1371/journal.pone.0269988

Vinette, B., Côté, J., El-Akhras, A., Mrad, H., Chicoine, G., & Bilodeau, K. (2022). Routes of administration, reasons for use, and approved indications of medical cannabis in oncology: A scoping review. *BMC Cancer*, *22*(1), 937. Advance online publication. DOI: 10.1186/s12885-022-09378-7 PMID: 35331185

Virginia Board of Pharmacy. (2023, July 17). *Regulations governing pharmaceutical processors.* https://register.dls.virginia.gov/details.aspx?id=10719

Volkow, N. D., Baler, R. D., Compton, W. M., & Weiss, S. R. B. (2014). Adverse health effects of marijuana use. *The New England Journal of Medicine*, *370*(23), 2219–2227. https://www.ncbi.nlm.nih.gov/pmc/articles/PMC4827335/. DOI: 10.1056/NEJMra1402309 PMID: 24897085

Volkow, N. D., Hampson, A. J., & Baler, R. D. (2017). Don't worry, be happy: Endocannabinoids and cannabis at the intersection of stress and reward. *Annual Review of Pharmacology and Toxicology*, *57*(1), 285–308. DOI: 10.1146/annurev-pharmtox-010716-104615 PMID: 27618739

Vyas, M. B., LeBaron, V. T., & Gilson, A. M. (2017). The use of cannabis in response to the opioid crisis: A review of the literature. *Nursing Outlook*, *66*(1), 56–65. DOI: 10.1016/j.outlook.2017.08.012 PMID: 28993073

Wade, D. T., & Halligan, P. W. (2017). The biopsychosocial model of illness: A model whose time has come. *Clinical Rehabilitation*, *31*(8), 995–1004. DOI: 10.1177/0269215517709890 PMID: 28730890

Wallace, M. S., Marcotte, T. D., Umlauf, A., Gouaux, B., & Atkinson, J. H. (2015). Efficacy of inhaled cannabis on painful diabetic neuropathy. *The Journal of Pain*, *16*(7), 616–627. DOI: 10.1016/j.jpain.2015.03.008 PMID: 25843054

Wang, Y., Boyd, A. E., Rountree, L., Ren, Y., Nyhan, K., Nagar, R., Higginbottom, J., Ranney, M. L., Parikh, H., & Mukherjee, B. (2025). *Towards enhancing data equity in public health data science.* Cornell University. https://doi.org//arXiv.2508.20301DOI: 10.48550

Wang, L., Hong, P. J., May, C., Rehman, Y., Oparin, Y., Hong, C. J., Hong, B. Y., AminiLari, M., Gallo, L., Kaushal, A., Craigie, S., Couban, R. J., Kum, E., Shanthanna, H., Price, I., Upadhye, S., Ware, M. A., Campbell, F., Buchbinder, R., & Busse, J. W. (2021). Medical cannabis or cannabinoids for chronic non-cancer and cancer-related pain: A systematic review and meta-analysis of randomised clinical trials. *BMJ (Clinical Research Ed.)*, *374*(1034), n1034. DOI: 10.1136/bmj.n1034 PMID: 34497047

Warf, B. (2014). High points: An historical geography of cannabis. *Geographical Review, 104*(4), 414–438. DOI: 10.1111/j.1931-0846.2014.12038.x

Wartko, P. D., Bobb, J. F., Boudreau, D. M., Matthews, A. G., McCormack, J., Lee, A. K., Qiu, H., Yu, O., Hyun, N., Idu, A. E., Campbell, C. I., Saxon, A. J., Liu, D. S., Altschuler, A., Samet, J. H., Labelle, C. T., Zare-Mehrjerdi, M., Stotts, A. L., Braciszewski, J. M., & Bradley, K. A. (2023). Nurse care management for opioid use disorder treatment: The PROUD cluster randomized clinical trial. *JAMA Internal Medicine, 183*(12), 1343–1354. DOI: 10.1001/jamainternmed.2023.5701 PMID: 37902748

Washington State House of Representatives. (2026, February 12). *House passes "Ryan's Law," restoring compassion and dignity to end-of-life care.* https://housedemocrats.wa.gov/blog/2026/02/12/house-passes-ryans-law-restoring-compassion-and-dignity-to-end-of-life-care/#:~:text=OLYMPIA%20%E2%80%94%20In%20the%20final%20chapter%20of,hospice%20facilities%20can%20access%20medical%20cannabis%20as

Watson Caring Science Institute. (n.d.). *The 10 Caritas Processes®*. In *Caring science theory*. Retrieved December 1, 2025, from https://www.watsoncaringscience.org/caring-science-theory/10-caritas-processes/

Watson, J. (2008). *Nursing: The philosophy and science of caring* (Rev. ed.). University Press of Colorado., https://upcolorado.com/university-press-of-colorado/item/1849-nursing-revised-edit

Weinstein, A., Brickner, O., Lerman, H., Greemland, M., Bloch, M., Lester, H., Chisin, R., Sarne, Y., Mechoulam, R., Bar-Hamburger, R., Freedman, N., & Even-Sapir, E. (2008). A study investigating the acute dose–response effects of 13 mg and 17 mg Δ9-tetrahydrocannabinol on cognitive-motor skills, subjective and autonomic measures in regular users of marijuana. *Journal of Psychopharmacology (Oxford, England), 22*(4), 441–451. DOI: 10.1177/0269881108088194 PMID: 18635724

What is a nurse administrator? Responsibilities & qualifications. (2024, September 11). Retrieved January 6, 2026, from https://www.carerev.com/blog/the-role-of-nurse-administrators

Whiting, P. F., Wolff, R. F., Deshpande, S., Di Nisio, M., Duffy, S., Hernández, A. V., Keurentjes, J. C., Lang, S., Misso, K., Ryder, S., Schmidlkofer, S., Westwood, M., & Kleijnen, J. (2015). Cannabinoids for medical use: A systematic review and meta-analysis. *Journal of the American Medical Association, 313*(24), 2456–2473. DOI: 10.1001/jama.2015.6358 PMID: 26103030

Wiese, J.L., Watson, T.M., Bozinoff, N., Rush, B., Stergiopoulos, V., Le Foll, B., & Rueda, S. (2024, December). "Like the Wild West": Health care provider perspectives on impacts of recreational cannabis legalization on patients and providers at a tertiary psychiatric hospital in Ontario, Canada. *Journal of Substance Use and Addiction Treatment 167*, 209487. https://doi.org/10.1016/j.josat.2024.209487

Wills, S. (1998). Cannabis use and abuse by man: an historical perspective. In *Cannabis* (pp. 16–46). CRC Press. DOI: 10.4324/9780203304228_chapter_1

Winkelman, M. (2010). *Shamanism: A biopsychosocial paradigm of consciousness and healing* (2nd ed.). Praeger., https://api.pageplace.de/preview/DT0400.9780313381829_A24399361/preview-9780313381829_A24399361.pdf DOI: 10.5040/9798216014133

Woodbridge, M., Sarma, N., & Vaillencourt, D. (2024). *Cannabis quality: The need for science-based global harmonization of standards.* U.S. Pharmacopeia. https://www.usp.org/sites/default/files/usp/document/our-work/DS/uspastm-cannabis-quality-recommendations.pdf

World Health Organization. (1948). *Constitution of the World Health Organization.* https://www.who.int/about/governance/constitution

World Health Organization. (2008). *Closing the gap in a generation: health equity through action on the social determinants of health - Final report of the commission on social determinants of health.* https://www.who.int/publications/i/item/WHO-IER-CSDH-08.1

World Health Organization. (2019). *WHO review of cannabis and cannabis related substances.* https://www.who.int/teams/health-product-and-policy-standards/controlled-substances/who-review-of-cannabis-and-cannabis-related-substances

World Health Organization. (2022). *Achieving well-being: A draft global framework for integrating well-being into public health utilizing a health promotion approach.* World Health Organization. https://www.who.int/publications/m/item/achieving-well-being

World Health Organization. (2023). *Cannabis and cannabinoids: Public health considerations.* WHO.

World Health Organization. (2024). *Global status report on alcohol and health and treatment of substance use disorders.* https://www.who.int/publications/i/item/9789240096745

World Health Organization. (2025). *State of the world's nursing 2025: investing in education, jobs, leadership and service delivery.* Geneva: World Health Organization. https://iris.who.int/server/api/core/bitstreams/a4173924-a18f-49b6-8bd1-9c2a4a098980/content

Worster, B., Ashare, R. L., Hajjar, E., Garber, G., Smith, K., & Kelly, E. L. (2023). Clinician attitudes, training, and beliefs about cannabis: An interprofessional assessment. *Cannabis and Cannabinoid Research, 8*(3), 547–556. DOI: 10.1089/can.2021.0022 PMID: 34978882

Worster, B., Hajjar, E. R., & Handley, N. (2022). Cannabis use in patients with cancer: A clinical review. *JCO Oncology Practice, 18*(11), 743–749. DOI: 10.1200/OP.22.00080 PMID: 35749680

Writer, C. (2024, July 16). *Can Nurses Legally Use Cannabis Across Different States?* Marijuana Packaging. https://marijuanapackaging.com/blogs/questions/can-nurses-legally-use-cannabis-across-different-states

Zalon, M. L., Ludwick, R., & Patton, R. M. (2024). Strengthening nurses' influence in health policy. *The American Journal of Nursing, 124*(9), 28–36. https://journals.lww.com/ajnonline/fulltext/2024/09000/strengthening_nurses__influence_in_health_policy.17.aspx. DOI: 10.1097/01.NAJ.0001028316.80475.bf PMID: 39115377

Zarhin, D., Negev, M., Vulfsons, S., & Sznitman, S. R. (2020). "Medical cannabis" as a contested medicine: Fighting over epistemology and morality. *Science, Technology & Human Values, 45*(3), 488–514. DOI: 10.1177/0162243919862866

Zehra, A., Burns, J., Liu, C. K., Manza, P., Wiers, C. E., Volkow, N. D., & Wang, G. J. (2018). Cannabis addiction and the brain: A review. *Journal of Neuroimmune Pharmacology, 13*(4), 438–452. DOI: 10.1007/s11481-018-9782-9 PMID: 29556883

Zeng, L., Lytvyn, L., Wang, X., Kithulegoda, N., Agterberg, S., Shergill, Y., Esfahani, M. A., Heen, A. F., Agoritsas, T., Guyatt, G. H., & Busse, J. W. (2021). Values and preferences toward medical cannabis among people living with chronic pain: A mixed-methods systematic review. *BMJ Open*, *11*(9), e050831. DOI: 10.1136/bmjopen-2021-050831 PMID: 34493521

Zeraatkar, D., Cooper, M. A., Agarwal, A., Vernooij, R. W., Leung, G., Loniewski, K., Dookie, J. E., Ahmed, M. M., Hong, B. Y., Hong, C., Hong, P., Couban, R., Agoritsas, T., & Busse, J. W. (2022). Long-term and serious harms of medical cannabis and cannabinoids for chronic pain: A systematic review of non-randomised studies. *BMJ Open*, *12*(8), e054282. DOI: 10.1136/bmjopen-2021-054282 PMID: 35926992

Zibrik, K., Laskin, J., & Ho, C. (2016). Integration of a nurse navigator into the triage process for patients with non-small-cell lung cancer: Creating systematic improvements in patient care. *Current Oncology (Toronto, Ont.)*, *23*(3), 280–283. DOI: 10.3747/co.23.2954 PMID: 27330366

Ziemianski, D., Capler, R., Tekanoff, R., Lacasse, A., Luconi, F., & Ware, M. A. (2015). Cannabis in medicine: A national educational needs assessment among Canadian physicians. *BMC Medical Education*, *15*(1), 52. DOI: 10.1186/s12909-015-0335-0 PMID: 25888752

Zolotov, Y. (2025). Developing Medical Cannabis Competencies a consensus statement. JAMA Network. https://jamanetwork.com/journals/jamanetworkopen/fullarticle/2839750

Zolotov, Y. (2025). Developing medical cannabis competencies: A consensus statement. *JAMA Network Open*. https://jamanetwork.com/journals/jamanetworkopen/fullarticle/2839750

Zolotov, Y. V. (2021). Medical cannabis education for health professionals: A systemic review. *Complementary Therapies in Medicine*, *56*, 102616.

Zolotov, Y., Grinstein Cohen, O., Findley, P. A., Reznik, A., Isralowitz, R., & Willard, S. (2021). Attitudes and knowledge about medical cannabis among Israeli and American nursing students. *Nurse Education Today*, *102*, 104929. https://www.sciencedirect.com/science/article/abs/pii/S0260691721000460. DOI: 10.1016/j.nedt.2021.104789 PMID: 33571928

Zolotov, Y., Mendoza Temple, L., Isralowitz, R., Gorelick, D. A., Abraham, R., Abrams, D. I., Barich, K., Boehnke, K. F., Dahmer, S., Friedman, J., Frye, P., Haramati, A., Isaac, J., Mathre, M. L., McNabb, M. E., Ring, M., Russo, E. B., Slawek, D. E., Temple, B. R., & Kogan, M. (2025). Developing medical cannabis competencies: A consensus statement. *JAMA Network Open*, *8*(1), e2839750. https://jamanetwork.com/journals/jamanetworkopen/fullarticle/2839750. DOI: 10.1001/jamanetworkopen.2025.35049 PMID: 41055914

Zolotov, Y., Metri, S., Calabria, E., & Kogan, M. (2021). Medical cannabis education among healthcare trainees: A scoping review. *Complementary Therapies in Medicine*, *58*, 102675. DOI: 10.1016/j.ctim.2021.102675 PMID: 33539943

Zolotov, Y., Temple, L. M., Isralowitz, R., Gorelick, D. A., Abraham, R., Abrams, D. I., Barich, K., Boehnke, K. F., Dahmer, S., Friedman, B. R., Wilson-King, G. S., Arnsten, J. H., & Kogan, M. (2025). Developing Medical Cannabis Competencies: A Consensus Statement. *JAMA Network Open*, *8*(10), e2535049.https://doi.org/10.1001/jamanetworkopen.2025.35049

Zolotov, Y., Vulfsons, S., Zarhin, D., & Sznitman, S. (2021). Medical cannabis: An oxymoron? Physicians' perceptions of medical cannabis. *The International Journal on Drug Policy*, *88*, 103–112. DOI: 10.1016/j.drugpo.2020.103112 PMID: 29653439

Zou, S., & Kumar, U. (2018). Cannabinoid receptors and the endocannabinoid system: Signaling and function in the central nervous system. *International Journal of Molecular Sciences*, *19*(3), 833. DOI: 10.3390/ijms19030833 PMID: 29533978

About the Contributors

Kathleen Pinto Araya is a Psychiatric Nurse Practitioner and brings over thirty years of experience in nursing, leadership, and higher education. She has spent her nursing career working in both New Jersey and Florida primarily in community health, neurology, and pediatrics, and continues to actively practice nursing. Dr. Pinto Araya has served in academia as a faculty member, and in leadership roles including Dean of Nursing, Program Chair, and Subject Matter Expert for undergraduate and graduate nursing students. Additionally, she held roles including Doctoral Advisor/Chair, and facilitator for Executive Leadership, Nursing Education, and Population Health. During her career, she has contributed to the nursing profession through her active research in debriefing following high fidelity simulation. In addition to her current research, Dr. Pinto Araya has presented on community health issues to several public and private organizations in the U.S. and internationally including the Global Council on Nursing and Health Education as a Scientific Committee Member and Keynote Speaker. She has been politically involved in the State Nurses Association as a forum committee member. She has also volunteered as a practicum mentor for nursing students at several local and national universities and has been recognized for excellence in practice and education by organizations including the National Society for Leadership and Success, Sigma Theta Tau, and Delta Mu Delta. Her research interests include Business, Research, Nursing, Administration, Education, Simulation, and Population/Community Health. Dr. Pinto Araya earned her PhD, Doctor of Philosophy in Nursing, Master of Science in Nursing, and Bachelor of Science in Nursing from the University of Phoenix. She earned her Psychiatric Nurse Practitioner Degree from Chamberlain University, Master of Business Administration, and Master of Healthcare Management from Capella University. Her undergraduate degree in Social Science was earned from Ocean County College and Diploma in Nursing from Ann May School of Nursing.

Rana Zeine, MD, PhD, MBA is Adjunct Faculty at Kean University, Biological Sciences (1/2020), and Union College of Union County STEM-Biology (9/2023-) Union, New Jersey, USA. She is associate editor for the Journal of Cannabis Research and guest editor for a collection with Springer-Nature. As Clinical Thematic Book Collection Editor with IGI Global Scientific Publishing, USA, she is editor of books on medical cannabis and psychedelics. She teaches Immunology, Neuroscience, Anatomy & Physiology, Microbiology, Cancer, Aging, Research, and formerly Pathology at Saint James School of Medicine. She serves on committees of the Society of Cannabis Clinicians. She received her B.S. Biology '83, Teaching Diploma '83, and M.D. '87 from American University of Beirut, Ph.D. in Experimental Medicine '93 from McGill University, Pathology Residency and Neuropathology Fellowship '04 from Albert Einstein College of Medicine, and M.B.A. '12 from Keller Graduate School of Management of DeVry College of New York.

Hasan H. Alsararatee is an Advanced Clinical Practitioner in Acute Medicine at Northampton General Hospital NHS Trust and a Senior Lecturer in Advanced Clinical Practice at Buckinghamshire New University. He is a member of the Editorial Board of the International Journal for Advancing Practice and a committee member of the Association of Advanced Practice Educators UK, contributing to national discussions on advanced practice education, capability development and workforce transformation. Hasan holds an MSc in Advanced Clinical Practice with distinction. His work aligns with national advanced practice frameworks and spans the four pillars of practice: clinical practice, leadership and management, education and research. His research and publications focus on acute medicine, frailty, end-of-life care, dermatological assessment, gastroenterology, pulmonary embolism, ethics and the development of AP roles. He has experience in leading research, audit and service evaluation projects, and has secured funding from the Royal College of Nursing and Buckinghamshire New University to support work on clinical supervision, advanced practice development and compassionate care within healthcare practice.

Carey S. (Clark) Cadieux, PhD, RN, AHN-BC, RYT, FAAN, has been a nurse for 31 years, with a wide range of practice experience including acute care, pediatrics, hospice care, and parish nursing. Dr. Cadieux is a Fellow of the American Academy of Nursing, an Associate Professor of Nursing at Binghamton University, and Past President of the American Cannabis Nurses Association (ACNA). Dr. Cadieux is the editor and author of the textbook Cannabis: A Handbook for Nurses (2021, Wolters-Kluwer), and she developed the first academic medical cannabis certificate in the US.

Mahima Choudhary is Research Scholar in Forensic Science at KR Mangalam University, India. She holds a Master's Degree in Forensic Science and her expertize area is Fingerprint and Forensic Chemistry. Her research focuses on pesticide residue detection with the help of gas sensor. She has also participated in international conferences and also in government recognized projects. She is committed to interdisciplinary research, innovation in forensic methodologies, and the application of scientific principles to strengthen the criminal justice system.

Thomas A. Clobes has over 16 years of experience in higher education and more than 20 years of diverse expertise in healthcare. He has made significant contributions to teaching, research, and service in health sciences, public health, and healthcare administration. Dr. Clobes is a dedicated educator recognized for his innovative approaches to teaching. His research focuses on emerging topics in medical cannabis, health policy, and equity in education, reflected in numerous peer-reviewed publications, conference presentations, and student-collaborated projects. He holds a Ph.D. in Health Sciences from Rutgers University, an M.S. in Medical Cannabis Sciences and Therapeutics from the University of Maryland, as well as an M.S. in Administration, a B.S. in Biology, and a B.S. in Psychology from California State University Bakersfield. His professional affiliations include the Society of Cannabis Clinicians and the American College of Healthcare Executives, further underscoring his dedication to advancing healthcare and education.

David Gordon, MD, IFMCP, ABoIM, is a board-certified physician in Internal and Integrative Medicine with nearly 25 years of clinical experience and more than a decade of focused work in medical cannabis. His clinical and educational efforts center on helping patients and practitioners use cannabis safely, intentionally, and effectively as part of broader integrative health strategies. Dr. Gordon has provided medical cannabis consultations for patients with diverse chronic health challenges, guiding them through the individualized use of cannabis within comprehensive health and wellness plans. His work emphasizes intentional use, careful monitoring, and ongoing reassessment to support meaningful improvements in quality of life while minimizing unintended harms, rather than reliance on fixed protocols. These clinical experiences form the foundation for his contributions to cannabis education and scholarship. He is the founder and owner of 4 Pillars Health & Wellness, an integrative medicine practice built on the principles of food, movement, relaxation, and community. For more than 15 years, Dr. Gordon operated a freestanding integrative primary care clinic and now focuses on consultative care, education, and clinical guidance at the intersection of integrative medicine and cannabis therapeutics. He also serves as Medical Director at Axon Integrative Health, where he provides clinical oversight and education within multidisciplinary integrative care settings. Dr. Gordon is an Adjunct Instructor in the Department of Cannabis Sciences at the Community College of Denver, where he teaches courses in cannabis physiology, pharmacology, and public health. His physiology-focused teaching emphasizes how cannabis interacts with human biological systems and how those interactions translate into both therapeutic potential and risk. In parallel, his public health course examines cannabis through a broader societal lens, exploring how history, policy, regulation, and social context shape patterns of use, access, and health outcomes. Together, these courses reflect his commitment to preparing students to think critically about cannabis at both the individual and population levels. Dr. Gordon received his medical degree and completed his residency training at the University of Colorado, where he remains affiliated with the clinical faculty. He is board-certified in Internal and Integrative Medicine and is a Certified Functional Medicine Practitioner through the Institute for Functional Medicine. Dr. Gordon lives in Denver, Colorado, with his family and continues to balance clinical practice, teaching, writing, and community engagement, with a focus on advancing responsible, patient-centered approaches to cannabis care.

Drudys Ledbetter, BSN, RN is a nurse executive, clinical systems strategist, author, and founder of Project Destigmatize HealTHCare, a nurse-led public health initiative advancing research, data infrastructure, and clinical integration at the intersection of healthcare and cannabis. She is also the principal of MAC Vernet Consulting, where she leads the development and implementation of Behavioral Risk Infrastructure (BRI), a system-level framework designed to capture, standardize, and integrate real-world behavioral exposure data into clinical decision-making, risk modeling, and health system performance. With over two decades of experience across critical care nursing, clinical operations, healthcare technology, and informatics, Drudys specializes in designing scalable, clinician-centered systems that bridge the gap between real-world patient behavior and clinical decision-making. Her work centers on signal integrity, behavioral risk visibility, and the operationalization of data that healthcare systems currently fail to capture. Her 2026 foundational paper, Behavioral Determinants of Health: From Invisible Risk to Clinical Intelligence, formally defines Behavioral Determinants of Health (BDOH) as an operational category of risk, identifies the Behavioral Visibility Gap as a structural limitation in healthcare systems, and introduces Behavioral Risk Infrastructure (BRI) as the framework required to make real-world behavior visible, measurable, and actionable in care . In 2020, she entered the legal cannabis industry as an operator, securing cultivation, manufacturing, and retail licenses. This experience exposed critical gaps in patient disclosure, documentation, and clinical guidance, ultimately informing her transition into full-time consulting, research, and policy innovation. Her work has since focused on addressing the cannabis disclosure gap and advancing infrastructure that enables healthcare systems to move from reactive interpretation of outcomes to proactive management of behavioral risk. Drudys is the creator of Cannaversations®, a registered media platform translating complex cannabis and healthcare topics for both clinical and consumer audiences, and a contributing columnist for CashColorCannabis Magazine. She has contributed to national policy and research conversations, including work with the Parabola Center for Law and Policy. She is the author of Truth & Triumph (2017), a foundational work reflecting her commitment to personal truth, resilience, and transformation—principles that continue to inform her leadership philosophy and approach to systems change. Her work sits at the intersection of clinical care, public health, policy, and emerging therapeutic markets, with a consistent focus on building infrastructure that reflects how people actually live, not only how systems are designed to function. She is a member of the American Cannabis Nurses Association and Cannabis Nurses of Color. Above all, she is a mother to Jayla Marie Anne and Jerome (RJ) Jr., whose lives continue to shape her commitment to building safer, more human-centered systems of care.

Elisabeth Mack, MBA, BSN, BA, RN, is a visionary nurse, educator, and entrepreneur redefining healing in the modern age. As the co-founder of Holistic Caring & The Green Nurse, and Bloom Hemp CBD, she bridges the gap between conventional healthcare and cannabis medicine through education, advocacy, and compassionate guidance. A seasoned healthcare and insurance executive turned cannabis nurse pioneer, Elisabeth helps patients and professionals navigate plant medicine with confidence—covering product selection, dosing, interactions, and timing. She is a licensed provider for the California Board of Registered Nursing and the author of the book Cannabis for Health: Become a Coach, and a groundbreaking curriculum that integrates cannabinoids into holistic and functional medicine. An active leader in the field, Elisabeth serves on the boards of LANORML and the Coachella Valley Cannabis Alliance Network (CVCAN), is a member of the Society of Cannabis Clinicians, and formerly served as Treasurer for the American Cannabis Nurses Association. She also co-hosts The Green Nurse Podcast: Clinical Conversations. Through her work, writing, and advocacy, Elisabeth empowers others to embrace wellness through truth, compassion, and the courage to heal—body, mind, and soul.

Sherri Mack, BSN-RN, is a pioneering visionary healthcare leader, registered nurse and cannabis nurse, serving as the co-founder of Holistic Caring and The Green Nurse, as well as the Chief Nursing Officer at Bloom Hemp CBD. Sherri leverages her extensive 35+ years of nursing experience to bridge the gap between patients, conventional medicine, and the plant medicine community. Holding a Bachelor of Science in Nursing from Boston College, Sherri holds key roles as a founding member of the Cannabis Nurses Network and the International Association of Psychedelic Nurses. She served on the Board of Directors for the American Cannabis Nurses Association and currently chairs the Health and Wellness Committee for the Coachella Valley Cannabis Alliance. A contributing author to the groundbreaking "Carey S. Clark's Handbook for Nurses," Sherri is also the primary author of Ask The Green Nurse on Substack and The Cannigma and hosts of the award-winning "The Green Nurse Podcast." Through her writing and the podcast, she shares inspiring healing stories and educates audiences on the transformative potential of plant-based medicine.

Janice Putnam is a registered nurse with 30 years of experience. She has dedicated 25 years to faculty service at the University of Central Missouri. Dr. Putnam earned her Ph.D. in Nursing from the University of Missouri. Her interests are tobacco and cannabis health policy issues, as well as their impact on higher education. At UCM, Dr. Putnam has been encouraged to blend her expertise in academia with administrative roles, including Associate Dean of the Graduate School, Interim Director of the Office of Sponsored Programs, and Senior Academic Policy and Compliance Specialist. She teaches courses including Drugs: Addiction to Recovery, Health Policy and Advocacy, and Health Equity, and serves on the Board of Directors for the American Cannabis Nurses Association.

Sameer Saharan currently serves as the Head of Department and Assistant Professor at Mody University of Science and Technology since September 2023, while also holding the position of Assistant Professor at Mody University. Prior to this, Dr. Saharan was an Assistant Professor at Mandsaur University for a brief period in 2023 and spent seven years at AMITY University Gurgaon as a Research Scholar and Visiting Faculty. Dr. Saharan holds a Doctor of Philosophy in Forensic Science and Technology from AMITY University Gurgaon, a Master's degree in Forensic Science from Kurukshetra University, and a Bachelor's degree from Maharshi Dayanand University.

Llewellyn Dawn Smith, MSN, RN CNEcl, is an accomplished nurse educator, researcher, and cannabis nursing advocate with more than four decades of clinical and academic experience. She began her nursing career as a graduate of Tidewater Community College (1985) and later earned her Master of Science in Nursing Education from Old Dominion University. Following her recent retirement from Sentara Obici Hospital, where she served as a staff nurse for many years, Llewellyn continues to advance nursing education as a Professor of Nursing at Paul D. Camp Community College. She teaches across the curriculum, integrating didactic instruction with clinical application. Her pedagogical approach is grounded in transparency, clinical rigor, and learner-centered engagement, earning her consistent recognition from students for her expertise, accessibility, and sound clinical judgment. Llewellyn has been an active leader in cannabis nursing for over a decade. She has served the American Cannabis Nurses Association (ACNA) in multiple leadership roles, including President (2022) and now Past President. She contributed significantly to the development of the Cannabis Nursing: Scope & Standards of Practice (2024), helping to formalize and advance this emerging specialty. Her scholarly work includes authorship of the foundational chapter "History of Cannabis and Prohibition" in Cannabis: A Handbook for Nurses (Clark, Ed., 2021), a text widely used in nursing education and professional development. In addition, her Magnet-recognized research study, "Effects of Cannabis Use on Sedation Requirements for Endoscopic Procedures," was published in Gastroenterology Nursing (July/August 2024), contributing valuable evidence to the clinical understanding of cannabis use and procedural sedation. Llewellyn also serves as Treasurer for both the Virginia Nurses Association and the Virginia Nurses Foundation (VNA/VNF), supporting statewide initiatives that strengthen nursing practice and leadership. She is the founder and owner of Smith Cannabis LLC 2016, a Portsmouth-based consulting practice through which she provides free cannabis nursing education, professional guidance, and patient-centered consultation

Deanna M. Sommers, PhD, MSN, RN, PNP-PC, is President of the American Cannabis Nurses Association (ACNA) and an accomplished nurse leader, educator, and scholar with more than three decades of experience in academic and healthcare environments. She holds a Doctor of Philosophy in Public Health with a specialization in Health Promotion and Community Education and a Master of Science in Nursing. Her clinical practice background includes intensive care, community health, and pediatric primary care, where she served as a Pediatric Nurse Practitioner for approximately 25 years. Dr. Sommers has held senior academic leadership positions, including Associate Dean and Director of a College of Nursing, contributing to curriculum development, faculty advancement, and student success. Her scholarly work includes doctoral research examining social ecological determinants of obesity and co-authorship of Chapter 3 (Cannabis Pharmacology) in Cannabis: A Handbook for Nurses. She also served as lead editor of Cannabis Nursing: Scope and Standards of Practice (2024), published by the American Nurses Association and the American Cannabis Nurses Association. Since joining ACNA in 2019, Dr. Sommers has provided sustained leadership in advancing cannabis nursing as a recognized specialty. As Chair of the ACNA Credentialing Committee, she led the writing subcommittee responsible for aligning ACNA's Scope and Standards with the American Nurses Association framework and coordinating development of the specialty recognition application and Scope of Practice statement. These efforts contributed to formal recognition of cannabis nursing as a specialty. In acknowledgment of this work, she received the ACNA Presidency Award. Dr. Sommers is an invited national speaker and has presented at the American Holistic Nurses Association Annual Conferences, Kaiser Permanente Grand Rounds, ACNA conferences and webinars, and interdisciplinary clinical forums. Her professional presentations address cannabis nursing fundamentals, clinical assessment, consumer safety, scope and standards of practice, and credentialing pathways. She serves as a featured guest on educational podcast episodes addressing cannabis nursing and public health topics. In her current role as ACNA President, Dr. Sommers provides organizational leadership in nursing education, credentialing development, governance, and policy advocacy. Her professional interests include advancing nurse-led, evidence-based cannabis care, strengthening professional infrastructure, promoting health equity, and supporting interdisciplinary collaboration.

Marie Michelle Zang is a registered nurse for over 20 years. She earned her Bachelor's Degree from the University of Nevada, Las Vegas School of Nursing and has been a Nurse Case Manager for over 10 years. She is a Certified Case Manager and a Certified Managed Care Nurse currently working as a Senior RN Case Manager for one of the leading health plan companies. She introduced one of the first hybrid Case Management Nursing and Cannabis Care Nursing program offered to health plan members and a pioneer in establishing this type of sub-specialty care. She received the March of Dimes Nurse of the Year Award for Case Management in 2015 and a recipient of the SAGES Center for Clinician Advancement in 2023 from United Health Group. She is a member of the American Cannabis Nurses Association and served in committees.

Index

A

B

C

D

P

R

S

T

W

www.ingramcontent.com/pod-product-compliance
Lightning Source LLC
LaVergne TN
LVHW060253011026
849161LV00011B/2707